Handbook of Drug Interactions

FORENSIC
SCIENCE AND MEDICINE

Steven B. Karch, MD, SERIES EDITOR

HANDBOOK OF DRUG INTERACTIONS: *A CLINICAL AND FORENSIC GUIDE,*
   edited by **Ashraf Mozayani and Lionel P. Raymon,** 2004

DIETARY SUPPLEMENTS: *TOXICOLOGY AND CLINICAL PHARMACOLOGY,*
   edited by **Melanie Johns Cupp and Timothy S. Tracy,** 2003

BUPRENOPHINE THERAPY OF OPIATE ADDICTION,
   edited by **Pascal Kintz and Pierre Marquet,** 2002

BENZODIAZEPINES AND GHB: *DETECTION AND PHARMACOLOGY,*
   edited by **Salvatore J. Salamone,** 2002

ON-SITE DRUG TESTING,
   edited by **Amanda J. Jenkins and Bruce A. Goldberger,** 2001

BRAIN IMAGING IN SUBSTANCE ABUSE: *RESEARCH, CLINICAL, AND FORENSIC APPLICATIONS,*
   edited by **Marc J. Kaufman,** 2001

TOXICOLOGY AND CLINICAL PHARMACOLOGY OF HERBAL PRODUCTS,
   edited by **Melanie Johns Cupp,** 2000

CRIMINAL POISONING: *INVESTIGATIONAL GUIDE FOR LAW ENFORCEMENT,*
      TOXICOLOGISTS, FORENSIC SCIENTISTS, AND ATTORNEYS,
   by **John H. Trestrail, III,** 2000

A PHYSICIAN'S GUIDE TO CLINICAL FORENSIC MEDICINE,
   edited by **Margaret M. Stark,** 2000

Handbook of Drug Interactions

A Clinical and Forensic Guide

Edited by

Ashraf Mozayani, PharmD, PhD
Harris County Medical Examiner Office, Houston, TX
and
Lionel P. Raymon, PharmD, PhD
University of Miami School of Medicine, Miami, FL

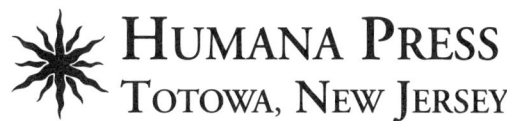

© 2004 Humana Press Inc.
999 Riverview Drive, Suite 208
Totowa, New Jersey 07512

www.humanapress.com

All rights reserved. No part of this book may be reproduced, stored in a retrieval system, or transmitted in any form or by any means, electronic, mechanical, photocopying, microfilming, recording, or otherwise without written permission from the Publisher.

The content, opinions, and points of view expressed in this book are the sole work of the authors and editors, who have warranted due diligence in the creation and issuance of their work. These views are not necessarily the views of the organizations with whom the authors are employed (or otherwise associated). The publisher, editors, and authors are not responsible for errors or omissions or for any consequences arising from the information or opinions presented in this book and make no warranty, express or implied, with respect to its contents.

Production Editor: Mark J. Breaugh.

Cover illustration: Two complementary views of drug interactions. The mathematical modeling of the drug is shown as a classic first order kinetic elimination curve and alteration in pharmacokinetics is amongst the best understood potential for undesired effects from combinations of two or more pharmaceuticals. But harder to grasp are the dynamic effects of drugs. The results of binding to target proteins, such as ion channels, can change the overall activity of cells, such as neurons, which in turn impinge on other target tissues. These pharmacodynamic interactions are complex and culminate in the symptomology observed in the patient. Any combination of chemicals in the body, endogenous or not, is a fluid game of competitions, synergies, or antagonisms at the metabolic and functional level. The results may go unseen, may be beneficial, may be harmful or, in some cases, lethal to the subject.

Cover design by Patricia F. Cleary.

Due diligence has been taken by the publishers, editors, and authors of this book to ensure the accuracy of the information published and to describe generally accepted practices. The contributors herein have carefully checked to ensure that the drug selections and dosages set forth in this text are accurate in accord with the standards accepted at the time of publication. Notwithstanding, as new research, changes in government regulations, and knowledge from clinical experience relating to drug therapy and drug reactions constantly occurs, the reader is advised to check the product information provided by the manufacturer of each drug for any change in dosages or for additional warnings and contraindications. This is of utmost importance when the recommended drug herein is a new or infrequently used drug. It is the responsibility of the health care provider to ascertain the Food and Drug Administration status of each drug or device used in their clinical practice. The publisher, editors, and authors are not responsible for errors or omissions or for any consequences from the application of the information presented in this book and make no warranty, express or implied, with respect to the contents in this publication.

For additional copies, pricing for bulk purchases, and/or information about other Humana titles, contact Humana at the above address or at any of the following numbers: Tel.: 973-256-1699; Fax: 973-256-8341; E-mail: humana@humanapr.com or visit our website: http://humanapress.com

This publication is printed on acid-free paper. ∞
ANSI Z39.48-1984 (American National Standards Institute) Permanence of Paper for Printed Library Materials.

Photocopy Authorization Policy:
Authorization to photocopy items for internal or personal use, or the internal or personal use of specific clients, is granted by Humana Press Inc., provided that the base fee of US $25.00 per copy, is paid directly to the Copyright Clearance Center at 222 Rosewood Drive, Danvers, MA 01923. For those organizations that have been granted a photocopy license from the CCC, a separate system of payment has been arranged and is acceptable to Humana Press Inc. The fee code for users of the Transactional Reporting Service is: [1-58829-211-8/04 $25.00].

Printed in the United States of America. 10 9 8 7 6 5 4 3 2 1

E-ISBN: 1-59259-654-1

Library of Congress Cataloging-in-Publication Data

Handbook of drug interactions : a clinical and forensic guide / [edited by] Ashraf Mozayani, Lionel P. Raymon.-- 1st ed.
   p. ; cm. -- (Forensic science and medicine)
Includes bibliographical references and index.
 ISBN 1-58829-211-8 (alk. paper)
 1. Drug interactions--Handbooks, manuals, etc. 2. Forensic pharmacology--Handbooks, manuals, etc.
  [DNLM: 1. Drug Interactions--Handbooks. 2. Forensic Medicine--methods--Handbooks. 3. Medication Errors--Handbooks. 4. Pharmacokinetics--Handbooks. QV 39 H23635 2003] I. Mozayani, Ashraf. II. Raymon, Lionel P. III. Series.
  RM302.H344 2003
  615'.7045--dc21
                            2003008434

Preface

Drug interactions and adverse drug effects have received much attention since studies published in daily newspapers have shown that they result in upwards of 100,000 Americans each year being hospitalized or remaining hospitalized longer than necessary, as well as leading to the death of a number of patients. Use of multiple drugs (8–12 on average in hospitalized patients) is common in a number of therapeutic regimens. In addition to multiple drug therapy, a patient may have access to several prescribers, and may have predisposing illnesses or age as risk factors for interactions. Drug interactions may occur between prescription drugs, but also between food and drug, and chemical and drug. Whereas some may be adverse, interactions may also be sought to decrease side effects or to improve therapeutic efficacy.

Combining drugs may cause pharmacokinetic and/or pharmacodynamic interactions. Pharmacokinetic mechanisms of interaction include alterations of absorption, distribution, biotransformation, or elimination. Absorption can be altered when drugs that alter pH or motility are co-administered, as seen with certain antiulcer or antidiarrheal medications, or when drugs are chelators or adsorbents (tetracyclines and divalent cations, cholestyramine, and anionic drugs). Distribution variations can result from competition for protein binding (sulfa drugs and bilirubin binding to albumin) or displacement from tissue-binding sites (digitalis and calcium channel blockers or quinidine). Induction of gene expression (slow), activation or inhibition (much quicker) of liver and extrahepatic enzymes such as P450, and conjugating enzymes have long found a place of choice in the literature describing the potential for adverse drug interactions resulting from altered metabolism. For example, induction is well described with the major anticonvulsant medications phenytoin, carbamazepine, and barbiturates, whereas inhibition can occur with antimicrobials from the quinolone, the macrolide, and the azole families. Finally, excretion can also be modified by drugs that change urinary pH, as carbonic anhydrase inhibitors do, or change secretion and reabsorption pathways, as probenecid does. Pharmacokinetic interactions in general result in an altered concentration of active drug or metabolite in the body, modifying the expected therapeutic response.

A second form of interaction has received little attention because of its modeling complexity and perhaps the poor understanding of basic physiological, biochemical, and anatomical substrates for drug action. Pharmacodynamic interactions involve additive (1 + 1 = 2), potentiating (0 + 1 = 2), synergistic (1 + 1 = 3), or antagonistic (1 + 1 = 0) effects at the level of receptors. Receptors are mainly proteins, such as enzymes (acetylcholinesterase, angiotensin-converting enzyme, for example), transport proteins (digitalis and Na$^+$/K$^+$ ATPase), structural proteins (colchicine and tubulin), or ion channels (Class I antiarrhythmics and voltage-dependent sodium channels). Large families of receptors to drugs involve signal transduction pathways and changes in intracellular second messenger concentrations (autonomic nervous system drugs and α, β, muscarinic receptors, for example). Finally, even less understood are interactions at the level of nucleic acids such as DNA and RNA, which can change the levels of expression of key proteins in target tissues (tolerance, tachyphylaxis of numerous central nervous system drugs).

Handbook of Drug Interactions: A Clinical and Forensic Guide addresses both types of drug interactions, emphasizing explanations when possible, and careful review of the general pharmacology. The result, we hope, will prove useful to health and forensic professionals as well as medical, pharmacy, nursing and graduate students alike.

Ashraf Mozayani
Lionel P. Raymon

Contents

Preface v
Contributors ix

PART I   CENTRAL NERVOUS SYSTEM DRUGS

Chapter 1: Drug Interactions with Benzodiazepines:
Epidemiologic Correlates with Other CNS Depressants and In Vitro Correlates with Inhibitors and Inducers of Cytochrome P450 3A4 3
David E. Moody

Chapter 2: Antiepileptic Drugs 89
Nathan L. Kanous II and Barry E. Gidal

Chapter 3: Opioids and Opiates 123
Seyed-Adel Moallem, Kia Balali-Mood, and Mahdi Balali-Mood

Chapter 4: Monoamine Oxidase Inhibitors and Tricyclic Antidepressants 149
Terry J. Danielson

Chapter 5: Selective Serotonin Reuptake Inhibitors 175
Mojdeh Mozayani and Ashraf Mozayani

Chapter 6: Antipsychotic Drugs and Interactions:
Implications for Criminal and Civil Litigation 187
Michael Welner

PART II   CARDIOVASCULAR DRUGS

Chapter 7: Cardiovascular Drugs 219
Johann Auer

PART III   ANTIBIOTICS

Chapter 8: Antimicrobial Drugs 295
Amanda J. Jenkins and Jimmie L. Valentine

Chapter 9: Drug Interactions with Medications Used for HIV/AIDS 319
Michael Frank

PART IV NONSTEROIDAL ANTIINFLAMMATORY DRUGS

Chapter 10: Nonsteroidal Antiinflammatory Drugs:
*Cyclooxygenase Inhibitors, Disease-Modifying
Antirheumatic Agents, and Drugs Used in Gout* 337
*Imad K. Abukhalaf, Daniel A. von Deutsch, Mohamed A. Bayorh,
and Robin R. Socci*

PART V ENVIRONMENTAL AND SOCIAL PHARMACOLOGY

Chapter 11: Food and Drug Interactions 379
Shahla M. Wunderlich

Chapter 12: Alcohol and Drug Interactions 395
A. Wayne Jones

Chapter 13: Nicotine and Tobacco 463
Edward J. Cone, Reginald V. Fant, and Jack E. Henningfield

Chapter 14: Anabolic Doping Agents 493
Daniel A. von Deutsch, Imad K. Abukhalaf, and Robin R. Socci

PART VI LEGAL ASPECTS

Chapter 15: Drug Interaction Litigation 599
Stephen A. Brunette

Chapter 16: Psychotropic Medications and Crime:
The Seasoning of the Prozac Defense 631
Michael Welner

Index 647

Contributors*

IMAD K. ABUKHALAF, PhD • Department of Pharmacology and Toxicology, NASA Space Medicine and Life Sciences Research Center; Clinical Research Center, Morehouse School of Medicine, Atlanta, GA; Department of Biotechnology and Genetic Engineering, Philadelphia University, Amman, Jordan.

JOHANN AUER, MD • Department of Cardiology and Intensive Care, General Hospital Wels, Wels, Austria

KIA BALALI-MOOD, PhD • Laboratory of Membrane Biophysics, Division of Pre Clinical Veterinary Sciences, The Vet School, College of Medicine & Veterinary Medicine, University of Edinburgh, Edinburgh, UK

MAHDI BALALI-MOOD, MD, PhD • Medical Toxicology Centre, Imam Reza Hospital, Mashad, Iran

MOHAMED A. BAYORH, PhD • Department of Pharmacology and Toxicology, NASA Space Medicine and Life Sciences Research Center; Cardiovascular-Alteration Team, National Space Biomedical Research Institute, Morehouse School of Medicine, Atlanta, GA

STEPHEN A. BRUNETTE, PC • Stephen A. Brunette, P. C., Colorado Springs, CO

EDWARD J. CONE, PhD • Pinney Associates, Bethesda, MD; Johns Hopkins University, Baltimore, MD

TERRY J. DANIELSON, PhD • Harris County Medical Examiner Office, Houston, TX

REGINALD V. FANT, PhD • Pinney Associates, Bethesda, MD

MICHAEL FRANK, MD • Division of Infectious Diseases, Medical College of Wisconsin, Milwaukee, WI

BARRY E. GIDAL, PharmD • Department of Neurology, School of Pharmacy, University of Wisconsin at Madison, Madison, WI

JACK E. HENNINGFIELD, PhD • Pinney Associates, Bethesda, MD; Department of Psychiatry and Behavioral Sciences, Johns Hopkins University School of Medicine, Baltimore, MD

AMANDA J. JENKINS, PhD • The Office of the Cuyahoga County Coroner, Cleveland, OH

A. WAYNE JONES, PhD, DSc • Department of Forensic Toxicology, University Hospital, Linköping, Sweden

NATHAN L. KANOUS II, PharmD • Pharmacy Practice Division, School of Pharmacy, University of Wisconsin at Madison, Madison, WI

SEYED-ADEL MOALLEM, PharmD, PhD • Department of Pharmacodynamy and Toxicology, School of Pharmacy, Mashhad University of Medical Sciences, Mashhad, Iran

DAVID E. MOODY, PhD • Center for Human Toxicology, Department of Pharmacology and Toxicology, University of Utah, Salt Lake City, UT

ASHRAF MOZAYANI, PharmD, PhD • Harris County Medical Examiner Office, Houston, TX

MOJDEH MOZAYANI, PharmD • Department of Pharmaceutical Services, Vanderbilt University Medical Center, Nashville, TN

LIONEL P. RAYMON, PharmD, PhD • Departments of Pathology, Pharmacology, Biochemistry, and Molecular Biology, Kaplan Medical Center; University of Miami School of Medicine, Miami, FL

ROBIN R. SOCCI, PhD • Department of Pharmacology and Toxicology, Morehouse School of Medicine, Atlanta, GA

JIMMIE L. VALENTINE, PhD • The Office of the Cuyahoga County Coroner, Cleveland, OH

DANIEL A. VON DEUTSCH, DDS, PhD, MSCR • Department of Pharmacology and Toxicology, NASA Space Medicine and Life Sciences Research Center, Clinical Research Center, Morehouse School of Medicine, Atlanta, GA

MICHAEL WELNER, MD • The Forensic Panel, NYU School of Medicine, New York, NY; Duquesne University School of Law, Pittsburgh, PA

SHAHLA M. WUNDERLICH, PhD, RD • Department of Human Ecology, Montclair State University, Upper Montclair, NJ

---

*The opinions or points of view expressed in this book are a consensus of the authors of the individual chapters. These views are not necessarily the views of the organizations with whom the authors are employed (or otherwise associated), nor the views of the authors of other chapters.

Part I
Central Nervous System Drugs

Chapter 1

Drug Interactions with Benzodiazepines

Epidemiologic Correlates with Other CNS Depressants and In Vitro Correlates with Inhibitors and Inducers of Cytochrome P450 3A4

David E. Moody, PhD

1. GENERAL INFORMATION ABOUT BENZODIAZEPINES

1.1. Introduction

The purpose of this chapter is to examine the drug interactions that occur with benzodiazepines and discuss the relevance of these interactions to the field of medicine in general with an emphasis on forensic toxicology. Because of the diverse nature of the benzodiazepines, some time has been taken to introduce this class of drugs. This introductory material has drawn upon some basic reference material and reviews [1–8], and is not otherwise referenced, except for specific points that did not come from these references. The primary literature will be more thoroughly cited in later sections presenting evidence of interactions with other central nervous system (CNS) depressants and specific enzyme involvement in the metabolism of benzodiazepines and drug interactions.

The benzodiazepines are a class of a relatively large number of drugs that share a common chemical structure and have anxiolytic to sedative action on the CNS. Chlordiazepoxide was first introduced in the 1960s, followed by diazepam, flurazepam, and

From: *Handbook of Drug Interactions: A Clinical and Forensic Guide*
A. Mozayani and L. P. Raymon, eds. © Humana Press Inc., Totowa, NJ

oxazepam. Since that time a number of benzodiazepines have been introduced. In the latest edition (1999) of Martindale *(7)*, at least 43 benzodiazepines were listed (Table 1). Most were found in the section on anxyolytic sedatives hypnotics and antipsychotics; one, clonazepam, was listed in the antiepileptics section. Of these 43 benzodiazepines only 12 are cross-listed in the latest edition (2002) of the *Physicians' Desk Reference* (Table 1; *8*); indicating their approval for use in the United States.

Many benzodiazepines are now made by more than one pharmaceutical house, or more than one subsidiary of a pharmaceutical house, and therefore have more than one trade name. A single example of trade names has been listed in Table 1, along with an associated manufacturer.

To understand the importance of drug interactions with benzodiazepines, a basic understanding of their pharmacodynamic action is required, along with the related therapeutic use. In addition, because many of the drug interactions are of a pharmacokinetic nature, the chemical structure and metabolism of the benzodiazepines must be appreciated.

1.2. Pharmacodynamics (Briefly), Uses, and Adverse Effects of Benzodiazepines

Most of the effects of benzodiazepines arise from their action on the CNS. Within the CNS the major molecular targets of the benzodiazepines are inhibitory neurotransmitter receptors directly activated by the amino acid, γ-aminobutyric acid (GABA). Benzodiazepines have been shown to bind and modulate the major GABA receptor in the brain, $GABA_A$, while $GABA_B$ receptors are not altered by benzodiazepines. The $GABA_A$ receptor is an integral membrane chloride channel that mediates most of the rapid inhibitory neurotransmission in the CNS. Benzodiazepines, unlike barbiturates that also bind $GABA_A$, act only in the presence of GABA. Typical benzodiazepine agonists increase the amount of chloride current generated by $GABA_A$ activation, potentiating the effect of GABA throughout the CNS. Bicuculline, an antagonist of $GABA_A$, reduces the behavioral and electrophysiological effects of benzodiazepines, and a benzodiazepine analog, flumazenil, that potently and selectively blocks the benzodiazepine binding site, is used clinically to reverse the effects of high doses of benzodiazepines *(4)*.

These CNS depressive effects result in anxiolytic, muscle relaxant, hypnotic, antigrade amnesia, anticonvulsant, and sedative effects that define the therapeutic uses of benzodiazepines (Table 2). Although the proper dose of any one benzodiazepine will produce many of these effects, some benzodiazepines are more appropriate for certain uses than others. In large part, this is dictated by the therapeutic half-life of the drug. Benzodiazepines are generally classified as short- (0–6 h), intermediate- (6–24 h), or long-acting (>24 h); some texts, however, will just use short- (0–24 h) and long-acting (>24 h) designations. Benzodiazepines used as anticonvulsants are long-acting and have rapid entry into the brain. Short- to intermediate-acting benzodiazepines are favored for treatment of insomnia. Short-acting benzodiazepines are used as preanesthia agents for sedation prior to surgery. Long-acting or multidose shorter-acting benzodiazepines are generally used as anxiolytics. The use of benzodiazepines listed in Martindale, along with their half-life, route(s) of administration, and normal range of doses, is presented in Table 3.

1. Drug Interactions with Benzodiazepines

Table 1
Benzodiazepines Listed in the 32nd Edition of Martindale (1999)

Generic Name	Representative Trade Name	Representative Manufacturer	CAS #
Adinazolam	None	Upjohn, USA	37115-32-5
Alprazolam[a]	Xanax (others)	Upjohn, USA	28981-97-7
Bentazepam	Tiadipona	Knoll, Sp	29462-18-8
Bromazepam	Lexotan (others)	Roche, UK	1812-30-2
Brotizolam	Lendormin	B.I., Ger	57801-81-7
Camazepam	Albego	Daker Farmasimos, Sp	36104-80-0
Chlordiazepoxide[a]	Librium (others)	Roche, USA	438-41-5
Cinolazepam	Gerodorm	Great, Aust	75696-02-5
Clobazam	Frisium	Hoechst, UK	22316-47-8
Clonazepam[a]	Klonopin (others)	Roche, USA	1622-61-3
Clorazepate[a]	Tranxene (others)	Abbott, USA	20432-69-3
Clotiazepam	Clozan (others)	Roerig, Belg	33671-46-4
Cloxazolam	Akton (others)	Excel, Belg	24166-13-0
Delorazepam	En	Ravizza, Ital	2894-67-9
Diazepam[a]	Valium (others)	Roche, USA	439-14-5
Estazolam[a]	Prosom (others)	Abbott, USA	29975-16-4
Ethyl Lorazepate	Victan (others)	Clin Midy, Fr	29177-84-2
Etizolam	Depas (others)	Fournier, Ital	40054-69-1
Fludiazepam	Erispan	Sumitomo, Jpn	3900-31-0
Flunitrazepam	Rohypnol (others)	Roche, UK	1622-62-4
Flurazepam[a]	Dalmane (others)	Roche, USA	1172-18-5
Halazepam	Paxipam (others)	Schering-Plough, Ital	23092-17-3
Haloxazolam	Somelin	Sankyo, Jpn	59128-97-1
Ketazolam	Solatran (others)	SmithKline Beecham, Sw	27223-35-4
Loprazolam	Dormonoct (others)	Hoechst Marian Russell, Belg	61197-73-7
Lorazepam[a]	Ativan (others)	Wyeth-Ayerst, USA	846-49-1
Lormetazepam	Loramet (others)	Wyeth, Sw	848-75-9
Medazepam	Rudotel	OPW, Ger	2898-12-6
Metaclazepam	Talis	Organon, Ger	65517-27-3
Mexazolam	Melex	Sankyo, Jpn	31868-18-5
Midazolam[a]	Versed	Roche, USA	59467-96-8
Nimetazepam	Ermin	Suitomo, Jpn	2011-67-8
Nitrazepam	Mogadon (others)	Roche, UK	146-22-5
Nordiazepam	Vegesan (others)	Mack, Sw	1088-11-5
Oxazepam[a]	Serax (others)	Wyeth-Ayerst, USA	604-75-1
Oxazolam	Serenal	Sankyo, Jpn	24143-17-7
Pinazepam	Domar (others)	Teoforma, Ital	52463-83-9
Prazepam	Demetrin (others)	Parke, Davis, Sw	2955-38-6
Quazepam	Doral (others)	Wallace, USA	36735-22-5
Temazepam[a]	Restoril (others)	Sandoz, USA	846-50-4
Tetrazepam	Myolastan (others)	Sanofi Winthrop, Fr	10379-14-3
Tofisopam	Grandaxin	Hung	22345-47-7
Triazolam[a]	Halcion	Upjohn, USA	28911-01-5

Note: Benzodiazepines listed in the 32nd edition of "Martindale The Complete Drug Reference, (1999)" (7). When more than one trade name was listed (noted as "other"), either the U.S. or most common one was chosen; a representative manufacturer was selected for listing.

[a]Also listed in the 2002 edition of the "Physicians Desk Reference" (2002) (8).

**Table 2
Uses of Benzodiazepines**

1. Anxiety (27)[a]	5. Alcohol Withdrawal (4)
2. Insomnia (26)	6. Muscle Spasms (3)
3. Presurgery / Sedation (8)	7. Panic Disorder (2)
4. Epilepsy / Seizures (7)	8. Depression (2)

[a]The number in parentheses represents the number of benzodiazepines listed in Martindale that are used to treat this disorder.

Drowsiness, sedation, and ataxia are the most frequent adverse effects of benzodiazepine use. They generally decrease on continued administration and arise from the CNS depressive effects of benzodiazepines. Less common adverse effects include vertigo, headache, mental depression, confusion, slurred speech, tremor, changes in libido, visual disturbances, urinary retention, gastrointestinal disturbances, changes in salivation, and amnesia. Rare events include paradoxical excitation leading to hostility and aggression, hypersensitivity reactions, jaundice, and blood disorders. With very high doses, hypotension, respiratory depression, coma, and occasionally death may occur.

Daily benzodiazepine use has been associated with dependence, tolerance, and after discontinuation, withdrawal symptoms in many individuals. Tolerance to the effects of benzodiazepines is a highly debated topic. It appears to occur in some individuals and may not occur in others. The likelihood of dependence appears higher in individuals with a history of drug or alcohol dependence and personality disorders. High doses and intravenous injection are used for their euphoric effects. Because development of dependence cannot be easily predicted, abrupt discontinuation of use is not recommended. Rather the dose should be tapered. Symptoms of withdrawal include anxiety, depression, impaired concentration, insomnia, headache, dizziness, tinnitus, loss of appetite, tremor, perspiration, irritability, perceptual disturbances, nausea, vomiting, abdominal cramps, palpitations, mild systolic hypertension, tachycardia, and orthostatic hypotension. If long-term use of benzodiazepines occurs, professional assisted withdrawal is recommended.

1.3. Basic Pharmacokinetics

The benzodiazepines are generally lipophilic drugs. Within the class, however, lipophilicity measured as the oil:water coefficient can differ over a 50-fold range. Due to their lipophilicity the benzodiazepines have relatively high plasma protein binding (70–99%) and relatively large volumes of distribution (0.3–22 L/kg) (Table 4). In general, the percent plasma protein binding and volume of distribution increase as does the oil:water partition coefficient.

The differences in lipophilicity can have a major impact on the pharmacokinetics of the benzodiazepine. Diazepam is regarded as a long-acting benzodiazepine. When diazepam is given as a single dose, however, it rapidly redistributes to nonplasma (lipid) compartments, the α elimination phase. It then slowly distributes back into the plasma compartment at subtherapeutic concentrations with a long terminal elimination half-life. Therefore, single doses of diazepam can be used as a short-term preanesthesia medication, whereas daily dosing will result in accumulation during the terminal elimination phase and provide long-acting therapy.

Table 3
Uses of Benzodiazepines Listed in Martindale

Generic Name	Half-Life (h)[a]	Route(s) of Administration	Usual Dose (mg)	Uses[b]
Adinazolam	short	—	—	1, 8
Alprazolam	11–15	oral	0.75–1.5	1, 8
Bentazepam	—	oral	25	1, 2
Bromazepam	12–32	oral	3–18	1, 2
Brotizolam	4–8	oral	0.25	2
Camazepam	—	oral	10	2
Chlordiazepoxide	5–30, 48–120[c]	oral, iv, im	25–100	1, 2, 3, 5, 6
Cinolazepam	—	—	—	2
Clobazam	18, 42[c]	oral	20–30	2, 4
Clonazepam	20–40	oral, iv	0.25–1	4, 7
Clorazepate	48–120[c]	oral, iv, im	15–90	1, 4, 5
Clotiazapam	4–18	oral	5–60	1, 2
Cloxazolam	long	oral, im	8–12	1, 3
Delorazepam	long	oral, im	0.5–6	1, 2, 3, 4
Diazepam	24–48, 48–120[c]	oral, iv, im	5–30	1, 2, 3, 4, 5, 6
Estazolam	10–24	oral	1–2	2
Ethyl Lorazepate	long	oral	1–3	1
Etizolam	short	oral	3	1, 2
Fludiazepam	short	oral	—	1
Flunitrazepam	16–35	oral, iv	0.5–2	2, 3
Flurazepam	47–100	oral	15–30	2
Halazepam	short	oral	20	1
Haloxazolam	short	oral	5	2
Ketazolam	long	oral	15–60	1
Loprazolam	4–15	oral	1–2	2
Lorazepam	10–20	oral, iv, sl	1–6	1, 2, 3, 4
Lormetazepam	11	oral	0.5–1.5	2
Medazepam	long	oral	10–20	1
Metaclazepam	short	oral	15	1
Mexazolam	—	oral	0.5	1
Midazolam	2–7	iv, im	2.5–7.5	3
Nimetazepam	short	oral	3	2
Nitrazepam	24–30	oral	5–10	2, 4
Nordiazepam	48–120	oral	15	1, 2
Oxazepam	4–15	oral	15–30	1, 2, 5
Oxazolam	long	oral	10	1
Pinazepam	long	oral	5–20	1, 2
Prazepam	48–120[c]	oral	30–60	1
Quazepam	39, 39–73[c]	oral	15	2
Temazepam	8–15	oral	10–40	1, 3
Tetrazepam	—	oral	25–50	6
Tofisopam	—	oral	150	1
Triazolam	1.5–5.5	oral	0.125–5	2

[a] If half-lives were not given, they were often referred to as short- or long-acting.
[b] See Table 2 for the number corresponding to different uses.
[c] Half-life for active metabolite.

Table 4
**The Percentage of Plasma Protein Binding
and Volume of Distribution (V_d) of Some Benzodiazepines**

Benzodiazepine	% Bound	V_d (l/kg)	Source
Alprazolam	71	0.7	a
Bromazepam	70	0.9	b
Chlordiazepoxide	96	0.3	a
Clobazam	85	1.0	b,c
Clonazepam	86	3.2	a
Clotiazepam	99	—	c
Diazepam	99	1.1	a
Estazolam	93	—	c
Flunitrazepam	78	3.3	a
Flurazepam	97	22.0	a
Halazepam	—	1.0	b
Lorazepam	91	1.3	a
Midazolam	95	1.1	a
Nitrazepam	87	1.9	a
Nordiazepam	98	0.8	a
Oxazepam	98	0.6	a
Prazepam	—	13.0	b
Quazepam	95	—	c
Temazepam	98	1.1	a
Triazolam	90	1.1	a

The source of information was: a = *(5)*; b = *(6)*; and c = *(7)*.

The benzodiazepines are well absorbed from the gastrointestinal tract, which allows for oral dosing of benzodiazepines (Table 3). As described in more detail in subheading 2.2, most will also undergo extensive first-pass metabolism, some to such an extent that parent drug is detected only at very low concentrations in blood (or blood-derived) samples. The plasma concentration benzodiazepines, or their primary pharmacodynamically active metabolites, correlates well with the dose of benzodiazepine administered (Fig. 1).

As a class, the benzodiazepines share many properties. There are structural differences between them, and these differences will affect the manner in which the benzodiazepine is metabolized, and thereby have an impact on their individual susceptibility to drug interactions.

2. CHEMISTRY AND METABOLISM OF BENZODIAZEPINES

2.1. Chemistry of Benzodiazepines

The classic structure of benzodiazepines (Fig. 2) consists of a benzene (A ring) fused to a seven-membered diazepine (B ring). In all but two of the commercially available benzodiazepines, the nitrogens in the diazepine ring are in the 1,4 position. Clobazam has nitrogens in the 1,5 position of the diazepine ring; tofisopam has nitrogens in the 2,3 position of the diazepine ring (Fig. 3). In addition, most commercially available

1. Drug Interactions with Benzodiazepines

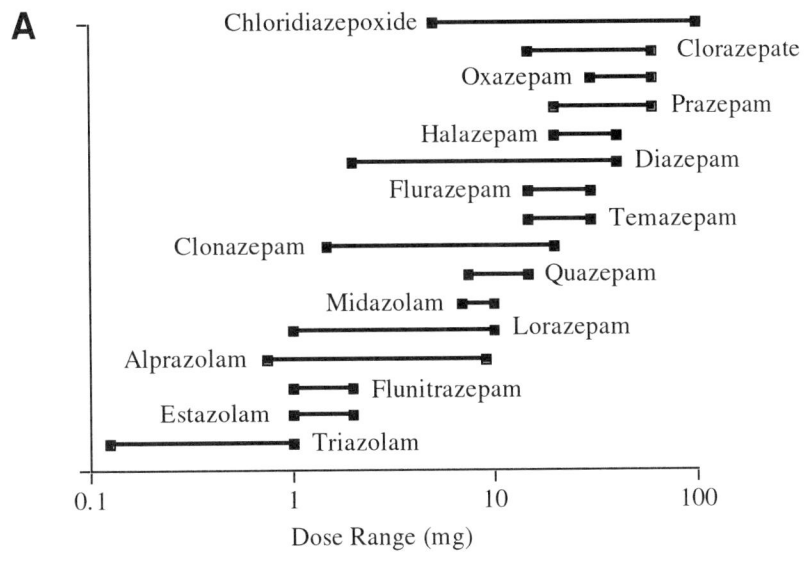

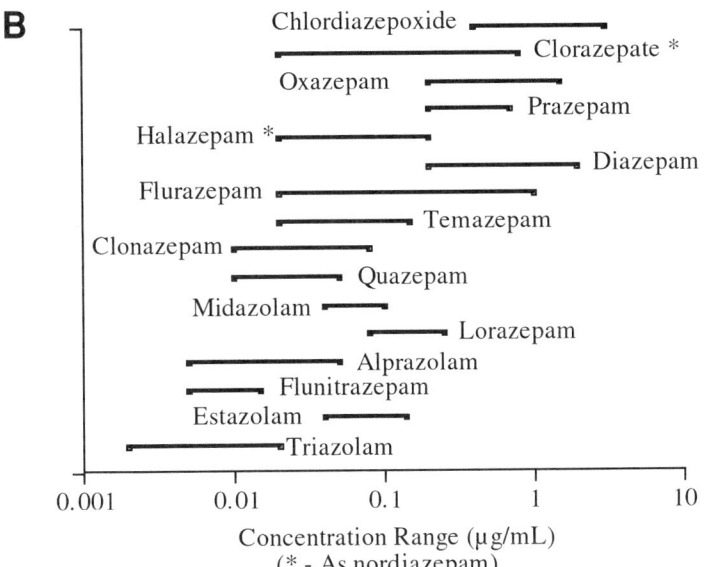

Fig. 1. The range of (**A**) therapeutic doses and (**B**) plasma concentrations of selected benzodiazepines. *In B, these concentrations are for the primary metabolite, nordiazepam.

benzodiazepines have an aryl substituent (C ring) at the 5 position of the diazepine ring. Therefore, with the exception of clobazam and tofisopam, these are 5-aryl-1,4-benzodiazepines.

Following the initial synthesis of chlordiazepoxide by Sternbach in 1957, and its introduction as a therapeutic agent in 1961, a number of benzodiazepines have been introduced onto the market. The initial modifications involved changes in the substituents on the diazepine ring. Modifications along this line first led to the development of diazepam, flurazepam, and oxazepam. These have continued through the years, leading

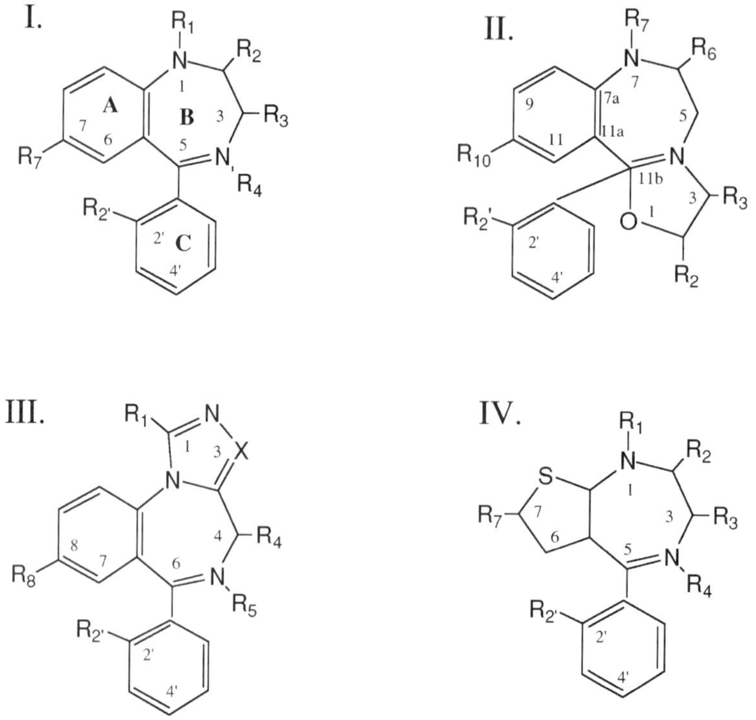

Fig. 2. Basic structure of the 5-aryl-1,4-benzodiazepines (I), 4,5-oxazolo-benzodiazepines (II), 1,2-triazolo- or 1,2-imidazo-benzodiazepines (III), and 1,4-thienodiazepines (IV).

to a number of 1,4-benzodiazepines (Table 5). Substitution of the benzene with a thieno group produced the 1,4-thienodiazepines (Figs. 2 and 3; Table 6). Annelation of an oxazolo (Fig. 2; Table 6) or oxazino group (ketazolam in Fig. 3; Table 6) at the 4,5 position of the diazepine has been used and the newer benzodiazepines have 1,2 anneled triazolo or imidazo groups (Fig. 2; Table 6). While most benzodiazepines have a phenyl substituent at the 5 position of the diazepine ring, bromazepam has a 2-pyridinyl substituent, and tetrazepam has a 1-cyclohexen-1-yl substituent at this position (Fig. 3; Table 6). Bentazepam, with a benzylthieno group fused to the diazepine ring, and brotizolam with both the thieno and triazolo groups are unique 1,4-thienodiazepines (Fig. 3; Table 6).

Structure activity studies have demonstrated some essential requirements for the benzodiazepine-mediated CNS effects. An electron-withdrawing group is required at the 7 position of the benzene (or thieno) group (R10 for oxazolo and R8 for triazolo or imidazo). These are generally the halides chloride, and occasionally bromide, or a nitroso group. An electron-withdrawing group at the 2' position of the 5-phenyl substituent is associated with increased potency and decreased half-life. Chloride or fluoride substituents have been used for this purpose.

2.2. Basic Metabolism of Benzodiazepines

Most of the 5-aryl-1,4-benzodiazepines are metabolized by N-dealkylation at the N-1 position and hydroxylation at the 3 position (Fig. 4). The N-dealkylation results

1. Drug Interactions with Benzodiazepines

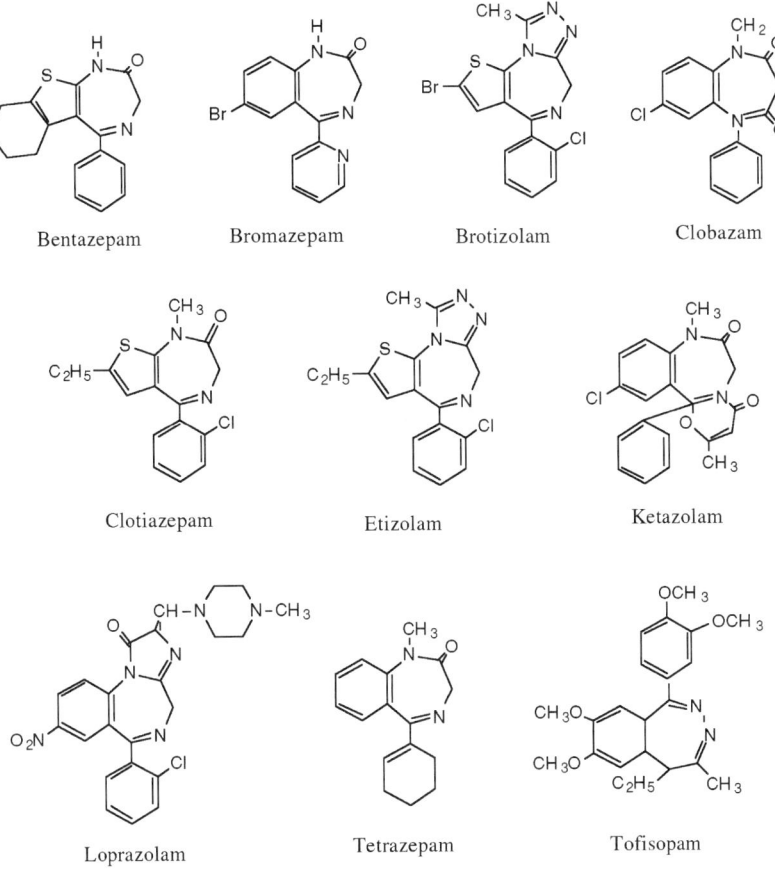

Fig. 3. Structure of "odd" benzodiazepines that could not easily be described in Tables 5 or 6.

in an active metabolite with a longer therapeutic half-life. In many cases the N-dealkyl metabolite is nordiazepam (N-desmethyldiazepam, nordiazam) (Fig. 4). Hydroxylation at the 3 position also results in an active metabolite. The 3-hydroxyl group is then conjugated, usually with glucuronide, resulting in an inactive metabolite. For benzodiazepines with a 3-hydroxyl group, such as temazepam, oxazepam (Fig. 4), lorazepam, and lormetazepam (not shown), conjugation of the 3-hydroxyl group is the major route of metabolism, even when other routes, such as N-dealkylation, may occur. These 3-hydroxyl benzodiazepines are consistently intermediate-acting drugs. Clorazepate is nonenzymatically decarboxylated to nordiazepam at the low pH of the stomach. The 4,5-oxazolo-benzodiazepines, such as ketazolam, oxazolam, and mexazolam, have the 4,5-oxazolo cleaved. It has been postulated by Ishigami et al. *(9)* that P450-mediated hydroxylation of the oxazolo-ring is followed by nonenzymatic cleavage of the ring, as shown for mexazolam (Fig. 5).

The 1,2-triazo- and 1,2-imidazo-benzodiazepines, alprazolam, triazolam, and midazolam, are metabolized by hydroxylation at the alpha (1') methyl group and at the 4 position (same as 3 position for other benzodiazepines). These metabolites are active until they are conjugated. 1'-Hydroxylation is the primary route for triazolam and mid-

Table 5
Structures of the 1,4-Benzodiazepines

Benzodiazipine	R_1	R_2	R_3	R_4	$R_{2'}$	R_7
I. 1,4-Benzodiazepines						
Camazepam	-CH$_3$	=O	-OCON(CH$_3$)$_2$	-H	-H	-Cl
Chlordiazepoxide	-H	-NHCH$_3$	-H	->O	-H	-Cl
Cinazolam	-CH$_2$CH$_2$CN	=O	-OH	-H	-F	-Cl
Clonazepam	-H	=O	-H	-H	-Cl	-NO$_2$
Clorazepate	-H	=O	-COO$^-$	-H	-H	-Cl
Delorazepam	-H	=O	-H	-H	-Cl	-Cl
Demoxepam	-H	=O	-H	->O	-H	-Cl
Diazepam	-CH$_3$	=O	-H	-H	-H	-Cl
Ethyl Lorazepate	-H	=O	-COOC$_2$H$_5$	-H	-F	-Cl
Fludiazepam	-CH$_3$	=O	-H	-H	-F	-Cl
Flunitrazepam	-CH$_3$	=O	-H	-H	-F	-NO$_2$
Flurazepam	-C$_2$H$_4$N(C$_2$H$_5$)$_2$	=O	-H	-H	-F	-Cl
Flutoprazepam	-CH$_2$CH=(CH$_2$CH$_2$)	=O	-H	-H	-F	-Cl
Halazepam	-CH$_2$CF$_3$	=O	-H	-H	-H	-Cl
Lorazepam	-H	=O	-OH	-H	-Cl	-Cl
Lormetazepam	-CH$_3$	=O	-OH	-H	-Cl	-Cl
Medazepam	-CH$_3$	-H	-H	-H	-H	-Cl
Metaclazepam	-CH$_3$	-CH$_2$OCH$_3$	-H	-H	-Cl	-Br
Nimetazepam	-CH$_3$	=O	-H	-H	-H	-NO$_2$
Nitrazepam	-H	=O	-H	-H	-H	-NO$_2$
Nordiazepam	-H	=O	-H	-H	-H	-Cl
Oxazepam	-H	=O	-OH	-H	-H	-Cl
Pinazepam	-CH$_2$C≡CH	=O	-H	-H	-H	-Cl
Prazepam	-CH$_2$-◁	=O	-H	-H	-H	-Cl
Quazepam	-CH$_2$CF$_3$	=S	-H	-H	-F	-Cl
Temazepam	-CH$_3$	=O	-OH	-H	-H	-Cl

azolam, while 4-hydroxylation is the primary route for alprazolam. Cleavage of the diazo-ring of alprazolam has also been described (Fig. 6). Adinazolam is successively N-demethylated at the 1-dimethylaminomethyl constituent to N-desmethyladinazolam and didesmethyladinazolam. The first N-demethyl product has a higher area under the curve than the parent drug and higher affinity for the central benzodiazepine receptors. Deamination of N-desmethyladinazolam with eventual 1-hydroxylation to 1-hydroxyalprazolam or side chain cleavage to estazoalm have been described in the mouse, but does not appear important in humans (10,11). Estazolam is hydroxylated to 1-oxoestazolam and to 4-hydroxyestazolam. Although both metabolites have minor activity, they are not formed in sufficient amounts to contribute to the pharmacologic activity of estazolam.

The 7-nitroso-benzodiazepines, clonazepam, flunitrazepam, and nitrazepam, are metabolized by successive reduction of the nitroso-group to the amine and subsequent N-acetylation of the amine to the corresponding acetamido-group (Fig. 7). These are

1. Drug Interactions with Benzodiazepines

Table 6
Structures of the Oxazolo-, 1,2-Triazo-, and 1,2-Imidazo- Benzodiazepines

II. Oxazolo-benzodiazepines	R_7	R_6	R_2	R_3	$R_{2'}$	R_{10}
Cloxazolam	-H	=O	-H	-H	-Cl	-Cl
Flutazolam	-CH$_2$CH$_2$OH	=O	-H	-H	-F	-Cl
Haloxazolam	-H	=O	-H	-H	-F	-Br
Metazolam	-H	=O	-H	-CH$_3$	-Cl	-Cl
Mexazolam	-H	=O	-CH$_3$	-H	-Cl	-Cl
Oxazolam	-H	=O	-CH$_3$	-H	-H	-Cl

III. 1,2-Triazo- or 1,2-Imidazo-Annelated-Benzodiazepines	R_1	X	R_4	R_5	$R_{2'}$	R_8
Adinazolam	-CH$_2$N(CH$_3$)$_2$	-N-	-H	-H	-H	-Cl
Alprazolam	-CH$_3$	-N-	-H	-H	-H	-Cl
Clinazolam	-CH$_3$	-CH-	-H	-H	-Cl	-Cl
Estazolam	-H	-N-	-H	-H	-H	-Cl
Midazolam	-CH$_3$	-CH-	-H	-H	-F	-Cl
Triazolam	-CH$_3$	-N-	-H	-H	-Cl	-Cl

V. Odd Structures (see Fig. 3)	
Bentazepam	Has thieno-cyclohexyl ring in place of benzyl A ring
Bromazepam	2-Pyridynyl ring at 5 position
Brotizolam	Has thieno ring in place of benzyl A ring along with 1,2-triazo fused ring
Clobazam	A 5-aryl-1,5-benzodiazepine
Clotiazepam	Has thieno ring in place of benzyl A ring
Etizolam	Has thieno ring in place of benzyl A ring along with 1,2-triazo fused ring
Ketazolam	Has a nonoxazolo 4,5-fused ring
Loprazolam	Has an imidazo fused ring with different N configuration / also 7-nitroso
Tetrazepam	Nonaromatic 6-membered ring at 5 position
Tofisopam	A 1-aryl-2,3-benzodiazepine

often the major metabolites present in urine and plasma and are devoid of activity at benzodiazepine receptors. N-Dealkylation at the 1 position of the diazo-ring is also a prominent route of metabolism for flunitrazepam. Clonazepam and flunitrazepam can also be hydroxylated at the 3 position of the diazoring. With nitrazepam, oxidative metabolism at the diazo ring results in ring cleavage; this can be followed by hydroxylation of the phenyl (B) ring (Fig. 7).

The routes of metabolism of other benzodiazepines, bromazepam (ring cleavage and 3-hydroxylation), clobazam (N-dealkylation and c-ring hydroxylation), clotiazepam (N-dealkylation and side chain hydroxylation), and loprazolam (N-dealkylation and spontaneous hydrolysis to polar compounds) have been described (Fig. 8). Metaclazepam has a methyl ether at the 2 position of the diazo-ring. This appears to block hydroxylation at the 3 position, with N- and O-demethylations forming the primary metabolites (Fig. 9; 12). Camazepam has a dimethylcarbamyl group at the 3 position of the diazo-ring. Successive hydroxylations of the methyl groups followed by N-hydroxymethy-

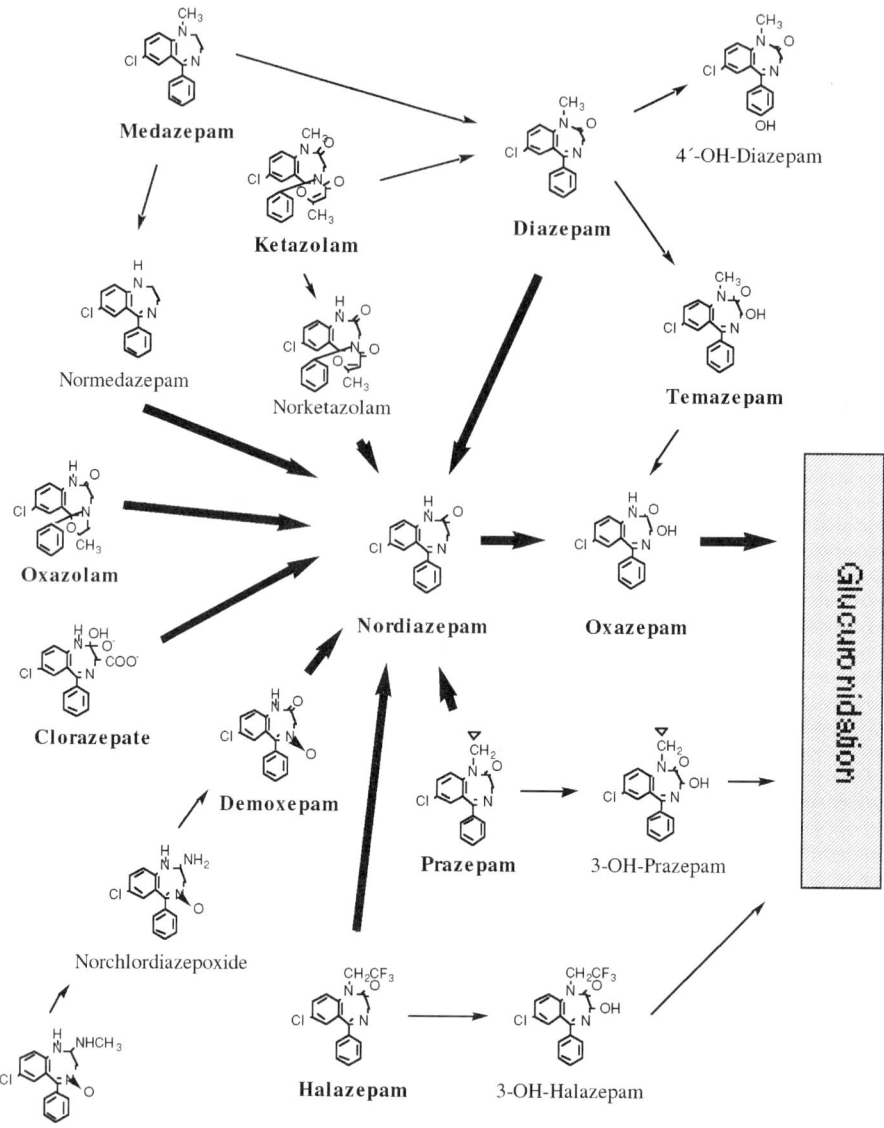

Fig. 4. Common metabolic pathways of 5-aryl-1,4-benzodiazepines. The compounds in bold type are pharmaceutical benzodiazepines. From *(401)*; reproduced from the *Journal of Analytical Toxicology* by permission of Preston Publications, a division of Preston Industries, Inc.

lations account for most of the metabolites, along with N-demethylation (Fig. 9; *13*). Tofisopam (tofizopam) is an unusual 2,3-diazepine with hydroxymethyl groups at four positions. O-Demethylation at the R1 and R4 positions has been described as the major routes of tofisopam's metabolism (Fig. 9; *14*). The metabolism of a number of other benzodiazepines has not been described. Based upon the principles discussed above, however, one can speculate on putative pathways of their metabolism (Table 7).

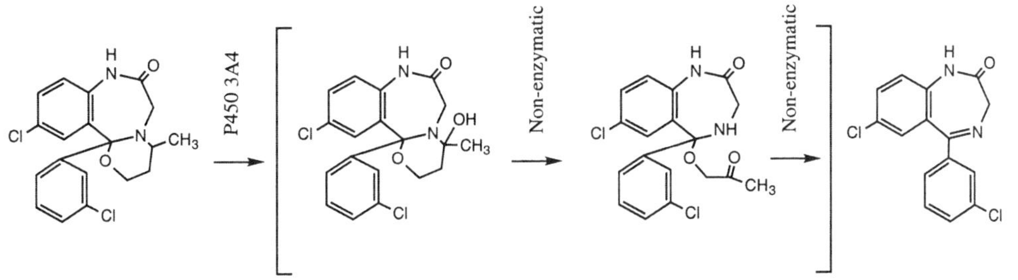

1. Drug Interactions with Benzodiazepines

Fig. 5. Metabolism of the 4,5-oxazolone ring as postulated for mexazolam by Ishigami et al. *(9)*.

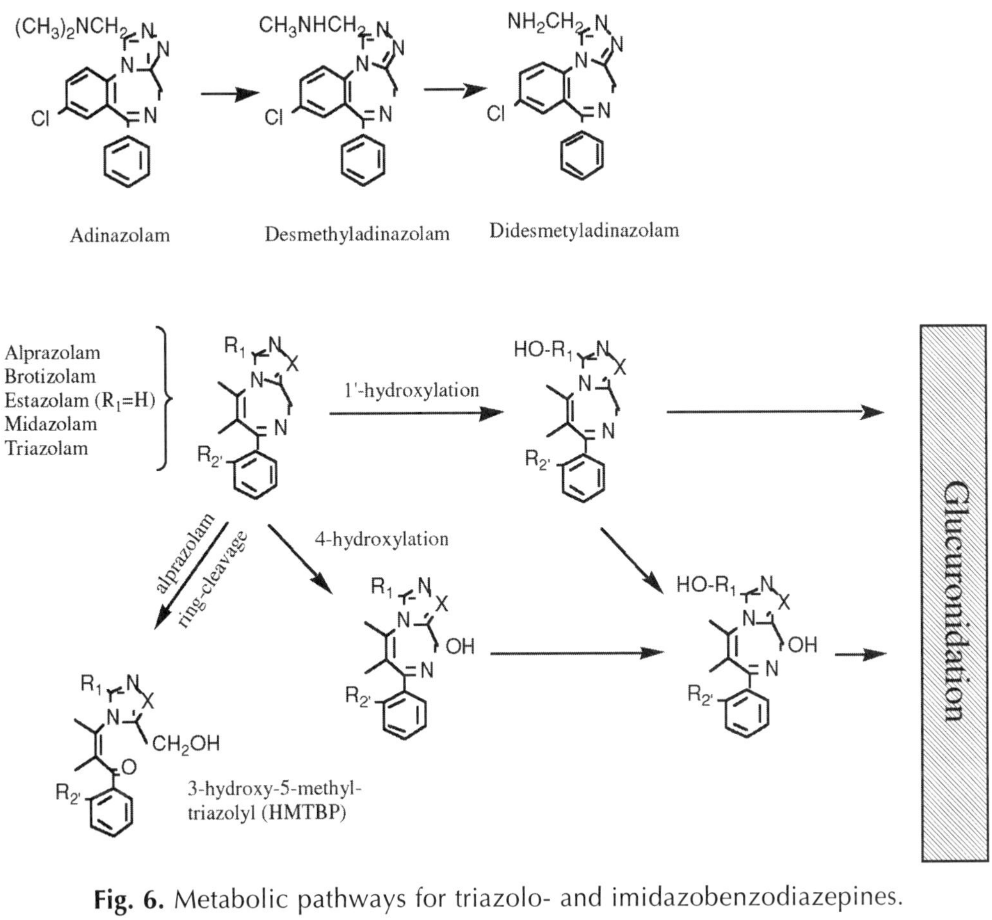

Fig. 6. Metabolic pathways for triazolo- and imidazobenzodiazepines.

2.3. The Role of Specific Enzymes in the Metabolism of Benzodiazepines

2.3.1. Methods Used to Determine Enzyme Involvement in the Metabolic Pathway

The methods for determination of the role of a specific enzyme in the pathway of a drug's metabolism have been developed most thoroughly for the cytochrome P450s

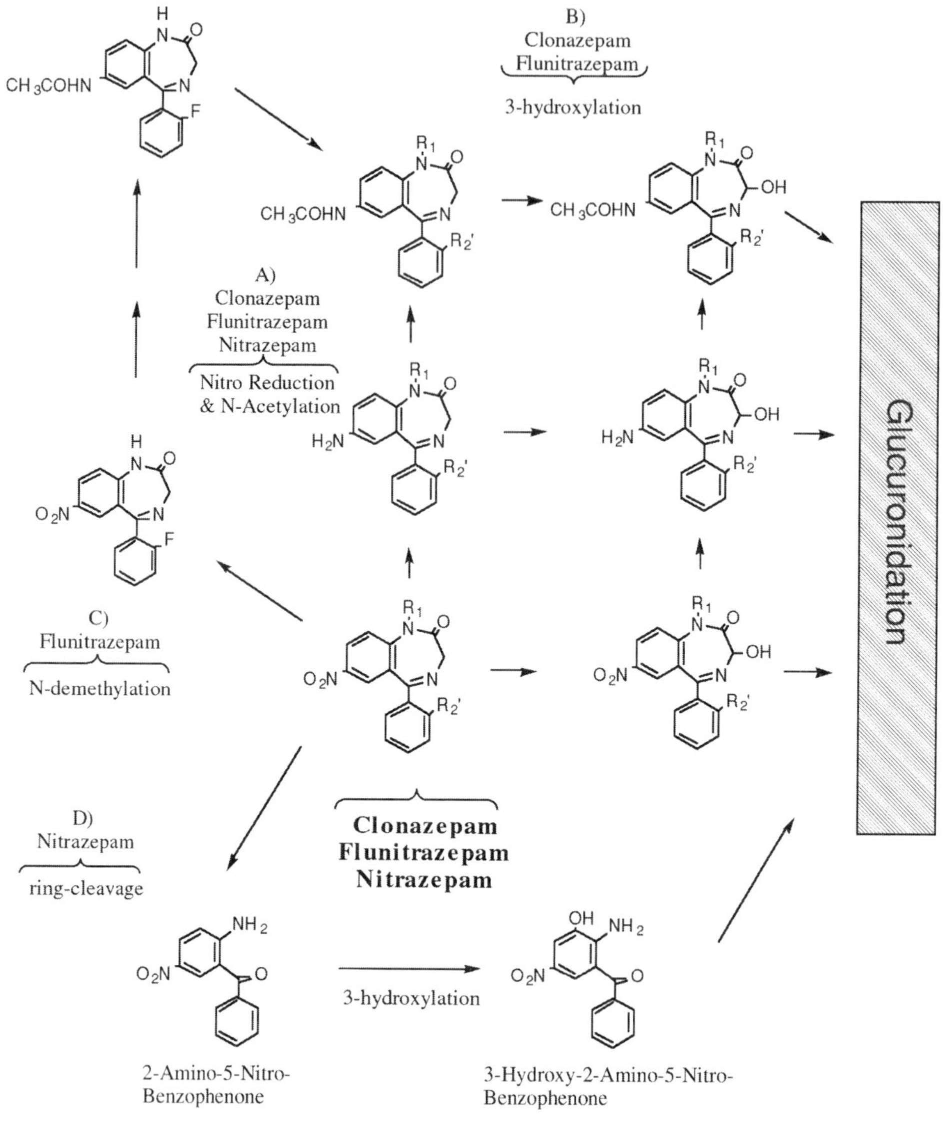

Fig. 7. Common metabolic pathways for 7-nitrobenzodiazepines. From *(401)*; reproduced from the *Journal of Analytical Toxicology* by permission of Preston Publications, a division of Preston Industries, Inc.

(P450s) *(15–19)*. Studies are done using human liver tissue that is now usually procured from donor tissue that is deemed unsuitable for transplantation. Most often studies utilize the microsomal cell fraction prepared from differential centrifugation of homogenates of liver tissue *(20)*, but cultured hepatocytes and liver slices are also being used. The methods used include the use of selective inhibitors, selective antibodies, correlation between P450 activities or contents in a number of human liver microsome (HLM) preparations with the pathway in question, and activities with cDNA-expressed P450s (Table 8). Each of these methods has certain strengths and weaknesses; the most convincing studies use most of them in an integrated approach (Table 8).

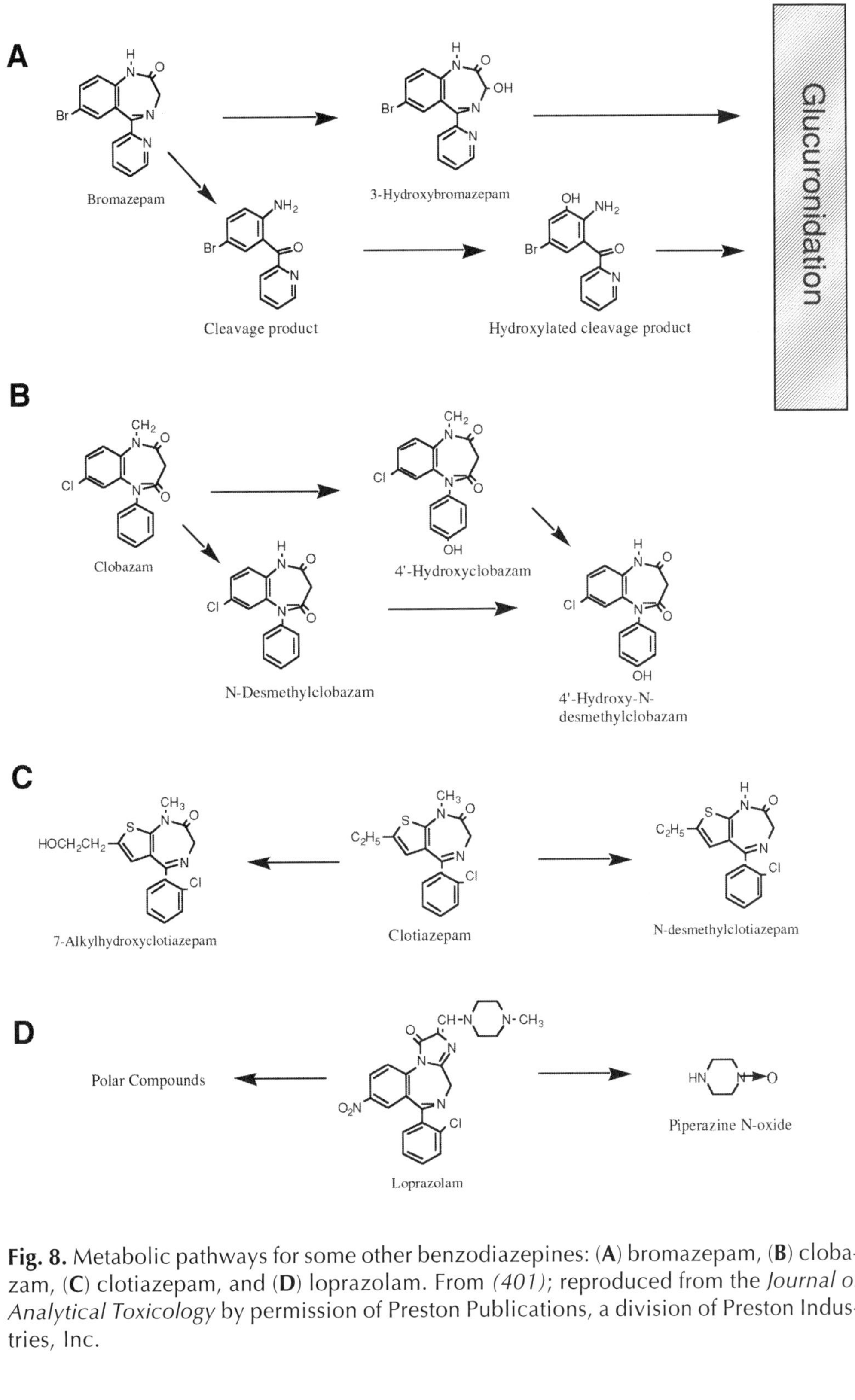

Fig. 8. Metabolic pathways for some other benzodiazepines: (**A**) bromazepam, (**B**) clobazam, (**C**) clotiazepam, and (**D**) loprazolam. From *(401)*; reproduced from the *Journal of Analytical Toxicology* by permission of Preston Publications, a division of Preston Industries, Inc.

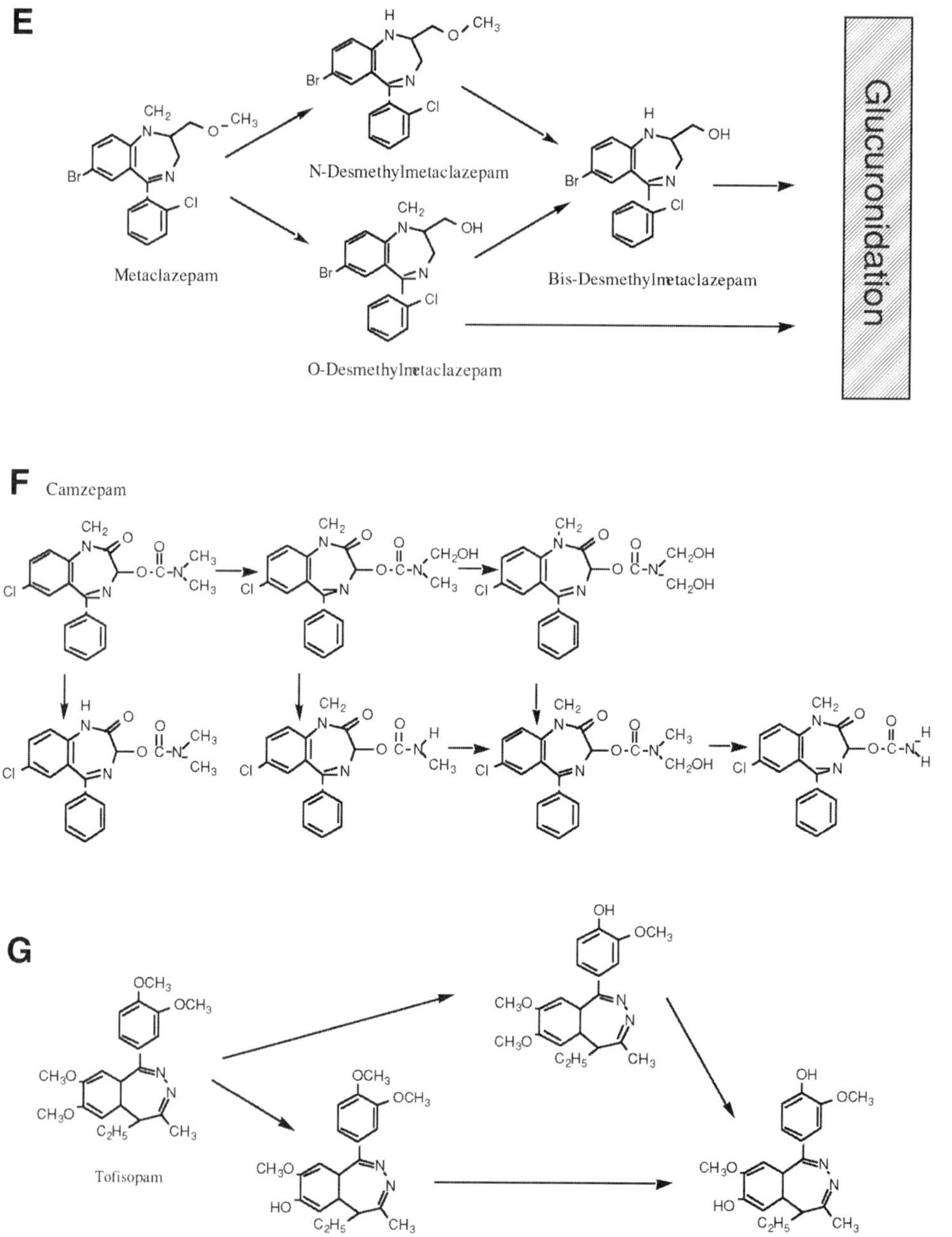

Fig. 9. Metabolic pathways for some other benzodiazepines (con'td.): (**E**) metaclazepam, (**F**) camazepem, and (**G**) tofisopam.

Selective inhibitors are often the easiest reagents to obtain and perform studies with. The results from their use, however, must be interpreted with care, as selectivity either is not complete, or is lost as the concentration of the inhibitor is increased. Recent studies have compared the ability of commonly used selective inhibitors to inhibit marker substrate P450 activities in either HLM or cDNA-expressed P450s *(21–23)*. A summary of their results is presented in Table 9. These comparisons can be useful in interpreting

Table 7
Speculation on Putative Metabolic Pathways for Benzodiazepines that Have Not Had Metabolites Defined

5-Aryl-1,4-Benzodiazepines	
Cinolazolam	conjugation of 3-hydroxyl; N-dealkylation
Delorazepam	3-hydroxylation → conjugation
Ethyl Lorazepate	3-ester hydrolysis → conjugation
Fludiazepam	3-hydroxylation → conjugation; N-dealkylation
Pinazepam	3-hydroxylation → conjugation; N-dealkylation
Tetrazepam	3-hydroxylation → conjugation; N-dealkylation

7-Nitroso-5-Aryl-1,4-Benzodiazepines	
Nimatazepam	amine reduction → N-acetylation
	3-hydroxylation → conjugation; N-dealkylation

4,5-Oxazolo-Benzodiazepines	
Cloxazolam	cleavage of 4,5-oxazolo-ring; 3-hydroxylation → conjugation
Haloxazolam	cleavage of 4,5-oxazolo-ring; 3-hydroxylation → conjugation
Mexazolam	cleavage of 4,5-oxazolo-ring; 3-hydroxylation → conjugation

1,2-Triazo-Benzodiazepine	
Etizolam	α-hydroxylation → conjugation; 4-hydroxylation

Table 8
Tools Used to Determine Involvement of Specific Enzymes in Xenobitotic Metabolism

1. Selective inhibitors
   - Relatively easy to get and most are relatively inexpensive
   - Selectivity is concentration dependent
   - Using titration can help determine % involvement in a pathway
   - Mechanism-based and metabolite intermediate complex inhibitors require 10–15 min preincubation before addition of test substrate

2. Selective antibodies
   - Either expensive or require collaboration with laboratory that produces them
   - Selectivity often limited to family of enzyme
   - Using titration can help determine % involvement in a pathway

3. Correlation
   - Requires a phenotyped HLM bank, the more HLM the better
   - Requires selective assays for all enzymes monitored
   - Selectivity is rarely perfect
   - If marker assay is not evenly distributed, high activity HLMs may bias result

4. cDNA-expressed enzymes
   - Excellent to determine if enzymes can carry out metabolism
   - Activities have improved over time
   - Newer studies are employing scaling techniques to help estimate % involvement. This requires a phenotyped liver bank

Table 9
Selectivity of P450 Inhibitors (% Inhibition)

Inhibitor	µM	1A2	2A6	2B6	2C8	2C9	2C19	2D6	2E1	3A4
Fur[a]	5[b]	90				—		—	15	—
	5[d]	20–90	—	—	—	—	—	—	—	—
	100[b]	90				—		—	15	—
	100[d]	30–95	—	20–30	—	15–30	15–30	—	0–15	0–25
	200[c]	90	—	—	45	30		65	30	50
7,8-BF	1[c]	95	—	—	20					
	10[b]	75				—		+20	+30	—
	100[b]	80				60		—	+90	30
α-NF	1[d]	20–95	—	—	+200	15	25			0–+50
	100[d]	90–95	0–65	—	+300	25–35	30–45			0–+1000
Orph	100[d]	—	—	0–20	0–25	—	—	0–70	—	0–25
	500[d]	0–70	—	70–75	65–70	25–30	0–65	55–90	30–40	35–70
Tran	1000[c]	60	100	100	80	90		—	60	65
Sulf	10[b]	—				65		—	—	—
	10[c]	—	—	—	100	90		15	—	—
	20[b]	—				75		20	—	—
	20[d]	0–20	—	—	—	90	—	—	—	10–30
	100[b]	—				85		—	—	—
	100[d]	0–30	—	20–35	20–30	90	—	—	15–25	20–25
Quin	0.5[c]	—	—	—	—	45		95	—	—
	0.5[d]	—	—	—	—	—	—	60–70	—	—
	1[b]	—				—		60	—	—
	10[b]	—				—		85	—	—
	10[d]	—	—	—	—	—	—	85–95	—	0–20
DDC	10[b]	—				—		—	50	—
	20[d]	—	20–35	—	—	15–35	0–50	—	35	—
	100[b]	20				20		30	75	20
	100[d]	10–30	50–70	10–40	15–45	30–60	35–80	20	70–75	20
	200[c]	—	90	30	35	40		50	90	25
3-MP	50[b]	—				—		65	70	—
	500[b]	35				40		80	75	20
	500[c]	—	20	50	—	60		75	80	35
Keto	1[d]	—	—	—	0–25	—	—	—	—	10–90
	2[b]	—				—		—	—	82
	5[d]	—	—	20–40	50–55	25	—	—	—	90–100
	10[c]	40	35	85	—	60		65	85	100
	50[b]	45				70		60	—	100

(continued)

1. Drug Interactions with Benzodiazepines

Table 9 (*continued*)

Inhibitor	µM	1A2	2A6	2B6	2C8	2C9	2C19	2D6	2E1	3A4
TAO	50[b]	—				—		—	—	80
	50[d]	—	—	—	—	—	—	—	—	25–50
	500[d]	—	0–20	0–20	20–30	—	—	—	15–30	75–80
	1000[c]	20	25	30	30	50		40	10	100

Note: "—" means less than 15% inhibition was observed; a blank spot indicates that P450 was not studied.

[a]The abbreviations used for inhibitors are listed along with the P450 it is commonly believed specific for in parentheses: Fur, furafylline (1A2); 7,8-BF, 7,8-benzoflavone (1A2); α-NF, α-naphthoflavone (1A2); Orph, orphenadrine (2B6); Tran, tranylcypromine (2C); Sulf, sulfaphenazole (2C9); Quin, quinidine (2D6); DDC, diethyldithiocarbamate (2E1); 3-MP, 3-methylpyrazole (2E1); Keto, ketoconazole (3A4); and TAO, troleandromycin (3A4).

[b]Data from Newton et al. *(21)*, who used four HLM with 15-min preincubation for studies with Fur, DDC, and TAO, and no preincubation for all other inhibitors.

[c]Data from Ono et al. *(22)*, who used cDNA-expressed P450s with 5-min preincubation for all inhibitors.

[d]Data from Sai et al. *(23)*, who used cDNA-expressed P450s with 10-min preincubation for Fur, DDC, and TAO, and 5-min preincubations for all other inhibitors.

results presented in this and other chapters of this book, and when researching the primary literature.

Selective antibodies are powerful tools, but their selectivity must be carefully determined. The most common limitation is their inability to distinguish P450s of the same family (e.g., 3A4 vs 3A5). A common feature of selective inhibitors and selective antibodies is that they can be used to titrate the activity in liver tissue preparations and provide an estimate of the percent involvement. Selective antibodies can also be used to quantitate the amount of a particular P450 or P450 family in liver tissue.

A common feature of liver tissue preparations is that there is usually large interindividual variation between preparations. This arises in part from true individual differences and from differences in tissue preparation. When a number of HLMs have been phenotyped by immunoquantitation and/or by determining P450 selective activities, they can be used for correlational studies. The metabolic pathway in question is measured in the different preparations and plotted as a scatter gram against the marker activities or contents. High and low correlation coefficients provide supportive evidence of the enzymes' positive or negative involvement, respectively. As with any correlation experiments the distribution of activities should be carefully examined to assure no heterogenous scatter is creating a biased result *(24)*.

cDNA-expressed P450s provide a means of measuring the pathway in question in a purified and reconstituted system. By themselves, they can only determine the ability of the enzyme to perform the reaction. Comparison of different P450s is complicated by differences in their membrane lipid contents, and the contents of the other enzymes involved in P450-mediated monooxygenations, NADPH cytochrome P450 reductase, and cytochrome b_5 *(18)*. In more recent experiments, scaling techniques have been employed to estimate the relative contributions of P450s using the results of experiments in cDNA-expressed P450s. The relative contribution of the enzyme (f_i) is calculated from: $f_i = [A_i v_i(s)] / [\Sigma A_i v_i(s)]$, where A_i is the relative abundance of the P450

Table 10
Involvement of Specific Enzymes in the Metabolism of Benzodiazepines

Drug	Pathway	P450	Level of Evidence[a]	References
Diazepam	3-Hydroxylation	3A4, 3A5 >> 2C19	1, 2, 4	*26–30*
	N-Demethylation	2C19, 3A4, 3A5 >> 2B6	1, 2, 4	*26–30*
Nordiazepam	3-Hydroxylation	3A4 >> 3A5	4	*27,28*
Temazepam	N-Dealkylation	3A4, 2C19 > 3A5 >> 2B6	4	*27,28*
Midazolam	1'-Hydroxylation	3A5 > 3A4 >> 2B6	1, 2, 3, 4	*31–42*
	4-Hydroxylation	3A4, 3A5 >> 2B6	1, 2, 3, 4	*32,33,35,37,38,41*
Triazolam	1'-Hydroxylation	3A	1, 2, 3	*32,41,207*
	4-Hydroxylation	3A	1, 2, 3	*32,41,207*
Alprazolam	1'-Hydroxylation	3A5 > 3A4	1, 2, 3, 4	*44,45*
	4-Hydroxylation	3A4, 3A5	1, 2, 3, 4	*43–45*
Adinozalam	N-Demethylation	3A4 > 2C19	1, 4	*46*
	2nd N-Demethylation	3A4 > 2C19	1, 4	*46*
Flunitrazepam	3-Hydroxylation	3A4	1, 2, 4	*47–49*
	N-demethylation	3A4, 2C19	1, 2, 4	*47–49*
Brotizolam	Utilization	3A4	4	*50*
	1'-Hydroxylation	3A4	1, 2	*50*
	4-Hydroxylation	3A4	1, 2	*50*
Mexazolam	Oxazolo-ring cleavage	3A4	2	*9*

[a]Level of evidence refers to the types of experiments with the same number listed in Table 8.

and $v_i(s)$ is the concentration velocity function of the P450. Abundance has been alternatively estimated from immunoquantitation of P450s in HLM *(25)* or from relative activity factors (RAFs) calculated from the ratio of activity of enzyme-specific pathways in HLM to that in cDNA-expressed P450s *(18)*. These methods are well described in the recent work of Venkatakrishnan et al. *(19)*.

2.3.2. Involvement of Specific P450s in the Metabolism of Benzodiazepines

The metabolism of a number of benzodiazepines has been studied using the methods described above. The results of these studies are summarized in Table 10. The P450 3A family has been implemented in all of these metabolic pathways that include: diazepam 3-hydroxylation and N-demethylation *(26–30)*, nordiazepam 3-hydroxylation *(27, 28)*, temazepam N-dealkylation *(27,28)*, midazolam 1'- and 4-hydroxylation *(31–42)*, alprazolam 1'- and 4-hydroxylation *(43–45)*, the first and second N-demethylations of adinozalam *(46)*, flunitrazepam 3-hydroxylation and N-demethylation *(47–49)*, brotizolam 1'- and 4-hydroxylation *(50)*, and the oxazolo-ring cleavage of mexazolam *(9)*.

In human liver there are two members of the 3A family, 3A4 and 3A5. P450 3A4 is the most abundant P450 in most livers, while 3A5 is detected in only approximately 20% of livers *(51)*. In a few of the studies cited above, 3A4 and 3A5 mediated activities have been compared. Equivalent activities were found for diazepam 3-hydroxylation and N-demethylation *(27,29)*, and for midazolam 4-hydroxylation *(33,35)*. P450 3A4 was more active than 3A5 for nordiazepam 3-hydroxylation and temazepam N-dealkylation *(27,28)*. In contrast, P450 3A5 was more active than 3A4 for midazolam 1'-hydroxylation *(33,35,42)*. Gorski et al. *(44)* indirectly suggest that 3A5 is more involved in the 1'-hydroxylation of alprazolam based upon correlation differences between livers that contain both 3A4 and 3A5 vs those containing only 3A4. As some differences have been observed in the response of 3A4 and 3A5 to inhibitors *(22)*, the differential metabolism of benzodiazepines by these two members of the 3A family may play a factor in susceptibility to certain drug interactions.

P450 2C19 appears to play a role in the N-demethylation of diazepam, temazepam, adinazolam, N-desmethyladinazolam, and flurazepam. For diazepam, this involvement has been confirmed from studies comparing extensive and poor 2C19 metabolisors *(52)*. For 3 poor metabolizers, compared to 13 extensive metabolizers, the clearance of diazepam was reduced by 50%, and the elimination half-life was increased twofold *(52)*. This study is consistent with the in vitro findings that show considerable diazepam N-demethylation activity with cDNA-expressed 2C19, inhibition of diazepam N-demethylation in HLM with omeprazole, and with anti-2C family antibodies *(26–30)*. In the same study, Bertilsson et al. *(52)* compared the elimination of nordiazepam in poor and extensive 2C19 metabolizers. With nordiazepam also, the clearance was reduced by 50%, and the elimination half-life was increased twofold *(52)*. This suggests that 2C19 can also be involved in some 3-hydroxylation reactions, which was not readily apparent from the results of the in vitro studies *(27)*.

P450 2B6 may have a minor role in the N-demethylations of diazepam and temazepam *(27–29)*, as well as the 1'- and 4-hydroxylations of midazolam *(39,41,42)*. Whether this role of 2B6 will have clinical significance has yet to be determined. In part, this will depend upon the relative content of 2B6 in human livers. Earlier studies on specific P450 content suggested that 2B6 did not exceed 1–2% of total P450 *(51)*, but a more recent one showed 100-fold variation in 2B6 content in 19 HLM from 0.7 to 71.1 pmol/mg protein. Assuming an average P450 content of 500 pmol/mg protein, this is a range of 0.14–14.2% of total P450. If high 2B6 content is coupled with low 3A4 and 3A5 content, then the likelihood of 2B6's contribution to the metabolism of some benzodiazepines may be increased.

In summary, P450 3A4 (and 3A5) are extensively involved in many pathways of oxidative metabolism of benzodiazepines. P450 2C19 is involved in many of the N-demethylation reactions, and may play a role in some other oxidative pathways. P450 2B6 may also have a role in certain oxidative pathways. Though a number of metabolic pathways of benzodiazepines have been studied, many have not. Little is known of the role of specific uridine diphosphate glucuronosyl transferases or sulfotransferases in conjugation of benzodiazepines or of the enzymes involved in reduction and subsequent acetylation of the nitroso-benzodiazepines.

3. BENZODIAZEPINE DRUG INTERACTIONS

3.1. General Considerations

Both pharmacodynamic and pharmacokinetic mechanisms have been observed for drug interactions concerning benzodiazepines. Most pharmacokinetic drug interactions involve either the inhibition or induction of specific P450s involved in the metabolism of benzodiazepines. They are the most common and the better documented of drug interactions with benzodiazepines. Most, however, result in either an increased (inhibitors) or decreased (inducers) activity of the benzodiazepine. When therapeutic doses are used these interactions may have clinical and forensic, if carried into driving or other machine-operating environments, but rarely lethal consequences. Pharmacokinetic drug interactions with benzodiazepines are specific for certain benzodiazepines depending upon the enzyme(s) involved in their metabolism. Some of these interactions were reviewed in the mid-1980s *(53,54)*. A more recent review was restricted to alprazolam, midazolam, and triazolam *(55)*.

Pharmacodynamic drug interactions with other CNS depressants are more likely to have lethal, as well as clinical and forensic, consequences. These drugs, which include ethanol, opioids, and barbiturates, also cause respiratory depression, and their combined use can have additive, and has been described in some cases, even synergistic effects. The potential for pharmacodynamic interactions exists for all benzodiazepines regardless of route of metabolism; synergistic interactions, however, may involve a combined pharmacodynamic and pharmacokinetic interaction that is specific for certain benzodiazepines. A number of reviews have considered the interactions of benzodiazepines and ethanol *(56–59)*. None were located addressing interactions with opioids or barbiturates.

The tables presenting pharmacokinetic and pharmacodynamic results of clinical studies (Tables 14–30) are structured in a similar format with consistent abbreviations. A key to these tables is presented at the end of the chapter in Table 31.

3.2. Epidemiological Occurrences of Benzodiazepines, Ethanol, and Opioids

3.2.1. The Occurrence of Other Drugs or Ethanol in Benzodiazepine-Associated Deaths

The epidemiologic record presents circumstantial evidence for the importance of drug interactions of benzodiazepines with ethanol and opioids. A number of studies have examined deaths linked to benzodiazepines. Those that investigated the involvement of other drugs and/or ethanol in the deaths are listed in Table 11A. In general, deaths linked to benzodiazepine use often, but not always, also have evidence of ethanol and/or other drug use. Some studies investigated only the involvement of ethanol *(60,61)*, or other drugs *(62)*, in addition to benzodiazepines. It is therefore difficult to get an exact estimate of how often only benzodiazepines were identified. In one study carried out in the United States and Canada that investigated deaths involving diazepam, only 2 of 914 deaths were identified with only diazepam *(63)*. In another study carried out in Sweden, benzodiazepines were identified in 144 of 702 deaths without other drugs or ethanol *(64)*. A sufficient dose of benzodiazepines can be lethal, but this appears to be exacerbated when other drugs are involved.

3.2.2. The Occurrence of Benzodiazepines in Opioid-Associated Deaths: The Buprenorphine Story

Benzodiazepines are also apparent in some opioid related deaths (Table 11B). Three studies were identified that investigated heroin-linked deaths. Benzodiazepines

1. Drug Interactions with Benzodiazepines

Table 11
The Presence of Alcohol and Other Drugs in Benzodiazepine Poisonings

Year	Population	Location	Reference
A) The occurrence of other drugs or ethanol in benzodiazepine-associated deaths			
1979	914 diazepam-positive fatalities 912 & other drug or EtOH; 51 EtOH; 295 EtOH and other drug; 566 other drug; propoxyphene > opiates > barbiturates	USA and Canada	63
1980	2723 overdoses 1071 benzo positive; 726 & other drugs (EtOH apparently not studied)	Toronto, Canada	62
1989	3430 overdoses 702 benzo positive; 144 benzo; 200 benzo & EtOH; 254 benzo & other drug; 104 benzo, other drug & EtOH	Stockholm, Sweden	64
1993	1576 benzodiazepine-associated deaths 891 single benzo; 591 single benzo & EtOH; 94 more than one benzo ± EtOH	Great Britain	60
1995	303 benzodiazepine-associated overdoses 303 total; 114 & EtOH	Newcastle, Australia	61
B) The occurrence of benzodiazepines in opioid-associated deaths			
1976	114 heroin-related deaths 9 benzo positives	Orange Co., CA	65
1977	268 heroin-related deaths 12 diazepam positive	Wayne Co., MI	66
1994	21 heroin-related deaths 2 benzo positive	Baltimore, MD	67
1998	Unknown no. of buprenorphine-related deaths 6 benzo positive cases	France	69

were also found in 5–10% of these deaths *(65–67)*. Opioids are well recognized for their respiratory depressant effects; that a combination with another CNS depressant that also causes respiratory depression may exacerbate the situation is not too suprising.

Buprenorphine has been used for years as an analgesic or for treatment of chronic pain at doses 0.3–0.8 mg. More recently, buprenorphine has been used in substitution therapy for opioid dependence. For the latter, doses of 8–32 mg are used. Buprenorphine is known as a partial µ agonist that appears to have ceiling effects in regard to its µ-activities such as respiratory depression *(68)*. Recently in France, however, six cases of deaths involving buprenorphine were also found to involve benzodiazepine use *(69;* Table 11B). That buprenorphine may interact with benzodiazepines was suggested in a series of letters to the editor in the journal *Anaesthesia*. Papworth *(70)* first reported four cases of prolonged somnolence and bradypnoea with combinations of buprenorphine and lorazepam. Forrest *(71)* then described a case, also with buprenorphine and lorazepam, that had prolonged somnolence, bradypnoea, and the need for assisted respiration. This was followed shortly thereafter by a report from Faroqui et al. *(72)* that found 11 subjects out of 64 that were premedicated with diazepam and had anesthesia induced with buprenorphine required assisted ventilation. This was not observed in 24 patients receiving diazepam and fentanyl.

This combined effect of buprenorphine and a benzodiazepine, midazolam, has now been reproduced in an animal model. Gueye et al. *(73)* have shown that rats given

Table 12
Benzodiazepine Use Among Opioid Users: Survey of Studies in 1990s

Year	Population	Location	Reference
1990	272 polydrug users (75% heroin) 28% were also using temazepam (use of other benzos not mentioned).	Northwest England	368
1990	249 male opiate addicts Greater than 50% used benzos, with flunitrazepam most common.	Penang, Malaysia	369
1991	323 methadone treatment subjects Daily, few times per week, and a few times per month benzo use was 14, 15, and 39% in those who did not share needles and 25, 18, and 24% in those who did share needles.	Philadelphia and New Jersey	370
1992	1245 injecting drug users 36.6% used benzos	Sydney, Australia	371
1992	103 methadone treatment subjects All had used heroin and benzodiazepines, relative liking of cocaine > cannabis >> stimulates ≈ benzos. Flunitrazepam and diazepam were the most favored.	Innsbruck, Austria	372
1993	313 applicants for methadone treatment 42% reported a benzo habit (37% of males; 56% of females).	Kensington, Australia	373
1993	973 admittees for inpatient opiate detoxiciation 80.2% history of benzo use; 68.5% current; 43.1% daily. Flunitrazepam > clorazepate > diazepam.	Barcelona, Spain	374
1993	222 methadone treatment subjects 36.5% use in the past month; 26.6% daily; and 11.3% five or more pills a day.	Kensington, Australia	375
1994	208 subjects (82.2% for opiate use) 90% had used benzos, 49% by injection.	clinics in seven cities in Britain	376

buprenorphine alone (30 mg/kg, iv) had a mild increase in $PaCO_2$ at 60 min. Rats given midazolam alone (160 mg/kg, ip) had a mild decrease in arterial pH at 90 min and increase in $PaCO_2$ at 60 min. When the doses were combined, there was a prolonged respiratory depression with the changes in blood pH and $PaCO_2$ noted within 20 min, with delayed hypoxia at 120 and 180 min.

This effect is apparently not due to an inhibition of the benzodiazepine metabolism. Kilicarslan and Sellers (74) have shown that metabolism of flunitrazepam to 3-hydroxyflunitrazepam in HLMs was not inhibited by norbuprenorphine, and while inhibited by buprenorphine, the K_i of 118 μM was suggestive of only 0.1–2.5% inhibition in vivo. The converse situation, inhibition of buprenorphine metabolism by benzodiazepines, has not yet been addressed.

Although the percentage of opioid-associated deaths that also show benzodiazepine use is relatively low (Table 11B), it is still a concern due to the potential for the pharmacodynamic interaction resulting in additive (or synergistic) effects on respiratory depression. Further epidemiological data substantiate the risk. Surveys conducted in the early 1990s in various parts of the world demonstrate that use of benzodiazepines is quite common in opioid-dependent subjects (Table 12). Regular benzodiazepine use ranged from 27 to 50%, whereas most had used benzodiazepines at one time. A great majority reported intravenous use of the benzodiazepines.

3.2.3. The Occurrence of Benzodiazepines, with or Without Ethanol or Other Drugs in Motor Vehicle Investigations

One other area in which epidemiological data point to potential interactions between benzodiazepines and ethanol or other drugs is within motor vehicle investigations. Studies that clearly indicated benzodiazepine and ethanol and/or other drug use were reveiwed and are listed in Table 13. These studies can be divided into three types: (a) studies on fatalities where in most studies drug use was determined in all cases, (b) studies on impaired driving where in most studies only cases with ethanol below a certain cutoff were tested for drugs, and (c) random testing where participants volunteered for inclusion in the drug-testing part of the study. These differnet protocols may have an impact on the drug findings.

In studies on driving fatalities, the presence of benzodiazepines ranged from 1.3 to 10.2%. Benzodiazepine positives were found in conjuction with ethanol in 25 to 78% of the cases. For impaired driving cases the presence of benzodiazepines ranged from 1 to 30% with the additional finding of ethanol ranging from 22 to 100%. Studies that focused on profession transportation reported very low incidences of benzodiazepine use. In a study on 168 track-driver fatalities, no benzodiazepines were detected *(75)*. In the two random studies, only commercial truck drivers were included. In one study, only 1 of 317 participants (88% compliance) was benzodiazepine positive and had a prescription for its use *(76)*. In the other study, none of the 822 (81% compliance) participants was positive for benzodiazepines *(77)*. In 1398 mandatory postaccident cases studied for the Federal Railroad Association, only 2 benzodiazepine positive cases were detected, 1 with prescription for its use *(78)*. Benzodiazepine use in vehicle-related investigations varies widely. This may be due in part to geographic and temporal differences in the studies. In 7 of the 10 studies that did not include commercial drivers, ethanol was a cofactor in greater than 50% of the cases.

Benzodiazepine-positive findings along with other drugs were described in a few of these studies. In a study of impaired drivers in California published in 1979, 14 of the 56 cases positive for chlordiazepoxide also had phenobarbital *(79)*. In a study of ethanol-negative-impaired drivers in St. Louis published in 1987, 10 and 8 of the 30 benzodiazepine-positive cases were also positive for barbiturates or opiate analgesics, respectively *(80)*. Two studies focused on cases positive for a specific drug(s). In a study in Sweden published in 2000 of 486 impaired drivers that had tested positive for codeine or dextropropoxyphene, 346 were also positive for a benzodiazepine *(81)*. In a study from Washington state published in 2001, 4 of 29 zolpidem-positive cases were also positive for benzodiazepines *(82)*. As with mixtures of benzodiazepines with ethanol, their mixture with other CNS depressant drugs is common in vehicle-irregularity-related studies.

3.3. Clinical Studies on Drug Interactions of Benzodiazepines with Other CNS Depressants

3.3.1. Pharmacodynamic and Pharmacokinetic Interactions with Analgesics and Anesthetics

Clinical studies on drug interactions between benzodiazepines and opioids, or other CNS depressants, have been mostly limited to interactions between the two benzodiaz-

Table 13
**The Occurrence of Benzodiazepines
with or Without Ethanol (or Other Drugs) in Motor Vehicle Investigations**

Year	Population	Location	Reference
A) Fatalities			
1977	127 driving fatalities 23 drug positive; 13 diazepam, 7 & EtOH	Dallas, Co., TX	*377*
1980	401 motor vehicle fatalities 64 drug positives; 15 benzos; 12 diazepam, 3 & EtOH, 4 & other drugs	Ontario, Canada	*378*
1986	1518 driving fatalities 32 benzo positive, 25 & EtOH	Alabama	*379*
1987	200 driving fatalities, survivors, or blood tested (resticted to EtOH < 0.05) 34 drug positive; 9 benzo, 7 & EtOH	Tasmania, Autralia	*380*
1993	168 trucker fatalities no benzos identified	USA	*75*
1996	318 driving fatalities 61 drug positive; 4 benzo, 2 & EtOH	Washington	*381*
B) Impaired situations			
1969	180 overt intoxication, but BAC ≤ 0.15% 38 drug positive; 2 chlordiazepoxide (BAC) 1 (0-< 0.05); 1 (0.10-0.15)	Santa Clara Co, CA	*382*
1979	765 drug positive-impaired driving 171 diazepam, 40 & EtOH; 56 chlordiazepoxide, 9 & EtOH, 14 & phenobarbital	California	*79*
1979	425 under influence (EtOH < 0.08 in 282) Drugs present in 115 cases; benzos in 90 (80 diazepam), 85 & EtOH	Northern Ireland	*383*
1981	71,937 impaired driving, but BAC ≤ 0.10% 684 benzos (571 dizepam), 310 & EtOH	Orange Co., CA	*384*
1984	56 impaired driving (saliva) 10 drug positive; 4 diazepam, 4 & EtOH	Ottawa, Canada	*385*
1987	184 impaired driving, negative EtOH 30 benzo positive; 10 & barbiturates, 8 & opiates analgesics	St. Louis, MO	*80*
1991	1398 mandatory railroad postaccident testing 85 drug positives; 2 benzos, 0 & EtOH	USA	*78*
1998	19,386 first road-traffic accidents Based on prescription data, use of benzos had a 1.52 risk factor (8.15 & EtOH) compared to 0.30 (1.0) with tricyclics and 0.51 (0.89) with SSRIs.	Tayside region, UK	*386*
2000	486 impaired drivers study restricted to dextropropoxyphene or codeine positive samples; 346 benzo	Sweden	*81*
2001	29 zolpidem positive impaired drivers 4 benzo positive; 1 & EtOH	Washington	*82*
C) Random testing			
1988	317 (88% compliance) random truck drivers 1 benzo positive with prescription	Tennessee	*76*
2002	822 (81% compliance) random truck drivers no benzos identified	Oregon/Washington	*77*

epines used as anesthetics, diazepam and midazolam, with other anesthetic or analgesic agents (Tables 14 and 15). One exception is a study on the effect of diazepam on methadone maintenance. In an initial paper, Preston et al. *(83)* demonstrated that a combination of diazepam and methadone produced subjective opioid effects greater than either drug alone (Table 14). In a follow-up report, these investigators studied the effect of

Table 14
Effect of Analgesics and Anesthetics on Benzodiazepine Pharmacodynamics

Benzodiazepine	Dose	Agent Dose	Agent Time	N	Reference
Methadone					
Diazepam	20 & 40, or	100 & 150% maintenance	0 h	5m	83
	40 mg diazepam and 150% maintenance dose induced changes in pupil constriction and subjective opioid effects greater than those by either drug alone.				
Papaveretum					
Midazolam	0.15–0.5/kg, iv	15–20 mg, im	0 h	37/29	86
	Sedative effect of midazolam was potentiated by opiate.				
Pethidine					
Midazolam	0.15–0.5/kg, iv	50–75 mg, im	0 h	47/29	86
	Sedative effect of midazolam was potentiated by opiate.				
Diazepam	10, iv	50–75 mg	0 h	50/50	87
	No difference in sedation noted, but patients more comfortable with procedure.				
Morphine					
Midazolam	0.01–0.03/kg, iv	0.006–0.12 mg/kg, iv	−10 min	5/dose	88
	Dose response: additive effect on visual analog determination of sedation.				
Fentanyl					
Diazepam	0–0.5/kg, iv	50 µg/kg	4 min	5/dose	90
	Dose response of diazepam: caused significant reduction in arterial pressure and systemic vascular resistance associated with decreases in (nor)epinephrine.				
Midazolam	≈0.35/kg, iv	50 µg, iv	−1 min	30/44	89
	Combination caused greater respiratory depression than midazolam alone.				
Midazolam	0.3/kg, iv	50 or 100 µg, iv	−2 min	52/100	91
	Fentanyl decreased onset time for midazolam anesthesia and % asleep at 3 min.				
Midazolam	0.05/kg, iv	2 µg/kg, iv	0 h	12m	92
	Synergistic increase in apnea and hypoxemia, no further reduction in fentanyl-reduction of ventilatory response to CO_2.				
Midazolam	0.02–0.37/kg, iv	1.9–8.5 µg/kg, iv	1 min	10f/dose	93
	Synergistic increase in inability to open eyes in response to command (anesthesia).				
Alfentanyl					
Diazepam	0.125/kg, iv	100 or 200 µg/kg, iv	5 min	10/dose	94
	Diazepam reduced the numbers responding to voice at 5 min (10 to 1, 5 to 1), increased heart rate, increased reductions in blood pressure, and increased number (1 to 5) with inadequate postoperative ventilation.				
Midazolam	0.3/kg, iv	150 or 300 µg, iv	−2 min	40/100	91
	Alfentanyl decreased onset time for midazolam anesthesia and % asleep at 3 min.				
Midazolam	0.07–0.35/kg, iv	0.02–0.18 mg/kg, iv	1 min	5/dose	95
	Dose response; found synergistic response of response to verbal command (sedation).				

(continued)

Table 14 (continued)

Benzodiazepine	Dose	Agent Dose	Agent Time	N	Reference
Alfentanyl *(continued)*					
Midazolam	0.023–0.2/kg, iv	0.016–0.15 mg/kg, iv	0 h	10/dose	96
	Dose response, response to verbal command (hypnosis), and response to tetanic stimulus (anesthesia) are synergistically enhanced.				
Naltrexone					
Diazepam	10, or	50 mg	–1.5 h	8f, 18m	103
	Negative mood states (sedation, fatique) were increased and positive mood states (friendliness, feeling high) were decreased by naltrexone.				
Propofol					
Midazolam	0.1–0.2/kg, iv	0.7–2.5 mg/kg, iv	0 h	10/dose	106
	Dose response: response to command was synergistically influenced; midazolam reduced dose of propofol required for response to tetanic stimuli.				
Midazolam	0.1–0.4/kg, iv	0.4–2.8 mg/kg, iv	2 min	10/dose	107
	Dose response: response to command was synergistically influenced.				
Thiopental					
Midazolam	0.03–0.37/kg, iv	0.7–3.6 mg/kg, iv	1 min	5/dose	104
	Dose response: response to command was synergistically influenced.				
Midazolam	0.04–0.2/kg, iv	0.7–4.5 mg/kg, iv	2.5 min	20/dose	105
	Dose response: response to command was synergistically influenced; midazolam reduced dose of thipopental required for response to electrical stimuli.				

Table 15
Effect of Analgesics and Anesthetics on the Pharmacokinetics of Benzodiazepines

Benzodiazepine	Dose	N	T_{max}	C_{max}	$t_{1/2}$	AUC	Cl	Reference
Methadone	100% of maintenance dose							
Diazepam	20, or	5m				0.95		84
Diazepam	40, or	5m				0.91		84
Methadone	150% of maintenance dose							
Diazepam	20, or	5m				1.28		84
Diazepam	40, or	5m				1.24		84
Propoxyphene	65 mg, 4/d, multidose							
Alprazolam	1, or	6f,2m	3.46	0.94	1.58*		0.62*	85
Diazepam	10, iv	2f,4m			1.14		0.87	85
Lorazepam	2, iv	1f,4m			0.99		1.10	85
Fentanyl	Patients undergoing orthopedic surgery ±200 µg, iv							
Midazolam	0.2/kg, iv	15/15			1.49*	1.54*	0.70*	97
Naltrexone	50 mg at –1.5h							
Diazepam	10, or	8f,18m	1.80*	0.93	1.05*	0.95		103
Propofol	Patients undergoing elective sugery ±2 mg/kg bolus, 9 mg/kg/h infusion							
Midazolam	0.2/kg, iv	12/12			1.61*	1.58*	0.63*	108

methadone on the pharmacokinetics of diazepam. Although not significant, a combination of 150% of the maintenance dose of methadone with either 20 or 40 mg oral diazepam resulted in an approximately 25% increase in the area under the curve (AUC) of diazepam (*84*; Table 15).

Propoxyphene is an extensively used analgesic; its coadministration with benzodiazepines would not be uncommon. In a single study, subjects took three different benzodiazepines, oral alprazolam and intravenous diazepam and lorazepam, each one twice. In one setting, no other drug was taken; in the other, propoxyphene was administered every 6 h from 12 h prior to the benzodiazepine and then for the duration of the study *(85)*. Coadministration of propoxyphene significantly inhibited the elimination of alprazolam; there was a slight, but nonsignificant inhibition of diazepam; and no effect on the pharmacokinetics of lorazepam (Table 15). No information was found on the in vitro inhibition of P450s by propoxyphene, but these data would support an inhibitory effect of propoxyphene on P450 3A4 that spares P450 2C19. No data were presented on the effect of propoxyphene on the pharmacodynamics of benzodiazepines.

When midazolam or diazepam is combined with the opioids papaveretum, pethidine, or morphine during anesthesia, potentiation of the sedative or subjective effects is consistently found *(86–88*; Table 14). Pharmacokinetic interactions between these drugs were not studied.

The combination of midazolam or diazepam with fentanyl has also been consistently found to result in potentiation of the sedative and in some cases respiratory depressant effects of the drugs *(89–93)*. In the latter two studies, which used midazolam, statistical evaluation of dose responses suggested that the drugs interacted in a synergistic manner *(92,93)*. A similar finding was found for combined use of diazepam or midazolam with alfentanil, including the synergistic response with midazolam (*91,94–96*; Table 14). With fentanyl it has been shown that its combination with midazolam results in a significant increase in the terminal elimination half-life ($t_{1/2}$) and AUC and significant decrease in the clearance of midazolam (*97*; Table 15). A similar pharmacokinetic study has not been done with alfentanil, but both are P450 3A4 substrates *(98–101)* and may have similar potential to inhibit midazolam metabolism, as has been found in vitro for fentanyl *(102)*.

The interaction between naltrexone, an opioid μ receptor antagonist, and diazepam is another exception to the studies between anesthetics. Naltrexone was found to increase the negative mood states such as sedation, and decrease the positive mood effects such as friendliness of diazepam (Table 14), with no effect on its pharmacokinetics (Table 15; *103*).

The interaction of the structurally unique anesthetic propofol or the barbiturate thiopental with midazolam has also been reported to have synergistic effects on the sedative effects of the drugs (Table 14; *104–107*). A pharmacokinetic study has been performed on the interaction of midazolam and propofol, and propofol was found to significantly increase the $t_{1/2}$ and AUC of midazolam (Table 15; *108*). This is consistent with the in vitro inhibition of midazolam metabolism by propofol *(109)*.

Clinical studies confirm that additive interactions occur between the opioids and other anesthetic agents. These have sometimes been found to be synergistic in their response. The synergistic response appears to occur when there is also a pharmacokinetic interaction resulting in the inhibition of the benzodiazepines' clearance.

Table 16
Effect of Ethanol on Benzodiazepine Pharmacodynamics

Benzodiazepine	Dose (mg)	Ethanol Dose	Ethanol Time	N	Reference
Alprazolam	0.5, or	0.8 g/kg	3 h	10m	*116*
	No effect on measures of side effects, tracking skills, angle recognition or free recall; diminished choice reaction time.				
Alprazolam	2, or	0.8 g/kg	3 h	10m	*116*
	No effect on measures of side effects, tracking skills, angle recognition, or free recall; diminished choice reaction time.				
Alprazolam	1, or	0.5 g/kg,	0.75 h	12/12	*110*
	Produced predictive additive effects on sedation, unsteadiness, dizziness, tiredness and psychomotor performance.				
Bromazepam	6, or 3/d × 14 d	0.5 g/kg	0 h	20m	*387*
	Enhanceed impairment of learning skills, but not short-term memory.				
Bromazepam	6, or 3/d × 14 d	0.5 g/kg	0 h	1f,16m	*113*
	No effect on reaction time or mistakes; enhanced effects on coordination skills, attention and propioception.				
Brotizolam	0.25, or	24 mL	0 h	13m	*120*
	Subjective perceptions of sedation were enhanced, but psychomotor performance was not.				
Chlordiazepoxide	5, or 3/d × 2 d	45 mL		6f,12m	*388*
	Subjects were tested on mental and then psychomotor performance starting at +1h. No significant difference ± ethanol.				
Chlordiazepoxide -lactam	10, or 3/d × 14 d	0.5 g/kg	0h	20	*115*
	No effect on reaction time; enhanced coordination mistakes at fixed and free speed and impairment of attention and propioception.				

(continued)

3.3.2. Pharmacodynamic and Pharmacokinetic Interactions with Ethanol

The effect of combined use of ethanol on pharmacodynamic end points has been studied with a large number of benzodiazepines (Table 16). In general, ethanol has a potentiating effect on some of the psychomotor and subjective measures, but rarely affects all such measures in any one study. In part because the studies were not designed to detect it, synergistic effects were not noted. Because of the diverse end points in the studies, there was no apparent general set of pharmacodynamic end points that ethanol consistently had an effect upon. For example, reaction time was a common end point. Ethanol was reported as enhancing impairment of reaction time for alprazolam *(110)*, clobazam *(111)*, diazepam *(112)*, and tofisopam *(112)*, whereas it had no effect on reaction time with bromazepam *(113)*, loprazolam *(114)*, oxazepam *(115)*, nordiazepam *(115)*, and temazepam *(115)*. Few of the studies compared benzodiazepines under the same conditions. It is therefore difficult to draw conclusions about some benzodiazepines being more susceptable to the interactive effects with ethanol.

Table 16 (*continued*)

Benzodiazepine	Dose (mg)	Ethanol Dose	Ethanol Time	N	Reference
Clobazam	20, or	77 g	0–1.5 h	8m	*111*
	Enhanced impairment of reaction errors and time, deviations of two-hand coordination and body sway.				
Clorazepate	20, or	1 g/kg		14m	*389*
	Enhance alcohol acute euphoric effects and decreased dysphoric effects in the following morning.				
Diazepam	5, or 3/d × 3 d	42 mL	0 h	20	*390*
	Measured ability for cancellation of letters, digit substition, addition and pegboard placement begining at +75 min. Performance under diazepam, ± EtOH, was slightly poorer than with placebo tablet.				
Diazepam	2, or 3/d × 2 d	45 mL		6f,12m	*388*
	Subjects were tested on mental and then psychomotor performance starting at +1 h. Ethanol enhanced the effects on two of nine mental tests; no effect on psychomotor tests.				
Diazepam	10, or /70 kg	0.75 mL/70 kg	0 h	8m	*129*
	Starting at +90 min, no effect on mirror tracing; slight enhancement of attention and time evaluation; significant with attempted letter cancellations, sorting, flicker fusion, complex coordination and clinical symptoms.				
Diazepam	10, or	0.5 g/kg		10/10	*117*
	Simulated driving by professional drivers from +30–70 min. Enhanced number of collsions and driving off the road instances.				
Diazepam	10, 20, or 40, or	0.5 g/kg	0 h	6m	*391*
	Markedly enhanced the effects on coordination and mood.				
Diazepam	10, or	0.8 g/kg	−0.5 h	10	*127*
	Enhanced impairment of tracking skills and oculo-motor coordination; enhanced nystagmus.				
Diazepam	10, iv	at 0.8–1.0 g/L	−1–8 h	6m	*128*
	Enhanced impairment of pursuit rotor performance and intoxication indices and visual analog scale.				
Diazepam	10, or/d × 2 d	0.8 g/kg		12m	*112*
	Enhanced impairment on coordination, reaction, flicker fusion, maddox wing and attention tests.				
Diazepam	10, or	at 0.5 g/L	−1.5–2.5 h	12m	*392*
	Produced additive effects on subjective alertness and measures of performance; synergistic effect on smooth pursuit eye movements.				
Diazepam	5, or	at 0.5 g/L	−1.5–4 h	8m	*393*
	Produced additive effects on adaptive tracking, smooth pursuit, DSST and body sway; did see supra-additive effects in 2 subjects.				
Diazepam	10, or	0.8 g/kg	3 h	10m	*116*
	No effect on measures of side effects, tracking skills, choice reaction time, angle recognition, or free recall.				
Flunitrazepam	2, or	0.8 g/kg	−0.5 h	12m	*124*
	Alcohol did not effect impairment of tracking skills at +1h, but did enhance impairment the following morning.				

(*continued*)

Table 16 (*continued*)

Benzodiazepine	Dose (mg)	Ethanol Dose	Ethanol Time	N	Reference
Flurazepam	30, or/d × 14 d	0.5 g/kg	10 h	7f,33m	394
	No effect on reaction time, reaction mistakes or attention; enhanced effects on coordination skills.				
Loprazolam	1, or	0.7 g/kg	0 h	8m	114
	No effects on simple reaction time; alleviated lopraz-impairment of manual dexterity; both alone impaired tracking, but not together; memory impaired by lopraz, improved by EtOH, not affected together.				
Oxazepam	10, 20, or 40, or	0.5 g/kg	0 h	6m	391
	Slightly enhanced the effects on coordination and mood.				
Oxazepam	15, or 3/d × 14 d	0.5 g/kg	0 h	20	115
	No effect on reaction time, attention or propioception; enhanced coordination mistakes at fixed and free speed.				
Midazolam	0.1/kg, iv	0.7 g/kg	4 h	16m	395
	Midazolam did not add to the +5h or +7h effects of EtOH.				
Nitrazepam	10, or/d × 14 d	0.5 g/kg	10 h	3f,17m	396
	No effect on reaction times; enhanced choice reaction and coordination mistakes and impaired attention.				
Nordiazepam	5, or 3/d × 14 d	0.5 g/kg	0 h	20	115
	No effect on reaction time, attention or propioception; enhanced coordination mistakes at fixed speed, no effect at free speed.				
Prazepam	20, or	0.5 g/kg	0 h	12m	125
	Enhanced impairment in auditory reaction and DSST; reduced reaction to auditory stimuli and cancellation test and enhanced drowsiness.				
Temazepam	20, or 3/d × 14 d	0.5 g/kg	0 h	20	115
	No effect on reaction time or attention; enhanced coordination mistakes at fixed speed, but not at free speed; enhanced impairment of propioception.				
Tofisopam	100, or × 3	0.8 g/kg		12m	112
	Enhanced impairment on coordination, reaction, flicker fusion, maddox wing and attention tests.				
Triazolam	0.25, or	at 0.8–0.95 g/L	−0.5–7.5 h	1f,6m	122
	Enhanced impairment of free recall, postural stability, and hand–eye coordination.				

The timing of the administration of ethanol was an important factor. When ethanol was given 3 h after alprazolam, only minimal effects were found *(116)*. When ethanol was given only 45 min after alprazolam, however, it had additive effects on most of the end points measured *(110)*. Similarly, combining ethanol with diazepam at the same time led to enhanced impairment of reaction time *(112)*, whereas giving the ethanol 3 h after diazepam did not *(116)*.

Ethanol, therefore, does appear to enhance the impairing effects of benzodiazepines in an additive fashion. In the one study that measured driving skills, diazepam and ethanol were taken together and the stimulated driving of professional drivers was

1. Drug Interactions with Benzodiazepines

Table 17
Effect of Ethanol on the Pharmacokinetics of Benzodiazepines in Nonalcoholics

Benzodiazepine	EtOH Dose	EtOH Dose	Time	N	T_{max}	C_{max}	$t_{1/2}$	AUC	Cl	Reference
Alprazolam	0.5, or	0.8 g/kg	+3 h	10m			no change			116
Alprazolam	2, or	0.8 g/kg,	+3 h	10m			no change			116
Brotizolam	0.25, or	24 mL	0 h	13m	0.95	1.23*	1.18*		0.84*	120
Chlordiazepoxide	25, or	0.8 g/kg	0 h	5m	1.67	1.48*				121
Clobazam	20, or	39 g		8m	1.00	1.59*		1.55*		111
Clotiazepam	5, or	24 mL	0 h	11			1.21		0.93	123
Diazepam	10, or	0.8 g/kg	0 h	5m	1.25	1.03				121
Diazepam	0.14/kg, or	0.75 mL/kg	0 h	8m	3.0	1.19				129
Diazepam	0.07/kg, iv	15 mL	0 h	1f,6m	1.42	1.58*				126
Diazepam	5, or	17 mL	0 h	2f,4m	2.27	0.94		1.00		130
Diazepam	10, or	0.8 g/kg (b)	−0.5 h	10	0.38	1.58*		1.15		127
Diazepam	10, ore	0.8 g/kg (wh)	−0.5 h	10	0.50	1.16		1.07		127
Diazepam	10, or	0.8 g/kg (wi)	−0.5 h	10	1.00	1.57*		1.21*		127
Diazepam	10, iv	0.8–1.0 g/L	−1–8 h	6m				1.31		128
Diazepam N-desmethyl	5, or	24 mL	−0.5 h	2f,4m	3.94 1.00	0.84 1.10	1.23	1.04 1.00		131
Diazepam N-desmethyl	5, or	24 mL	0 h	2f,4m	2.11 1.12	0.87 1.00	1.21	1.07 0.94		131
Diazepam	10, or	0.8 g/kg	3 h	10m	≈ 35% higher					116
Diazepam	10, or	0.5 g/L	−1.5–2.5 h	12m	1.23	1.15		1.12		392
Flunitrazepam	2, or	0.8 g/kg	−0.5 h	12m	0.98	1.02	0.81	1.05		124
Prazepam	20, or	0.5 g/kg	0 h	12m	0.83	1.09		0.92		125
Triazolam	0.25, or	0.8–0.95 g/L	−0.5–7.5 h	1f,6m		1.08	1.22*	0.84*		122

Table 18
Effect of Ethanol on the Pharmacokinetics of Benzodiazepines in Chronic Alcoholics

Benzodiazepine	Dose	Condition	N	T_{max}	C_{max}	$t_{1/2}$	AUC	Cl	Reference
Chlordiazepoxide N-desmethyl	50, or	acute vs 7 d abst	5	1.87 2.60	1.01 0.71	1.52	2.35		133
Chlordiazepoxide N-desmethyl	50, im	acute vs 7 d abst	5	2.41 1.70	1.94 1.02	1.85	3.35		133
Chlordiazepoxide N-desmethyl demoxepam	25, or (md)	2 vs 6 d abst	6		2.1ss* 1.91ss* 0.15ss*				134
Diazepam	10, or	1–11 d abst	11/14	1.00	0.43*				135
Diazepam N-desmethyl	10, iv	1–3 d abst	14/13				0.71* 0.65*		136
Diazepam	6	1 d vs 6 d abst	7			0.83		0.67	137

studied. The combined use of ethanol and diazepam resulted in increased numbers of collisions and driving off the road instances *(117)*.

Ethanol is known to affect the metabolism of many drugs. In general, acute use of ethanol is associated with the inhibition of drug metabolism; chronic use induces metabolism *(118,119)*. Therefore, examination of the effect of ethanol on benzodiazepine pharmacokinetics should differentiate between studies on acute exposure in nonalcoholics (Table 17) and studies in alcoholics (Table 18).

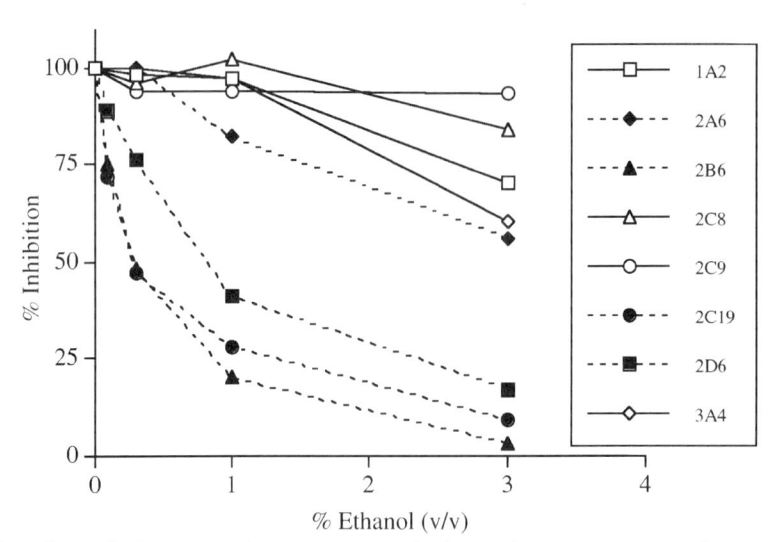

Fig. 10. The effect of ethanol on the in vitro metabolism of cDNA-expressed P450s. Adapted from data presented by Busby et al. *(132)*. Note that experiments were designed to test ethanol as a solvent for addition of substrates. The two lower concentrations, 0.1 and 0.3% (v,v) would equate to 0.079 and 0.237 g/100 mL, respectively.

Acute exposure to ethanol was found to inhibit the clearance of a number of benzodiazepines as seen from increased C_{maxs}, $t_{1/2}$s, AUCs, and/or decreased clearance. Thus is the case for brotizolam *(120)*, chlordiazepoxide *(121)*, clobazam *(111)*, and triazolam *(122)*. With some benzodiazepines, however, ethanol did not have any effect on their pharmacokinetics; these include alprazolam *(116)*, clotiazepam *(123)*, flunitrazepam *(124)*, and prazepam (*125*; Table 17). For the latter studies, either the 3-h interval between alprazolam and ethanol administration, or the ability of non-P450-dependent pathways to metabolize flunitrazepam may explain the negative findings. Such is not the case, however, for clotiazepam and prazepam, which require P450 for either hydroxylation or N-dealkylation reactions. For these two benzodiazepines the effect was not significant, but could be considered suggestive of impaired elimination. Diazepam interactions with ethanol were the subject of numerous studies that showed varying results. An inhibition of clearance was reported in some studies *(126–128)*, whereas only a prolongation of the C_{max} was found in some studies *(121,129–131)*. In general, the former studies administered ethanol 30–60 min prior to diazepam, whereas the latter administered the two drugs at the same time.

The results from these clinical studies indicate that acute ethanol, taken either with or shortly before, may interfere with the elimination of many, but not all benzodiazepines. Although this would appear to arise from the inhibition of P450-dependent metabolism of the benzodiazepines, some inconsistencies exist. A single study was found on the in vitro inhibition of different forms of human liver P450s *(132)*. At concentrations close to 0.10 g/100 mL, only P450s 2C19 and 2D6 were partially inhibited. Cytochrome P450 3A4, which is associated with the metabolism of many benzodiazepines, was fairly resistant to the inhibitory effects of ethanol for the marker substrate studied (Fig. 10; *132*). Due to the complex nature of the P450 3A4 substrate binding

1. Drug Interactions with Benzodiazepines

site(s), however, it has become apparent that some substrates may show different responses to inhibitors.

The study of benzodiazepine pharmacokinetics in chronic alcoholics entering treatment programs has been used to support the theory that chronic ethanol induces the metabolism of benzodiazepines *(56)*. The studies were designed in two ways (Table 18). Either a comparison within the subjects at 1–2 d after initiation of treatment vs 6–7 d later, or comparison of the subjects to control subjects. With the former design, administration of oral, intramuscular or intravenous chlordiazepoxide had longer $t_{1/2}$s of higher steady-state concentrations at the beginning of the study *(133,134)*. It was suggested that these results arose from an initial inhibition of chlordiazepoxide from residual ethanol in the first sesssion with unmasking of an induced state in the later session *(56)*. This is supported by studies on diazepam where abstinent alcoholics were compared to nonalcoholic controls (Table 18). With oral or intravenous administration of diazepam, elimination was greater in the alcoholics *(135,136)*. One study was contradictory. When seven subjects entering a detoxification ward were given intravenous diazepam on d 1 and again 4–20 d later, the $t_{1/2}$ and clearance were higher in the latter session, but not significantly due to large intrasubject variations *(137)*. An inductive effect of ethanol pretreament on the metabolism of diazepam was also found in rats *(136)*. A rationale for this inductive effect was found from a report that ethanol induces P450 3A, as well as 2E, in cultured human hepatocytes *(138)*.

3.4. The Interaction Between Benzodiazepines and Other Drugs

With most of the other drugs for which interactions have been described with the benzodiazepines, they are dependent upon whether the benzodiazepine is metabolized by P450. For this reason, in the applicable subsections some time has been spent to summarize the P450 inhibitory or inductive activity of the class of drugs being discussed. This will generally take the course of examining the in vitro potency of the drugs as inhibitors.

3.4.1. Benzodiazepines and Gastrointestinal Agents

3.4.1.1. BENZODIAZEPINES, ANTACIDS, AND MISCELLANEOUS GASTROINTESTINAL AGENTS

Benzodiazepines have an acidic pKa, and changes in the pH of the gastrointestinal tract may influence their rate of absorption. Some of the earliest drug interaction studies focused on the effect of antacids on the pharmacokinetics of benzodiazepines (Table 19). In 1976, Nair et al. *(139)* gave 10 mg oral diazepam alone or in combination with aluminum hydroxide, magnesium trisilicate, or sodium citrate to 200 women undergoing minor gynecological procedures. Aluminum hydroxide and sodium citrate were reported to hasten the onset of the soporific effect of diazepam, with no apparent effect on its pharmacokinetics. Magnesium trisilicate was found to delay the effect; it also prolonged the T_{max} and decreased the C_{max}. In contrast to the findings of Nair et al. *(139)* with magnesium trisilicate and diazepam, Elliot et al. *(140)* found no effect on the pharmacokinetics of temazepam or midazolam.

The mixture of aluminum and magnesium hydroxides (Maalox) were found to prolong the T_{max} and decrease the C_{max} for chlordiazepoxide *(141)*, clorazepate *(142,143)*, and diazepam *(144)*. The mixture of aluminum hydroxide and magnesium trisilicate

Table 19
Drug Interactions with Antacids and Miscellaneous Gastrointestinal Agents

Inhibitor/Benzo	Dose	N	T$_{max}$	C$_{max}$	t$_{1/2}$	AUC	Cl	PhDyn	Reference
Antacids									
AlOH	40 mL								
Diazepam	10, or	20/17	1.00	0.94				+	139
MgOH/AlOH	30 mL × 2, 100 mL (chlor)								
Chlordiazepoxide	25, or	10m	2.13	0.93	1.03	0.97			141
Clorazepate	15, or	15m	2.00	0.80*	0.96	0.94			142
Clorazepate	15, or	5f,5m	1.56*	0.69*		0.90*		+	143
Diazepam	5, or	9	1.40	0.66*		0.98			144
MgOH/AlOH	30 mL, multidose								
Clorazepate	7.5, or (md)	4f,6m		0.95ss					146
Mg trisilicate/AlOH	30 mL × 2								
Diazepam	5, or	9	1.30	0.74*		0.96			144
Mg trisilicate	30 mL								
Diazepam	10, or	15/17	1.50	0.78				+	139
Midazolam	15, or	5m	0.86	1.13	1.23	1.37	0.86		140
Temazepam	20, or	1f,4m	0.95	1.04	0.93	1.00	1.00		140
Sodium citrate	9 µmol at 0 h								
Diazepam	10, or	15/17	1.00	0.91				+	139
Sodium bicarbonate	enough to maintain pH 6 for 2h								
Clorazepate	15, or	4m	1.11	0.81					145
N-desmethyl			14.0*	0.28*		0.55*			
AlOH gel	3600 mg pretreatment in dialysis patients								
Temazepam	30, or	11	1.30	1.00	1.13	1.08*		0	147
Triazolam	0.5, or	11	0.93	1.58*	0.99	1.28*	0.74*		148
Other gastrointestinal agents									
Misoprostol	200 µg, 4/d, multidose								
Diazepam	10, or/d (md)	6m		1.02	1.01	1.03		0	149
N-desmethyl				1.00	0.89	1.00			
Cisapride	8 mg, iv at −8 min								
Diazepam	10, or	8	0.72*	1.18*		0.92		++ (early)	150

(Gelusil) had a similar effect on diazepam *(144)*. In one of the studies on clorazepate and Maalox, this was found to be associated with reduced pharmacodynamic effects *(143)*. For clorazepate, not only is the absorption of the drug dependent upon pH, so is its conversion to nordiazepam. Abruzzo et al. *(145)* showed that maintenance of the stomach pH at 6 with sodium bicarbonate greatly prolonged and reduced the peak of plasma nordiazepam from clorazepate. After multidose treatment with both clorazepate and Maalox, however, steady-state concentrations of the metabolite nordiazepam were not affected *(146)*, which suggests that antacids will have no effect under multidosing schemes.

    Aluminum hydroxides are also taken by patients on dialysis to bind dietary phosphates. Kroboth et al. *(147)* found that this treatment had no effect on the absorption of temazepam. In another study, however, they found that the elimination of triazolam

1. Drug Interactions with Benzodiazepines

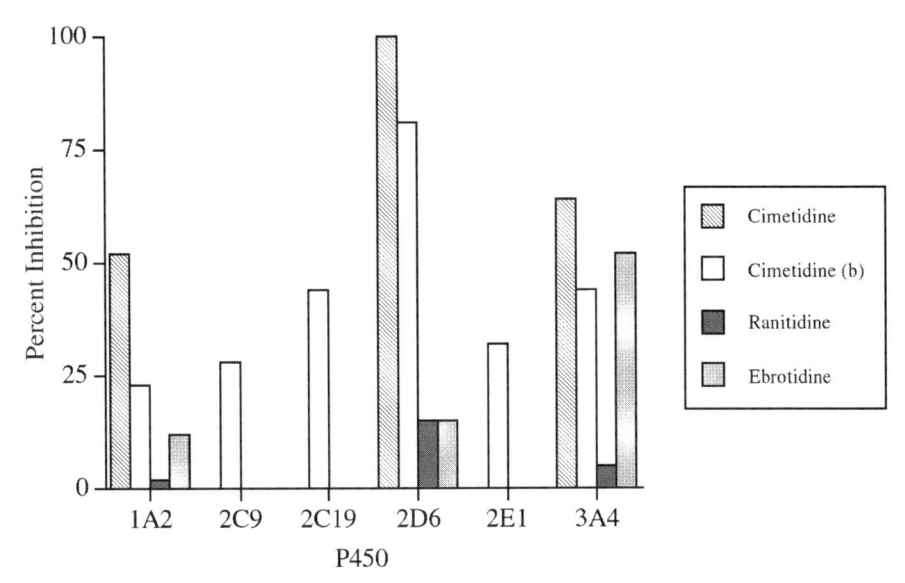

Fig. 11. A summary of in vitro experiments on the inhibition of P450-selective substrates in HLMs with H_2-receptor antagonists. The data on cimetidine (b) is from Knodell et al. *(153)*, where the marker reactions were: 1A2, ethoxyresorufin deethylase; 2C9, tobultamide hydroxylase; 2C19, hexobarbital hydroxylase; 2D6, bufuralol hydroxylase; 2E1, aniline hydroxylase; 3A4, an average of responses of nifedipine oxidase and erythromycin demethylase. The other data are from Martinez et al. *(154)*, where the marker reactions are: 1A2, caffeine N-demethylation to paraxanthine; 2D6, dextromethorphan O-demethylation; and 3A4, dextromethorphan N-demethylation.

was reduced in dialysis patients taking aluminum hydroxide *(148)*. The renal disease enhanced elimination of triazolam, so the net effect of aluminum hydroxide was to return the pharmacokinetic parameters toward those noted in matched controls *(148;* Table 19).

Misoprostal is a novel synthetic prostaglandin E1 analog with antisecretroy properties. When misoprostal was given in combination with oral diazepam it did not have any effect on diazepam pharmacokinetics *(149)*. Cisapride increases gastric motility. Intravenous cisapride was found to enhance the absorption of oral diazepam with consequent increased impairment in early (45 min) tests on reaction time *(150)*.

3.4.1.2. Interactions with H_2-Receptor Antagonists

The H_2-receptor antagonists are widely used for treatment of gastrointentinal ulcers. Cimetidine was the first H_2-receptor antagonist and was followed by ranitidine, famotidine, oxmetidine, nizatidine, and ebrotidine. Among these drugs, cimetidine is well known to cause drug–drug interactions with a number of drugs due to its inhibitory effects on several P450s *(151,152)*. The other H_2-receptor antagonists are relatively mild inhibitors. Knodell et al. *(153)* studied the effect of cimetidine on a number of P450-selective activities and found inhibition was greatest for 2D6 > 2C19, 3A4 > 2E1 > 2C9, 1A2 (Fig. 11). Martinez et al. *(154)* directly compared the in vitro effects of cimetidine, ranitidine and ebrotidine on a number of P450-selective activities (Fig. 11). In brief, cimetidine was found to have significant inhibitory effects on P450 2D6 >

1A2 and 3A4. Ranitidine and ebrotidine had some, but relatively fewer inhibitory effects on these P450s.

Klotz et al. *(155)* compared the spectral dissociation constants of the H$_2$-receptor antagonists with HLMs and determined the following K$_s$ values: oxmetidine, 0.2 mM; cimetidine, 0.87 mM; ranitidine, 5.1 mM; famotidine and nizatidine, no effect up to 4 mM. In another in vitro comparison of the effect of cimetidine and nizatidine on the 1'-hydroxylation of midazolam in HLMs, Wrighton and Ring *(36)* determined K$_i$s of 268 and 2860 µM, respectively. For comparative purposes, the K$_i$s of ketoconazole and nifedipine, known 3A4 inhibitors, were 0.11 and 22 µM. With the exception of oxmetidine, for which only a single clinical study was performed, these in vitro findings will favorably describe the interactions seen between the H$_2$-receptor antagonists and benzodiazepines that rely upon P450-mediated metabolism for their elimination.

Coadministration of multiple doses of cimetidine has been found to diminish the elimination of a number of benzodiazepines (Table 20), that include: adinazolam *(156)*, alprazolam *(157,158)*, bromazepam *(159)*, chlordiazepoxide *(160)*, clobazam *(161)*, clorazepate *(162)*, diazepam *(149,163–168)*, flurazepam *(169)*, midazolam *(140,170)*, nitrazepam *(171)*, nordiazepam *(172)*, and triazolam *(157,158,173)*. Single doses of cimetidine seem to have milder effect, but have been found to diminsih the elimination of diazepam *(174)* and midazolam *(154,175,176)* in a dose-dependent fashion (Table 20). In all studies, but one, that monitored pharmacodynamic effects these were mildly diminished also (Table 20). Gough et al. *(165)* found inhibition of diazepam pharmacokinetics without any change in the monitored pharmacodynamic measures. Lorazepam *(166,169,174,177)* and oxazepam *(169,172,177)*, which are exclusively glucuronidated, and temazepam *(140,178)*, which can be glucuronidated without further metabolism, were resistant to the effects of cimetidine. The outlier in this scheme is clotiazepam, which appears to require P450-dependent metabolism, but was unaffected by cimetidine. It was also resistant to inhibitory effects by ethanol *(123)*.

Multidose ranitidine inhibited the elimination of oral diazepam *(179)*, midazolam *(140,170,180)*, and triazolam *(181)*, but was inaffective against intravenous doses of these benzodiazepines *(179,181–183)*, intravenous lorazepam *(182)*, and oral temazepam *(140)*. A single dose of ranitidine had no effect on oral adinazolam *(184)*, oral midazolam *(154)*, or infused midazolam *(175)*. Multidose famotidine *(155,185,186)*, oxmetidine *(155)*, and nizatidine *(155)* had no effect on the pharmacokinetics of intravenous diazepam. A single dose of ebrotidine had no effect on oral midazolam *(154;* Table 20).

Vanderveen et al. *(181)* found that ranitidine diminished the elimination of oral, but not intravenous triazolam. They hypothesized that the increase in pH caused by ranitidine was responsible for the diminished elimination of oral triazolam. The basis of their hypothesis was that at acidic pH triazolam is in equilibrium with its more poorly absorbed benzophenone (Fig. 12). With increased pH, less benzophenone is formed and more triazolam is absorbed *(181)*. The prior findings of Cox et al. *(173)*, however, seem to dispute this hypothesis. They administered intraduodenal infusions of triazolam in solutions at pH 2.3, where 47% was the benzophenone, and pH 6.0, with negligible benzophenone, and found no difference in the pharmacokinetics. Ranitidine does appear to inhibit the metabolism of some benzodiazepines. This appears to be limited to first-pass metabolism within either the gastrointestinal tract or the liver.

1. Drug Interactions with Benzodiazepines

Table 20
Drug Interactions with H₂-Receptor Antagonists

Inhibitor/Benzo	Dose	N	T$_{max}$	C$_{max}$	t$_{1/2}$	AUC	Cl	PhDyn	Reference
Cimetidine	800–1000 mg/d in divided doses, multidose								
Adinazolam	20/d, or (md)	6f,6m	1.33	1.39*	1.08	1.45*	0.67*	++	156
N-desmethyl			1.44	1.19	1.08	1.43*			
Adinazolam	40/d, or (md)	6f,6m	1.09	1.21*	1.18	1.44*	0.73*	++	156
N-desmethyl			1.00	1.25*	0.95	1.27*			
Adinazolam	60/d, or (md)	6f,6m	1.06	1.26*	1.35*	1.36*	0.75*	++	156
N-desmethyl			1.25	1.25*	1.00	1.32*			
Alprazolam	1, or	9	1.00	1.03	1.34*		0.63*		157
Alprazolam	0.5, 3/d, or (md)	4f,4m	0.90	1.85*	1.16	1.73*	0.59*		158
Bromazepam	6, or	2f,6m	1.91	1.22	1.26*		0.50*		159
Chlordiazepoxide	0.6/kg, iv	4f,4m			2.36*		0.37*		160
Clobazam	30, or	9m	1.12	0.91	1.11*	1.17*			397
N-desmethyl			0.98	1.03		1.11			
Clobazam	30, or	6	0.59	1.16	1.39*	1.59			161
N-desmethyl			1.54	1.29*	1.90*	1.57*			
N-Desmethylclob	30, or	5	1.68	1.04	1.24*	1.37*			161
Clorazepate	15, or	3 young			1.62*		0.67*		162
Clorazepate	15, or	5 elderly			1.71*		0.53*		162
Clotiazepam	5, or	11			0.97		0.95		123
Diazepam	0.1/kg, iv	2f,4m			1.53*		0.57*	++	163
Diazepam	5, or (md)	6		1.38ss*	2.56*		0.67*		164
Diazepam	10, or	3f,4m			1.33*	1.76*	0.50*	0	165
Diazepam	10, iv	8			1.47*		0.76*		166
Diazepam	5–30, or (md)	3f,7m		1.39ss*				++	167
N-desmethyl				1.38ss*					
Diazepam	10, iv	11m			1.32*	1.20*	0.73*		186
N-desmethyl						1.19*			
Diazepam	0.1/kg, iv	12m			1.39*	1.53*	0.58*		168
N-desmethyl						0.81*			
Diazepam	10, or (md)	6m		1.57*	1.81*	1.83*			149
N-desmethyl				1.59*	1.49*	1.59*			
Flurazepam	30, or	6m	1.43	1.10	1.50*	1.46			169
Lorazepam	2, iv	4f,4m			0.90		1.21		177
Lorazepam	2, iv	8			1.10		0.96		166
Lorazepam	2, or	6m	0.81	0.88	1.00	0.97			169
Midazolam	15, or	5m	0.72	2.38*	1.20	2.02*	0.52*		140
Midazolam	15, or	1f,7m			1.07	1.35*			170
Midazolam	0.07/kg, iv	10m						+++	398
Nitrazepam	5–10, or	6m	0.81	1.00	1.25*		0.83*		171
Nordiazepam	20, or	2f,3m			1.40*		0.72*	++	172
Oxazepam	50, or	2f,3m			0.90		0.87	0	172
Oxazepam	45, or	2f,2m			0.78		1.37		177
Oxazepam	30, or	4f,4m	1.41	0.95	1.04	1.11*			169
Temazepam	20, or	1f,4m	0.74	0.87	0.84	0.99	0.85		140
Temazepam	30, or	9	0.95	0.89	1.15		1.01		178
Triazolam	0.5, or	9	1.06	1.20	0.97	1.54*	0.66*		157
Triazolam	0.5, or (md)	2f,6m	1.40	1.51*	1.68*	2.22*	0.45*		158
Triazolam	0.5, or	4m	1.06	1.51*	1.01	1.54*			173

(continued)

Table 20 (*continued*)

Inhibitor/Benzo	Dose	N	T_max	C_max	t_1/2	AUC	Cl	PhDyn	Reference
Cimetidine	400 (mid b) 800 mg (mid a,c), 200 (dia a, lor a), 400 iv (dia b, lor b) single dose								
Diazepam a	10, or	5/5	1.00	1.26					*174*
Diazepam b	10, or	5/5	0.50	1.34*					*174*
Lorazepam a	2.5, or	7/7	1.00	1.12					*174*
Lorazepam b	2.5, or	6/7	1.00	1.24					*174*
Midazolam a	0.025/kg/h	8m		1.26ss*				0	*175*
Midazolam b	15, or	6	0.81	1.37*	1.61	1.36*		+++	*176*
Midazolam c	7.5, or	8m			1.46*	1.50*	0.68*		*154*
Ranitidine	150 mg 2/d, multidose								
Diazepam	5, or (md)	6		0.74*	1.06		1.33*		*179*
Diazepam	0.1/kg, iv	4			1.04		1.04		*179*
Diazepam	10, iv	10m			0.89		0.93		*182*
Diazepam	10, iv	9			1.04		1.04		*183*
Lorazepam	2, iv	10m			0.97		1.09		*182*
Midazolam	15, or	5m		1.53*		1.66*		+	*180*
Midazolam	15, or	5m	0.93	1.52*	1.00	1.66*	0.59		*140*
Midazolam	10, or	32f/32f						++	*399*
Midazolam	15, or	1f,7m			1.21*	1.23*			*170*
Midazolam	0.07/kg, iv	8/10						0	*398*
Temazepam	20, or	1f,4m	1.10	0.95	1.20	1.15	0.85		*140*
Temazepam	20, or	20/20						0	*399*
Triazolam	0.25, or	12m	1.00	1.30	0.97	1.27*			*181*
Triazolam	0.25, iv	12m		0.79	1.01	0.99	1.01		*181*
Ranitidine	300 mg, single dose								
Adinazolam	30, or	12m	0.86	1.03	1.00	0.99	1.01	0	*184*
N-desmethyl			0.75	1.01	1.07	1.02			
Midazolam	0.05/kg inf	8m		1.08ss					*175*
Midazolam	7.5, or	8m			1.29	1.32	0.82		*154*
Famotidine	40 mg 2/d, multidose								
Diazepam	0.1/kg, iv	8m			0.86		1.11	0	*185*
Diazepam	10, iv	11m			0.96	0.97	1.01		*186*
N-desmethyl						1.02			
Diazepam	10, iv	8			0.86		1.14		*155*
Oxmetidine	800 mg/d, multidose								
Diazepam	10, iv	8			1.12		0.94		*155*
Nizatidine	300 mg/d, multidose								
Diazepam	10, or	9			1.07		0.95		*183*
Ebrotidine	400 mg								
Midazolam	7.5, or	8m			0.79	1.07	0.85		*154*

3.4.1.3. Interactions with H^+-K^+ ATPase Inhibitors (Proton Pump Inhibitors)

The H^+-K^+ ATPase, or proton pump, inhibitors suppress gastric acid secretion and are used to treat gastric ulcer, duodenal ulcer, gastroesophageal reflux, and other hypersecretory states. Omeprazole has been best characterized as an inhibitor of P450 2C19, and can cause drug interactions with drugs that are 2C19 substrates. In vitro, both omeprazole and lansoprazole inhibit 2C19 with K_is 10-fold lower than those for inhibition of other P450s (Fig. 13; *187,188*). Data on the in vitro inhibition of P450s by

1. Drug Interactions with Benzodiazepines 43

Fig. 12. The equilibrium reaction between triazolam and its benzophenone. Formation of the benzophenone is favored at pH < 4. As the benzophenone would not be absorbed as effectively as triazolam, it was postulated that agents that increase stomach pH would decrease the amount of the benzophenone and thereby increase the absorption of the benzodiazepine. Whereas this conversion is useful for the gas chromatographic detection of many benzodiazepines, as explained in the text, it does not appear to impact drug interactions involving agents that change stomach pH.

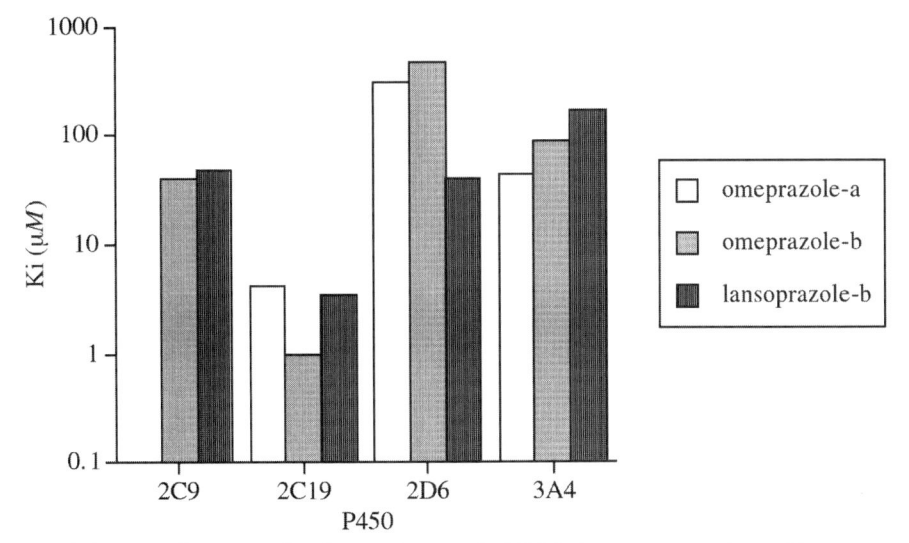

Fig. 13. Inhibition of P450-selective pathways in HLMs by omeprazole and lansoprazole. Omeprazole-a is from *(187)*, where the pathways were: 2D6, bufuralol 1'-hydroxylation; 2C19, S-mephenytoin 4'-hydroxylation; and 3A4, midazolam 1'-hydroxylation. Omeprazone-b and lansoprazole-b are from *(188)*, where the pathways were: 2D6, dextromethorphan O-demethylation; 2C9, tolbutamide 4-methylhydroxylation; 2C19, S-mephenytoin 4'-hydroxylation; and 3A4, dextromethorphan N-demethylation. Note the log scale on the Y-axis.

pantoprazole were not found. In vivo, omeprazole is the only consistent inhibitor of P450 2C19 *(189,190)*. This is seen with its effects on diazepam pharmacokinetics (Table 21). In four different studies, omeprazole was found to inhibit elimination of either intravenous or oral diazepam *(168,191–193)*. Andersson et al. further demonstrated that omeprazole did not affect diazepam pharmacokinetics in 2C19 poor metabolizers *(192)*. Caraco et al. *(193)* demonstrated that omeprazole was a more potent inhibitor in Caucasian than in Chinese extensive metabolizers. Lansoprazole *(194)* and pantoprazole *(195)* had no effect on the pharmacokinetics of diazepam (Table 21).

Table 21
Drug Interactions with H⁺-K⁺ ATPase Inhibitor Antisecretory Agents

Inhibitor/Benzo	Dose	N	T_{max}	C_{max}	$t_{1/2}$	AUC	Cl	PhDyn	Reference
Omeprazole	20 mg/d (dia b, c), 40 mg/d (dia a, d), multidose								
Diazepam a	0.1/kg, iv	8m			2.30*		0.45*		*191*
Diazepam b	0.1/kg, iv	12m			1.36*	1.39*	0.73*		*168*
Diazepam c	0.1/kg, iv	6 2C19em			1.20*	2.34*	0.74*		*192*
Diazepam c	0.1/kg, iv	4 2C19pm			0.95	1.10	0.90		*192*
Diazepam d	10, or	8m Chi,em			0.95		0.76*		*193*
N-desmethyl					1.03	1.24*			
Diazepam d	10, or	7m Cau, em			1.34*		0.61*		*193*
N-desmethyl					1.58*	1.41*			
Lansoprazole	60 mg/d, multidose								
Diazepam	0.1/kg, iv	12m			1.11	1.12	0.91		*194*
Pantoprazole	240 mg, iv/d, multidose								
Diazepam	0.1/kg, iv	7f,5m			0.91	0.99	1.01		*195*

3.4.2. Interactions with Imidazole Antifungal Agents

The imidazole antifungal agents are well known for their ability to inhibit P450-mediated drug metabolism *(196)*. Ketoconazole is the prototype, and is an often used 3A4-selective inhibitor. Most studies comparing the effects of the imidazole antifungal agents on different P450s have utilized ketoconazole *(21–23,197)*. These demonstrate that ketoconazole can inhibit many P450s, but that its ability to inhibit 3A4 at concentrations of ≈1 μ*M* make it 10–100 times more specific for this P450 gene product (Fig. 14A). Studies comparing the inhibitory ability of the other imidazole antifungal agents are limited. That by Maurice et al. *(197)*, who studied inibition of cyclosporin oxidase suggests a ranking of: clotrimazole, ketoconazole > miconazole >> fluconazole > secnidazole > metronidazole (Fig. 14B). von Moltke et al. *(38,198)* found a similar ranking: ketoconazole > itraconazole > fluconazole for the inhibition of midazolam α- and 4-hydroxylation and for triazolam α- and 4-hydroxylation (not shown). Jurima-Romet at al. *(199)* studied another 3A4 substrate, terfenadine, and found ketoconazole, itraconazole, and fluconazole had almost equivalent K_is. When studying the inhibition of 2C9 using tolbutamide as the substrate, Back et al. *(200)* found miconazole, with an IC_{50} of 0.85 μ*M*, was the most potent inhibitor of 2C9, with a relative ranking of miconazole > clotrimazole > ketoconazole, fluconazole > terconazole > metronidazole (Fig. 14B). Tassaneeyakul et al. *(201)* studied the effect of the azoles on 2E1 mediated 4-nitrophenol hydroxylation. Whereas fluconazole, itraconazole, and ketoconazole were without effect, miconazole, bifonazole, clotrimazole, and econazole inhibited the activity with K_is of 4, 7, 12, and 25 μ*M* (not shown).

In clinical studies on drug interactions between benzodiazepines and the imidazole antifungal agents, the responses appear to follow inhibition of P450 3A4 potencies (Table 22). Ketoconazole has been found to inhibit the elimination of alprazolam *(202,203)*, chlordiazepoxide *(204)*, midazolam *(205)*, and triazolam *(202,206,207;* Table 22). Fluconazole has been found to inhibit the elimination of midazolam *(208, 209)* and triazolam *(210)*, but not bromazepam *(211)*. Itraconazole has been found to inhibit the elimination of alprazolam *(212)*, diazepam *(213)*, midazolam *(205,208,214)*,

1. Drug Interactions with Benzodiazepines

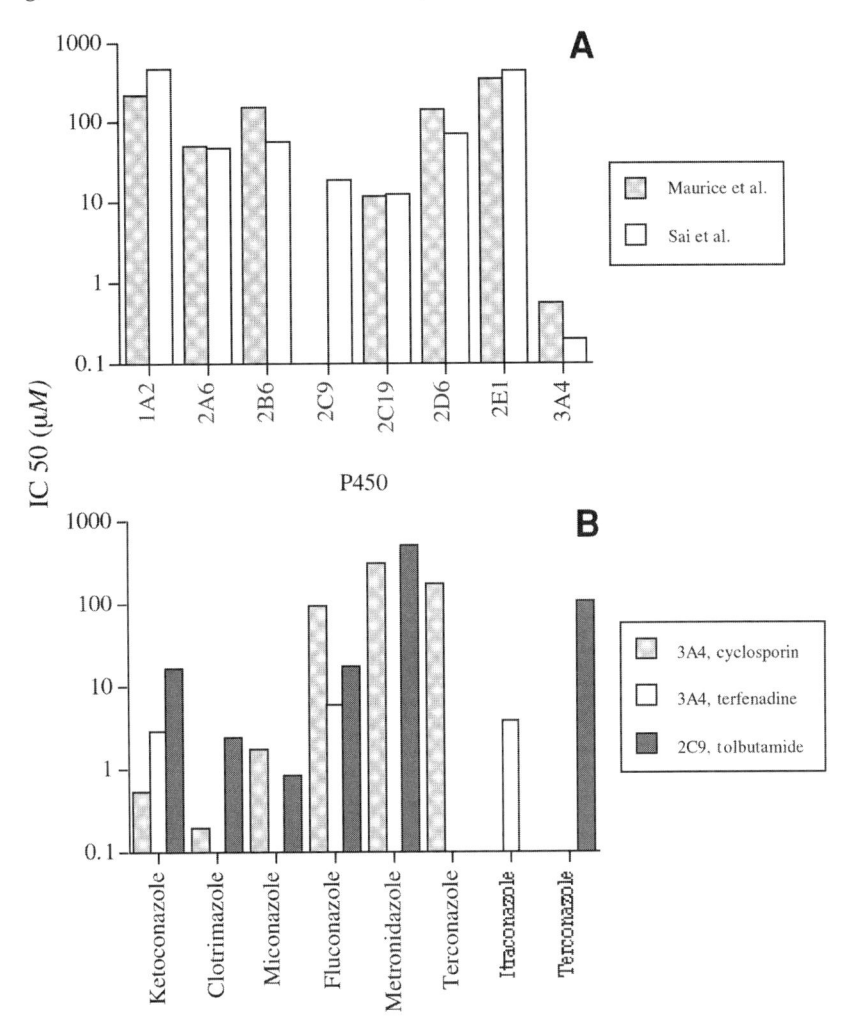

Fig. 14. Inhibition of human liver P450s by imidazole antifungal agents. (**A**) The inhibition of different P450s by ketoconazole in HLMs from Maurice et al. *(197)* where the marker activities are: 1A2, phenacetin O-deethylase; 2A6, coumarin 7α-hydroxylase; 2B6, benzphetamine demethylase; 2C19, mephenytoin 4-hydroxylase; 2D6, debrisoquine 4-hydroxylase; 2E1, aniline hydroxylase; and 3A4, cyclosporin oxidase, and in cDNA-expressed P450s from Sai et al. *(23)*. (**B**) Inhibition of P450 3A4 and 2C9 in HLMs by different imidazoles. The cyclosporin data are from Maurice et al. *(197)*, the terfenadine data are from Jurima-Romet et al. *(199)*, and the tolbutamide data are from Back et al. *(200)*. Note the log scale on the Y-axis.

and triazolam *(206,215)*. Metronidazole had no effect on the elimination of alprazolam *(216)*, diazepam *(217)*, lorazepam *(216)*, or midazolam *(218)*. The same was true for the nonimidazole antifungal agent, terbinafine, on midazolam *(214)* and triazolam (*219*; Table 21). The increases in AUC for midazolam were 15.9, 10.8, and 3.59 following ketoconazole, itraconazole, and fluconazole, respectively. A similar potency was seen with triazolam of 13.7, 8.15, and 3.65 (Table 22).

Table 22
Drug Interactions with Antifungal Agents

Inhibitor/Benzo	Dose	N	T$_{max}$	C$_{max}$	t$_{1/2}$	AUC	Cl	PhDyn	Reference
Ketoconazole	200 mg 2/d, 400 mg 1/d (chlor, mid, tri a), multidose								
Alprazolam	1, or	7m	1.07	1.10	3.88*	3.98*	0.31*	+++	202
Alprazolam	1, or	9	0.83	1.08	1.45*	1.76*	0.54*		203
Chlordiazepoxide	0.6/kg, iv	6m			1.82*	1.54*	0.62*		204
N-desmethyl							0.64*		
demoxepam							0.70*		
Midazolam	7.5, or	7f,2m	1.84*	4.09*	3.11*	15.9*		+++	205
Triazolam a	0.25, or	6f,3m	1.67*	3.07*	6.45*	8.15*		+++	206
Triazolam b	0.125, or	2f,7m	1.45	2.27*	3.97*	9.16*	0.12*	+++	207
Triazolam c	0.25, or	7m	1.58	2.08*	6.10*	13.7*	0.09	+++	202
Fluconazole	50 mg/d (tri b), 100 mg/d (bro, tri a,c), 200 mg/d (tri d, mid a) multidose, single 400 mg (mid c) vs iv (mid b)								
Bromazepam	3, or	12m	1.60	0.99	1.00	1.09	0.89	0	211
Bromazepam	3, rectal	12m	0.92	0.98	1.00	1.09	0.86	0	211
Midazolam a	0.05/kg, iv	5f,7m			1.52*		0.49*	++	208
Midazolam a	7.5, or	5f,7m	1.70	1.74*	2.14*	3.59*		++	208
Midazolam b	7.5, or	4f,5m	2.00	1.79*	2.23*	3.08*		++	209
1-hydroxy				1.24	2.42*	1.50*			
Midazolam c	7.5, or	4f,5m	2.00	2.30*	2.23*	3.41*		++	209
1-hydroxy				1.11	2.57*	1.56*			
Triazolam a	0.25, or	10f,2m	1.11*	1.25*	1.84*	2.46*		+++	219
Triazolam b	0.25, or	5f,3m	1.15	1.47*	1.29*	1.59*		0	210
Triazolam c	0.25, or	5f,3m	1.92*	1.40*	1.77*	1.99*		++	210
Triazolam d	0.25, or	5f,3m	1.54*	2.33*	2.26*	3.65*		++++	210
Itraconazole	200 mg/d,100 mg/d (mid b) multidose, 200 mg once at −3h (tri b)								
Alprazolam	0.8, or	10m	1.94	1.29	2.57*	1.62*	0.39*	++	212
Diazepam	5, or	5f,5m	0.81	1.06	1.34*	1.34*		0	213
N-desmethyl				0.99		0.97			
Midazolam a	7.5, or	7f,2m	1.54	3.41*	2.82*	10.8*		+++	205
Midazolam b	7.5, or	8f,4m	0.80	2.56*	2.08*	5.74*		+++	214
Midazolam c	7.5, or	5f,7m	1.80	2.51*	3.59*	6.64*		+	208
Midazolam d	0.05/kg, iv (md)	5f,7m			2.41*		0.31*	+	208
Triazolam a	0.25, or	4f,3m	2.67*	2.80*	6.76*	8.15*		++++	206
Triazolam b	0.25, or	4f,6m	1.94*	1.76*	3.11*	2.83*		++	215
Metronidazole	400 mg, 2/d, multidose								
Alprazolam	1, or	4f,6m	0.79	1.05	0.94		1.18		216
Diazepam	0.1/kg, iv	3f,3m			1.00		1.23		217
Lorazepam	2, iv	4f,4m			0.85		1.15		216
Midazolam	15, or	6f,4m	1.25	0.94	1.10	0.91		0	218
1-hydroxy			1.00	1.00	0.76	0.88			
Terbinafine	250 mg/d, multidose								
Midazolam	7.5, or	8f,4m	0.8	0.82	0.92	0.75		0	214
Triazolam	0.25, or	10f,2m	0.83*	0.85	0.86	0.81		0	219

For studies that followed the pharmacodynamic effects of benzodiazepines, the imidazole antifungal agents were found to enhance these in all cases (Table 22). Their ability to do this followed the same potency ranking as with their effects on the pharmacokinetics, ketoconazole > itraconazole > fluconazole. Indeed, multiple doses of ketoconazole strongly enhanced the pharmacodynamic effects of triazolam and midazolam;

1. Drug Interactions with Benzodiazepines

triazolam was also strongly enhanced by itraconazole and fluconazole. These imidazole antifungals were some of the most potent inhibitors found during the research for this review.

3.4.3. Interactions with Serotonin Selective Reuptake Inhibitors

The serotonin selective reuptake inhibitors (SSRIs) are fairly potent inhibitors of human liver P450s (Fig. 15). They are most active against P450 2D6, where they have relative potency of paroxetine > flouxetine > sertraline, fluvoxamine > citalopram > venlafaxine, nefazodone, with K_is ranging from 0.07 to 33 μM (Fig. 15A; *220–223*). Their inhibitory action, however, is not limited to P450 2D6. P450 3A4–dependent metabolism of alprazolam is inhibited with K_is ranging from 10 to 83 μM (fluvoxamine > nefazodone, sertraline > paroxetine > fluoxetine); 2C19 metabolism of mephenytoin with K_is ranging from 1.1 to 87 μM and 2C9 metabolism of phenytoin with K_is ranging from 6 to 66 μM (Fig. 15B; *222–224*). Of particular importance for this class of drugs is that the initial metabolite often has equal inhibitory potency to the parent drug (Fig. 15). This is seen with midazolam where the substrate inhibition constant for α-hydroxylation was 1.4 and 11.5 μM for norfluoxetine and fluoxetine; those for 4-hydroxylation were 17 and 67 μM *(38)*.

Since benzodiazepines that undergo oxidative metabolism are primarily P450 3A4 (or 2C19) substrates, they are not affected by SSRI comedication to the extent of some P450 2D6 substrates. Pharmacokinetically significant drug interactions have, however, been identified (Table 23). Fluoxetine was found to inhibit the elimination of alprazolam *(225,226)* and diazepam *(227)*, but was reported as without effect on clonazepam *(226)* and triazolam *(228)*.

During one of the studies on alprazolam, Greenblatt et al. *(226)* demonstrated the clinical relevance of the inhibition by the metabolite, norfluoxetine. Subjects were randomly allocated to either the placebo-fluoxetine or fluoxetine-placebo order of study, with a 14-d washout period between sessions. For subjects that took placebo first, the inhibition of alprazolam elimination was significant; for those that took fluoxetine first, it was not. The reason for this was that in subjects that took fluoxetine first, norfluoxetine plasma concentrations were still quite high *(226)*. During the 8 d of active treatment with fluoxetine, mean norfluoxetine concentrations rose from 25 to 80 ng/mL. During the 14 to 31 d after sessation of treatment they went from 55 to 45 ng/mL *(226)*. Further discussion on the effect of long half-life of SSRI metabolites can be found in the relevant chapter in this monograph.

Fluvoxamine was found to inhibit the elimination of diazepam *(229)* and midazolam *(230)*. Nefazodone was found to inhibit the elimination of alprazolam and triazolam *(231–233)*, but not lorazepam *(231,234)*. Sertraline had no effect on clonazepam *(235)* or diazepam *(236)*. Venlafaxine actually enhanced the elimination of alprazolam *(237)* and diazepam (*238*; Table 23).

Where studied, the effects of the SSRIs on the pharmacodynamics of the benzodiazepine reflected their effect on its pharmacokinetics (Table 23). Nefazodone had greater inhibitory effect on alprazolam than did fluoxetine, and in turn enhanced the pharmacokinetics of alprazolam to a greater extent *(225,231,232)*. The pharmacodynamics of lorazepam and clonazepam were not effected by nefazodone or sertraline, respectively; nor were their pharmacokinetics *(231,234,235)*. The enhanced elimination of

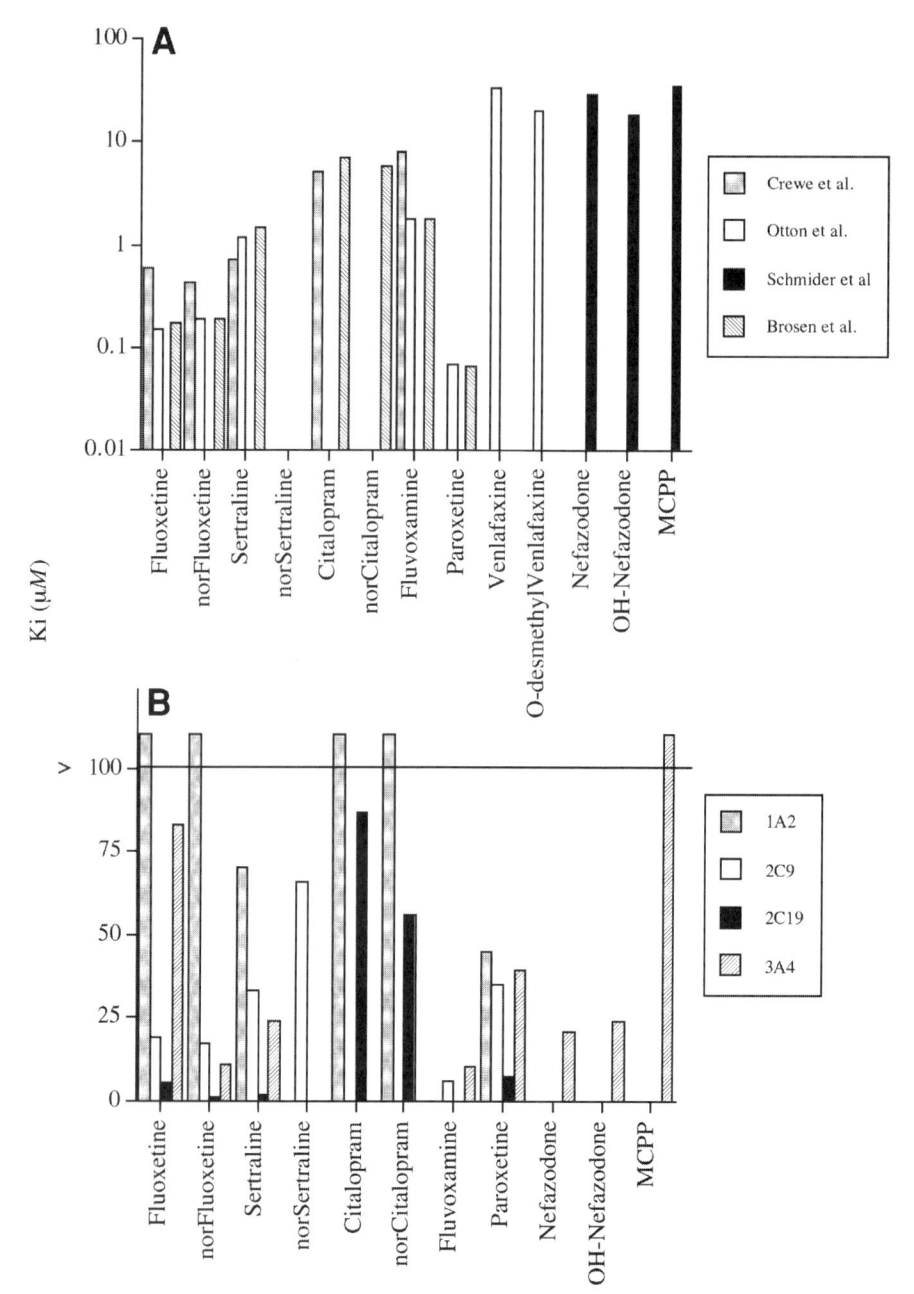

Fig. 15. Inhibition of human liver P450s by the selective seratonin reuptake inhibitors. (**A**) Inhibition of P450 2D6 activities (note the log scale on the Y-axis). The data are from: Crewe et al. *(220)* using sparteine 2-dehydrogenation; and Otton et al. *(221)*, Schmider at al. *(222)*, and Brosen et al. *(223)* using dextromethorphan O-demethylation. (**B**) Inhibition of other P450s. The 1A2, 2C19, and 3A4 (except nefazodone and metabolites) data are from Brosen et al. *(223)* using paracetamol, S-mephenytoin, and alprazolam as the respective substrates. The 3A4 inhibition by nefazodone and metabolites is from Schmider et al. *(222)* using dextromethorphan N-demethylation, and the 2C9 data are from Schmider at al. *(224)* using phenytoin p-hydroxylation.

1. Drug Interactions with Benzodiazepines

Table 23
Drug Interactions with Antidepressants

Inhibitor/Benzo	Dose	N	T_{max}	C_{max}	$t_{1/2}$	AUC	Cl	PhDyn	Reference
Fluoxetine	60 mg/d (tria, alp a), 20 mg 2/d (clon, alp b) multidose								
Alprazolam a	1, or (md)	20/20		1.33ss*	1.27*			++	225
Alprazolam b	1, or	6m	0.71	1.46	1.17*	1.26*	0.79*		226
Clonazepam	1, or	6m	0.46*	1.22*	0.93	0.99	1.01		226
Diazepam	10, or	6m			1.50*	1.48*	0.62*	0	227
N-desmethyl						0.65*			
Triazolam	0.25, or	19	0.71	1.10	1.01	1.02	0.93		228
Fluvoxamine	titrated up to 150 mg/d, multidose								
Diazepam	10, or	4f,4m	1.33	1.32	2.31*	2.80*	0.35*		229
N-desmethyl				3.32*	1.15		1.41*		
Midazolam	0.025/kg, iv	10f,10m					0.67*		230
Nefazodone	200 mg 2/d, multidose								
Alprazolam	1, or (md)	12/12	1.14	1.60*	2.05*	1.98*		+++	231,232
1'-hydroxy			2.00	1.00					
4-hydroxy			2.00	0.64*		0.72*			
Lorazepam	2, or (md)	12/12	0.88	0.99	0.91	1.02		0	231,234
Triazolam	0.25, or	12m	2.20	1.66*	4.59*	3.90*		+++	231,233
Sertraline	100 mg 1/d (clon), 50 increased to 200 mg 1/d (dia), multidose								
Clonazepam	1, or (md)	8f,8m			0.96		1.10	0	235
7-amino					0.78*	1.05			
Diazepam	10, iv	10/10			0.88		0.92		236
N-desmethyl			1.23	1.26		1.13			
Venlafaxine	37.5 mg 2/d (alp), 50 mg 3/d (dia), multidose								
Alprazolam	2, or	1f,15m	0.80	0.94	0.79*	0.71*	1.37*	--	237
Diazepam	10, or	18m	0.86	1.07		0.84*	1.08*	-	238
N-desmethyl			0.88	0.93		0.91	1.02		

alprazolam and diazepam caused by venlafaxine was associated with diminished pharmacodynamics. An exception was the study on diazepam and fluoxetine, where a pharmacokinetic interaction was found, but there was no effect on the pharmacodynamic measures in the study (227; Table 23).

3.4.4. Interactions with Oral Contraceptives

The oral contraceptives are known to interfere with the elimination of a number of drugs (239). Oral contraceptives vary in their composition, but in general they contain an estrogen and a progestin. These can be given in combination or in sequence. In most oral contraceptives the estrogen is ethinylestradiol. Ethinylestradiol is a mechanism-based inhibitor of P450 3A4 (240). A number of progesterones are used including, norethindrone, norgestrel, levonorgestrel, ethynodiol diacetate, norethisterone, desogestrel, 3-keto-desogestrel, gestodene, and norgestmate. In a study by Back et al. (241) the progestins studied were found to inhibit a number of P450s (3A4, 2C19, and 2C9), but with IC_{50}s in the 25 to > 100 µM range (Fig. 16). In combination with the inhibition of P450-mediated reactions, oral contraceptives are also inducers of glucuronidation.

A number of studies compared the pharmacokinetics of benzodiazepines in woman who did vs woman who did not use oral contraceptives (Table 24). Inhibition

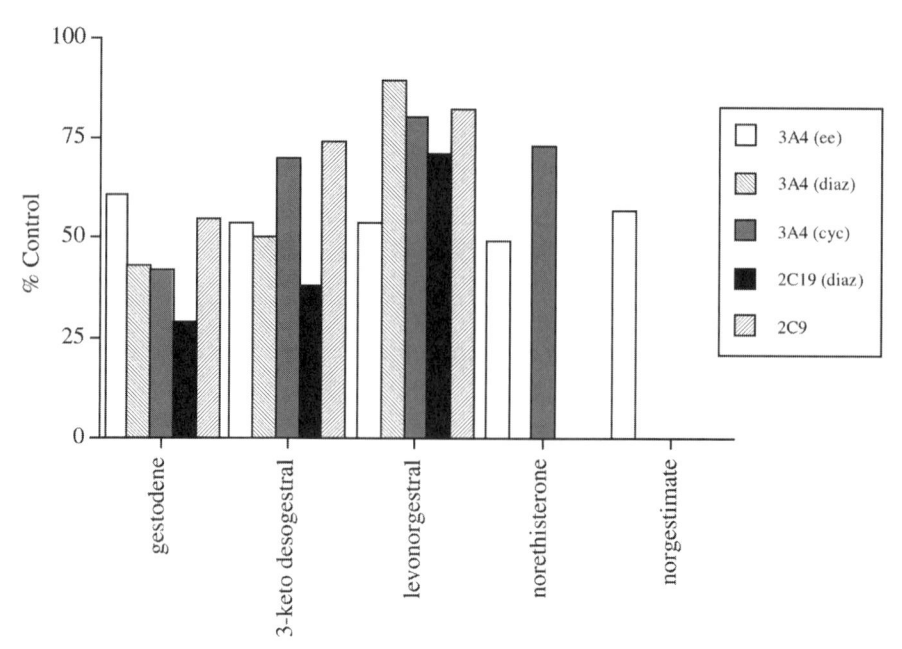

Fig. 16. Inhibition of human liver P450s by progestogens. Data are taken from Back et al. *(241)* where marker assays were performed in HLMs after coincubation with the progestogens. The values shown are the % of control after use of the highest concentration of the progestogen. The substrates and concentration of progestogens were: 3A4 (ee), ethinylestradiol, 100 μ*M*; 3A4 (diaz), diazepam hydroxylation, 100 μ*M*; 3A4 (cyc), cyclosporin hydroxylation, 50 μ*M*; 2C19 (diaz), diazepam N-demethylation, 100 μ*M*; and 2C9 (tol), tolbutamide, 25 μ*M*.

of the elimination of benzodiazepines primarily metabolized by P450 has been found for alprazolam *(242)*, chlordiazepoxide *(243,244)*, clotiazepam *(123)*, diazepam *(245, 246)*, midazolam *(247)*, nitrazepam *(248)*, and triazolam *(242)*. No effect was found in another study on alprazolam *(249)*, for bromazepam *(159)*, with intramuscular midazolam *(250)*, or in a study that compared unlabeled intravenous midazolam to $_{13}N^3$-labeled oral midazolam *(251)*. In contrast, the elimination of benzodiazepines depending primarily on glucuronidation was enhanced as found for lorazepam *(242,244,252)*, oxazepam *(244,252)*, and temazepam *(242)*.

In a study on conjugated estrogens and medroxyprogesterone at doses used for estrogen replacement therapy, no or minimal effect was found on the pharmacokinetics of midazolam *(253;* Table 23).

The changes in woman taking oral contraceptives were not dramatic. In studies on the pharmacodynamic responses no effect was found for midazolam *(247,251)* or temazepam *(254)*. Interestingly, Kroboth et al. *(254)* found minimal stimulation to the benzodiazepine effect in woman taking oral contraceptives along with alprazolam, triazolam, and lorazepam. The finding for lorazepam was contrary to the pharmacokinetic response. In a subsequent study, Kroboth and McAuley *(255)* discuss these findings in light of the ability of a progesterone metabolite 3α-5α-tetrahydroprogesterone to bind to the GABA receptor and enhance binding of benzodiazepines. Pretreatment with

1. Drug Interactions with Benzodiazepines

Table 24
Drug Interactions with Oral Contraceptives

Inhibitor/Benzo	Dose	N	T$_{max}$	C$_{max}$	t$_{1/2}$	AUC	Cl	PhDyn	Reference
Regular therapeutic doses of low-dose estrogen oral contraceptives									
Alprazolam	1, or	10/10	0.71	1.18	1.29*	1.35*	0.79*	+	242,254
Alprazolam	1, or	16/23			1.03	1.07	1.02		249
Bromazepam	6, or	11/7	0.91	1.14	1.06		0.99		159
Chlordiazepoxide	0.6/kg, iv	7/11			1.64		0.66		243
Chlordiazepoxide	0.6/kg, iv	6/6			1.77*		0.40*		244
Clotiazepam	5, or	6/8			2.27		1.01		123
Diazepam	10, iv	5/10			1.83*		0.51*		245
Diazepam	10, iv	8/8			1.47*		0.60*		246
Lorazepam	2, iv	15/15			0.93		1.20		252
Lorazepam	2, iv	7/8			0.43*		3.73*		244
Glucuronide			6.00*	1.50*					
Lorazepam	2, or	11/9	0.86	1.06	0.78*	0.94	1.12	+	242,254
Midazolam	7.5, im	8/7	1.17	0.78	1.61	0.84	1.11		250
1-hydroxy			0.94	0.88	0.94	0.89			
Midazolam	7.5, or	9f	1.00	1.16	1.10	1.20*		0	247
1-hydroxy			1.00	1.25	1.30	1.43*			
Midazolam	0.05/kg, iv	9f			1.09	0.93	1.08	0	251
$^{13}N_3$-Midazolam	3, or	9f	0.78	1.06	0.89	1.10	0.92	0	251
Nitrazepam	5, or	6/6	1.19	1.17	1.00		0.82		248
Oxazepam	30, or	17/14			0.94		1.27		252
Oxazepam	45, or	5/6			0.64		2.57*		244
Temazepam	30, or	10/10	0.89	0.82	0.60*	0.61*	1.62*	0	242,254
Triazolam	0.5, or	10/10	1.50	1.06	1.16	1.44	1.47	+	242,254
Conjugated estrogens (0.625 mg) ± medroxyprogesterone (5 mg)									
Midazolam	3, or	10/10			1.20	1.18	0.89		253

progesterone was found to enhance the pharmacodynamic effects of triazolam. These findings suggest that the progesterones used in oral contraceptives and estrogen replacement therapy may stimulate the action of benzodiazepines despite their actions on the pharmacokinetics of the benzodiazepine.

3.4.5. Interactions with Anticonvulsants

The anticonvulsants include many medications that are known to induce P450s, including P450 3A4. In an in vitro study using primary cultures of human hepatocytes, Pichard et al. *(256)* were able to produce induction of both P450 3A4 content measured immunochemically and the 3A4-mediated activity, cyclosporin oxidase, with the anticonvulsants phenobarbital and phenytoin (Fig. 17). Carbamazepine induced 3A4 content, but reduced its activity. This reduction was not found in HLMs, and was attributed by the authors to cellular toxicity at the doses used in the induction study *(256)*.

Clinical studies following epileptic patients who use a mixture of anticonvulsants that include carbamazepine and/or phenytoin when compared to nonmedicated controls have shown that anticonvulsant treatment enhances the elimination of clobazam *(257)*, diazepam *(258)*, and midazolam *(259;* Table 25). In a study comparing patients taking noninducing anticonvulsants, inducing anticonvulsants and inducing anticonvulsants that included felbamate, the ratio of N-desmethylclobazam to clobazam were

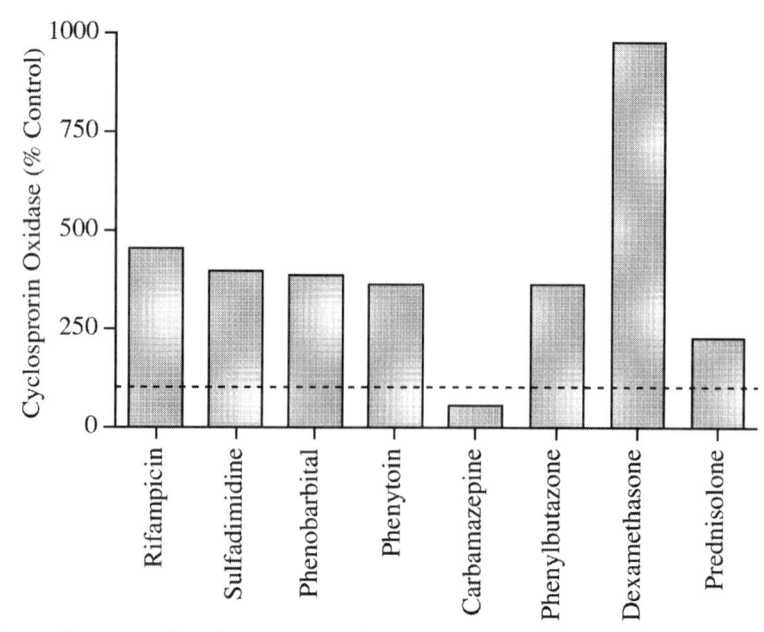

Fig. 17. The induction of cyclosporin oxidase activity, a marker for P450 3A4, in primary cultures of human hepatocytes. The data are from Pichard et al. *(256)*; the dashed line shows 100% control activity.

greatest in the latter group, suggesting the inductive properties of felbamate *(260)*. The clearance of clorazepate was greater in epileptic patients taking phenytoin and/or phenobarbital than for literature values for nonmedicated subjects *(261)*.

Controlled studies in healthy volunteers with carbamazepine alone have demonstrated its ability to enhance the elimination of alprazolam *(262)*, clobazepam *(263)*, and clonazepam *(264;* Table 25). The effect of carbamazepine on alprazolam is consistent with a case report on decreased alprazolam plasma concentrations coinciding with decreased effectiveness in a patient with atypical bipolar disorder once he was started on carbamazepine treatment *(265)*.

Valproic acid was found to increase the clearance of diazepam without any effect on its $t_{1/2}$; this was attributed to the ability of valproic acid to displace diazepam from its plasma protein binding sites *(266,267)*. Valproic acid also decreases the elimination of lorazepam, with decreases in clearance and increased $t_{1/2}$ *(268,269)*. This was shown to be due to inhibition of lorazepam glucuronide formation *(268;* Table 25).

In the study on carbamazepine and/or phenytoin on midazolam, the AUC and C_{max} of midazolam were greatly reduced, to 5.7 and 7.4% of nontreated controls, and the pharmacodynamic measures were significantly reduced *(259)*. When alprazolam was given along with carbamazepine, only minimal diminution of the pharmacodynamic effects were observed. The authors attributed this to the sedative nature of carbamazepine *(262)*, which would be greater in these nontolerant volunteer subjects than in the epileptic patients used for the midazolam study. Sedation scales were only minimally affected during the study on the interaction between valproic acid and lorazepam *(269)*.

1. Drug Interactions with Benzodiazepines

Table 25
Drug Interactions with Anticonvulsants

Inhibitor/Benzo	Dose	N	T_{max}	C_{max}	$t_{1/2}$	AUC	Cl	PhDyn	Reference
Anticonvulsants	Several, but including carbamazepine and/or phenytoin								
Clobazam	30, or	6/6				0.43*			257
N-desmethyl						2.90*			
Diazepam	10, iv	9/6				0.39*	2.58*		258
N-desmethyl			0.71*	1.50*					
Midazolam	15, or	6/7	1.00	0.07*	0.42*	0.06*		---	259
Carbamazepine	100 mg 3/d (alp), 200 mg 2/d (clob), 200 mg 1/d (clon), multidose								
Alprazolam	0.8, or	7m	0.62	1.11	0.45*		2.22*	-	262
Clobazam	20, or (md)	2f,4m		0.38ss*	0.37*		2.58*		263
N-desmethyl				1.44*	0.59*				
Clonazepam	1, or (md)	2f,5m		0.29ss*	0.70*				264
Valproic acid	250 or 500 mg 2/d (lor), 500 mg 3/d (diaz), multidose								
Diazepam	10, iv	6m			0.99	0.69*	1.45*		267
Lorazepam	2, iv	8m		(effect in 6 of 8)			0.60*		268
Glucuronide							0.42*		
Lorazepam	1, or	16m	1.05	1.08*	1.35*	1.20	0.69*	±	269

3.4.6. Interactions with Cardiovascular Agents

Drug interactions of benzodiazepines have been found with a number of cardiovascular agents, particularly the β-adrenoreceptor antagonists and the calcium channel blockers. Information on the in vitro interactions of these drugs with P450s is essentially limited to the calcium channel blockers (Fig. 18). Early studies found only moderate to weak inhibitory action on P450 3A4 metabolism by calcium channel blockers; the percent inhibition of cyclosporin oxidation using 50 μM nicardipine, nifedipine, verapamil, and diltiazem was 81, 17, 29, and 20, respectively, when the inhibitor was added at the start of the reaction *(270)*. More recently, Sutton et al. *(271)* found that the N-desmethyl- and N,N-didesmethyl- metabolites of diltiazem were much more potent inhibitors of 3A4 activity (respective IC_{50}s of 11 and 0.6 μM) than the parent compound (IC_{50} of 120 μM). When diltiazem was preincubated with microsomes and NADPH prior to addition of substrate its effective inhibitory potential greatly increased due to metabolite formation. In a subsequent study, Ma et al. *(272)* tested the ability of a number of calcium channel blockers to inhibit 3A4, 2D6, and 2C9 activities (Fig. 18). For all, except mibefradil and nifedipine, inhibition of 3A4 was enhanced with preincubation in the presence of NADPH; this did not have any effect on inhibition of 2C9 or 2D6 activities. Whether the preincubation effect was due to generation of more active metabolites, or some other mechanism-based or metabolite intermediary complex formation route of inhibition has not been determined except for diltiazem. While metabolites of propranolol are known to bind to microsomes *(273)*, no studies were found on P450 selective inhibition by this or other β-adrenoreceptor antagonists, even though they have been found to cause drug interactions.

Propranolol has mixed effects on benzodiazepines in clinical studies (Table 26). It enhanced the elimination of alprazolam *(274)*, it inhibited the elimination of bromazepam *(159)* and diazepam *(274,275)*, and it had no effect on the elimination of

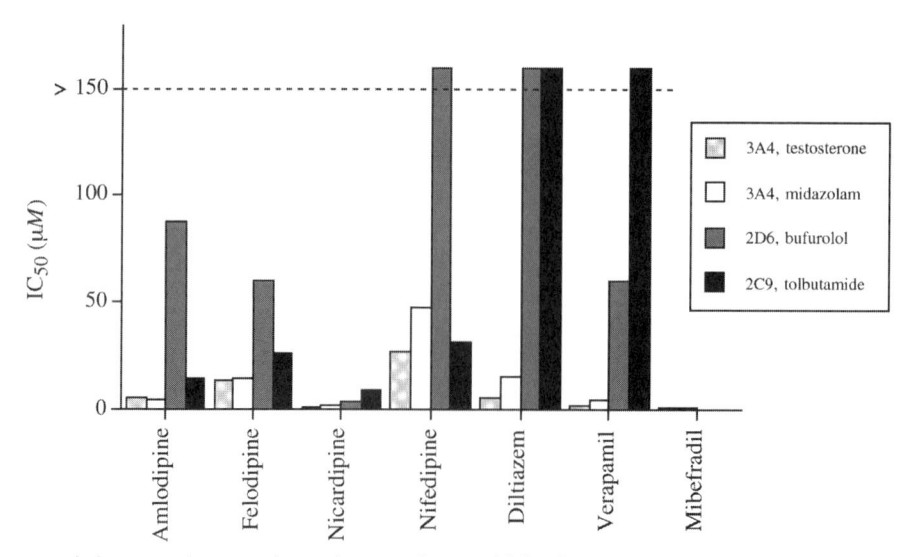

Fig. 18. Inhibition of P450s by calcium channel blockers. Data are from Ma et al. (272) using the results after preincubation of the inhibitor with HLMs and NADPH prior to addition of substrate. Preincubation decreased the IC$_{50}$s for all 3A4 inhibition except for mibefradil and nifedipine. Preincubation had no effect on inhibition of 2D6 or 2C9. Bars extending above the dashed line had IC$_{50}$s greater than 150 µM (100 µM for verapamil and 2C9).

lorazepam *(274)* or oxazepam *(276)*. Metoprolol also inhibited the elimination of bromazepam *(277)* and diazepam *(275,278)* with no effect on lorazepam *(277)*. Atenolol and labetalol had no effect on the pharmacokinetics of diazepam *(275)* and oxazepam *(276)*, respectively. In the aforementioned studies, the inhibition of elimination was only slight to mild, and where studied *(275,276,278)* there were only slight or no effects on the pharmacodynamics of the benzodiazepines (Table 26).

Diltiazem has been shown to inhibit the elimination of intravenous *(279)* and oral *(280)* midazolam, and oral triazolam *(281,282)*. Verapamil inhibits the elimination of midazolam *(280)*, and mibefradil the elimination of triazolam *(283)*. Isradipine was without effect on triazolam *(283)*. The inhibitory calcium channel blockers had significant enhancing effects on the pharmacodynamics of the benzodiazepines *(280–283;* Table 26).

3.4.7. Interactions with Antibiotics

Among the antibiotics, the antitubular agent rifampin (rifampicin) is well known for its ability to induce drug metabolism *(284)*, as can also be seen in in vitro systems (Fig. 17). The macrolide antibiotics are well-known inhibitors of P450 3A4 *(285)*. The specificity of the macrolide antibiotics is exemplified by troleandomycin, which is commonly used as a selective inhibitor of 3A4 (Table 9). Yamazaki and Shimada *(286)* have also demonstrated that erythromycin, roxithromycin, and the M1, M2 and M3 metabo-

Table 26
Drug Interactions with Cardiovascular Agents

Inhibitor/Benzo	Dose	N	T$_{max}$	C$_{max}$	t$_{1/2}$	AUC	Cl	PhDyn	Reference
Propranolol	80 mg, 2–3/d, multidose								
Alprazolam	1, or	6	1.50	0.79*	0.86		1.38		274
Bromazepam	6, or	2f,5m	0.97	1.19	1.20*		0.79		159
Diazepam	5, or (md)	12m	1.31	1.16		1.19		+	275
Diazepam	5, iv	8			1.20		0.83*		274
Lorazepam	2, iv	9			1.04		0.98		274
Propranolol	80 mg, at 0h								
Oxazepam	15, or	2f,4m	0.91	0.84	0.93		1.09	±	276
Metoprolol	100 mg, 2/d, multidose								
Bromazepam	6, or	12m	0.98	1.17	0.92	1.35	0.87	0	277
Diazepam	5, or (md)	12m	1.15	1.21*		1.25*		+	275
Diazepam	0.1/kg, iv	6m			1.27		0.81	+	278
Lorazepam	2, or	12m	1.14	0.93	0.92	1.01	0.97	0	277
Atenolol	25 mg, 2/d, multidose								
Diazepam	5, or (md)	12m	1.23	1.08		1.06		0	275
N-desmethyl						1.00			
Labetalol	200 mg, at 0 h								
Oxazepam	15 mg, or	2f,4m	1.00	0.91	0.95		0.90	0	276
Diltiazem	60 mg, plus 0.1 mg/kg/h infusion during anethesia								
Midazolam	0.1/kg, iv	15/15			1.43	1.15*			279
Diltiazem	60 mg, 3/d, multidose								
Midazolam	15, or	9f	1.09	2.05*	1.49*	3.75*		++	280
Triazolam	0.25, or	7f,3m	1.50*	1.86*	2.35*	2.83*		++	281
Triazolam	0.25, or	7m	1.19	1.71*	1.85*	2.28*		++	282
Verapamil	80 mg, 3/d, multidose								
Midazolam	15, or	9f	0.64	1.97*	1.41*	2.92*		++	280
Mibefradil	50 mg, 1/d, multidose								
Triazolam	0.25, or	5f,2m	2.00*	1.89*	4.62*	8.36*		+++	283
Isradipine	5 mg, multidose								
Triazolam	0.25, or	5f,2m	1.00	0.94	0.78*	0.77*		0	283

lites of roxithromycin inhibit P450 3A4 with no effect on activities selective for 1A2 or 2C9. In a similar study Zhao et al. *(287)* demonstrated that erythromycin, clarithromycin, rokitamycin, and the rokitamycin metabolite, LMA7, inhibit 3A4 selective activity with no effect on 1A2, 2C9, or 2D6 activities. The macrolide antibiotics form metabolite intermediate complexes with human liver microsomal P450 *(286,288)*. This should be taken into consideration when comparing studies on the in vitro inhibition with these compounds, as lower IC$_{50}$ or K$_i$ values will be obtained when the inhibitor is preincubated with the microsomes and a source of NADPH prior to addition of substrate (Fig. 19). A number of studies have compared the ability of the macrolide antibiotics to inhibit P450 3A4 selective activities *(287,289,290)*. From these studies the relative inhibitory potency of the macrolide antibiotics can be ranked as josamycin, troleandomycin > rokitamycin > erythromycin, clarithromycin > roxithromycin >> azithromycin, spiramycin, the latter two having no inhibitory effect at concentrations up to 250 μ*M* (Fig. 19). The clinical studies discussed below also address drug interactions with isoniazid. A recent study found isoniazid was a mechanism-based inhibitor of P450 1A2, 2A6,

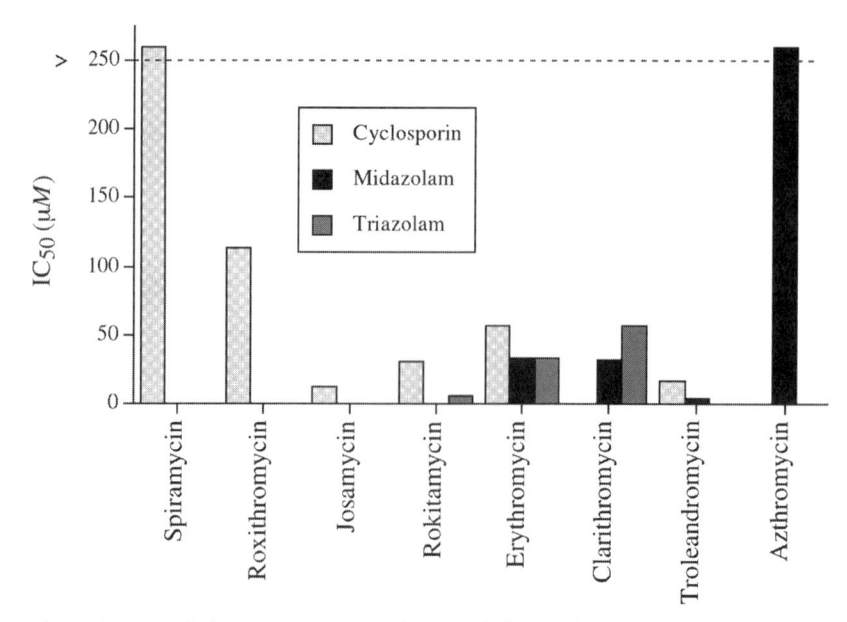

Fig. 19. The relative inhibitory potency of macrolide antibiotics toward P450 3A4 activities in HLMs. The data for cyclosporin (oxidase) are from Marre et al. *(289)*. These incubations were performed without preincubation of the inhibitors, which generally results in higher IC$_{50}$s. The data for midazolam (α-hydroxylation) and triazolam (α-hydroxylation) are from Greenblatt et al. *(290)* and Zhao et al. *(287)*, respectively. Both of these studies preincubated the microsomes with the macrolide antibiotics prior to addition of substrate.

2C19, and 3A4 (respective K$_i$s of 56, 60, 10, and 36 µ*M*), with little or no effect on 2D6 and 2E1 *(291)*. The fluoroquinolone antibiotics that include ciprofloxacin are also addressed and are know to inhibit P450 1A2 activities both in vivo *(292)* and in vitro *(293,294)*. Their selectivity for that P450, however, has not been established.

Generalized antitubucular treatment that included a combination of rifampin, ethambutol, and isoniazid was found to result in significantly enhanced elimination of diazepam (*295*; Table 27). In the same study, ethambutol was found to have no significant effect on diazepam elimination, whereas isoniazid actually inhibited the elimination of diazepam *(295)*. This strongly suggested that the induction of diazepam elimination was due to rifampin, which was subsequently confirmed by Ohnhaus et al. *(296)*. Isoniazid has also been found to inhibit the elimination of triazolam *(297)*, whereas it had no effect on oxazepam *(297)* or clotiazepam *(123)*. Rifampin has also been shown to induce the elimination of alprazolam *(203)*, midazolam *(298,299)*, nitrazepam *(300)*, and triazolam *(301)*; it had no or only a slight inductive effect on temazepam *(300)*. In the studies on midazolam *(298,299)* and triazolam *(301)*, the induction of drug elimination almost negated any pharmacodynamic effect of the benzodiazepine.

Erythromycin has been found to inhibit the elimination of alprazolam *(302)*, diazepam *(303)*, flunitrazepam *(303)*, midazolam *(304–306)*, and triazolam *(290,307)*. It had little or no effect on the pharmacokinetics of temazepam *(308)*. Olkkola et al. *(305)*

Table 27
Drug Interactions with Antibiotics

Inhibitor/Benzo	Dose	N	T_{max}	C_{max}	$t_{1/2}$	AUC	Cl	PhDyn	Reference
Generalized antitubucular treatment (isoniazid, rifampin and ethambutol) for at least 2 wk									
Diazepam	5–7.5, iv	7/7			0.25*		4.05*		295
Ethambutol	25 mg/kg, iv, 1/d, multidose in newly diagnosed tubucular patients								
Diazepam	5–7.5, iv	6/6			1.15		0.78		295
Isoniazid	90 mg, 2/d, multidose								
Clotiazepam	5, or	11			1.27		1.17		123
Diazepam	5–7.5, iv	6f,3m			1.33*		0.74*		295
Oxazepam	30, or	5f,4m	0.74	1.03	1.11	0.98	1.09		297
Triazolam	0.5, or	2f,4m	1.16	1.20	1.31*	1.46*	0.58*		297
Rifampin	1200 mg, 1/d, multidose								
Diazepam	10, or	7m	0.76	0.69*	0.28*	0.27*	3.72*		296
N-desmethyl						0.42*	3.18r*		
3-hydroxy						0.52*	2.68r*		
oxazepam						0.77*	1.29r*		
Rifampin	600 mg, 1/d, multidose								
Alprazolam	1, or	4	0.75	0.64*	0.18*	0.12*	7.54*		203
Diazepam	10, or	7m	1.18	0.80	0.30*	0.23*	4.27*		296
N-desmethyl						0.51*	1.48r*		
3-hydroxy						0.57*	1.88r*		
oxazepam						0.87	1.20r*		
Midazolam	15, or	5f,5m	1.25	0.06*	0.42*	0.04*		----	298
Midazolam	15, or	5f,4m	0.67	0.05*	0.20*	0.02*		----	299
Nitrazepam	5, or	8	0.75	0.96	0.61*		1.83*		300
Temazepam	10, or	8	0.86	0.90	0.86		1.11		300
Triazolam	0.5, or	4f,6m	1.00	0.12*	0.46*	0.06*		----	301
Erythromycin	750 mg, at –1 h								
Midazolam	10, or	5m	0.50*	1.20*				++	304
Erythromycin	500 mg (diaz, flun, tem, mid, triaz b) 400 mg (alp), 333 mg (triaz a), 3/d, multidose								
Alprazolam	0.8, or	12m	2.63*	1.18	2.52*	1.61*	0.40*	0	302
Diazepam	5, or	5f,1m	0.62	1.21	1.72	1.07*		0	303
N-desmethyl						0.81			
Flunitrazepam	1, or	3f,12m	2.00	1.17	1.56*	1.28*		0	303
Midazolam	0.05/kg, iv	4f,2m			1.77*		0.46*	+	305
Midazolam	15, or	9f,3m	0.66	2.79*	2.38*	4.42*		+++	305
Midazolam	15, or	8f,4m	1.00	2.71*	2.19*	3.81*		+++	306
Temazepam	20, or	6f,4m	0.87	1.13	1.00			0	308
Oxazepam			1.05	0.96	1.07				
Triazolam a	0.5, or	16m	0.90	1.46*	1.54*	2.06*	0.48*		307
Triazolam b	0.125, or	6f,6m	1.00	1.77*	2.25*	3.80*	0.35*	+++	290
Troleandomycin	1 g, 2/d, multidose								
Triazolam	0.25, or	7m	1.57*	2.08*	3.58*	3.76*	0.26*	+++	309
Roxithromycin	300 mg, 1/d, multidose								
Midazolam	15, or	5f,5m	0.94	1.37	1.29*	1.47*		+	310
Azithromycin	500 mg, 3/d (mid), 2/d (triaz), multidose								
Midazolam	15, or	8f,4m	1.00	1.29	1.09	1.26		0	306
Triazolam	0.125, or	6f,6m	1.00	1.14	0.94	1.02	1.01	±	290
Clarithromycin	500 mg, 2/d, multidose								
Triazolam	0.125, or	6f,6m	1.22	1.97*	3.07*	5.25*	0.23*	++++	290
Ciprofloxacin	500 mg, 2/d, multidose								
Diazepam	10, iv	10m			1.18	1.16	0.91		312
Diazepam	5, iv	6f,6m			1.94*	1.50*	0.63*	0	311

demonstrated that the effect of erythromycin was more potent for oral than intravenous midazolam. For oral midazolam, the erythromycin interaction produced significantly enhanced pharmacodynamic reactions *(304–306)*, whereas the interaction of erythromycin with alprazolam *(302)*, diazepam *(303)*, flunitrazepam *(303)*, and intravenous midazolam *(305)* had little or no effect on the pharmacodynamics of the drugs (Table 26). Troleandomycin *(309)* and clarithromycin *(290)* inhibit the elimination of triazolam; the interaction with troleandomycin being associated with a significant effect on its pharmacodynamics. Roxithromycin had a small but significant effect on the pharmacokinetics and pharmacodynamics of midazolam *(310)*. Azithromycin had no effect on the pharmacokinetics and pharmacodynamics of midazolam (*290,306*; Table 27).

The fluoroquinolone antibiotic ciprofloxacin was found to inhibit the elimination of 5 mg intravenous diazepam in one study *(311)*, with little or no pharmacodynamic effect. In another study, ciprofloxacin had little or no effect on the elimination of 10 mg intraveneous diazepam (*312*; Table 26). Possibly higher doses of diazepam overcome a weak inhibitory action of ciprofloxacin.

3.4.8. Interactions with Antiretroviral Agents

The antiretroviral agents, particularly the protease inhibitors and nonnucleoside reverse transcriptase inhibitors, are an emerging group of potent inhibitors, and, in some cases, inducers of drug-metabolizing enzymes *(313–315)*. In vitro, the protease inhibitors are particularly potent inhibitors of P450 3A4, with 2C9 and 2C19 also inhibited by some (Fig. 20A). The relative potency for inhibition of 3A4 is ritonavir > indinavir > saquinavir *(316–321*; Fig. 20A). Saqinavir has variously been found equipotent to nelfinavir *(318)*, less potent than nelfinavir *(319,320)*, and more potent than nelfinavir *(321)*. In a single study on amphenavir, it was found to inhibit 3A4 with a potency similar to indinavir *(320)*. A single study comparing the inhibitory potency of the nonnucleoside reverse transcriptase inhibitors suggests that their relative ability to inhibit P450 3A4 is delaviridine > efanvirenz >> nevirapine *(322)*. P450s 2C9 and 2C19 are also susceptible to inhibition by delaviridine and efanvirenz (Fig. 20B; *322*).

The antiretroviral agents are given in combination. Much of what is currently know about their ability to induce drug metabolism comes from clinical studies on the combination of two or more of these drugs. From these studies the protease inhibitors, ritonivar, nelfinavir, amprenavir, and the nonnucleoside reverse transcriptase inhibitors, efavirenz and nevirapine, have all shown the potential to induce drug metabolism *(313,315)*. They also inhibit the metabolism of some of the other antiretroviral agents.

Studies on the interactions of antiretroviral agents with benzodiazepines are currently limited (Table 28), but will probably grow based on the clinical significance of these drugs. Ritonavir, after 2 or 3 d of treatment, has been found to inhibit the elimination of triazolam *(323)* and alprazolam *(324)*. The inhibition of triazolam is quite significant with major effects on the pharmacokinetics of this benzodiazepine. The effects on alprazolam are also significant, but did not have as great an impact on its pharmacodynamics. In the paper concerning ritonavir and alprazolam *(324)*, the authors cite an abstract that was unavailable for review. The abstracted study apparently tested the interaction between ritonavir and alprazolam after 10 d of ritonavir treatment and found no significant effect. Greenblatt et al. *(324)* speculate that the longer treatment with rito-

1. Drug Interactions with Benzodiazepines

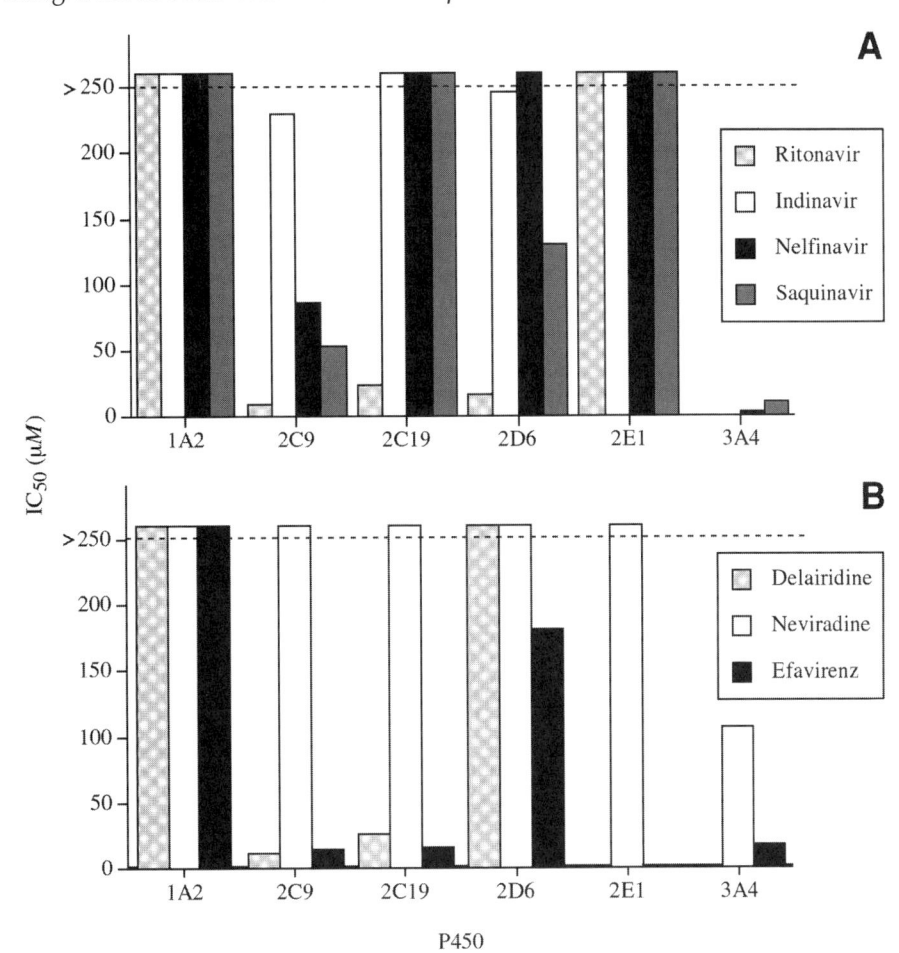

Fig. 20. The relative inhibitory potency of (**A**) protease inhibitor and (**B**) non-nucleoside reverse transcriptase inhibitor antiretroviral agents toward selective P450 activities in HLMs. The data for the protease inhibitors are from von Moltke et al. *(319)*, except for the effect of saquinavir on P450 2C9, which are from Eagling et al. *(316)*. The data for the non-nucleoside reverse transcriptase inhibitors are from von Moltke et al. *(322)*, except for the effect of nevirapine on P450 2E1, which are from Erickson et al. *(402)*.

navir is coupled with greater induction of metabolism, such that the mixed inhibition-induction of alprazolam has an end effect of no result.

The interaction of midazolam with saquinavir has also been studied. Three- or 5-d treatment with saquinavir causes a significant inhibition of the elimination of oral midazolam associated with a significant enhancement of its pharmacokinetics. Saquanivar also inhibited the elimination of intravenous midazolam, but to a lesser extent (*325;* Table 28). The mixed inductive and inhibitory nature of the protease inhibitors and the nonnucleoside reverse transcriptase inhibitors may make it more difficult to predict when drug interactions will occur. Further studies may shine more light on the matter.

Table 28
Drug Interactions with Antiretroviral Agents

Inhibitor/Benzo	Dose	N	T_{max}	C_{max}	$t_{1/2}$	AUC	Cl	PhDyn	Reference
Ritonavir	200 mg, 2/d, four doses (triaz at +1 h after 3rd dose; alpraz at +1 h after 2nd dose)								
Triazolam	0.125, or	6m	1.80*	1.87*	13.6*	20.4*	0.04*	++++	323
Alprazolam	1.0, or	8	1.50	1.04	2.23*	2.48*	0.41*	++	324
Saquinavir	1200 mg, 3/d, 5d (midaz on d3 or d5)								
Midazolam	7.5, or	6f,6m	1.33	2.35*	2.53*	5.18*		+++	325
α-hydroxy-			1.33	0.62*		0.19*			
Midazolam	0.05/kg, iv	6f,6m		0.90ss	2.31*	2.49*	0.44	+	325
α-hydroxy-			1.00	0.57*		0.42*			

3.4.9. Interactions with Grapefruit Juice

In a seminal study reported in 1991, Baily et al. *(326)* demonstrated that grapefruit juice, but not orange juice, significantly increased the bioavailability of oral felodipine and nifedipine, both P450 3A4 substrates. In combination with studies demonstrating grapefruit juice had no effect on intravenously administered drugs, and since the AUCs and C_{max}s were often increased but not $t_{1/2}$s, it was concluded that grapefruit juice had its main impact on bioavailability at the level of the gastrointestinal system. P450 3A4 is also the major P450 in the gastrointestinal system *(327,328)*, and the drugs affected by grapefruit juice are 3A4 substrates *(329,330)*. This connection was highlighted when it was shown that ingestion of grapefruit juice in human volunteers was associated with a loss of 3A4 content, but not mRNA *(331,332)*. Efforts to determine the components of grapefruit juice responsible for its inhibitory effects therefore centered on P450 3A4 inhibitors.

A major unique component of grapefruit juice is the flavonoid, naringen. It can make up to 10% of the dry weight of the juice and is responsible for the bitter taste. The initial study on inhibition of P450 3A4 found that naringen was essentially ineffective; the aglycone of naringen, naringenen, however, did inhibit nifedipine oxidation with an IC_{50} of 100 μ*M (333)*. In the same study, it was shown that other aglycone flavonoids unique to grapefruit, quercetin, kaempferol, apegenin, and hesperetin, also inhibited nifedipine oxidation with respective approximate IC_{50}s of 80, 90, 300, and 300 μ*M* (Fig. 21). Additional studies confirmed the ability of these flavonoids to inhibit 3A4 specific activities, including nifedipine oxidation *(334)*, midazolam α-hydroxylation *(37,335)*, quinidine 3-hydroxylation *(335)*, 17β-estradiol metabolism *(336)*, and saquinavir metabolism *(337)*. Two clinical studies examined the relative inhibitory action of quercetin vs grapefruit juice on nifedipine pharmacokinetics *(338)* and naringen vs grapefruit juice on felodipine pharmacokinetics *(339)*. Neither flavoniod when administered at doses comparable to those in the grapefruit juice caused any effect on the bioavailability of the drug *(338,339)*.

Examination of the inhibitory capacity of HPLC fractions of extracts of grapefruit juice pointed to the furanocoumarin components of grapefruit juice as other inhibitors of P450 3A4 *(337,340–342)*. Their inhibitory capacity for 3A4-related substrates was one to two orders of magnitude greater than the flavonoids (Fig. 21). Subsequent

1. Drug Interactions with Benzodiazepines

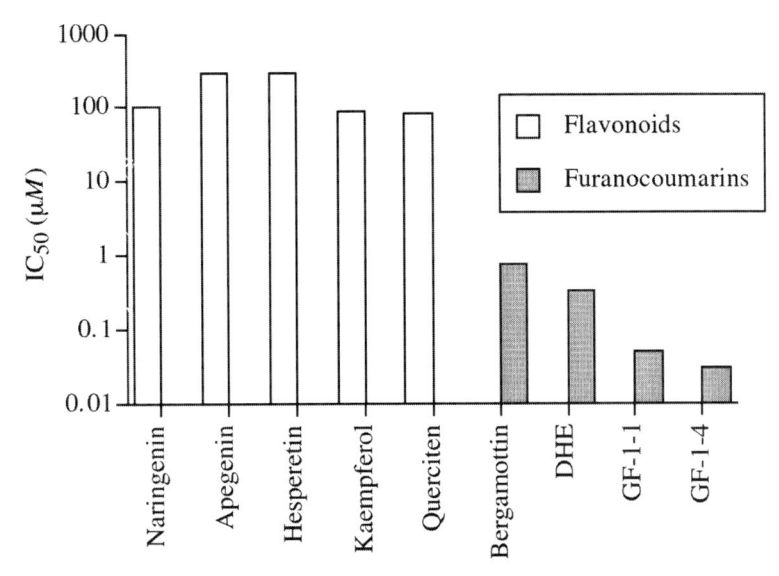

Fig. 21. The relative potency of components of grapefruit juice to inhibit P450 3A4 activities. The data for the flavonoids are for nifedipine oxidation and are from Guengerich and Kim *(333)*. Data for the furocoumarins, bergamottin, and 6',7'-dihydroxybergamottin (DHB) are for saquinavir metabolism and are from Eagling et al. *(337)*. The data for the HPLC fractions containing furocoumarins designated GF-1-1 and GF-1-4 are K_is for inhibition of testosterone 6β-hydroxylation and are from Fukuda et al. *(342)*. Note the log scale on the Y-axis.

studies demonstrated that the furanocoumarins were mechanism-based inhibitors of P450 3A4 *(332,343)*, which was consistent with the loss of 3A4 content in enterocytes. With only limited amounts of the furanocoumarins available, there has not yet been a clinical study to indicate they can substitute for grapefruit juice in causing drug interactions. Their role in grapefruit juice drug interactions therefore has not yet been established.

The effect of grapefruit juice may not be limited to 3A4 substrates; one of the furanocoumarins, bergamottin, was shown to inhibit activies selective for P450s 2A6, 2C9, 2D6, 2E1, and 3A4 all with IC_{50}s in the 2–6 μ*M* range *(344)*. In addition, Fuhr et al. *(345)* found that grapefruit juice decreases the oral clearance of caffeine, a P450 1A2 substrate. Grapefruit juice also effects P-glycoprotein-mediated transport, increasing the basolateral to apical flux *(337,346,347)*. The relative role the transporter and P450 3A4 have on the bioavailability of a drug may also be important in determining the active component in the effect of grapefruit juice. For benzodiazepines undergoing oxidative metabolism, P450 3A4 appears to be more important.

Coadministration of grapefruit juice was found to increase the AUC of oral, but not intravenous, midazolam *(348,349)*, oral triazolam *(350)*, and oral alprazolam *(351;* Table 29). In normal subjects, the effect was modest, and accompanied with no or only minor effects on the pharmacodynamics of the benzodiazepines *(348,350–352)*. In a study performed on subjects with cirrhosis of the liver, the effect of grapefruit

Table 29
Drug Interactions with Juices

Inhibitor/Benzo	Dose	N	T$_{max}$	C$_{max}$	t$_{1/2}$	AUC	Cl	PhDyn	Reference
Grapefruit juice	250–400 mL								
Midazolam	10, or	13/12						+	352
Midazolam	5, iv	8m			1.00	1.04	0.95	0	348
1-hydroxy			0.89	1.19	1.00	1.06			
Midazolam	15, or	8m			0.98	1.52*	0.96	++	348
1-hydroxy			2.05*	1.00	1.00	1.30*			
Midazolam	15, or	3f,7m[a]	1.24	1.16	1.00	2.31*			349
1-hydroxy			1.73	0.27*	1.06	0.38*			
Triazolam	0.25, or	13/12						0	352
Triazolam	0.25, or	4f,6m	1.67	1.25*	1.18	1.47*		+	350
Grapefruit juice	200 mL 3/d, multidose								
Alprazolam	0.8, or	6m	0.83	1.08	1.38*	1.18*		+	351
Tangerine juice	100 mL at –0.25 h and 100 mL at 0 h								
Midazolam	15, or	4f,4m	2.00*	0.82	1.00	0.86		delay	353
1-hydroxy			1.25*	0.70*	0.95	0.87			

[a]Subjects had liver cirrhosis.

juice was much greater, and a related decrease in the C$_{max}$ and AUC of the 1-hydroxy-metabolite was found that was not seen in normal subjects (*349*). This suggests that cirrhotics are more dependent upon intestinal metabolism of midazolam. In a study on other juices, tangerine juice was found to delay the absoprtion of midazolam and slightly delay its pharmacodynamic effects (*353*; Table 29).

3.4.10. Interactions with Miscellaneous Agents

Clinical studies concerning potential drug interactions with benzodiazepines have been performed with a number of drugs for which either only a single drug in its class was studied, or there was no explicit connection with an aspect of drug metabolism. These studies will be considered in this section.

3.4.10.1. INTERACTIONS WITH METHYLXANTHINES

Intravenous aminophylline, a prodrug of theophylline, was tested as a potential antagonist of diazepam. It produces a slight, but insignificant decrease in the T$_{max}$ and C$_{max}$ of diazepam, with no effect on the AUC. It did produce a significant decrease in the pharmacodynamic measures of diazepam (*354*; Table 30). The effect of chronic theophylline on alprazolam was compared in subjects with chronic obstructive pulmonary disease that were or were not taking theophylline. Following 7 d of 1/d alprazolam, the pharmacokinetics were compared in the two groups; in the group taking theophylline a significant decrease in the steady-state level and AUC of alprazolam was observed (*355*). Caffeine was found to have no effect on the pharmacokinetics of diazepam (*356*) or alprazolam (*203*); but caffeine did slightly diminsh the pharmacodynamic measures for diazepam (*356*; Table 30).

3.4.10.2. INTERACTIONS WITH ANTIPYRINE

Antipyrine has long been known to be an inducer of drug metabolism in humans. In an initial study, Ohnhaus et al. (*357*) demonstrated that a 7-d treatment with antipy-

1. Drug Interactions with Benzodiazepines

Table 30
Drug Interactions with Miscellaneous Agents

Inhibitor/Benzo	Dose	N	T$_{max}$	C$_{max}$	t$_{1/2}$	AUC	Cl	PhDyn	Reference
Aminophylline	5.6 mg/kg, iv								
Diazepam	0.25/kg, or	8m	0.75	0.86		1.00		---	354
Theophylline	chronic for obstructive pulmonary disease								
Alprazolam	0.5, or, 7 d	6/5		0.25ss*		0.32*			355
Caffeine	6 mg/kg (diaz) 100 mg (alpr) at 0 h								
Diazepam	0.3/kg, or	3f,3m	1.00	1.00				-	356
Alprazolam	1, or	9	1.08	1.03	1.22	1.07	0.82		203
Antipyrine	600 mg, 2/d, multidose								
Diazepam	10, or	2f,5m	1.09	0.95	0.49*		1.93*		357
N-desmethyl					0.42*	0.46*			
Diazepam	10, or	7	0.82	1.01	0.59*	0.51	2.02*		296
N-desmethyl						0.84	1.40r		
3-hydroxy						0.82	1.28r		
oxazepam						1.06	0.87r		
Disulfiram	500 mg, 1/d, multidose								
Chlordiazepoxide	50, iv	6			1.84*		0.46*		358
Diazepam	0.143/kg, or	6	0.85	0.97	1.37*		0.59*		358
Oxazepam	0.429/kg, or	5	1.00	0.83	1.17		1.02		358
Disulfiram	chronic treatment of alcoholics								
Alprazolam	2, or	5f,6m	1.19	0.88	0.92	0.94			359
Diflunisal	500 mg, 2/d, multidose								
Oxazepam	30, or	6m	0.96	0.62*	1.13	0.84	1.48*		400
glucuronide			1.20	1.34	1.30*	1.70*	0.62r*		
Glucocorticoid	chronic treatment								
Midazolam	0.2/kg, iv	8/10			0.96	0.64	1.27		360
1-hydroxy					0.60*	0.67			
Dexamethasone	1.5 mg, 1/d, multidose								
Triazolam	0.5, or	8f,2m	1.00	1.15	1.05	0.82		0	361
Paracetamol	1g/d from –1 d to +3 d								
Diazepam	10, or	1f,2m	1.00	1.01	1.12		0.94		362
Probenecid	2 g, at –2h (adin) or 500 mg, 4/d (lor) or 500 mg 1/d (tem, nit) multidose								
Adinazolam	60, or	16m	0.67	1.37*	1.06	1.13*	0.84*	++	364
N-desmethyl			1.92*	1.49*	0.90	1.77*			
Lorazepam	2, iv	9			2.31*		0.55*		363
Nitrazepam	5, or	8	1.20	1.08	1.21*		0.75*		300
Temazepam	10, or	8	1.09	0.93	1.06		0.90		300
Modafinal	200 mg/d, 7 d; 400 mg/d, 21d								
Triazolam	0.125, or	16f	1.43*	0.56*	0.65*	0.38*			366
Herbal dietary supplements									
Garlic oil	500 mg, 3/d, 28 d								
Midazolam	8, or	6f,6m		1.00	(1-h 1'-OH/midazolam)				367
Panax ginseng	500 mg, 3/d, 28 d (5% ginseosides)								
Midazolam	8, or	6f,6m		1.00	(1-h 1'-OH/midazolam)				367
Ginkgo biloba	60 mg, 4/d, 28 d (24% flavone glycosides; 6% terpene lactones)								
Midazolam	8, or	6f,6m		1.00	(1-h 1'-OH/midazolam)				367
Hypericum perforatum (St. John's wort) 300 mg, 3/d, 28 d (0.3% hypericin)									
Midazolam	8, or	6f,6m		1.98*	(1-h 1'-OH/midazolam)				367

rine significantly decreased the AUC and t$_{1/2}$ of oral diazepam. In this study, the AUC and t$_{1/2}$ of N-desmethyldiazepam were also significantly decreased. In a follow-up study comparing the effects of antipyrine and rifampin on the elimination of diazepam, 7-d pretreatment with antipyrine had similar effects on the parent drug; the AUCs of the N-desmethyl-, 3-hydroxy-, and oxazepam metabolites were not suppressed as much suggesting relative induction of these pathways (*296*; Table 30).

3.4.10.3. INTERACTIONS WITH DISULFIRAM

Both disulfiram and certain benzodiazepines are used to treat alcoholism. Chronic disulfiram treatment was found to diminsh the elimination of chlordiazepoxide and diazepam, but not that of oxazepam in normal subjects (Table 30). The clearance and $t_{1/2}$ of the three benzodiazepines in chronic alcoholics who had received chronic disulfiram treatment were similar to those in the disulfirma-treated normal subjects *(358)*. In a study with 11 chronic alcoholics, alprazolam was given prior to initiation of disulfiram treatment and again after 2 wk of disulfiram; no change in the pharmacokinetics of alprazolam was noted *(359)*.

3.4.10.4. INTERACTION WITH DIFLUNISAL

Diflunisal is a salicyclic-derived nonsteroidal antiinflammatory agent. Like oxazepam it is primarily elimated after glucuronidation, and both are highly protein bound. When oxazepam was given before and after 7 d of 2/d treatment with diflunisal, the C_{max} of oxazepam was decreased and its oral clearance increased. Significant increases were also found in the $t_{1/2}$ and AUC, and a decrease in the clearance of the oxazepam glucuronide (Table 30). The authors conclude that the interaction resulted from the displacement of oxazepam from its protein-binding sites and by inhibition of the tubular secretion of the oxazepam glucuronide.

3.4.10.5. INTERACTIONS WITH GLUCOCORTICOIDS

The effect of glucocorticoids (primarily predonisolone) on the pharmacokinetics of midazolam was studied by comparing surgery patients receiving intravenous midazolam who were on chronic glucocorticoid therapy to those who were not *(360)*. There was a decrease in the AUC of midazolam and 1'-hydroxymidazolam and increase in the clearance of midazolam in the glucocorticoid group, but the changes did not reach significance. The $t_{1/2}$ of 1'-hydroxymidazolam was significantly decreased and the renal clearance of its glucuronide significantly increased. The authors concluded that these findings were consistent with the induction of P450 and/or glucuronidation *(360)*. Five daily "small" doses of dexamethasone were found to have no significant effect on the pharmacokinetics or pharmacodynamics of triazolam in normal volunteers *(361*; Table 30).

3.4.10.6. INTERACTION WITH PARACETAMOL

When paracetamol was taken 1 d before and 3 d following a single oral dose of diazepam, there was no effect on the plasma phamacokinetics of diazepam (Table 30). The authors did detect a significant decrease in the percentage of diazepam plus metabolites excreted in urine over a 96-h period *(362)*. The findings suggest that paracetamol may decrease the glucuronidation of diazepam metabolites.

3.4.10.7. INTERACTIONS WITH PROBENECID

Probenecid is well known for its ability to inhibit renal tubular secretion of organic acids. The effect of probenecid on the elimination of benzodiazepines was first studied

1. Drug Interactions with Benzodiazepines

**Table 31
Key to Drug Interaction Tables**

Interacting drug	The route is oral, unless stated otherwise. An indication of the duration of treament is given, and when different the benzodiazepines considered are noted separately in parentheses (e.g., triaz a, triaz b).
Benzodiazepines	The benzodiazepine of interest is indented 1/4 inch; if a metabolite was also studied, it is listed directly below with a 1/2-inch indentation.
Dose	All doses are in mg. The abbreviations for route of administration are: or, oral; iv, intravenous; im, intramuscular.
N	For cross-over studies only one group of subject numbers are provided; if gender was specified, females are noted with an "f"; males with an "m" (e.g., 8 or 4f,4m). For comparisons between groups, a '/' separates the groups; the one receiving the interactant is listed first (50/40, refers to a study where 50 subjects recieved the interactant and 40 did not).
Pharmacokinetics	Are presented as the ratio of the interactant to the control group. Findings presented as significant by the authors are noted with an asterisk "*".
T_{max}	Time to maximal plasma (serum or blood) concentration.
C_{max}	Maximum plasma (serum or blood) concentration. If ratio is followed by "ss," this was a steady-state measurement.
$t_{1/2}$	Terminal elimination half-life.
AUC	Area under the time versus concentration curve. If the AUC for both the actual time of measurement and one extrapolated to infinity were presented, the former was used.
Cl	Clearance for iv administration; apparent oral clearance for oral administration. If followed by an "r," this refers to renal clearance.
PhDyn	A qualitative assessment of the results of pharmacodynamic measures recorded in the study. This was both an assessment of the degree of change and the number of measures that changed: 0 – no effect; - to ----, a diminution in the pharmacodynamics ranging from slight to loss of all effect; + to ++++, an enhancement of the pharmacodynamics ranging from slight to toxic.

with lorazepam. Abernethy et al. *(363)* gave probenecid 4/d from 12 h before a single intravenous dose of lorazepam. The $t_{1/2}$ of lorazepam was significantly increased and its clearance significantly decreased. This result suggested not just inhibition of excretion, but also inhibition of glucuronide formation *(363)*. Brockmeyer et al. *(300)* studied the pharmacokinetics of nitrazepam and temazepam both before and after 7 d treatment with probenecid. With nitrazepam, there was a moderate increase in $t_{1/2}$ and decrease in clearance. With temazepam there was no significant effect on plasma pharmacokinetics, but there was reduced urinary content of the temazepam glucuronide *(300)*. When adinazolam was given with probenecid *(364)*, there were increases in the C_{max} and AUC for both adinazolam and its N-desmethyl metabolite, more so for the metabolite. This was associated with potentiation of the psychomotor effects of the benzodiazepine (Table 30). The authors suggest that the major effect is on the elimination of the metabolite *(364)*. Probenecid does effect the renal elimination of many benzodiazepines; it may also have an effect on glucuronidation and possibly P450 mediated reactions.

3.4.10.8. INTERACTION WITH MODAFINAL

Modafinal is a novel wake-promoting agent used to treat excessive daytime sleepiness. In HLMs, modafinal inhibited P450 2C19, with no significant effect on the other P450 activities studied. In cultured human hepatocytes, it induced P450s 1A2, 2B6, and 3A4/5 *(365)*. The effect of modafinal on the pharmacokintics of triazolam (and ethinyl estradiol) was studied in females taking daily birth control medication containing ethinyl estradiol *(366)*. In a group of woman given triazolam before and after 28 d of treatment with modafinal, there was a significant induction of the elimination of triazolam (Table 30).

3.4.10.9. INTERACTIONS WITH HERBAL DIETARY SUPPLEMENTS

Gurley and coworkers *(367)* studied the effect on 28-d use of various herbal supplements (St. John's wort, garlic oil, *Panax ginseng, Ginkgo biloba*) on a P450 phenotyping "cocktail" designed to measure 1A2, 2D6, 2E1, and 3A4 activities. The ratio of 1'-OH-midazolam to midazolam in 1-h serum samples was used to monitor P450 3A4. Individuals had the phenotyping cocktail before and after a 28-d period of use of the supplement; each supplement use was separated by a 30-d washout period. St. John's wort (*Hypericum perforatum*) was found to increase the 1'-OH/midazolam almost 98%, indicating induction of its metabolism. None of the other supplements affected the P450 3A4 phenotype ratio (Table 29). St. John's wort also induced P450 2E1, whereas garlic oil decreased 2E1 *(367)*.

4. CONCLUSIONS

A number of drugs and some dietary substances are known to interact with the benzodiazepines. Other CNS depressants including ethanol, opioids, and anesthetics have an additive effect on the pharmacodynamics of the benzodiazepine that is unrelated to the route of benzodiazepine metabolism. When an inhibition of metabolism is also encountered, the effect may be synergistic. Interactions with other drugs and dietary substances are generally based upon an interaction at the site of metabolism. Most often this reflects the involvement of P450 3A4, but in some instances the involvement of 2C19 in diazepam metabolism, and glucuronidation are also sites of interaction. A few examples of displacement from protein binding and inhibition of renal tubular secretion also exist. These metabolic interactions can vary from having little or no effect on the pharmacodynamics to inhibitions that produce toxic side effects and inductions that essentially negate the pharmacodynamics of the benzodiazepine. These studies, however, have been conducted at "normal" therapeutic doses. A misadventure with either or both interactant is likely to magnify the end result.

ACKNOWLEDGMENTS

This review grew from an earlier review of benzodiazepines by Center for Human Toxicology faculty, and materials gathered for a workshop on benzodiazepines at the Society of Forensic Toxicology 2000 meeting, Milwaukee, WI. This work was supported in part by U.S. Public Health Service grant R01 DA10100. Though I have tried to achieve a thorough review of the peer-reviewed literature, many papers were not available. Authors who feel I have missed their studies are asked to send the pertinent reprints. Should this article be updated in the future, I will make my best effort to include those studies at that time.

REFERENCES

1. Greenblatt DJ, Shader RI, and Abernethy DR. Drug therapy. Current status of benzodiazepines. First of two parts. N Engl J Med 309:354–358 (1983).
2. Greenblatt DJ, Shader RI, and Abernethy DR. Drug therapy. Current status of benzodiazepines. Second of two parts. N Engl J Med 309:410–416 (1983).
3. Jones GR and Singer PP. The newer benzodiazepines. In: Baselt RC, ed. Analytical toxicology, vol. 2. Chicago: Year Book Medical Publishers, 1989:1–69.
4. Hobbs WR, Rall TW, and Verdoorn TA. Hypnotics and sedatives: ethanol. In: Hardman JG, Limbird LE, Molinoff PB, Ruddon RW, and Gilman AG, eds. Goodman & Gilman's The pharmacological basis of therapeutics. New York: McGraw-Hill, 1996:361–396.
5. Benet LZ, Oie S, and Schwartz JB. Design and optimization of dosage regimes: pharmacokinetic data. In: Hardman JG, Limbird LE, Molinoff PB, Ruddon RW, and Gilman AG, eds. Goodman & Gilman's The pharmacological basis of therapeutics. New York: McGraw-Hill, 1996:1707–1792.
6. Baselt RC and Cravey RH. Disposition of toxic drugs and chemicals in man. Foster City, CA: Chemical Toxicology Institute, 1995.
7. Parfitt K. Martindale the complete drug reference, 1999.
8. Murray L. Physicians' desk reference. (2002).
9. Ishigami M, Honda T, Takasaki W, Ikeda T, Komai T, Ito K, and Sugiyama Y. A comparison of the effects of 3-hydroxy-3-methylglutaryl-coenzyme a (HMG-COA) reductase inhibitors on the CYP3A4-dependent oxidation of mexazolam in vitro. Drug Metab Dispos 29: 282–288 (2001).
10. Sethy VH, Collins RJ, and Daniels EG. Determination of biological activity of adinazolam and its metabolites. J Pharm Pharmacol 36:546–548 (1984).
11. Fleishaker JC and Phillips JP. Adinazolam pharmacokinetics and behavioral effects following administration of 20–60 mg doses of its mesylate salt in volunteers. Psychopharmacology 99:34–39 (1989).
12. Borchers F, Achtert G, Hausleiter HJ, and Zeugner H. Metabolism and pharmacokinetics of metaclazepam (Talis®), Part III: Determination of the chemical structure of metabolites in dogs, rabbits and men. Eur J Drug Metab Pharmacokinet 9:325–346 (1984).
13. Lu X-L and Yang SK. Enantiomer resolution of camazepam and its derivatives and enantioselective metabolism of camazepam by human liver microsomes. J Chromatogr A 666: 249–257 (1994).
14. Tomori E, Horvath G, Elekes I, Lang T, and Korosi J. Investigation of the metabolites of tofizopam in man and animals by gas-liquid chromatography-mass spectrometry. J Chromatogr A 241:89–99 (1982).
15. Wrighton SA, Vandenbranden M, Stevens JC, Shipley LA, Ring BJ, Rettie AE, and Cashman JR. In vitro methods for assessing human drug metabolism: their use in drug development. Drug Metab Rev 25:453–484 (1993).
16. Rodrigues AD. Use of in vivo human metabolism studies in drug development: an industrial perspective. Biochem Pharmacol 48:2147–2156 (1994).
17. Guengerich FP. In vitro techniques for studying drug metabolism. J Pharmacokin Biopharm 24:521–533 (1996).

18. Crespi CL and Miller VP. The use of heterologously expressed drug metabolizing enzymes—state of the art and prospects for the future. Pharmacol Ther 84:121–131 (1999).
19. Venkatakrishnan K, Von Moltke LL, Court MH, Harmatz JS, Crespi CL, and Greenblatt DJ. Comparison between cytochrome P450 (CYP) content and relative activity approaches to scaling from cDNA-expressed CYPs to human liver microsomes: ratios of accessory proteins as sources of discrepancies between approaches. Drug Metab Dispos 28:1493–1504 (2000).
20. Nelson AC, Huang W, and Moody DE. Variables in human liver microsome preparation: impact on the kinetics of l-α-acetylmethadol (LAAM) N-demethylation and dextromethorphan O-demethylation. Drug Metab Dispos 29:319–325 (2001).
21. Newton DJ, Wang RW, and Lu AYH. Cytochrome P450 inhibitors: evaluation of specificities in the in vitro metabolism of therapeutic agents by human liver microsomes. Drug Metab Dispos 23:154–158 (1995).
22. Ono S, Hatanaka T, Hotta H, Satoh T, Gonzalez FJ, and Tsutsui M. Specificity of substrate and inhibitor probes for cytochrome P450s: evaluation of in vitro metabolism using cDNA-expressed human P450s and human liver microsomes. Xenobiotica 26:681–693 (1996).
23. Sai Y, Dai R, Yang TJ, Krausz KW, Gonzalez FJ, Gelboin HV, and Shou M. Assessment of specificity of eight chemical inhibitors using cDNA-expressed cytochromes P450. Xenobiotica 30:327–343 (2000).
24. Moody DE, James JL, Clawson GA, and Smuckler EA. Correlations among changes in hepatic microsomal components after intoxication with alkyl halides. Mol Pharmacol 20:685–693 (1981).
25. Shimada T, Tsumura F, and Yamazaki H. Prediction of human liver microsomal oxidations of 7-ethoxycoumarin and chlorzoxazone with kinetic parameters of recombinant cytochrome P-450 enzymes. Drug Metab Dispos 27:1274–1280 (1999).
26. Andersson T, Miners JO, Veronese ME, and Birkett DJ. Diazepam metabolism by human liver microsomes is mediated by both S-mephenytoin hydroxylase and CYP3A isoforms. Br J Clin Pharmacol 38:131–137 (1994).
27. Ono S, Hatanaka T, Miyazawa S, Tsutsui M, Aoyama T, Gonzalez FJ, and Satoh H. Human liver microsomal diazepam metabolism using cDNA-expressed cytochrome P450s: role of CYP2B6, 2C19 and the 3A subfamily. Xenobiotica 26:1155–1166 (1996).
28. Yang TJ, Shou M, Korzekwa KR, Gonzalez FJ, Gelboin HV, and Yang SK. Role of cDNA-expressed human cytochromes P450 in the metabolism of diazepam. Biochem Pharmacol 55:889–896 (1998).
29. Yang TJ, Krausz KW, Sai Y, Gonzalez FJ, and Gelboin HV. Eight inhibitory monoclonal antibodies define the role of individual P-450s in human liver microsomal diazepam, 7-ethoxycoumarin, and imipramine metabolism. Drug Metab Dispos 27:102–109 (1999).
30. Shou MG, Lu T, Krausz KW, Sai Y, Yang TJ, Korzekwa KR, et al. Use of inhibitory monoclonal antibodies to assess the contribution of cytochromes P450 to human drug metabolism. Eur J Pharmacol 394:199–209 (2000).
31. Fabre G, Rahmani R, Placidi M, Combalbert J, Covo J, Cano J-P, et al. Characterization of midazolam metabolism using hepatic microsomal fractions and hepatocytes in suspension obtained by perfusing whole human livers. Biochem Pharmacol 37:4389–4397 (1988).
32. Kronbach T, Mathys D, Umeno M, Gonzalez FJ, and Meyer UA. Oxidation of midazolam and triazolam by human liver cytochrome P450IIIA4. Mol Pharmacol 36:89–96 (1989).
33. Gorski JC, Hall SD, Vandenbranden M, Wrighton SA, and Jones DR. Regioselective biotransformation of midazolam by members of the human cytochrome p450 3A (CYP3A) subfamily. Biochem Pharmacol 47:1643–1653 (1994).

34. Thummel KE, Shen DD, Podoll TD, Kunze KL, Trager WF, Hartwell PS, et al. Use of midazolam as a human cytochrome P450 3 probe: in vitro–in vivo correlations in liver transplant patients. J Pharmacol Exp Ther 271:54956 (1994).
35. Wandel C, Bocker R, Bohrer H, Browne A, Rugheimer E, and Martin E. Midazolam is metabolized by at least three different cytochrome P450 enzymes. Br J Anaesth 73:658–661 (1994).
36. Wrighton SA and Ring BJ. Inhibition of human CYP3A catalyzed 1'-hydroxy midazolam formation by ketoconazole, nifedipine, erythromycin, cimetidine, and nizatidine. Pharm Res 11:921–924 (1994).
37. Ghosal A, Satoh H, Thomas PE, Bush E, and Moore D. Inhibition and kinetics of cytochrome P4503A activity in microsomes from rat, human, and cDNA-expressed human cytochrome P450. Drug Metab Dispos 24:940–947 (1996).
38. von Moltke LL, Greenblatt DJ, Schmider J, Duan SX, Wright CE, Harmatz JS, and Shader RI. Midazolam hydroxylation by human liver microsomes in vitro: inhibition by fluoxetine, norfluoxetine, and by azole antifungal agents. J Clin Pharmacol 36:783–791 (1996).
39. Ekins S, Vandenbranden M, Ring BJ, Gillespie JS, Yang TJ, Gelboin HV, and Wrighton SA. Further characterization of the expression in liver and catalytic activity of CYP2B6. J Pharmacol Exp Ther 286:1253–1259 (1998).
40. Wandel C, Bocker RH, Bohrer H, deVries JX, Hofman W, Walter K, et al. Relationship between hepatic cytochrome P450 3A content and activity and the disposition of midazolam administered orally. Drug Metab Dispos 26:110–114 (1998).
41. Perloff MD, von Moltke LL, Court MH, Kotegawa T, Shader RI, and Greenblatt DJ. Midazolam and triazolam biotransformation in mouse and human liver microsomes: relative contribution of CYP3A and CYP2C isoforms. J Pharmacol Exp Ther 292:618–628 (2000).
42. Hamaoka N, Oda Y, Hase I, and Asada A. Cytochrome P4502B6 and 2C9 do not metabolize midazolam: kinetic analysis and inhibition study with monoclonal antibodies. Brit J Anaesth 86:540–544 (2001).
43. Schmider J, Greenblatt DJ, von Moltke LL, Harmatz JS, Duan SX, Karsov D, and Shader RI. Characterization of six in vitro reactions mediated by human cytochrome P450: application to the testing of cytochrome P450-directed antibodies. Pharmacology 52:125–134 (1996).
44. Gorski JC, Jones DR, Hamman MA, Wrighton SA, and Hall SD. Biotransformation of alprazolam by members of the human cytochrome P4503A subfamily. Xenobiotica 29:931–944 (1999).
45. Hirota N, Ito K, Iwatsubo T, Green CE, Tyson CA, Shimada N, et al. In vitro/in vivo scaling of alprazolam metabolism by CYP3A4 and CYP3A5 in humans. Biopharm Drug Dispos 22:53–71 (2001).
46. Venkatakrishnan K, von Moltke LL, Duan SX, Fleishaker JC, Shader RI, and Greenblatt DJ. Kinetic characterization and identification of the enzymes responsible for hepatic biotransformation of adinazolam and N-desmethyladinazolam in man. J Pharm Pharmacol 50:265–274 (1998).
47. Coller JK, Somogyi AA, and Bochner F. Flunitrazepam oxidative metabolism in human liver microsomes: involvement of CYP2C19 and CYP3A4. Xenobiotica 29:973–986 (1999).
48. Hesse LM, Venkatakrishnan K, von Moltke LL, Shader RI, and Greenblatt DJ. CYP3A4 is the major CYP isoform mediating the in vitro hydroxylation and demethylation of flunitrazepam. Drug Metab Dispos 29:133–140 (2001).
49. Kilicarslan T, Haining RL, Rettie AE, Busto U, Tyndale RF, and Sellers EM. Flunitrazepam metabolism by cytochrome P450s 2C19 and 3A4. Drug Metab Dispos 29:460–465 (2001).

50. Senda C, Kishimoto W, Sakai K, Nagakura A, and Igarashi T. Identification of human cytochrome P450 isoforms involved in the metabolism of brotizolam. Xenobiotica 27:913–922 (1997).
51. Shimada T, Yamazaki H, Mimura M, Inui Y, and Guengerich FP. Interindividual variations in human liver cytochrome P-450 enzymes involved in the oxidation of drugs, carcinogens and toxic chemicals: studies with liver microsomes of 30 Japanese and 30 Caucasians. J Pharmacol Exp Ther 270:414–423 (1994).
52. Bertilsson L, Henthorn TK, Sanz E, Tybring G, Sawe J, and Villen T. Importance of genetic factors in the regulation of diazepam metabolism: relationship to S-mephenytoin, but not debrisoquin, hydroxylation phenotype. Clin Pharmacol Ther 45:348–355 (1989).
53. Abernethy DR, Greenblatt DJ, Ochs HR, and Shader RI. Benzodiazepine drug-drug interactions commonly occurring in clinical practice. Curr Med Res Opin 8(Suppl 4):80–93 (1984).
54. Abernethy DR, Greenblatt DJ, and Shader RI. Benzodiazepine hypnotic metabolism: drug interactions and clinical implications. Acta Psychiatr Scand 74(Suppl 332):32–38 (1986).
55. Yuan R, Flockhart DA, and Balian JD. Pharmacokinetic and pharmacodynamic consequences of metabolism-based drug interactions with alprazolam, midazolam, and triazolam. J Clin Pharmacol 39:1109–1125 (1999).
56. Sellers EM and Busto U. Benzodiazepines and ethanol: assessment of the effects and consequences of psychotropic drug interactions. J Clin Psychopharmacol 2:249–262 (1982).
57. Chan AWK. Effects of combined alcohol and benzodiazepine: a review. Drug Alcohol Depend 13:315–341 (1984).
58. Linnoila MI. Benzodiazepines and alcohol. J Psychiat Res 24(Suppl 2):121–127 (1990).
59. Tanaka E. Toxicological interactions between alcohol and benzodiazepines. Clin Toxicol 40:69–75 (2002).
60. Serfaty M and Masterton G. Fatal poisonings attributed to benzodiazepines in Britain during the 1980s. Br J Psychiatry 163:386–393 (1993).
61. Buckley NA, Dawson AH, Whyte IM, and O'Connell DL. Relative toxicity of benzodiazepines in overdose. Br Med J 310:219–221 (1995).
62. Busto U, Kaplan HL, and Sellers EM. Benzodiazepine-associated emergencies in Toronto. Am J Psychiatry 137:224–227 (1980).
63. Finkle BS, McCloskey KL, and Goodman LS. Diazepam and drug-associated deaths: a survey in the United States and Canada. J Am Med Assoc 242:429–434 (1979).
64. Hojer J, Baehrendtz S, and Gustafsson L. Benzodiazepine poisoning: experience of 702 admissions to an intensive care unit during a 14-year period. J Int Med 226:117–122 (1989).
65. Richards RG, Reed D, and Cravey RH. Death from intravenously administered narcotics: a study of 114 cases. J Forensic Sci 21:467–482 (1976).
66. Monforte JR. Some observations concerning blood morphine concentrations in narcotic addicts. J Forensic Sci 22:718–724 (1977).
67. Goldberger BA, Cone EJ, Grant TM, Caplan YH, Levine BS, and Smialek JE. Disposition of heroin and its metabolites in heroin-related deaths. J Anal Toxicol 18:22–28 (1994).
68. Walsh SL, Preston KL, Stitzer ML, Cone EJ, and Bigelow GE. Clinical pharmacology of buprenorphine: ceiling effects at high doses. Clin Pharmacol Ther 55:569–580 (1994).
69. Reynaud M, Tracqui A, Petit G, Potard D, and Courty P. Six deaths linked to misuse of buprenorphine-benzodiazepine combinations. Am J Psychiatry 155:448–449 (1998).
70. Papworth DP. High dose buprenorphine for postoperative analgesia. Anaesthesia 38:163 (1983).
71. Forrest AL. Buprenorphine and lorazepam. Anaesthesia 38:598 (1983).
72. Faroqui MH, Cole M, and Curran J. Buprenorphine, benzodiazepines and respiratory depression. Anaesthesia 38:1002–1003 (1983).

73. Gueye PN, Borron SW, Risede P, Monier C, Buneaux F, Debray M, and Baud FJ. Buprenorphine and midazolam act in combination to depress respiration in rats. Toxicol Sci 65: 107–114 (2002).
74. Kilicarslan T and Sellers EM. Lack of interaction of buprenorphine with flunitrazepam metabolism. Am J Psychiatry 157:1164–1166 (2000).
75. Crouch DJ, Birky MM, Gust SW, Rollins DE, Walsh JM, Moulden JV, et al. The prevalence of drugs and alcohol in fatally injured truck drivers. J Forensic Sci 38:1342–1353 (1993).
76. Lund AK, Preusser DF, Blomberg RD, and Williams AF. Drug use by tractor-trailer drivers. J Forensic Sci 33:648–661 (1988).
77. Couper FJ, Pemberton M, Jarvis A, Hughes M, and Logan BK. Prevalence of drug use in commercial tractor-trailer drivers. J Forensic Sci 47:562–567 (2002).
78. Moody DE, Crouch DJ, Andrenyak DM, Smith RP, Wilkins DG, Hoffman AM, and Rollins DE. Mandatory post-accident drug and alcohol testing for the Federal Railroad Administration: a comparison of results for two consecutive years. NIDA Res Mono 100:79–96 (1991).
79. Lundberg GD, White JM, and Hoffman KI. Drugs (other than or in addition to ethyl alcohol) and driving behavior: a collaborative study of the California Association of Toxicologists. J Forensic Sci 24:207–215 (1979).
80. Poklis A, MaGinn D, and Barr JL. Drug findings in "driving under the influence of drugs" cases: a problem of illicit drug use. Drug Alcohol Depend 20:57–62 (1987).
81. Jonasson U, Jonasson B, Saldeen T, and Thuen F. The prevalence of analgesics containing dextropropoxyphene or codeine in individuals suspected of driving under the influence of drugs. Forensic Sci Int 112:163–169 (2000).
82. Logan BK and Couper FJ. Zolpidem and driving impairment. J Forensic Sci 46:105–110 (2001).
83. Preston KL, Griffiths RR, Stitzer ML, Bigelow GE, and Liebson IA. Diazepam and methadone interactions in methadone maintenance. Clin Pharmacol Ther 36:534–541 (1984).
84. Preston KL, Griffiths RR, Cone EJ, Darwin WD, and Gorodetzky CW. Diazepam and methadone blood levels following concurrent administration of diazepam and methadone. Drug Alcohol Depend 18:195–202 (1986).
85. Abernethy DR, Greenblatt DJ, Morse DS, and Shader RI. Interaction of propoxyphene with diazepam, alprazolam and lorazepam. Br J Clin Pharmacol 19:51–57 (1985).
86. Gamble JAS, Kawar P, Dundee JW, Moore J, and Briggs LP. Evaluation of midazolam as an intravenous induction agent. Anaesthesia 36:868–873 (1981).
87. Boldy DAR, English JSC, Lang GS, and Hoare AM. Sedation for endoscopy: a comparison between diazepam, and diazepam plus pethidine with naloxone reversal. Br J Anaesth 56:1109–1111 (1984).
88. Tverskoy M, Fleyshman G, Ezry J, Bradley EL, and Kissin I. Midazolam-morphine sedative interaction in patients. Anesth Analges 68:282–285 (1989).
89. Kanto J, Sjovall S, and Vuori A. Effect of different kinds of premedication on the induction properties of midazolam. Br J Anaesth 54:507–511 (1982).
90. Tomicheck RC, Rosow CE, Philbin DM, Moss J, Teplick RS, and Scheider RC. Diazepam-fentanyl interaction—hemodynamic and hormonal effects in coronary artery surgery. Anesth Analg 62:881–884 (1983).
91. Dundee JW, Halliday NJ, McMurray TJ, and Harper KW. Pretreatment with opioids: the effect on thiopentone induction requirements and on the onset of action of midazolam. Anaesthesia 41:159–161 (1986).
92. Bailey PL, Pace NL, Ashburn MA, Moll JWB, East KA, and Stanley TH. Frequent hypoxemia and apnea after sedation with midazolam and fentanyl. Anesthesiology 73:826–830 (1990).

93. Ben-Shlomo I, Abd-El-Khalim H, Ezry J, Zohar S, and Tverskoy M. Midazolam acts synergistically with fentanyl for induction of anaesthesia. Br J Anaesth 64:45–47 (1990).
94. Silbert BS, Rosow CE, Keegan CR, Latta WB, Murphy AL, Moss J, and Philbin DM. The effect of diazepam on induction of anesthesia with alfentanyl. Anesth Analg 65:71–77 (1986).
95. Vinik HR, Bradley EL, and Kissin I. Midazolam-alfentanyl synergism for anesthetic induction in patients. Anesth Analg 69:213–217 (1989).
96. Short TG, Plummer JL, and Chui PT. Hypnotic and anaesthetic interactions between midazolam, propofol and alfentanyl. Br J Anaesth 69:162–167 (1992).
97. Hase I, Oda Y, Tanaka K, Mizutani K, Nakamoto T, and Asada A. I.v. fentanyl decreases the clearance of midazolam. Br J Anaesth 79:740–743 (1997).
98. Yun CH, Wood M, Wood AJJ, and Guengerich FP. Identification of the pharmacogenetic determinants of alfentanil metabolism: cytochrome P-450 3A4. An explanation of the variable elimination clearance. Anesthesiology 77:467–474 (1992).
99. Labroo RB, Thummel KE, Kunze KL, Podoll T, Trager WF, and Kharasch ED. Catalytic role of cytochrome P4503A4 in multiple pathways of alfentanil metabolism. Drug Metab Dispos 23:490–496 (1995).
100. Tateishi T, Krivoruk Y, Ueng YF, Wood AJJ, Guengerich FP, and Wood M. Identification of human liver cytochrome p-450 3A4 as the enzyme responsible for fentanyl and sufentanil n-dealkylation. Anesth Analg 82:167–172 (1996).
101. Guitton J, Buronfosse T, Desage M, Flinois J-P, Perdrix J-P, Brazier J-L, and Beaune P. Possible involvement of multiple human cytochrome P450 isoforms in the liver metabolism of propofol. Br J Anaesth 80:788–795 (1998).
102. Oda Y, Mizutani K, Hase I, Nakamoto T, Hamaoka N, and Asada A. Fentanyl inhibits metabolism of midazolam: competitive inhibition of CYP3A4 in vitro. Brit J Anaesth 82:900–903 (1999).
103. Swift R, Davidson D, Rosen S, Fitz E, and Camara P. Naltrexone effects on diazepam intoxication and pharmacokinetics in humans. Psychopharmacology 135:256–262 (1998).
104. Tverskoy M, Fleyshman G, Bradley EL, and Kissin I. Midazolam-thiopental anesthetic interaction in patients. Anesth Analg 67:342–345 (1988).
105. Short TG, Galletly DC, and Plummer JL. Hypnotic and anaesthetic action of thiopentone and midazolam alone and in combination. Br J Anaesth 66:13–19 (1991).
106. Short TG and Chui PT. Propofol and midazolam act synergistically in combination. Br J Anaesth 67:539–545 (1991).
107. McClune S, McKay AC, Wright PMC, Patterson CC, and Clarke RSJ. Synergistic interaction between midazolam and propofol. Br J Anaesth 69:240–245 (1992).
108. Hamaoka N, Oda Y, Hase I, Mizutani K, Nakamoto T, Ishizaki T, and Asada A. Propofol decreases the clearance of midazolam by inhibiting CYP3A4: an in vivo and in vitro study. Clin Pharmacol Ther 66:110–117 (1999).
109. Miller E and Park GR. The effect of oxygen on propofol-induced inhibition of microsomal cytochrome P450 3A4. Anaesthesia 54:320–322 (1999).
110. Bond A, Silveira JC, and Lader M. Effects of single doses of alprazolam and alcohol alone and in combination on psychological performance. Hum Psychopharmacol 6:219–228 (1991).
111. Taeuber K, Badian M, Brettel HF, Royen T, Rupp W, Sittig W, and Uihlein M. Kinetic and dynamic interaction of clobazam and alcohol. Br J Clin Pharmacol 7:91S–97S (1979).
112. Seppala T, Palva ES, Mattila MJ, Kortilla K, and Shrotriya RC. Tofisopam, a novel 3,4-benzodiazepine: multiple-dose effects on psychomotor skills and memory. Comparison with diazepam and interactions with ethanol. Psychopharmacology 69:209–218 (1980).

113. Saario I. Psychomotor skills during subacute treatment with thioridazine and bromazepam, and their combined effects with alcohol. Ann Clin Res 8:117–123 (1976).
114. McManus IC, Ankier SI, Norfolk J, Phillips M, and Priest RG. Effects of psychological performance of the benzodiazepine, loprazolam, alone and with alcohol. Br J Clin Pharmacol 16:291–300 (1983).
115. Palva ES and Linnoila M. Effect of active metabolites of chlordiazepoxide and diazepam, alone or in combination with alcohol, on psychomotor skills related to driving. Eur J Clin Pharmacol 13:345–350 (1978).
116. Linnoila M, Stapleton JM, Lister R, Moss H, Lane E, Granger A, and Eckardt MJ. Effects of single doses of alprazolam and diazepam, alone and in combination with ethanol, on psychomotor and cognitive performance and on automatic nervous system reactivity in healthy volunteers. Eur J Clin Pharmacol 39:21–28 (1990).
117. Linnoila M and Hakkinen S. Effects of diazepam and codeine, alone and in combination with alcohol, on simulated driving. Clin Pharmacol Ther 15:368–373 (1974).
118. Sellers EM, Frecker RC, and Romach MK. Drug metabolism in the elderly: confounding of age, smoking, and ethanol effects. Drug Metab Rev 14:225–250 (1983).
119. de la Maza MP, Hirsch S, Petermann M, Suazo M, Ugarte G, and Bunout D. Changes in microsomal activity in alcoholism and obesity. Alcohol Clin Exp Res 24:605–610 (2000).
120. Scavone JM, Greenblatt DJ, Harmatz JS, and Shader RI. Kinetic and dynamic interaction of brotizolam and ethanol. Br J Clin Pharmacol 21:197–204 (1986).
121. Linnoila M, Otterstrom S, and Antilla M. Serum chlordiazepoxide, diazepam and thioridazine concentrations after the simultaneous ingestion of alcohol or placebo drink. Ann Clin Res 6:4–6 (1974).
122. Dorian P, Sellers EM, Kaplan HL, Hamilton C, Greenblatt DJ, and Abernethy D. Triazolam and ethanol interaction: kinetic and dynamic consequences. Clin Pharmacol Ther 37:558–562 (1985).
123. Ochs HR, Greenblatt DJ, Verburg-Ochs B, Harmatz JS, and Grehl H. Disposition of clotiazepam: influence of age, sex, oral contraceptives, cimetidine, isoniazid and ethanol. Eur J Clin Pharmacol 26:55–59 (1984).
124. Linnoila M, Erwin CW, Brendle A, and Loque P. Effects of alcohol and flunitrazepam on mood and performance in healthy young men. J Clin Pharmacol 21:430–435 (1981).
125. Girre C, Hirschhorn M, Bertaux L, Palombo S, and Fournier PE. Comparison of performance of healthy volunteers given prazepam alone or combined with ethanol. Relation to drug plasma concentrations. Int Clin Psychopharmacol 6:227–238 (1991).
126. Hayes SL, Pablo G, Radomoki T, and Palmer RG. Ethanol and oral diazepam absorption. N Engl J Med 296:186–189 (1977).
127. Laisi U, Linnoila M, Seppala T, Himberg J-J, and Mattila MJ. Pharmacokinetic and pharmacodynamic interactions of diazepam with different alcoholic beverages. Eur J Clin Pharmacol 16:263–270 (1979).
128. Sellers EM, Naranjo CA, Giles HG, Frecker RC, and Beeching M. Intravenous diazepam and oral ethanol interaction. Clin Pharmacol Ther 28:638–645 (1980).
129. Morland J, Setekleiv J, Haffner JFW, Stromsaether CE, Danielsen A, and Wethe GH. Combined effects of diazepam and ethanol on mental and psychomotor functions. Acta Pharmacol Toxicol 34:5–15 (1974).
130. Greenblatt DJ, Shader RI, Weinberger DR, Allen MD, and MacLaughlin DS. Effect of a cocktail on diazepam absorption. Psychopharmacology 57:199–203 (1978).
131. Divoll M and Greenblatt DJ. Alcohol does not enhance diazepam absorption. Pharmacology 22:263–268 (1981).

132. Busby WF, Ackermann JM, and Crespi CL. Effect of methanol, ethanol, dimethyl sulfoxide, and acetonitrile on in vitro activities of cDNA-expressed human cytochromes P-450. Drug Metab Dispos 27:246–249 (1999).
133. Perry PJ, Wilding DC, Fowler RC, Helper CD, and Caputo JF. Absorption of oral and intramuscular chlordiazepoxide by alcoholics. Clin Pharmacol Ther 23:535–541 (1978).
134. Sellers EM, Greenblatt DJ, Zilm DH, and Degani N. Decline in chlordiazepoxide plasma levels during fixed-dose therapy of alcohol withdrawal. Br J Clin Pharmacol 6:370–372 (1978).
135. Sellman R, Pekkarinen A, Kangas L, and Raijola E. Reduced concentrations of plasma diazepam in chronic alcoholic patients following an oral administration of diazepam. Acta Pharmacol Toxicol 36:25–32 (1975).
136. Sellman R, Kanto J, Raijola E, and Pekkarinen A. Human and animal study on elimination from plasma and metabolism of diazepam after chronic alcohol intake. Acta Pharmacol Toxicol 36:33–38 (1975).
137. Pond SM, Phillips M, Benowitz NL, Galinsky RE, Tong TG, and Becker CE. Diazepam kinetics in acute alcohol withdrawal. Clin Pharmacol Ther 25:832–836 (1979).
138. Kostrubsky VE, Strom SC, Wood SG, Wrighton SA, Sinclair PR, and Sinclair JF. Ethanol and isopentanol increase CYP3A and CYP2E in primary cultures of human hepatocytes. Arch Biochem Biophys 322:516–520 (1995).
139. Nair SG, Gamble JAS, Dundee JW, and Howard PJ. The influence of three antacids in the absorption and clinical action of oral diazepam. Br J Anaesth 48:1175–1180 (1976).
140. Elliot P, Dundee JW, Elwood RJ, and Collier PS. The influence of H2 receptor antagonists on the plasma concentration of midazolam and temazepam. Eur J Anesth 1:245–251 (1984).
141. Greenblatt DJ, Shader RI, Harmatz JS, Franke K, and Koch-Weser J. Influence of magnesium and aluminum hydroxide mixture on chlordiazepoxide absorption. Clin Pharmacol Ther 19:234–239 (1976).
142. Chun AHC, Carrigan PJ, Hoffman DJ, Kershner RP, and Stuart JD. Effect of antacids on absorption of clorazepate. Clin Pharmacol Ther 22:329–335 (1977).
143. Shader RI, Georgotas A, Greenblatt DJ, Harmatz JS, and Allen MD. Impaired absorption of desmethyldiazepam from clorazepate by magnesium aluminum hydroxide. Clin Pharmacol Ther 24:308–315 (1978).
144. Greenblatt DJ, Allen MD, MacLaughlin DS, Harmatz JS, and Shader RI. Diazepam absorption: effect of antacids and food. Clin Pharmacol Ther 24:600–609 (1978).
145. Abruzzo CW, Macasieb T, Weinfeld R, Rider AJ, and Kaplan SA. Changes in the oral absorption characteristics in man of dipotassium clorazepate at normal and elevated gastric pH. J Pharmacokinet Biopharm 5:377–390 (1977).
146. Shader RI, Ciraulo DA, Greenblatt DJ, and Harmatz JS. Steady-state plasma desmethyldiazepam during long-term clorazepate use: effect of antacids. Clin Pharmacol Ther 31: 180–183 (1982).
147. Kroboth PD, Smith RB, Rault R, Silver MR, Sorkin MI, Puschett JB, and Juhl RP. Effects of end-stage renal disease and aluminum hydroxide on temazepam kinetics. Clin Pharmacol Ther 37:453–459 (1985).
148. Kroboth PD, Smith RB, Silver MR, Rault R, Sorkin MI, Puschett JB, and Juhl RP. Effects of end stage renal disease and aluminium hydroxide on triazolam pharmacokinetics. Br J Clin Pharmacol 19:839–842 (1985).
149. Lima DR, Santos RM, Werneck E, and Andrade GN. Effect of orally administered misoprostol and cimetidine on the steady state pharmacokinetics of diazepam and nordiazepam in human volunteers. Eur J Drug Metab Pharmacokinet 16:161–170 (1991).
150. Bateman DN. The action of cispride on gastric emptying and the pharmacodynamics and pharmacokinetics of diazepam. Eur J Clin Pharmacol 30:205–208 (1986).

1. Drug Interactions with Benzodiazepines

151. Dal Negro R. Pharmacokinetic drug interactions with anti-ulcer drugs. Clin Pharmacokinet 35:135–150 (1998).
152. Flockhart DA, Desta Z, and Mahal SK. Selection of drugs to treat gastro-oesophageal reflux disease—the role of drug interactions. Clin Pharmacokinet 39:295–309 (2000).
153. Knodell RG, Browne DG, Gwozdz GP, Brian WR, and Guengerich FP. Differential inhibition of individual human liver cytochromes P-450 by cimetidine. Gastroenterology 101:1680–1691 (1991).
154. Martinez C, Albet C, Agundez JAG, Herrero E, Carrillo JA, et al. Comparative in vitro and in vivo inhibition of cytochrome P450 CYP1A2, CYP2D6, and CYP3A by H_2-receptor antagonists. Clin Pharmacol Ther 65:369–376 (1999).
155. Klotz U, Arvela P, Pasanen, Kroemer H, and Pelkonen O. Comparative effects of H_2-receptor antagonists on drug metabolism *in vitro* and *in vivo*. Pharmacol Ther 33:157–161 (1987).
156. Hulhoven R, Desager JP, Cox S, and Harvengt C. Influence of repeated administration of cimetidine on the pharmacokinetics and pharmacodynamics of adinazolam in healthy subjects. Eur J Clin Pharmacol 35:59–64 (1988).
157. Abernethy DR, Greenblatt DJ, Divoll M, Moschitto LJ, Harmatz JS, and Shader RI. Interaction of cimetidine with triazolobenzodiazepines alprazolam and triazolam. Psychopharmacology 80:275–278 (1983).
158. Pourbaix S, Desager JP, Hulhoven R, Smith RB, and Harvengt C. Pharmacokinetic consequences of long term coadministration of cimetidine and triazolobenzodiazepines, alprazolam and triazolam, in healthy subjects. Int J Clin Pharmacol Ther Toxicol 23:447–451 (1985).
159. Ochs HR, Greenblatt DJ, Friedman H, Burstein ES, Locniskar A, Harmatz JS, and Shader RI. Bromazepam pharmacokinetics: influence of age, gender, oral contraceptives, cimetidine and propranolol. Clin Pharmacol Ther 41:562–570 (1987).
160. Desmond PV, Patwardhan RV, Schenker S, and Speeg KV. Cimetidine impairs elimination of chlordiazepoxide (Librium) in man. Ann Intern Med 93:266–268 (1980).
161. Pullar T, Edwards D, Haigh JRM, Peaker S, and Feely MP. The effect of cimetidine on the single dose pharmacokinetics of oral clobazam and N-desmethylclobazam. Br J Clin Pharmacol 23:317–321 (1987).
162. Divoll M, Greenblatt DJ, Abernethy DR, and Shader RI. Cimetidine impairs clearance of antipyrine and desmethyldiazepam in the elderly. J Am Geriatr Soc 30:684–689 (1982).
163. Klotz U and Reimann I. Delayed clearance of diazepam due to cimetidine. N Engl J Med 302:1012–1014 (1980).
164. Klotz U and Reimann I. Elevation of steady-state diazepam levels by cimetidine. Clin Pharmacol Ther 30:513–517 (1981).
165. Gough PA, Curry SH, Araujo OE, Robinson JD, and Dallman JJ. Influence of cimetidine on oral diazepam elimination with measurement of subsequent cognitive change. Br J Clin Pharmacol 14:739–742 (1982).
166. Abernethy DR, Greenblatt DJ, Divoll M, Ameer B, and Shader RI. Differential effect of cimetidine on drug oxidation (antipyrine and diazepam) vs. conjugation (acetaminophen and lorazepam): prevention of acetaminophen toxicity by cimetidine. J Pharmacol Exp Ther 224:508–513 (1983).
167. Greenblatt DJ, Abernethy DR, Morse DS, Harmatz JS, and Shader RI. Clinical importance of the interaction of diazepam and cimetidine. N Engl J Med 310:1639–1643 (1984).
168. Andersson T, Andren K, Cederberg C, Edvardsson G, Heggelund A, and Lundborg P. Effect of omeprazole and cimetidine on plasma diazepam levels. Eur J Clin Pharmacol 39:51–54 (1990).
169. Greenblatt DJ, Abernethy DR, Koepke HH, and Shader RI. Interaction of cimetidine with oxazepam, lorazepam, and flurazepam. J Clin Pharmacol 24:187–193 (1984).

170. Fee JPH, Collier PS, Howard PJ, and Dundee JW. Cimetidine and ranitidine increase midazolam bioavailability. Clin Pharmacol Ther 41:80–84 (1987).
171. Ochs HR, Greenblatt DJ, Gugler R, Muntefering G, Locniskar A, and Abernethy DR. Cimetidine impairs nitrazepam clearance. Clin Pharmacol Ther 34:227–230 (1983).
172. Klotz U and Reimann I. Influence of cimetidine on the pharmacokinetics of desmethyldiazepam and oxazepam. Eur J Clin Pharmacol 18:517–520 (1980).
173. Cox SR, Kroboth PD, Anderson PH, and Smith RB. Mechanism for the interaction between triazolam and cimetidine. Biopharm Drug Dispos 7:567–575 (1986).
174. McGowan WAW and Dundee JW. The effect of intravenous cimetidine on the absorption of orally administered diazepam and lorazepam. Br J Clin Pharmacol 14:201–211 (1982).
175. Klotz U, Arvela P, and Rosenkranz B. Effect of single doses of cimetidine and ranitidine on the steady-state plasma levels of midazolam. Clin Pharmacol Ther 38:652–655 (1985).
176. Salonen M, Aantaa E, Aaltonen L, and Kanto J. Importance of the interaction of midazolam and cimetidine. Acta Pharmacol Toxicol 58:91–95 (1986).
177. Patwardhan RV, Yarborough GW, Desmond PV, Johnson RF, Schenker S, and Speeg KV Jr. Cimetidine spares the glucuronidation of lorazepam and oxazepam. Gastroenterology 79:912–916 (1980).
178. Greenblatt DJ, Abernethy DR, Divoll M, Locniskar A, Harmatz JS, and Shader RI. Noninteraction of temazepam and cimetidine. J Pharm Sci 73:399–401 (1984).
179. Klotz U, Reimann IW, and Ohnhaus EE. Effect of ranitidine on the steady state pharmacokinetics of diazepam. Eur J Clin Pharmacol 24:357–360 (1983).
180. Elwood RJ, Hildebrand PJ, Dundee JW, and Collier PS. Ranitidine influences the uptake of oral midazolam. Br J Clin Pharmacol 15:743–745 (1983).
181. Vanderveen RP, Jirak JL, Peters GR, Cox SR, and Bombardt PA. Effect of rantidine on the disposition of orally and intravenously administered triazolam. Clin Pharmacy 10:539–543 (1991).
182. Abernethy DR, Greenblatt DJ, Eshelman FN, and Shader RI. Ranitidine does not impair oxidative or conjugative drug metabolism: noninteraction with antipyrine, diazepam, and lorazepam. Clin Pharmacol Ther 35:188–192 (1984).
183. Klotz U, Gottlieb W, Keohane PP, and Dammann HG. Nocturnal doses of ranitidine and nizatidine do not affect the disposition of diazepam. J Clin Pharmacol 27:210–212 (1987).
184. Suttle AB, Songer SS, Dukes GE, Hak LJ, Koruda M, Fleishaker JC, and Brouwer KLR. Ranitidine does not alter adinazolam pharmacokinetics or pharmacodynamics. J Clin Psychopharmacol 12:282–287 (1992).
185. Klotz U, Arvela P, and Rosenkranz B. Famotidine, a new H_2-receptor antagonist, does not affect hepatic elimination of diazepam or tubular secretion of procainamide. Eur J Clin Pharmacol 28:671–675 (1985).
186. Locniskar A, Greenblatt DJ, Harmatz JS, Zinny MA, and Shader RI. Interaction of diazepam with famotidine and cimetidine, two H_2-receptor antagonists. J Clin Pharmacol 26:299–303 (1986).
187. VandenBranden M, Ring BJ, Binkley SN, and Wrighton SA. Interaction of human liver cytochromes P450 in vitro with LY307640, a gastric proton pump inhibitor. Pharmacogenetics 6:81–91 (1996).
188. Ko J-W, Sukhova N, Thacker D, Chen P, and Flockhart DA. Evaluation of omeprazole and lansoprazole as inhibitors of cytochrome P450 isoforms. Drug Metab Dispos 25:853–862 (1997).
189. Tucker GT. The interaction of proton pump inhibitors with cytochromes P450. Aliment Pharmacol Ther 8(Suppl 1):33–38 (1994).

190. Andersson T. Pharmacokinetics, metabolism and interactions of acid pump inhibitors: focus on omeprazole, lansoprazole and pantoprazole. Clin Pharmacokinet 31:9–28 (1996).
191. Gugler R and Jensen JC. Omeprazole inhibits oxidative drug metabolism. Gastroenterology 89:1235–1241 (1985).
192. Andersson T, Cederberg C, Edvardsson G, Heggelund A, and Lundborg P. Effect of omeprazole treatment on diazepam plasma levels in slow versus normal rapid metabolizers of omeprazole. Clin Pharmacol Ther 47:79–85 (1990).
193. Caraco Y, Tateishi T, and Wood AJJ. Interethnic difference in omeprazole's inhibition of diazepam metabolism. Clin Pharmacol Ther 58:62–72 (1995).
194. Lefebvre RA, Flouvat B, Karola-Tamisier S, Moerman E, and Van Ganse E. Influence of lansoprazole treatment on diazepam plasma concentrations. Clin Pharmacol Ther 52:458–463 (1992).
195. Gugler R, Hartmann M, Rudi J, Brod I, Huber R, Steinijans VW, et al. Lack of pharmacokinetic interaction of pantoprazole with diazepam in man. Br J Clin Pharmacol 42:249–252 (1996).
196. Venkatakrishnan K, von Moltke LL, and Greenblatt DJ. Effects of the antifungal agents on oxidative drug metabolism—clinical relevance. Clin Pharmacokinet 38:111–180 (2000).
197. Maurice M, Pichard L, Daujat M, Fabre I, Joyeux H, Domergue J, and Maurel P. Effects of imidazole derivatives on cytochromes P450 from human hepatocytes in primary culture. FASEB J 6:752–758 (1992).
198. von Moltke LL, Greenblatt DJ, Duan SX, Harmatz JS, and Shader RI. Inhibition of triazolam hydroxylation by ketoconazole, itraconazole, hydroxyitraconazole and fluconazole in vitro. Pharm Pharmacol Commun 4:443–445 (1998).
199. Jurima-Romet M, Crawford K, Cyr T, and Inaba T. Terfenadine metabolism in human liver: in vitro inhibition by macrolide antibiotics and azole antifungals. Drug Metab Dispos 22:849–857 (1994).
200. Back DJ, Tjia JF, Karbwang J, and Colbert J. *In vitro* inhibition studies of tolbutamide hydroxylase activity of human liver microsomes by azoles, sulphonamides and quinilines. Br J Clin Pharmacol 26:23–29 (1988).
201. Tassaneeyakul W, Birkett DJ, and Miners JO. Inhibition of human hepatic cytochrome P4502E1 by azole antifungals, CNS-active drugs and non-steroidal anti-inflammatory agents. Xenobiotica 28:293–301 (1998).
202. Greenblatt DJ, Wright CE, von Moltke LL, Harmatz JS, Ehrenberg BL, Harrel LM, et al. Ketoconazole inhibition of triazolam amd alprazolam clearance: differential kinetic and dynamic consequences. Clin Pharmacol Ther 64:237–247 (1998).
203. Schmider J, Brockmoller J, Arold G, Bauer S, and Roots I. Simultaneous assessment of CYP3A4 and CYP1A2 activity in vivo with alprazolam and caffeine. Pharmacogenetics 9:725–734 (1999).
204. Brown MW, Maldonado AL, Meredith CG, and Speeg KV. Effect of ketoconazole on hepatic oxidative metabolism. Clin Pharmacol Ther 37:290–297 (1985).
205. Olkkola KT, Backman JT, and Neuvonen PJ. Midazolam should be avoided in patients receiving the systemic antimycotics ketoconazole or itraconazole. Clin Pharmacol Ther 55:481–485 (1994).
206. Varhe A, Olkkola KT, and Neuvonen PJ. Oral triazolam is potentially hazardous to patients receiving systemic antimycotics ketoconazole or itraconazole. Clin Pharmacol Ther 56:601–607 (1994).
207. von Moltke LL, Greenblatt DJ, Harmatz JS, Duan SX, Harrel LM, Cotreau-Bibbo MM, et al. Triazolam biotransformation by human liver microsomes in vitro: effects of metabolic inhibitors and clinical confirmation of a predicted interaction with ketoconazole. J Pharmacol Exp Ther 276:370–379 (1996).

208. Olkkola KT, Ahonen J, and Neuvonen PJ. The effect of systemic antimycotics, itraconazole and fluconazole, on the pharmacokinetics and pharmacodynamics of intravenous and oral midazolam. Anesth Analges 82:511–516 (1996).
209. Ahonen J, Olkkola KT, and Neuvonen PJ. Effect of route of administration of fluconazole on the interaction between fluconazole and midazolam. Eur J Clin Pharmacol 51:415–419 (1997).
210. Varhe A, Olkkola KT, and Neuvonen PJ. Effect of fluconazole dose on the extent of fluconazole-triazolam interaction. Br J Clin Pharmacol 42:465–470 (1996).
211. Ohtani Y, Kotegawa T, Tsutsumi K, Morimoto T, Hirose Y, and Nakano S. Effect of fluconazole on the pharmacokinetics and pharmacodynamics of oral and rectal bromazepam: an application of electroencephalography as the pharmacodynamic method. J Clin Pharmacol 42:183–191 (2002).
212. Yasui N, Kondo T, Otani K, Furukori H, Kaneko S, Ohkubo T, Nagasaki T, and Sugawara K. Effect of itraconazole on the single oral dose pharmacokinetics and pharmacodynamics of alprazolam. Psychopharmacology 139:269–273 (1998).
213. Ahonen J, Olkkola KT, and Neuvonen PJ. The effect of the antimycotic itraconazole on the pharmacokinetics and pharmacodynamics of diazepam. Fund Clin Pharmacol 10:314–318 (1996).
214. Ahonen J, Olkkola KT, and Neuvonen PJ. Effect of itraconazole and terbinafine on the pharmacokinetics and pharmacodynamics of midazolam in healthy volunteers. Br J Clin Pharmacol 40:270–272 (1995).
215. Neuvonen PJ, Varhe A, and Olkkola KT. The effect of ingestion time interval on the interaction betwen itraconazole and triazolam. Clin Pharmacol Ther 60:326–331 (1996).
216. Blyden GT, Scavone JM, and Greenblatt DJ. Metronidazole impairs clearance of phenytoin but not of alprazolam or lorazepam. J Clin Pharmacol 28:240–245 (1988).
217. Jensen JC and Gugler R. Interaction between metronidazole and drugs eliminated by oxidative metabolism. Clin Pharmacol Ther 37:407–410 (1985).
218. Wang JS, Backman JT, Kivisto KT, and Neuvonen PJ. Effects of metronidazole on midazolam metabolism in vitro and in vivo. Eur J Clin Pharmacol 56:555–559 (2000).
219. Varhe A, Olkkola KT, and Neuvonen PJ. Fluconazole, but not terbinafine, enhances the effects of triazolam by inhibiting its metabolism. Br J Clin Pharmacol 41:319–323 (1996).
220. Crewe HK, Lennard MS, Tucker GT, Woods FR, and Haddock RE. The effect of selective serotonin re-uptake inhibitors on Cytochrome P4502D6 (CYP2D6) activity in human liver microsomes. Br J Clin Pharmacol 34:262–265 (1992).
221. Otton SV, Ball SE, Cheung SW, Inaba T, Rudolph RL, and Sellers EM. Venlafaxine oxidation in vitro is catalysed by CYP2D6. Br J Clin Pharmacol 41:149–156 (1996).
222. Schmider J, Greenblatt DJ, von Moltke LL, Harmatz JS, and Shader RI. Inhibition of cytochrome P450 by nefazodone in vitro: studies of dextromethorphan O- and N-demethylation. Br J Clin Pharmacol 41:339–343 (1996).
223. Brosen K and Naranjo CA. Review of the pharmacokinetic and pharmacodynamic interaction studies with citalopram. Eur Neuropsychopharmacol 11:275–283 (2001).
224. Schmider J, Greenblatt DJ, von Moltke LL, Karsov D, and Shader RI. Inhibition of CYP2C9 by selective serotonin reuptake inhibitors in vitro: studies of phenytoin p-hydroxylation. Br J Clin Pharmacol 44:495–498 (1997).
225. Lasher TA, Fleishaker JC, Steenwyk RC, and Antal EJ. Pharmacokinetic pharmacodynamic evaluation of the combined administration of alprazolam and fluoxetine. Psychopharmacology 104:323–327 (1991).
226. Greenblatt DJ, Preskorn SH, Cotreau MM, Horst WD, and Harmatz JS. Fluoxetine impairs clearance of alprazolam but not of clonazepam. Clin Pharmacol Ther 52:479–486 (1992).

227. Lemberger L, Rowe H, Bosomworth JC, Tenbarge JB, and Bergstrom RF. The effect of fluoxetine on the pharmacokinetics and psychomotor responses of diazepam. Clin Pharmacol Ther 43:412–419 (1988).
228. Wright CE, Lasher-Sisson TA, Steenwyk RC, and Swanson CN. A pharmacokinetic evaluation of the combined administration of triazolam and fluoxetine. Pharmacotherapy 12:103–106 (1992).
229. Perucca E, Gatti G, Cipolla G, Spina E, Barel S, Soback S, et al. Inhibition of diazepam metabolism by fluvoxamine: a pharmacokinetic study in normal volunteers. Clin Pharmacol Ther 56:471–476 (1994).
230. Kashuba ADM, Nafziger AN, Kearns GL, Leeder JS, Gotschall R, Rocci ML, et al. Effect of fluvoxamine therapy on the activities of CYP1A2, CYP2D6, and CYP3A as determined by phenotyping. Clin Pharmacol Ther 64:257–268 (1998).
231. Kroboth PD, Folan MM, Lush RM, Chaikin PC, Shukla UA, Barbhaiya R, and Salazar DE. Coadministration of nefazodone and benzodiazepines: I. Pharmacodynamic assessment. J Clin Psychopharmacol 15:306–319 (1995).
232. Greene DS, Salazar DE, Dockens RC, Kroboth PD, and Barbhaiya RH. Coadministration of nefazodone and benzodiazepines: III. A pharmacokinetic interaction study with alprazolam. J Clin Psychopharmacol 15:399–408 (1995).
233. Barbhaiya RM, Shukla UA, Kroboth PD, and Greene DS. Coadministration of nefazodone and benzodiazepines: II. A pharmacokinetic interaction study with triazolam. J Clin Psychopharmacol 15:320–326 (1995).
234. Greene DS, Salazar DE, Dockens RC, Kroboth PD, and Barbhaiya RH. Coadministration of nefazodone and benzodiazepines: IV. A pharmacokinetic interaction study with lorazepam. J Clin Psychopharmacol 15:409–416 (1995).
235. Bonate PL, Kroboth PD, Smith RB, Suarez E, and Oo C. Clonazepam and sertraline: absence of drug interaction in a multiple-dose study. J Clin Psychopharmacol 20:19–27 (2000).
236. Gardner MJ, Baris BA, Wilner KD, and Preskorn SH. Effect of sertraline on the pharmacokinetics and protein binding of diazepam in healthy volunteers. Clin Pharmacokinet 32 (Suppl 1):43–49 (1997).
237. Amchin J, Zarycranski W, Taylor KP, Albano D, and Klockowski PM. Effect of venlafaxine on the pharmacokinetics of alprazolam. Psychopharmacology Bull 34:211–219 (1998).
238. Troy SM, Lucki I, Peirgies AA, Parker VD, Klockowski PM, and Chiang ST. Pharmacokinetic and pharmacodynamic evaluation of the potential drug interaction between venlafaxine and diazepam. J Clin Pharmacol 35:410–419 (1995).
239. Shenfield GM and Griffin JM. Clinical pharmacokinetics of contraceptive steroids: an update. Clin Pharmacokinet 20:15–37 (1991).
240. Guengerich FP. Oxidation of 17α-ethynylestradiol by human liver cytochrome P-450. Mol Pharmacol 33:500–508 (1988).
241. Back DJ, Houlgrave R, Tjia JF, Ward S, and Orme MLE. Effect of the progestogens, gestodene, 3-keto desogestral, levonorgestrel, norethisterone and norgestimate on the oxidation of ethyloestradiol and other substrates by human liver microsomes. J Ster Biochem Mol Biol 38:219–225 (1991).
242. Stoehr GP, Kroboth PD, Juhl RP, Wender DB, Phillips JP, and Smith RB. Effect of oral contraceptives on triazolam, temazepam, alprazolam, and lorazepam kinetics. Clin Pharmacol Ther 36:683–690 (1984).
243. Roberts RK, Desmond PV, Wilkinson GR, and Schenker S. Disposition of chlordiazepoxide: sex differences and effects of oral contraceptives. Clin Pharmacol Ther 25:826–831 (1979).
244. Patwardhan RV, Mitchell MC, Johnson RF, and Schenker S. Differential effects of oral contraceptive steroids on the metabolism of benzodiazepines. Hepatology 3:248–253 (1983).

245. Giles HG, Sellers EM, Naranjo CA, Frecker RC, and Greenblatt DJ. Disposition of intravenous diazepam in young men and women. Eur J Clin Pharmacol 20:207–213 (1981).
246. Abernethy DR, Greenblatt DJ, Divoll M, Arendt R, Ochs HR, and Shader RI. Impairment of diazepam metabolism by low-dose estrogen containing oral contraceptive steroids. N Engl J Med 306:791–792 (1982).
247. Palovaara S, Kivisto KT, Tapanainen P, Manninen P, Neuvonen PJ, and Laine K. Effect of an oral contraceptive preparation containing ethinylestradiol and gestodene on CYP3A4 activity as measured by midazolam 1'-hydroxylation. Brit J Clin Pharmacol 50:333–337 (2000).
248. Jochemsen R, Van der Graaff M, Boeijinga JK, and Breimer DD. Influence of sex, menstrual cycle and oral contraception on the disposition of nitrazepam. Br J Clin Pharmacol 13:319–324 (1982).
249. Scavone JM, Greenblatt DJ, Locniskar A, and Shader RI. Alprazolam pharmacokinetics in women on low-dose oral contraceptives. J Clin Pharmacol 28:454–457 (1988).
250. Holazo AA, Winkler MB, and Patel IH. Effects of age, gender and oral contraceptives on intramuscular midazolam pharmacokinetics. J Clin Pharmacol 28:1040–1045 (1988).
251. Belle DJ, Callaghan JT, Gorski JC, Maya JF, Mousa O, Wrighton SA, and Hall SD. The effects of an oral contraceptive containing ethinyloestradiol and norgestrel on CYP3A activity. Br J Clin Pharmacol 53:67–74 (2002).
252. Abernethy DR, Greenblatt DJ, Ochs HR, Weyers D, Divoll M, Harmatz JS, and Shader RI. Lorazepam and oxazepam kinetics in women on low-dose oral contraceptives. Clin Pharmacol Ther 33:628–632 (1983).
253. Gorski JC, Wang ZQ, Heahner-Daniels BD, Wrighton SA, and Hall SD. The effect of hormone replacement therapy on CYP3A activity. Clin Pharmacol Ther 68:412–417 (2000).
254. Kroboth PD, Smith RB, Stoehr GP, and Juhl RP. Pharmacodynamic evaluation of the benzodiazepine-oral contraceptive interaction. Clin Pharmacol Ther 38:525–532 (1985).
255. Kroboth PD and McAuley JW. Progesterone: does it affect response to drug. Psychopharmacology Bull 33:297–301 (1997).
256. Pichard L, Fabre I, Domergue J, Saint Aubert B, Mourad G, and Maurel P. Cyclosporin A drug interactions: screening for inducers and inhibitors of cytochrome P-450 (cyclosporin A oxidase) in primary cultures of human hepatocytes and in liver microsomes. Drug Metab Dispos 18:595–606 (1990).
257. Jawad S and Richens A. Single dose pharmacokinetic study of clobazam in normal volunteers and epileptic patients. Br J Clin Pharmacol 18:873–877 (1984).
258. Dhillon S. Pharmacokinetics of diazepam in epileptic patients and normal volunteers following intravenous administration. Br J Clin Pharmacol 12:841–844 (1981).
259. Backman JT, Olkkola KT, Ojala M, Laaksovirta H, and Neuvonen PJ. Concentrations and effects of oral midazolam are greatly reduced in patients treated with carbamazepine or phenytoin. Epilepsia 37:253–257 (1996).
260. Contin M, Riva R, Albani F, and Baruzzi A. Effect of felbamate on clobazam and its metabolite kinetics in patients with epilepsy. Ther Drug Monit 21:604–608 (1999).
261. Wilensky AJ, Levy RH, Troupin AS, Moretti-Ojemann L, and Friel P. Clorazepate kinetics in treated epileptics. Clin Pharmacol Ther 24:22–30 (1978).
262. Furukori H, Otani K, Yasui N, Kondo T, Kaneko S, Shimoyama R, et al. Effect of carbamazepine on the single oral dose pharmacokinetics of alprazolam. Neuropsychopharmacology 18:364–369 (1998).
263. Levy RH, Lane EA, Guyot M, Brachet-Liermain A, Cenraud B, and Loiseau P. Analysis of parent drug-metabolite relationship in the presence of an inducer: application to the carbamazepine-clobazam interaction in normal man. Drug Metab Dispos 11:286–292 (1983).

264. Lai AA, Levy RH, and Cutler RE. Time-course of interaction between carbamazepine and clonazepam in normal man. Clin Pharmacol Ther 24:316–323 (1978).
265. Arana GW, Epstein S, Molloy M, and Greenblatt DJ. Carbamazepine-induced reduction of plasma alprazolam concentrations: a clinical case report. J Clin Psychiatry 49:448–449 (1988).
266. Dhillon S and Richens A. Serum protein binding of diazepam and its displacement by valproic acid in vitor. Br J Clin Pharmacol 12:591–592 (1981).
267. Dhillon S and Richens A. Valproic acid and diazepam interactions in vivo. Br J Clin Pharmacol 13:553–560 (1982).
268. Anderson GD, Gidal BE, Kantor ED, and Wilensky AJ. Lorazepam-valproate interaction: studies in normal subjects and in isolated perfused rat liver. Epilepsia 35:221–225 (1994).
269. Samara EE, Granneman RG, Witt GF, and Cavanaugh JH. Effect of valproate on the pharmacokinetics and pharmacodynamics of lorazepam. J Clin Pharmacol 37:442–450 (1997).
270. Tija JF, Back DJ, and Breckenridge AM. Calcium channel antagonists and cyclosporin metabolism: in vitro studies with human liver microsomes. Br J Clin Pharmacol 28:362–365 (1989).
271. Sutton D, Butler AM, Nadin L, and Murray M. Role of CYP3A4 in human hepatic diltiazem N-demethylation: inhibition of CYP3A4 activity by oxidized diltiazem metabolites. J Pharmacol Exp Ther 282:294–300 (1997).
272. Ma B, Prueksaritanont T, and Lin JH. Drug interactions with calcium channel blockers: possible involvement of metabolite-intermediate complexation with CYP3A. Drug Metab Dispos 28:125–130 (2000).
273. Shaw L, Lennard MS, Tucker GT, Bax NDS, and Woods HF. Irreversible binding and metabolism of propranolol by human liver microsomes—relationship to polymorphic oxidation. Biochem Pharmacol 36:2283–2288 (1987).
274. Ochs HR, Greenblatt DJ, and Verburg-Ochs B. Propranolol interactions with diazepam, lorazepam, and alprazolam. Clin Pharmacol Ther 36:451–455 (1984).
275. Hawksworth GM, Betts T, Crowe A, Knight R, Nyemitei-Addo I, Parry K, et al. Diazepam /β-adrenoceptor antagonist interactions. Br J Clin Pharmacol 17:69S–76S (1984).
276. Sonne J, Dossing M, Loft S, Olesen KL, Vollmer-Larsen A, Victor MA, et al. Single dose pharmacokinetics and pharmacodynamics of oral oxazepam during concomitant administration of propranolol and labetalol. Br J Clin Pharmacol 29:33–37 (1990).
277. Scott AK, Cameron GA, and Hawksworth GM. Interaction of metoprolol with lorazepam and bromazepam. Eur J Clin Pharmacol 40:405–409 (1991).
278. Klotz U and Reimann IW. Pharmacokineitc and pharmacodynamic interaction study of diazepam and metoprolol. Eur J Clin Pharmacol 26:223–226 (1984).
279. Ahonen J, Olkkola KT, Salmenpera M, Hynynen M, and Neuvonen PJ. Effect of diltiazem on midazolam and alfentanil disposition in patients undergoing coronary artery bypass grafting. Anesthesia 85:1246–1252 (1996).
280. Backman JT, Olkkola KT, Aranko K, Himberg J-J, and Neuvonen PJ. Dose of midazolam should be reduced during diltiazem and verapamil treatments. Br J Clin Pharmacol 37: 221–225 (1994).
281. Varhe A, Olkkola KT, and Neuvonen PJ. Diltiazem enhances the effects of triazolam by inhibiting its metabolism. Clin Pharmacol Ther 59:369–375 (1996).
282. Kosuge K, Nishimoto M, Kimura M, Umemura K, Nakashima M, and Ohashi K. Enhanced effect of triazolam with diltiazem. Br J Clin Pharmacol 43:367–372 (1997).
283. Backman JT, Wang J-S, Wen X, Kivisto KT, and Neuvonen PJ. Mibefradil but not isradipine substantially elevates the plasma concentrations of the CYP3A4 substrate triazolam. Clin Pharmacol Ther 66:401–407 (1999).

284. Venkatesan K. Pharmacokinetic drug interactions with rifampicin. Clin Pharmacokinet 22:47–65 (1992).
285. Westphal JF. Macrolide-induced clinically relevant drug interactions with cytochrome P-450A (CYP) 3A4: an update focused on clarithromycin, azithromycin and dirithromycin. Brit. J Clin Pharmacol 50:285–295 (2000).
286. Yamazaki H and Shimada T. Comparative studies of in vitro inhibition of cytochrome P450 3A4-dependent testosterone 6β-hydroxylation by roxithromycin and its metabolites, troleandomycin, and erythromycin. Drug Metab Dispos 26:1053–1057 (1998).
287. Zhao XJ, Koyama E, and Ishizaki T. An in vitro study on the metabolism and possible drug interactions of rokitamycin, a macrolide antibiotic, using human liver microsomes. Drug Metab Dispos 27:776–785 (1999).
288. Lindstrom TD, Hanssen BR, and Wrighton SA. Cytochrome P-450 complex formation by dirithromycin and other macrolides in rat and human livers. Antimicrob Agents Chemother 37:265–269 (1993).
289. Marre F, de Sousa G, Orloff AM, and Rahmani R. In vitro interaction between cyclosporin A and macrolide antibiotics. Br J Clin Pharmacol 35:447–448 (1993).
290. Greenblatt DJ, von Moltke LL, Harmatz JS, Counihan M, Graf JA, Durol ALB, et al. Inhibition of triazolam clearance by macrolide antimicrobial agents: in vitro correlates and dynamic consequences. Clin Pharmacol Ther 64:278–285 (1998).
291. Wen X, Wang J-S, Neuvonen PJ, and Backman JT. Isoniazid is a mechanism-based inhibitor of P_{450} 1A2, 2A6, 2C19 and 3A4 isoforms in human liver microsomes. Eur J Clin Pharmacol 57:799–804 (2002).
292. Edwards DJ, Bowles SK, Svensson CK, and Rybak MJ. Inhibition of drug metabolism by quinolone antibiotics. Clin Pharmacokinet 15:194–204 (1988).
293. Fuhr U, Wolff T, Harder S, Schymanski P, and Staib AH. Quinolone inhibition of cytochrome P-450-dependent caffeine metabolism in human liver microsomes. Drug Metab Disposit 18:1005–1010 (1990).
294. Sarkar M, Polk RE, Guzelian PS, Hunt C, and Karnes HT. In vitro effect of fluoroquinolones on theophylline metabolism in human liver microsomes. Antimicrob Agents Chemother 34:594–599 (1990).
295. Ochs HR, Greenblatt DJ, Roberts GM, and Dengler HJ. Diazepam interaction with antituberculous drugs. Clin Pharmacol Ther 29:671–678 (1981).
296. Ohnhaus EE, Brockmeyer N, Dylewicz P, and Habicht H. The effect of antipyrine and rifampin on the metabolism of diazepam. Clin Pharmacol Ther 42:148–156 (1987).
297. Ochs HR, Greenblatt DJ, and Knuchel M. Differential effect of isoniazid on triazolam oxidation and oxazepam conjugation. Br J Clin Pharmacol 16:743–746 (1983).
298. Backman JT, Olkkola KT, and Neuvonen PJ. Rifampin drastically reduces plasma concentrations and effects of oral midazolam. Clin Pharmacol Ther 59:7–13 (1996).
299. Backman JT, Kivisto KT, Olkkola KT, and Neuvonen PJ. The area under the plasma concentration-time curve for oral midazolam is 400-fold larger during treatment with itraconazole than with rifampicin. Eur J Clin Pharmacol 54:53–58 (1998).
300. Brockmeyer NH, Mertins L, Klimek K, Goos M, and Ohnhaus EE. Comparative effects of rifampin and/or probenecid on the pharmacokinetics of temazepam and nitrazepam. Int J Clin Pharmacol Ther Toxicol 28:387–393 (1990).
301. Villikka K, Kivisto KT, Backman JT, Olkkola KT, and Neuvonen PJ. Triazolam is ineffective in patients taking rifampin. Clin Pharmacol Ther 61:8–14 (1997).
302. Yasui N, Otani K, Kaneko S, Ohkubo T, Osanai T, Sugawara K, et al. A kinetic and dynamic study of oral alprazolam with and without erythromycin in humans: in vivo evidence for the involvement of CYP3A4 in alprazolam metabolism. Clin Pharmacol Ther 59:514–519 (1996).

303. Luurila H, Olkkola KT, and Neuvonen PJ. Interaction between erythromycin and the benzodiazepines diazepam and flunitrazepam. Pharmacol Toxicol 78:117–122 (1996).
304. Vanakoski J, Mattila MJ, Vainio P, Idanpaan-Heikkila JJ, and Tornwall M. 150 mg fluconazole does not substantially increase the effects of 10 mg midazolam or the plasma midazolam concentrations in healthy subjects. Int J Clin Pharmacol Ther Toxicol 33:518–523 (1995).
305. Olkkola KT, Aranko K, Luurila H, Hiller A, Saarnivaara L, Himberg J-J, and Neuvonen PJ. A potentially hazardous interaction between erythromycin and midazolam. Clin Pharmacol Ther 53:298–305 (1993).
306. Zimmermann T, Yeates RA, Laufen H, Scharpf F, Leitold M, and Wildfeuer A. Influence of the antibiotics erythromycin and azithromycin on the pharmacokinetics and pharmacodynamics of midazolam. Arsch-Forsch Drug Metab 46:213–217 (1996).
307. Phillips JP, Antal EJ, and Smith RB. A pharmacokinetic drug interaction between erythromycin and triazolam. J Clin Psychopharmacol 6:297–299 (1986).
308. Luurila H, Olkkola KT, and Neuvonen PJ. Lack of interaction of erythromycin with temazepam. Ther Drug Monit 16:548–551 (1994).
309. Warot D, Bergougnan L, Lamiable D, Berlin I, Benison G, Danjou P, and Puech AJ. Troleandomycin-triazolam interaction in healthy volunteers: pharmacokinetic and psychometric evaluation. Eur J Clin Pharmacol 32:389–393 (1987).
310. Backman JT, Aranko K, Himberg J-J, and Olkkola KT. A pharmacokinetic interaction between roxithromycin and midazolam. Eur J Clin Pharmacol 46:551–555 (1994).
311. Kamali F, Thomas SHL, and Edwards C. The influence of steady-state ciprofloxacin on the pharmacokinetics and pharmacodynamics of a single dose of diazepam. Eur J Clin Pharmacol 44:365–367 (1993).
312. Wijnands WJA, Trooster JFG, Teunissen PC, Cats HA, and Vree TB. Ciprofloxacin does not impair the elimination of diazepam in humans. Drug Metab Dispos 18:954–957 (1990).
313. Barry M, Mulcahy F, Merry C, Gibbons S, and Back D. Pharmacokinetics and potential interactions amongst antiretroviral agents used to treat patients with HIV infection. Clin Pharmacokinet 36:289–304 (1999).
314. Li XL and Chan WK. Transport, metabolism and elimination mechanisms of anti-HIV agents. Advan Drug Delivery Rev 39:81–103 (1999).
315. Tseng AL and Foisy MM. Significant interactions with new antiretrovirals and psychotic drugs. Ann Pharmacother 33:461–473 (1999).
316. Eagling VA, Back DJ, and Barry MG. Differential inhibition of cytochrome P450 isoforms by the protease inhibitors, ritonavir, saquinavir and indinavir. Br J Clin Pharmacol 44:190–194 (1997).
317. Inaba T, Fischer NE, Riddick DS, Stewart DJ, and Hidaka T. HIV protease inhibitors, saquinavir, indinavir and ritonavir: inhibition of CYP3A4-mediated metabolism of testosterone and benzoxazinorifamycin, KRM-1648, in human liver microsomes. Toxicol Lett 93:215–219 (1997).
318. Lillibridge JH, Liang BH, Kerr BM, Webber S, Quart B, Shetty BV, and Lee CA. Characterization of the selectivity and mechanism of human cytochrome P450 inhibition by the human immunodeficiency virus-protease inhibitor nelfinavir mesylate. Drug Metab Dispos 26:609–616 (1998).
319. von Moltke LL, Greenblatt DJ, Grassi JM, Granda BW, Duan SX, Fogelman SM, et al. Protease inhibitors as inhibitors of human cytochromes P450: high risk associated with ritonavir. J Clin Pharmacol 38:106–111 (1998).
320. Decker CJ, Laitinen LM, Bridson GW, Raybuck SA, Tung RD, and Chaturvedi PR. Metabolism of amprenavir in liver microsomes: role of CYP3A4 inhibition for drug interactions. J Pharm Sci 87:803–807 (1998).

321. Zalma A, von Moltke LL, Granda BW, Harmatz JS, Shader RI, and Greenblatt DJ. In vitro metabolism of trazodone by CYP3A: inhibition by ketoconazole and human immunodeficiency viral protease inhibitors. Biol Psychiat 47:655–661 (2000).
322. von Moltke LL, Greenblatt DJ, Granda BW, Giancarlo GM, Duan SX, Daily JP, et al. Inhibition of human cytochrome P450 isoforms by nonnucleoside reverse transcriptase inhibitors. J Clin Pharmacol 41:85–91 (2001).
323. Greenblatt DJ, von Moltke LL, Harmatz JS, Durol ALB, Daily JP, Graf JA, et al. Differential impairment of triazolam and zolpidem clearance by ritonavir. J Acq Immune Defic Syndr 24:129–136 (2000).
324. Greenblatt DJ, von Moltke LL, Harmatz JS, Durol ALB, Daily JP, Graf JA, et al. Alprazolam-ritonavir interaction: implications for product labeling. Clin Pharmacol Ther 67:335–341 (2000).
325. Palkama VJ, Ahonen J, Neuvonen PJ, and Olkkola KT. Effect of saquinavir on the pharmacokinetics and pharmacodynamics of oral and intravenoud midazolam. Clin Pharmacol Ther 66:33–39 (1999).
326. Bailey DG, Spence JD, Munoz C, and Arnold JMO. Interaction of citrus juices with felodipine and nifedipine. Lancet 337:268–269 (1991).
327. Watkins PB, Wrighton SA, Schuetz EG, Molowa DT, and Guzelian PS. Identification of glucocortisol-inducible cytochrome P-450 in the intestinal mucosa of rats and man. J Clin Invest 80:1029–1036 (1987).
328. Kolars JC, Schmiedlin-Ren P, Schuetz JD, Fang C, and Watkins PB. Identification of rifampin-inducible P450IIIA4 (CYP3A4) in human small bowel enterocytes. J Clin Invest 90:1871–1878 (1992).
329. Bailey DG, Malcolm J, Arnold O, and Spence JD. Grapefruit juice-drug interactions. Br J Clin Pharmacol 46:101–110 (1998).
330. Greenblatt DJ, Patki KC, von Moltke LL, and Shader RI. Drug interactions with grapefruit juice: an update. J Clin Psychopharmacol 21:357–359 (2001).
331. Lown KS, Bailey DG, Fontana RJ, Janardan SK, Adair CH, Fortlage LA, et al. Grapefruit juice increases felodipine oral bioavailability in humans by decreasing intestinal CYP 3A protein expression. J Clin Invest 99:1–9 (1997).
332. Schmiedlin-Ren P, Edwards DJ, Fitzsimmons ME, He K, Lown KS, Woster PM, et al. Mechanisms of enhanced oral availability of CYP3A substrates by grapefruit constituents: decreased enterocyte CYP3A4 concentration and mechanism-based inactivation by furanocoumarins. Drug Metab Dispos 25:1228–1233 (1997).
333. Guengerich FP and Kim D-H. In vitro inhibition of dihydropyridine oxidation and aflatoxin B_1 activation in human liver microsomes by naringenin and other flavonoids. Carcinogenesis 11:2275–2279 (1990).
334. Miniscalco A, Lundahl J, Regardh CG, Edgar B, and Eriksson UG. Inhibition of dihydropyridine metabolism in rat and human liver microsomes by flavonoids found in grapefruit juice. J Pharmacol Exp Ther 261:1195–1199 (1991).
335. Ha HR, Chen J, Leuenberger PM, Freiburghaus AU, and Follath F. In vitro inhibition of midazolam and quinidine metabolism by flavonoids. Eur J Clin Pharmacol 48:367–371 (1995).
336. Schubert W, Eriksson U, Edgar B, Cullberg G, and Hedner T. Flavonoids in grapefruit juice inhibit the in vitro hepatic metabolism of 17 beta-estradiol. Eur J Drug Metab Pharmacokinet 20:219–224 (1995).
337. Eagling VA, Profit L, and Back DJ. Inhibition of the CYP3A4-mediated metabolism and P-glycoprotein-mediated transport of the HIV-I protease inhibitor saquinavir by grapefruit juice components. Br J Clin Pharmacol 48:543–552 (1999).

338. Rashid J, McKinstry C, Renwick AG, Dirnhuber M, Waller DG, and George CF. Quercetin, an *in vitro* inhibitor of CYP3A, does not contribute to the interaction between nifedipine and grapefruit juice. Br J Clin Pharmacol 36:460–463 (1993).
339. Bailey DG, Arnold JMO, Munoz C, and Spence JD. Grapefruit juice-felodipine interaction—mechanism, predictability, and effect of naringin. Clin Pharmacol Ther 53:637–642 (1993).
340. Edwards DJ, Bellevue FH, and Woster PM. Identification of 6',7'-dihydroxybergamottin, a cytochrome P-450 inhibitor in grapefruit juice. Drug Metab Dispos 24:1287–1290 (1996).
341. Fukuda K, Ohta T, and Yamazoe Y. Grapefruit component interacting with rat and human P450 CYP3A: possible involvement of non-flavonoid components in drug interaction. Biol Pharm Bull 20:560–564 (1997).
342. Fukuda K, Ohta T, Oshima Y, Ohashi N, Yoshikawa M, and Yamazoe Y. Specific CYP3A4 inhibitors in grapefruit juice: furocoumarins dimers as components of drug interaction. Pharmacogenetics 7:391–396 (1997).
343. Guo L-Q, Fukuda K, Ohta T, and Yamazoe Y. Role of furanocoumarin derivatives on grapefruit juice-mediated inhibition of human CYP3A activity. Drug Metab Dispos 28:766–771 (2000).
344. He K, Iyer KR, Hayes RN, Sinz MW, Woolf TF, and Hollenberg PF. Inactivation of cytochrome P450 3A4 by bergamottin, a component of grapefruit juice. Chem Res Toxicol 11:252–259 (1998).
345. Fuhr U, Klittich K, and Staib AH. Inhibitory effect of grapefruit juice and its bitter principal, naringenin, on CYP1A2 dependent metabolism of caffeine in man. Br J Clin Pharmacol 35:431–436 (1993).
346. Edwards DJ, Fitzsimmons ME, Schuetz EG, Yasuda K, Ducharme MP, Warbasse LH, et al. 6',7'-Dihydroxybergamottin in grapefruit juice and Seville orange juice: effects on cyclosporine disposition, enterocyte CYP3A4, and P-glycoprotein. Clin Pharmacol Ther 65:237–244 (1999).
347. Soldner A, Christians U, Susanto M, Wacher VJ, Silverman JA, and Benet LZ. Grapefruit juice activates P-glycoprotein-mediated drug transport. Pharm Res 16:478–485 (1999).
348. Kupersmchmidt HHT, Ha HR, Ziegler WH, Meier PJ, and Krahenbuhl S. Interaction between grapefruit juice and midazolam in humans. Clin Pharmacol Ther 58:20–28 (1995).
349. Andersen V, Pedersen N, Larsen N-E, Sonne J, and Larsen S. Intestinal first pass metabolism of midazolam in kiver cirrhosis—effect of grapefruit juice. Br J Clin Pharmacol 54:120–124 (2002).
350. Hukkinen SK, Varhe A, Olkkola KT, and Neuvonen PJ. Plasma concentrations of triazolam are increased by concomitant ingestion of grapefruit juice. Clin Pharmacol Ther 58:127–131 (1995).
351. Yasui N, Kondo T, Furukori H, Kaneko S, Ohkubo T, Uno T, et al. Effects of repeated ingestion of grapefruit juice on the single and multiple oral-dose pharmacokinetics and pharmacodynamics of alprazolam. Psychopharmacology 150:185–190 (2000).
352. Vanakoski J, Mattila MJ, and Seppala T. Grapefruit juice does not enhance the effects of midazolam and triazolam in man. Eur J Clin Pharmacol 50:501–508 (1996).
353. Backman JT, Maenpaa J, Belle DJ, Wrighton SA, Kivisto KT, and Neuvonen PJ. Lack of correlation between in vitro and in vivo studies on the effects of tangeretin and tangerine juice on midazolam hydroxylation. Clin Pharmacol Ther 67:382–390 (2000).
354. Henauer SA, Hollister LE, Gillespie HK, and Moore F. Theophylline antagonizes diazepam-induced psychomotor impairment. Eur J Clin Pharmacol 25:743–747 (1983).
355. Tuncok Y, Akpinar O, Guven H, and Akkoclu A. The effects of theophylline on serum alprazolam levels. Int J Clin Pharmacol Ther 32:642–645 (1994).

356. Ghoneim MM, Hinrichs JV, Chiang C-K, and Loke WH. Pharmacokinetic and pharmacodynamic interations between caffeine and diazepam. J Clin Psychopharmacol 6:75–80 (1986).
357. Ohnhaus EE, Park BK, Colombo JP, and Heizmann P. The effect of enzyme induction on diazepam metabolism in man. Br J Clin Pharmacol 8:557–563 (1979).
358. MacLeod SM, Sellers EM, Giles HG, Billings BJ, Martin PR, Greenblatt DJ, and Marshman JA. Interaction of disulfiram with benzodiazepines. Clin Pharmacol Ther 24:583–589 (1978).
359. Diquet B, Gujadhur L, Lamiable D, Warot D, Hayoun H, and Choisy H. Lack of interaction between disulfiram and alprazolam. Eur J Clin Pharmacol 38:157–160 (1990).
360. Nakajima M, Suzuki T, Sasaki T, Yokoi T, Hosoyamada A, Yamamoto T, and Kuroiwa Y. Effects of chronic administration of glucocorticoid on midazolam pharmacokinetics in humans. Ther Drug Monit 21:507–513 (1999).
361. Villikka K, Kivisto KT, and Neuvonen PJ. The effect of dexamethasone on the pharmacokinetics of triazolam. Pharmacol Toxicol 83:135–138 (1998).
362. Mulley BA, Potter BI, Rye RM, and Takeshita K. Interactions between diazepam and paracetamol. J Clin Pharmacy 3:25–35 (1978).
363. Abernethy DR, Greenblatt DJ, Ameer B, and Shader RI. Probenecid impairment of acetaminophen and lorazepam clearance: direct inhibition of ether glucuronide formation. J Pharmacol Exp Ther 234:345–349 (1985).
364. Golden PL, Warner PE, Fleishaker JC, Jewell RC, Millikin S, Lyon J, and Brouwer KLR. Effects of probenecid on the pharmacokinetics and pharmacodynamics of adinazolam in humans. Clin Pharmacol Ther 56:133–141 (1994).
365. Robertson P, Decory HH, Madan A, and Parkinson A. In vitro inhibition and induction of human hepatic cytochrome P450 enzymes by modafinil. Drug Metab Dispos 28:664–671 (2000).
366. Robertson P, Hellriegel ET, Arora S, and Nelson M. Effect of modafinal on the pharmacokinetics of ethinyl estradiol and triazolam in healthy volunteers. Clin Pharmacol Ther 71:46–56 (2002).
367. Gurley BJ, Gardner SF, Hubbard MA, Williams DK, Gentry WB, Cui Y, and Ang CYW. Cytochrome P450 phenotype ratios for predicting herb–drug interactions in humans. Clin Pharmacol Ther 72:276–287 (2002).
368. Klee H, Faugier J, Hayes C, Boulton T, and Morris J. AIDS-related risk behavior, polydrug use and temazepam. Br J Addict 85:1125–1132 (1990).
369. Navaratnam V and Foong K. Adjunctive drug use among opiate addicts. Curr Med Res Opin 11:611–619 (1990).
370. Metzger D, Woody G, De Philippis D, McLellan AT, O'Brien CP, and Platt JJ. Risk factors for needle sharing among methadone-treated patients. Am J Psychiatry 148:636–640 (1991).
371. Darke S, Hall W, Ross M, and Wodak A. Benzodiazepine use and HIV risk-taking behaviour among injecting drug users. Drug Alcohol Depend 31:31–36 (1992).
372. Barnas C, Rossmann M, Roessler H, Riemer Y, and Fleishchhacker WW. Benzodiazepines and other psychotropic drugs abused by patients in a methadone maintenance program: familiarity and preferance. J Clin Psychopharmacol 12:397–402 (1992).
373. Hall W, Bell J, and Carless J. Crime and drug use among applicants for methadone maintenance. Drug Alcohol Depend 31:123–129 (1993).
374. San L, Tato J, Torrens M, Castillo C, Farre M, and Cami J. Flunitrazepam consumption among heroin addicts admitted for in-patient detoxification. Drug Alcohol Depend 32:281–286 (1993).
375. Darke S, Swift W, Hall W, and Ross M. Drug use, HIV risk-taking and psychosocial correlates of benzodiazepine use among methadone maintenance clients. Drug Alcohol Depend 34:67–70 (1993).

376. Strang J, Griffiths P, Abbey J, and Gossop M. Survey of injected benzodiazepines among drug users in Britain. BMJ 308:1082 (1994).
377. Garriott JC, DiMaio VJM, Zumwalt RE, and Petty CS. Incidence of drugs and alcohol in fatally injured motor vehicle drivers. J Forensic Sci 22:383–389 (1977).
378. Warren R, Simpson H, Hilchie J, Cimbura G, Lucas D, and Bennett R. Drugs detected in fatally injured drivers in the province of Ontario. Alcohol Drugs Traffic Safety 1:203–217 (1980).
379. Fortenberry JC, Brown DB, and Shelvin LT. Analysis of drug involvement in traffic fatalities in Alabama. Am J Drug Alcohol Abuse 12:257–267 (1986).
380. McLean S, Parsons RS, Chesterman RB, Johnson MG, and Davies NW. Drugs, alcohol and road accidents in Tasmania. Med J Aust 147:6–11 (1987).
381. Logan BK and Schwilke EW. Drug and alcohol use in fatally injured drivers in Washington state. J Forensic Sci 41:505–510 (1996).
382. Finkle BS, Biasotti AA, and Bradford LW. The occurrence of some drugs and toxic agents encountered in drinking driver investigations. J Forensic Sci 13:236–245 (1968).
383. Robinson TA. The incidence of drugs in impaired driving specimens in Northern Ireland. J Forensic Sci Soc 19:237–241 (1979).
384. White JM, Clardy DO, Graves MH, Kuo MC, MacDonald BJ, Wiersema SJ, and Fitzpatrick G. Testing for sedative-hypnotic drugs in the impaired driver: a survey of 72,000 arrests. Clin Toxicol 18:945–957 (1981).
385. Peel HW, Perrigo BJ, and Mikhael NZ. Detection of drugs in saliva of impaired drivers. J Forensic Sci 29:185–189 (1984).
386. Barbone F, McMahon AD, Davey PG, Morris AD, Reid IC, McDevitt DG, and MacDonald TM. Association of road-traffic accidents with benzodiazepine use. Lancet 352:1331–1336 (1998).
387. Liljequist R, Linnoila M, Mattila MJ, Saario I, and Seppala T. Effect of two weeks' treatment with thioridazine, chlorpromazine, sulpiride and bromazepam, alone or in combination with alcohol, on learning and memory in man. Psychopharmacologia 44:205–208 (1975).
388. Hughes FW, Forney RB, and Richards AB. Comparative effect in human subjects of chlordiazepoxide, diazepam, and placebo on mental and physical performance. Clin Pharmacol Ther 6:139–145 (1965).
389. Staak M, Raff G, and Strohm H. Pharmacopsychological investigation of changes in mood induced by dipotassium chlorazepate with and without simultaneous alcohol administration. Int J Clin Pharmacol Ther Toxicol 18:283–291 (1980).
390. Lawton MP and Cahn B. The effects of diazepam (Valium®) and alcohol on psychomotor performance. J Nerv Ment Dis 136:550–554 (1963).
391. Molander L and Duvhok C. Acute effects of oxazepam, diazepam and methylperone, alone and in combination with alcohol on sedation, coordination and mood. Acta Pharmacol Toxicol 38:145–160 (1976).
392. van Steveninck AL, Gieschke R, Schoemaker RC, Roncari G, Tuk B, Pieters MSM, et al. Pharmacokinetic and pharmacodynamic interactions of bretazenil and diazepam with alcohol. Br J Clin Pharmacol 41:565–573 (1996).
393. van Steveninck AL, Gieschke R, Schoemaker HC, Pieters MSM, Kroon JM, Breimer DD, and Cohen AF. Pharmacodynamic interactions of diazepam and intravenous alcohol at pseudo steady state. Psychopharmacology 110:471–478 (1993).
394. Saario I and Linnoila M. Effect of subacute treatment with hypnotics, alone or in combination with alcohol, on psychomotor skills related to driving. Acta Pharmacol Toxicol 38: 382–392 (1976).
395. Lichter JL, Korttila K, Apfelbaum J, Rupani G, Ostman P, Lane B, et al. Alcohol after midazolam sedation: does it really matter. Anesth Analges 70:S 237 (1990).

396. Saario I, Linnoila M, and Maki M. Interaction of drugs with alcohol on human psychomotor skills related to driving: effect of sleep deprivation or two weeks' treatment with hypnotics. J Clin Pharmacol 15:52–59 (1975).
397. Grigoleit HG, Hajdu P, Hundt HKL, Koeppen D, Malerczyk V, Meyer BH, et al. Pharmacokinetic aspects of the interaction between clobazam and cimetidine. Eur J Clin Pharmacol 25:139–142 (1983).
398. Sanders LD, Whitehead C, Gildersleve CD, Rosen M, and Robinson JO. Interaction of H_2-receptor antagonists and benzodiazepine sedation. Anaesthesia 48:286–292 (1993).
399. Wilson CM, Robinson FP, Thompson EM, Dundee JW, and Elliot P. Effect of pretreatment with ranitidine on the hypnotic action of single doses of midazolam, temazepam and zopiclone. Br J Anaesth 58:483–486 (1986).
400. Van Hecken AM, Tjandramaga TB, Verbesselt R, and De Schepper PJ. The influence of diflunisal on the pharmacokinetics of oxazepam. Br J Clin Pharmacol 20:225–234 (1985).
401. Huang W and Moody DE. Immunoassay detection of benzodiazepines and benzodiazepine metabolites in blood. J Anal Toxicol 19:333–342 (1995).
402. Erickson DA, Mather G, Trager WF, Levy RH, and Keirns JJ. Characterization of the in vitro biotransformation of the HIV-1 reverse transcriptase inhibitor nevirapine by human hepatic cytochromes P-450. Drug Metab Dispos 27:1488–1495 (1999).

Chapter 2

Antiepileptic Drugs

Nathan L. Kanous II, PharmD and Barry E. Gidal, PharmD

1. INTRODUCTION

1.1. Epidemiology of Epilepsy

Epilepsy is a chronic neurologic disorder characterized by recurrent seizures. Estimates indicate that approximately 120 in 100,000 people in the United States seek medical attention each year as the result of experiencing a seizure. Though not every patient that has a seizure has epilepsy, approximately 125,000 new cases of epilepsy are diagnosed every year *(1–3)*.

The incidence of epilepsy in the general population is highest in newborn and young children with a second peak occurring in patients older than 65 years. It has been suggested that there may be some genetic predisposition to the development of seizures and epilepsy. Although the incidence of epilepsy is higher among patients with mental retardation and cerebral palsy, neither condition is synonymous with epilepsy *(1)*.

1.2. Etiology

Epilepsy is recognized as a syndrome of disturbed electrical activity in the brain that can be caused by a variety of stimuli. This disturbed electrical activity leads to the development of seizures. Seizures occur because of the abnormal discharge of neurons within the central nervous system (CNS). Even slight abnormal discharges can destabilize the electrical homeostasis of neurons, thus increasing the propensity for other abnormal activity and the propagation of seizure activity *(3)*.

Precipitation of seizures in predisposed patients can occur as the result of a variety of inciting factors. Hyperventilation, sleep, sleep deprivation, and sensory and emotional stimuli have all been implicated. Hormonal changes associated with menses and several prescription drugs and drug classes may also influence the onset or frequency of seizure activity in patients with epilepsy. In addition, many antiepileptic drugs (AEDs) are known to cause seizures at excessive concentrations *(3)*.

From: *Handbook of Drug Interactions: A Clinical and Forensic Guide*
A. Mozayani and L. P. Raymon, eds. © Humana Press Inc., Totowa, NJ

2. MEDICATIONS UTILIZED IN THE TREATMENT OF EPILEPSY

AEDs act within the central nervous system in one of two ways: by reducing pathologic electrical discharges or by inhibiting the propagation of aberrant electrical activity. This may occur through effects on specific ion channels, inhibitory neurotransmitters, or excitatory neurotransmitters. Though multiple neurophysiological effects of AEDs have been theorized and hypothesized, it is important to recognize that the true mechanisms of action of these agents are poorly understood and may be multifactorial (4).

Testing to determine the serum concentration of AEDs is commonly employed. The widespread availability of this technology makes the determination of serum concentrations an attractive method for use in forensic science. For most AEDs there is poor correlation between maintenance doses and their resulting serum concentrations (5). In addition there is important interindividual variability in both therapeutic and toxic response to medications (5–7). Therefore, knowledge of the pharmacokinetics of AEDs is essential for understanding and interpreting serum concentrations of AEDs. This includes issues related to all aspects of drug disposition: absorption, distribution, metabolism, and excretion.

This situation is further complicated by the fact that AEDs are subject to pharmacokinetic interactions with one another and many other drugs and foods (5). Interactions with other drugs may lead to loss of efficacy or toxic effects from either the AED or the other interacting drug. This can be particularly important with the initiation or discontinuation of either drug and careful attention should be paid to the time course of initiation or discontinuation of any drug in the interpretation of the effects of drugs and serum drug concentrations (8).

AEDs are well known for causing side effects. Side effects are generally classified as acute or chronic. Further, these effects may be described as being concentration dependent or idiosyncratic. Concentration-dependent effects are usually relatively common and well characterized. Allergic reactions are typically mild but may be severe in some cases. Other idiopathic reactions are rare but can be serious and life threatening (9). Knowledge of the mechanism(s) of the toxic effects of AEDs and their relationship to serum concentration data are also important for the practicing forensic scientist.

Last, it is important to recognize that many AEDs are frequently employed for off-label use. The majority of off-label use involves the treatment of psychiatric disorders, particularly bipolar affective disorder or manic depressive disorder (10). Other off-label uses include such things as migraine prophylaxis, attention-deficit disorder, and neuropathic pain.

2.1. Phenytoin and Fosphenytoin

2.1.1. Chemistry

Phenytoin is a hydantoin anticonvulsant medication that is structurally related to the barbiturates. Although similar, the monoacylurea structure of phenytoin makes it a much weaker organic acid than the barbiturates (11). This results in very poor aqueous solubility of phenytoin.

Parenteral phenytoin must be formulated as a highly alkaline aqueous solution to maintain adequate solubility. This is accomplished through the use of an aqueous vehi-

2. Antiepileptic Drugs

cle consisting of 40% propylene glycol and 10% ethanol in water buffered with sodium hydroxide to a pH of 12. Parenteral phenytoin is incompatible with dextrose-based intravenous solutions. Preparation of intravenous phenytoin in dextrose-based solutions results in immediate precipitation of the free acid *(12)*.

Oral phenytoin is available in a variety of formulations as the free acid or sodium salt in both immediate- and extended-release formulations.

Fosphenytoin is a phenytoin prodrug. This drug was developed and formulated specifically to improve the solubility of phenytoin for parenteral use. Fosphenytoin is a disodium phosphate ester of phenytoin. As such, fosphenytoin is freely soluble in aqueous solution and is rapidly and completely converted to phenytoin in vivo through the action of serum phosphatase enzymes *(13)*.

2.1.2. Pharmacology

Phenytoin and fosphenytoin are effective at reducing seizure frequency and severity without causing generalized central nervous system depression. This action is mediated through effects on voltage-activated Na^+ channels in neuronal cell membranes *(11)*.

Depolarization of the neuronal cell membrane triggers the voltage-activated Na^+ channel to open, thus facilitating transmission of the action potential down the axon and, ultimately, from cell to cell. After opening, these voltage-activated Na^+ channels will spontaneously close. This is termed inactivation of the Na^+ channel. This inactivation is thought to cause the refractory period, a period of time after an action potential during which another action potential cannot be evoked *(11)*.

These drugs effectively limit repetitive firing of action potentials by prolonging inactivation, thus slowing the rate of repolarization of neuronal cells. At therapeutic concentrations, only neuronal cells that have been depolarized are protected from repetitive firing with no effect on spontaneous firing or responses to γ-aminobutyric acid (GABA) or glutamate *(14)*. This effectively limits the propagation of the aberrant electrical discharges that characterize epilepsy.

2.1.3. Pharmacokinetics

The pharmacokinetics of phenytoin (and also fosphenytoin) are strongly influenced by its limited aqueous solubility and saturable enzymatic elimination. The inactivation of these drugs by cytochrome P450 isozymes predisposes them to the influence of drug interactions.

2.1.3.1. Absorption

Because of its broad effectiveness in the management of epilepsy and the nature of epilepsy as a clinical disorder, phenytoin is available in a variety of formulations. Differences in physicochemical properties of the various formulations results in significant variability in both the rate and extent of absorption from each preparation.

Several factors including pK_a and lipid solubility, pH of the dissolution medium, solubility in the medium, and phenytoin concentration influence the rate and extent of absorption in the gastrointestinal tract. These factors are commonly altered by the presence of food or drugs in the gastrointestinal tract and the individual formulation *(12,13,15)*.

Phenytoin is poorly absorbed in the stomach due to the low pH of gastric juice (approximately 2.0), which renders it insoluble even though it may be present in a nonionized form. The duodenum serves as the primary site of absorption with its higher pH increasing the solubility of the drug. Absorption slows within the jejunum and ileum and is again poor in the colon *(12,13,15)*.

Also because of poor solubility, intramuscular administration of phenytoin results in drug precipitation and the formation of an insoluble mass. This effect, coupled with the pain associated with intramuscular injection of a high-pH solution, mandate that phenytoin be administered intravenously when a parenteral route is necessary *(16)*.

Because of its improved solubility profile, fosphenytoin can be administered either intramuscularly or intravenously. Comparison of area under the curve measures for total or free phenytoin concentrations between fosphenytoin and phenytoin sodium are nearly identical, indicating complete bioavailability of fosphenytoin by either route *(13)*.

In an effort to facilitate simple and rapid utilization of parenteral fosphenytoin for the more problematic phenytoin, fosphenytoin is packaged and dosed as milligram phenytoin equivalents (mPEs) *(13)*. Although this facilitates accurate conversion between parenteral dosage forms, this conversion is less accurate when converting oral phenytoin to parenteral mPEs. This is because oral phenytoin is formulated as a sodium salt. Thus, a 100-mg capsule of phenytoin sodium delivers only 92 mg of actual phenytoin *(13)*. This represents an approximately 9% difference in total dose when oral phenytoin is converted to parenteral fosphenytoin or phenytoin. This may result in increased serum concentrations of phenytoin after conversion, particularly in light of the unpredictable nonlinear kinetics of phenytoin metabolism.

2.1.3.2. Distribution

Phenytoin is approximately 90% protein bound in the plasma, primarily to albumin. The remaining 10% is unbound or "free" phenytoin and is pharmacologically active because that which is bound to plasma proteins is unable to cross the blood–brain barrier. Because of the passive diffusion of phenytoin into the cerebrospinal fluid (CSF), the concentration of phenytoin in the CSF is considered equivalent to the unbound plasma concentration *(15)*.

The generally recognized therapeutic range for phenytoin is 10–20 µg/mL, which includes both bound and unbound drug. The 10% of phenytoin which remains unbound corresponds to an equivalent unbound therapeutic range of 1–2 µg/mL *(17)*.

Protein binding of phenytoin is dependent upon albumin concentration and can also be influenced by a variety of clinical conditions and situations. Low-serum albumin, renal failure, or concomitant use of other protein-bound drugs may change the protein binding and serum concentration of phenytoin *(17,18)*.

2.1.3.3. Metabolism

Phenytoin is extensively metabolized via the cytochrome P450 system. This occurs primarily through the 2C19 and 2C9 isozymes and accounts for the involvement of phenytoin in a variety of drug interactions *(12)*. Of note is the fact that the metabolism of phenytoin involves the intermediate formation of an arene oxide. This arene oxide intermediate has been implicated as the source of various toxicities and teratogenicity associated with the use of phenytoin *(19)*.

Phenytoin is also known for its nonlinear pharmacokinetics. At low doses, phenytoin exhibits a first-order dose-dependent kinetic profile. As the dose of phenytoin

2. Antiepileptic Drugs

increases, OH-phenytoin begins to inhibit CYP450D6, which is responsible for its own formation. This suicide inhibition leads to disproportionate and dramatic increases in serum concentration with relatively small changes in dosing rate *(12)*. In most patients, the usual therapeutic range exceeds the concentration at which metabolism is half-maximal, which causes phenytoin to exhibit a nonlinear profile in the majority of patients. A variety of situations such as concurrent illness, medications, pregnancy, age, or genetics may influence the maximal rate of metabolism and thus may alter the pharmacokinetic profile of phenytoin in a given patient *(20)*.

2.1.3.4. EXCRETION

Approximately 95% of an administered dose is excreted in the urine or feces as metabolites *(12,20)*.

2.1.4. Adverse Reactions

With initial therapy, the CNS depressant effects of phenytoin are most prominent and may cause lethargy, fatigue, incoordination, blurred vision, and drowsiness (Table 1). Slow-dose titration can minimize these effects *(9)*.

At high serum concentrations (greater than 20 µg/mL) many patients exhibit lateral gaze nystagmus. Other adverse effects known to occur at excessive plasma concentrations include ataxia, mental-status changes, and coma. Further, phenytoin has the ability to precipitate seizures or status epilepticus at extreme concentrations.

Chronic adverse effects include gingival hyperplasia, which can occur in up to 50% of patients receiving long-term therapy. Other long-term effects include hirsutism, acne, coarsening of facial features, vitamin D deficiency, osteomalacia, folic acid deficiency (with resultant macrocytosis), hypothyroidism, and peripheral neuropathy.

2.1.5. Contraindications and Precautions

Patients with hypersensitivity reactions to any hydantoin AED may react to other hydantoin AEDs such as phenytoin. In addition, some patients exhibit cross-sensitivity to other compounds with similar chemical structures such as barbiturates, succinimides, and oxazolidinediones.

Prenatal exposure to hydantoin AEDs may result in the development of cleft palate, cleft lip, cardiac malformations, and a constellation of physical abnormalities referred to as the fetal anticonvulsant syndrome: prenatal growth deficiency, microcephaly, hypophasia of the fingernails, and craniofacial abnormalities *(21)*.

The use of parenteral phenytoin can alter automaticity of cardiac tissue and may result in the development of ventricular arrhythmias and should only be used with extreme caution in patients with second- or third-degree arterio venous (AV) blockade, bradycardia, or significant cardiac disease *(22)*.

Because of the risk of myelosuppression, the use of phenytoin in immunosuppressed patients or patients with blood dyscrasias may increase the risk of infection or exacerbation of the hematologic abnormality.

The metabolism of phenytoin may be impaired in patients with active liver disease or active alcoholism with subsequent toxic effects associated with elevated serum concentrations *(6,12,23)*.

Table 1
Antiepileptic Drug Side Effects

AED	Acute Side Effects – Concentration Dependent	Acute Side Effects – Idiosyncratic	Chronic Side Effects
Phenytoin	Ataxia Nystagmus Behavioral changes Dizziness Headache Incoordination Sedation Lethargy Cognitive Impairment Fatigue Visual Blurring	Blood dyscrasias Rash Immunologic reactions	Behavior changes Cerebellar syndrome Connective tissue changes Skin thickening Folate deficiency Gingival hyperplasia Hirsutism Coarsening of facial features Acne Cognitive impairment Metabolic bone disease Sedation
Carbamazepine	Diplopia Dizziness Drowsiness Nausea Unsteadiness Lethargy	Blood dyscrasias Rash	Hyponatremia
Lamotrigine	Diplopia Dizziness Unsteadiness Headache	Rash	Not established
Valproic Acid Sedation	GI upset Acute pancreatitis Unsteadiness Tremor Thrombocytopenia	Acute hepatic failure	Polycystic ovary-like syndrome Alopecia Weight gain Hyperammonemia
Ethosuximide	Ataxia Drowsiness GI distress Unsteadiness Hiccoughs	Blood dyscrasias Rash	Behavior changes Headache

(continued)

2.1.6. Drug Interactions

Phenytoin is involved in many drug interactions (Tables 2 and 3). These interactions are well characterized and phenytoin may be the target or cause of interactions. Pharmacokinetic drug interactions affecting absorption, metabolism, or excretion have the potential to either increase or decrease the plasma concentration of phenytoin. Though food may slightly alter the rate of absorption of phenytoin, it is well recognized that enteral feedings can dramatically decrease the bioavailability of phenytoin suspension when administered via a feeding tube *(24)*.

Although phenytoin is highly protein bound, protein-binding interactions are generally of minimal significance. As phenytoin is displaced from plasma proteins, the free

2. Antiepileptic Drugs

Table 1 (continued)

AED	Acute Side Effects - Concentration Dependent	Acute Side Effects - Idiosyncratic	Chronic Side Effects
Gabapentin	Dizziness Fatigue Somnolence Ataxia		Weight gain
Topiramate	Difficulties concentrating Psychomotor slowing Speech or language problems Somnolence, fatigue Dizziness Headache	Not established	Kidney stones
Felbamate	Anorexia Nausea Vomiting Insomnia Headache	Aplastic anemia Acute hepatic failure	Not established
Vigabatrin	Sedation Fatigue	Visual field defects Agitation Irritability Depression Psychosis	Not established
Levetiracetam	Sedation Behavioral Disturbance	Not established	Not established
Zonisamide	Sedation Dizziness Cognitive impairment Nausea	Rash Oligohydrosis	Kidney stones

From *(99)* with permission.

fraction of phenytoin increases. This is followed by an increase in the clearance of phenytoin, a decrease in total phenytoin concentration, and subsequent reestablishment of baseline free phenytoin concentration *(17)*. It is important that clinicians understand the mechanism of this interaction and do not react to decreases in total concentration without considering the possibility that free concentrations remain therapeutic.

Long-term use of phenytoin decreases folic acid absorption *(9)*. Replacement of folic acid effectively increases the clearance of phenytoin and thereby decreases phenytoin concentrations. Supplementation of folic acid, alone or as a vitamin, has the potential to decrease plasma phenytoin concentrations and subsequently decrease seizure control *(25)*.

2.2. Carbamazepine and Oxcarbazepine

2.2.1. Chemistry

The chemical structure of carbamazepine (CBZ) is tricyclic in nature, with two benzene rings flanking one azepine ring that contains a double bond. This structure is

Table 2
Interactions Between Antiepileptic Drugs*

AED	Added Drug	Effect[a,b]
Phenytoin (PHT)	Carbamazepine	Decr. PHT
	Felbamate	Incr. PHT
	Methosuximide	Incr. PHT
	Phenobarbital	Incr. or decr. PHT
	Valproic acid	Decr. Total PHT
	Vigabatrin	Decr. PHT
Carbamazepine (CBZ)	Felbamate	Incr. 10, 11 epoxide
	Felbamate	Decr. CBZ
	Phenobarbital	Decr. CBZ
	Phenytoin	Decr. CBZ
Oxcarbazepine	Carbamazepine	Decr. MHD
	Phenytoin	Decr. MHD
	Phenobarbital	Decr. MHD
Lamotrigine (LTG)	Carbamazepine	Decr. LTG
	Phenobarbital	Decr. LTG
	Phenytoin	Decr. LTG
	Primidone	Decr. LTG
	Valproic Acid	Incr. LTG
Valproic Acid (VPA)	Carbamazepine	Decr. VPA
	Lamotrigine	Decr. VPA
	Phenobarbital	Decr. VPA
	Primidone	Decr. VPA
	Phenytoin	Decr. VPA
Ethosuximide (ETX)	Carbamazepine	Decr. ETX
	Valproic acid	May incr. ETX
Gabapentin	No known interactions	
Topiramate (TPM)	Carbamazepine	Decr. TPM
	Phenytoin	Decr. TPM
	Valproic acid	Decr. TPM
Tiagabine (TGB)	Carbamazepine	Decr. TGB
	Phenytoin	Decr. TGB
Felbamate (FBM)	Carbamazepine	Decr. FBM
	Phenytoin	Decr. FBM
	Valproic acid	Incr. FBM
Vigabatrin	Phenytoin	Incr. PHT
Levetiracetam	No known interactions	
Zonisamide	Carbamazepine	Decr. zonisamide
	Phenytoin	Decr. zonisamide
	Phenobarbital	Decr. zonisamide

*From (99) with permission.
[a]Incr., increased; Decr., decreased.
[b]MHD, 10-hydroxy-oxcarbazepine.

2. Antiepileptic Drugs

Table 3
Interactions with Other Drugs*

AED	Altered by	Result[a]	Alters	Result[a]
Phenytoin (PHT)	Antacids	Decr. absorption of PHT	Oral contraceptives (OC)	Decr. efficacy of OC
	Cimetidine	Incr. PHT	Bishydroxycoumarin	Decr. anticoagulation
	Chloramphenicol	Incr. PHT	Folic acid	Decr. folic acid
	Disulfiram	Incr. PHT	Quinidine	Decr. quinidine
	Ethanol (acute)	Incr. PHT	Vitamin D	Decr. vitamin D
	Fluconazole	Incr. PHT		
	Isoniazid	Incr. PHT		
	Propoxyphene	Incr. PHT		
	Warfarin	Incr. PHT		
	Alcohol (chronic)	Decr. PHT		
Carbamazepine (CBZ)	Cimetidine	Incr. CBZ	Oral contraceptives (OC)	Decr. efficacy of OC
	Erythromycin	Incr. CBZ		
	Fluoxetine	Incr. CBZ	Doxycycline	Decr. doxycycline
	Isoniazid	Incr. CBZ	Theophylline	Decr. theophylline
	Propoxyphene	Incr. CBZ	Warfarin	Decr. warfarin
Oxcarbazepine			Oral contraceptives (OC)	Decr. efficacy of OC
Valproic Acid (VPA)	Cimetidine	Incr. VPA	Oral contraceptives (OC)	Decr. efficacy of OC
	Salicylates	Incr. free VPA		
Gabapentin	Cimetidine	Incr. gabapentin		
	Aluminum-containing antacids	Decr. gabapentin		
Topiramate (TPM)			Oral contraceptives (OC)	Decr. efficacy of OC
Tiagabine (TGB)	Cimetidine	Incr. TGB		
Felbamate (FBM)			Warfarin	Incr. warfarin

*From (99) with permission.
[a]Incr. increased; Decr. decreased.

most closely related to antipsychotic and antidepressant drugs such as chlorpromazine, imipramine, and maprotiline. CBZ differs from other heterocyclic AEDs by being tricyclic, lacking an amide group in the heterocyclic ring, and not possessing a saturated carbon atom in the cyclic structure *(26)*.

CBZ is insoluble in water although easily soluble in many organic solvents including benzene, chloroform, and dichloromethane. This lipophilicity strongly influences drug transport across biological membranes.

Oxcarbazepine, a biological prodrug, is a keto analog of CBZ. This change in structure alters the solubility of the compound and renders it only slightly soluble in chloroform, dichloromethane, acetone, and methanol whereas it is practically insoluble in water ethanol and ether *(27)*.

2.2.2. Pharmacology

CBZ enhances the inactivation voltage-activated Na^+ channels by slowing their recovery. This results in a net decrease in high-frequency repetitive firing of action potentials. These effects are evident and selective at serum concentrations within the therapeutic range *(28)*. No effect of carbamazepine on exogenously administered GABA or glutamate have been identified. The 10,11 epoxycarbamazepine metabolite also contributes a similar therapeutic effect *(29)*.

The pharmacologic effect of oxcarbazepine is due to a principal metabolite, 10-hydroxy-oxcarbazepine *(27)*. The mechanism of action is similar to that of carbamazepine but may also include increased potassium conduction and modulation of high-voltage calcium channels *(30,31)*.

2.2.3. Pharmacokinetics

It is well known that absorption of CBZ varies significantly from one dosage form to another *(32)*. Further, the effects of CBZ on the cytochrome P450 isozyme system warrants close assessment of the pharmacokinetics of this drug in clinical use.

2.2.3.1. Absorption

CBZ tablets are incompletely and erratically absorbed. The time to maximal serum concentration (t_{max}) is 8 or more h for tablets but 3–5 h for the suspension *(33)*. That means that the full effects of a given oral dose of carbamazepine tablets may not be recognized until 8 or more h after the dose has been ingested, whereas a similar dose of the suspension reaches maximal concentration in just 3–5 h and may influence the interpretation of serum concentration data. In addition to delayed absorption of carbamazepine from tablets, it has also been recognized that tablet formulations can be adversely affected by humidity and moisture content, thus further delaying or decreasing absorption *(34)*.

CBZ exhibits both zero-order and first-order absorption characteristics. Approximately 35% of an oral dose is absorbed in zero-order fashion (no effect of dose on absorption) whereas the remainder of the dose is absorbed according to a first-order kinetics. At doses greater than 20 mg/kg, an inverse relationship between dose and absorption begins to occur *(35)*.

Absolute bioavailability of CBZ is approximately 75% of the dose administered. This is similar between all dosage forms.

2. Antiepileptic Drugs

2.2.3.2. Distribution

CBZ is highly protein bound with 75 to 80% bound to albumin and other plasma proteins with an apparent volume of distribution of 0.8 to 2 L/kg. Unbound concentrations of CBZ vary inversely with the concentration of α_1-acid glycoprotein *(36)*.

CBZ is readily distributed into cerebrospinal fluid and these concentrations vary linearly with plasma levels. Although there may be wide variability in CBZ concentration between patients, the ratio of plasma:CSF concentration is relatively constant between patients *(37)*.

CBZ is also readily distributed into amniotic fluid and breast milk *(38)*. Although the use of CBZ is not contraindicated among pregnant women, it must be recognized that the newborn may be susceptible to adverse effects associated with exposure to CBZ.

Consistent with its lower lipid solubility, 10,11 epoxycarbamazepine has a lower apparent volume of distribution and increased fraction unbound of 48 to 53% *(39)*. The commonly accepted therapeutic range for CBZ in adults is 4 to 12 µg/mL *(40)*. To date, no accepted therapeutic range for the use of oxcarbazepine in treating epilepsy has been established *(41)*. Clinical trials in patients treated for neurologic pain have reported serum 10-hydroxy-carbazepine concentrations between 50 and 100 µg/mL *(42)*.

2.2.3.3. Metabolism

CBZ is essentially completely metabolized in humans through both oxidative and conjugative pathways. The primary metabolite, carbamazepine epoxide, is pharmacologically active and may accumulate in patients using CBZ over long periods of time *(36)*. This may potentially lead to the development of toxicity in a patient who manifests no change in plasma CBZ level after an increase in daily CBZ dose.

A comparison of patients reveals a lower ratio of CBZ epoxide to CBZ among patients receiving monotherapy when compared to those receiving multiple AEDs *(43)*.

2.2.3.3.1. Autoinduction. After initial dosing, CBZ induces its own metabolism significantly leading to increased clearance, decreased serum half-life, and a subsequent decline in plasma concentration over time. Studies have shown that whereas the elimination half-life of CBZ in single-dose studies varied from 20 to 65 h, the half-life was decreased by approximately 50% after multiple dosing for 10 to 20 d *(44,45)*.

There is a time dependence of CBZ kinetics secondary to this phenomenon of autoinduction. As the autoinduction progresses, changes in daily dose are required to maintain adequate plasma concentrations. Autoinduction is expected to be complete within 20 to 30 d and is dependent upon CBZ dose *(44,45)*.

2.2.3.4. Excretion

Approximately 72% of a given dose of CBZ is eliminated as metabolites in the urine. The remaining 28% is eliminated in the feces.

2.2.4. Adverse Reactions

The most common side effects of CBZ include dizziness, drowsiness, ataxia, dyskinesia, diplopia, and headache (Table 1). These effects are typically dose related and may resolve with continued administration only to recur with significant increases in plasma concentration *(9)*.

Idiopathic reactions to CBZ include blood dyscrasias and hypersensitivity reactions. Aplastic anemia, agranulocytosis, and pancytopenia have been reported to occur rarely with the use of CBZ and more often when CBZ is used in combination with other medications. Leukopenia is reported to occur in nearly 10% of patients. Though somewhat common, there appears to be no association between the presence of leukopenia and an increased incidence of infection. This has been hypothesized to occur as a result of white blood cell (WBC) redistribution *(9)*.

Hypersensitivity manifests most commonly as the development of an eczematous rash, which can progress in some patients to Stevens-Johnson syndrome *(46)*.

Dilutional hyponatremia and the syndrome of inappropriate antidiuretic hormone have been reported. The incidence of this phenomenon may increase with the age of the patient and appears somewhat dose related although low-dose therapy does not preclude the development of hyponatremia *(47)*.

2.2.5. Contraindications and Precautions

Some patients with a history of hypersensitivity to tricyclic antidepressants may be sensitive to CBZ and should only be treated with CBZ when the potential benefit outweighs the risk of hypersensitivity.

The use of CBZ in patients with absence seizures has been associated with worsening of seizures while using CBZ and should be avoided. Similarly, CBZ is considered ineffective for the treatment of Lennox-Gastaut syndrome *(11)*.

Congenital abnormalities have been reported to occur in infants of mothers who take CBZ. Current evidence indicates a higher risk of malformations with combination therapy, which may result in higher plasma CBZ concentrations *(48)*.

2.2.6. Drug Interactions

CBZs metabolic fate and its influence on the cytochrome p450 system make CBZ the subject of many significant drug interactions (Tables 2 and 3; *5*). Interestingly, valproic acid can effectively increase the plasma concentration of the 10,11-epoxide metabolite without changing the concentration of CBZ. Erythromycin inhibits the metabolism of CBZ resulting in clinically significant increases in plasma CBZ concentration. CBZ can induce the metabolism of many other drugs potentially leading to loss of therapeutic effect. Several examples include valproic acid, theophylline, warfarin, and ethosuximide.

2.3. Lamotrigine

2.3.1. Chemistry

Lamotrigine is a phenyltriazine AED unrelated to other currently available AEDs. As a tertiary amine, lamotrigine is only very slightly soluble in water, and slightly soluble in 0.1 M HCl *(49)*.

2.3.2. Pharmacology

Lamotrigine effectively inhibits the reactivation of voltage-activated Na$^+$ channels, similar to phenytoin and CBZ. Further, this action appears greater during repetitive activation, such as may occur during an epileptic seizure (double check that). However, unlike CBZ and phenytoin, lamotrigine also competitively blocks high-voltage

2. Antiepileptic Drugs

Ca^+ flux, by blocking presynaptic-type Ca^+ channels. Lamotrigine is also effective at inhibiting the release of glutamate and GABA from neurons, although this effect is much more pronounced for glutamate than for GABA *(49)*.

2.3.3. Pharmacokinetics

The pharmacokinetics of lamotrigine are unique when compared to other AEDs in that although it is not a subject of drug interactions related to oxidative metabolism through the cytochrome P-450 system, it is subject to interaction with drugs that may alter its glucuronide conjugation.

2.3.3.1. Absorption

Lamotrigine is readily and completely absorbed from the gastrointestinal system. The bioavailability is 98%. Plasma concentrations peak 1–3 h after oral administration and absorption appears to be linearly related to dose up to approximately 700 mg. Food does not alter the absorption of lamotrigine and systemic absorption can occur with rectal administration although to a more limited extent than with oral dosing *(50)*.

2.3.3.2. Distribution

Lamotrigine is approximately 56% bound to plasma proteins, which remains constant throughout the range of concentrations from 1 to 10 µg/mL. The apparent volume of distribution is 0.9–1.2 L/kg and is independent of dose administered. Although lamotrigine serum concentrations can be determined, no therapeutic range has been established for this drug and it is advised that treatment decisions be guided by therapeutic response without concern for serum concentration *(51)*.

2.3.3.3. Metabolism

Lamotrigine undergoes hepatic metabolism by uridine diphosphate (UDP)-glucuronosyl-transferase (UGT 1A4). Metabolism can occur at either heterocyclic nitrogen atom to form one of two glucuronide conjugates. These glucuronide conjugates are pharmacologically inactive *(51)*.

The half-life of lamotrigine is approximately 24–29 h in healthy volunteers. Though some evidence suggests that lamotrigine may undergo autoinduction, the relatively slow onset of autoinduction and the slow, tapered dosing schedule make this autoinduction clinically insignificant.

2.3.3.4. Excretion

Single-dose studies indicate that approximately 70% of a given dose is eliminated in the urine, almost entirely as glucuronide conjugates. Less than 10% of an administered dose is renally eliminated as unchanged drug *(51)*.

2.3.4. Adverse Reactions

Lamotrigine can cause a number of CNS side effects including drowsiness, ataxia, diplopia, and headache (Table 1). These effects occur significantly less frequently when compared to other AEDs *(52)*.

A hallmark side effect of lamotrigine is the development of a rash. Though several types of rash have been reported, the most common is a generalized erythematous morbilliform rash that is typically mild to moderate in severity. Case reports of the development of Stevens-Johnson syndrome have been reported. Rash appears to occur more frequently in patients receiving concomitant valproic acid (VPA) and with rapid dose escalation *(53)*.

2.3.5. Contraindications and Precautions

Dermatologic reactions to lamotrigine appear to be more frequent in children when compared to adults. Safety and efficacy in patients up to the age of 16 years has not been proven. As noted previously the development of rash is more common among patients receiving valproic acid.

Significant interindividual differences in pharmacokinetics of lamotrigine have been observed in patients with renal dysfunction and careful consideration should be given that the benefits outweigh the risks of treatment in this patient population *(51)*.

2.3.6. Drug Interactions

Since lamotrigine is not metabolized by the cytochrome P450 system, it is not involved in precipitating cytochrome P450-based drug interactions. However, lamotrigine clearance is increased by phenytoin and CBZ. VPA decreases lamotrigine clearance and increases its half-life (Table 2). Conversely, the addition of lamotrigine to VPA can decrease VPA concentrations by as much as 25% *(51)*.

2.4. Valproate

2.4.1. Chemistry

Valproate is a short-chain branched fatty acid with low water solubility. Clinically, this compound is available as a sodium salt (valproate sodium Depakene®) with high water solubility and also as a complex of valproic acid and sodium valproate (divalproate Depakote®). This complex rapidly dissociates in the gastrointestinal tract to two molecules of valproate.

2.4.2. Pharmacology

Similar to phenytoin and carbamazepine, VPA prolongs the recovery of voltage-activated Na^+ channels. This effectively reduces propagation of rapid-firing action potentials. Some evidence exists to suggest that VPA blocks calcium currents in T-type calcium channels similar to that seen with ethosuximide *(54)*.

VPA has no direct modulatory effect on GABAergic neurotransmission. However, VPA may alter CNS GABA concentrations via two mechanisms. First, VPA may stimulate glutamic acid decarboxylase, thus increasing GABA synthesis. Second, valproic acid may inhibit the action of GABA transaminase and succinic semialdehyde dehydrogenase, therefore decreasing the degradation of GABA in the CNS. In either case, the net result is an increase in the concentration of GABA in the CNS *(54)*.

2.4.3. Pharmacokinetics

VPA is a widely used AED and is available in multiple formulations for oral and parenteral administration. Oral formulations include capsules, tablets, and syrup with immediate-release characteristics, enteric-coated tablets of sodium valproate or divalproex sodium, and enteric-coated sprinkles of divalproex sodium. Knowledge of the differences in pharmacokinetics between formulations is important.

2. Antiepileptic Drugs

2.4.3.1. ABSORPTION

Oral VPA is essentially 100% bioavailable. However, because of difficulties associated with gastric irritation, enteric-coated and delayed-release formulations have been developed to improve tolerability *(54)*. Multiple oral formulations of VPA are available: immediate-release capsules, tablets, and syrup; enteric-coated tablets; and sprinkles of divalproex sodium. The rate of absorption of VPA differs among the various formulations *(54)*.

Immediate-release formulations are rapidly absorbed with peak concentrations reached within 2 h. Enteric-coated tablets delay absorption but remain rapid once the tablet reaches the small intestine. The time of onset for absorption of delayed-release formulations is dependent upon the state of gastric emptying with peak plasma concentrations occurring between 3 and 8 h after oral administration. In patients taking delayed-release VPA, true trough concentrations may not occur until after administration of a morning dose. No difference in bioavailabilty has been noted between immediate- or delayed-release formulations *(54)*.

2.4.3.2. DISTRIBUTION

VPA is highly bound to plasma proteins with an apparent volume of distribution of 0.13–0.19 L/kg for adults and 0.2–0.3 L/kg in children. Protein binding is saturable at therapeutic concentrations and the free fraction of VPA increases with increasing total concentration. This effect can be quite dramatic with a threefold increase in total concentration leading to a near 10-fold increase in the concentration of free VPA *(5)*.

Serum concentrations of VPA are expected to be above 50 µg/mL to achieve therapeutic response. However, some controversy exists as to what the maximum concentration of the therapeutic range is. The most commonly cited maximal concentration of VPA is 100 µg/mL *(5)*. Though some reports have linked the emergence of adverse effects to concentrations greater than 80 µg/mL, higher concentrations may be required and tolerated in the management of difficult to control patients.

2.4.3.3. METABOLISM

VPA is metabolized extensively by the liver with a glucuronide conjugate and a 3-oxo-VPA metabolite accounting for over 70% of an administered dose. One metabolite, a 4-ene-VPA causes marked hepatotoxicity in rats and may be responsible for reports of hepatotoxicity in humans although this has not been entirely substantiated. It should also be noted that higher concentrations of the 4-ene-VPA may be present in patients taking enzyme-inducing drugs such as phenobarbital *(54)*.

2.4.3.4. EXCRETION

The majority of VPA (70–80%) is excreted in the urine as metabolites. In addition, portions of VPA are excreted in bile (7%) and through the lung (2–18%) *(5)*.

2.4.4. Adverse Reactions

The most common side effects encountered with the use of VPA are mild and gastrointestinal in nature: nausea, vomiting, gastrointestinal distress, and anorexia (Table 1). CNS-related side effects such as drowsiness, ataxia, and tremor appear to be dose related. Any of these dose-related side effects may recur with changes in plasma concentration.

Hair loss is occasionally seen early in therapy but generally resolves with continued use *(5,9)*.

The most serious idiosyncratic effect of VPA is hepatotoxicity. Risk factors for death due to hepatotoxicity include age less than 2 years, mental retardation, and use of multiple AEDs. These events also occurred early in therapy *(55)*. Hyperammonemia is a very common finding among patients using VPA but is not considered to be a consequence of hepatic damage *(9,55)*. Pancreatitis is very rare.

Thrombocytopenia and other blood dyscrasias have been commonly reported to occur in patients receiving VPA but rarely lead to drug discontinuation. Bleeding can occur in some patients as a result *(56)*.

Excessive weight gain is a common side effect associated with chronic use of VPA *(9)*.

2.4.5. Contraindications and Precautions

Valproate crosses the placenta and observational studies have revealed that first-trimester use of valproate is associated with an increased risk of neural tube defects. Careful consideration of the use of this medication during pregnancy is warranted *(57)*.

Pediatric use of VPA is associated with an increased risk of hepatotoxicity. Risk factors include age less than 2 years, multiple-AED use, and mental retardation. In addition, VPA should not be used in patients with current hepatic disease *(9,55)*.

VPA does alter platelet aggregation *(9)*. Caution should be exercised when using VPA with other drugs that may affect platelet aggregation and by patients with a history of thrombocytopenia and other risk factors for bleeding.

The use of VPA in combination with lamotrigine significantly increases the risk of dermatologic reactions to lamotrigine and caution is warranted *(52)*.

2.4.6. Drug Interactions

Because VPA is extensively metabolized, alterations in liver enzyme function can change the clearance of VPA. Common enzyme-inducing drugs such as phenytoin, CBZ, primidone, and phenobarbital increase VPA metabolism (Table 2). Highly protein-bound drugs such as aspirin and phenytoin have a propensity to displace VPA from binding sites and may change plasma VPA concentrations (Table 3; *5*).

VPA inhibits the metabolism of phenobarbital resulting in a significant decrease in phenobarbital clearance and subsequent toxic effects. As mentioned previously, VPA has the potential to increase the concentration of the 10,11 epoxide metabolite of CBZ without altering the concentration of CBZ *(5)*.

2.5. Ethosuximide

Ethosuximide is indicated for the treatment of absence seizures. In this capacity, it is considered the drug of first choice. Combination therapy with VPA is indicated in patients with difficult to control absence seizures despite monotherapy with ethosuximide.

2.5.1. Chemistry

Ethosuximide is a monocyclic AED that contains a five-member ring structure with two carbonyl oxygen atoms flanking a ring nitrogen. This compound is considered

2. Antiepileptic Drugs

soluble in ethanol or ether, freely soluble in water or chloroform, and only very slightly soluble in hexane *(58)*. Though containing a chiral center, ethosuximide is utilized clinically as a racemic mixture of the two compounds.

2.5.2. Pharmacology

Ethosuximide exhibits antiseizure activity by reducing low-threshold Ca^{++} currents in the thalamic region. There is no effect on recovery of voltage-activated Na^+ channels and thus no change in sustained repetitive firing. Ethosuximide has no influence on the action or concentration of GABA in the CNS. As a result of this unique mechanism of action, the use of ethosuximide is limited to the treatment of absence seizures *(59)*.

2.5.3. Pharmacokinetics

2.5.3.1. ABSORPTION

Absorption of ethosuximide is rapid and nearly complete (90 to 95%) and does not appear to be effected by long-term administration. Peak concentrations are reached within 1 to 4 h after oral administration *(5,59)*. Although the rate of absorption of oral syrup may be faster than that of oral tablets, the formulations are considered bioequivalent.

2.5.3.2. DISTRIBUTION

Ethosuximide distributes widely and homogeneously throughout the body. Based on this phenomenon, several studies have concluded that saliva concentrations of ethosuximide can be evaluated in lieu of plasma concentrations for therapeutic monitoring *(59,60)*.

The apparent volume of distribution is 0.62–0.65 L/kg in adults and 0.69 L/kg in children. Protein binding of ethosuximide is very low, ranging from 0 to 10% in humans *(60)*.

Serum concentrations of ethosuximide can be useful in monitoring therapy. The generally accepted therapeutic range is 40 to 100 µg/mL *(5,59)*.

2.5.3.3. METABOLISM

Ethosuximide is extensively metabolized via hepatic oxidation with 80–90% of an administered dose transformed to inactive metabolites. Biotransformation is catalyzed through the action of CYP3A in a first-order fashion. Ethosuximide does not induce hepatic microsomal enzymes or the uridine diphosphate glucuronosyl transferase (UDPGT) system *(5,59)*.

2.5.3.4. EXCRETION

Approximately 10–20% of an administered dose of ethosuximide is renally eliminated with nonrenal routes accounting for the majority of elimination. The apparent half-life of the parent compound is 30–60 h in adults and 30–40 h in children *(58)*.

2.5.4. Adverse Reactions

Adverse reactions from use of ethosuximide are relatively benign when compared to other AEDs (Table 1). Most of these effects are dose related, predictable, and resolve with a decrease in dose. Nausea and vomiting occur in up to 40% of patients taking ethosuximide. CNS side effects such as drowsiness, dizziness, fatigue, lethargy, and hiccups are also relatively common. Various behavioral changes have been reported but are not well correlated with ethosuximide use *(9,59)*.

Episodes of psychosis have been reported to occur in young adults with a history of mental disorders who are treated with ethosuximide. These psychotic reactions typically occur after the onset of seizure control and resolve after discontinuation of the drug and recurrence of seizures. This phenomenon is called forced normalization *(61)*.

Dermatologic adverse effects are the most common idiosyncratic reactions and range from mild dermatitis and rash to erythema multiforme and Stevens-Johnson syndrome *(62)*. Other rare effects include systemic lupus erythematosus, a lupus-like syndrome, and various blood dyscrasias *(63)*.

2.5.5. Contraindications and Precautions

Although teratogenic effects in humans have not been documented with the use of ethosuximide, caution is warranted as birth defects have been associated with the use of other AEDs.

Patients with active hepatic or renal disease may be at increased risk of side effects because of altered pharmacokinetics of ethosuximide.

2.5.6. Drug Interactions

Few drug interactions have been reported with ethosuximide. CBZ may induce the metabolism of ethosuximide resulting in loss of seizure control (Table 2). When ethosuximide metabolism reaches saturation, VPA may interfere by inhibiting the metabolism of ethosuximide and prolonging its half-life *(5)*.

2.6. Gabapentin

2.6.1. Chemistry

The chemical structure of gabapentin is that of GABA covalently bound to a cyclohexane ring. The inclusion of a lipophilic cyclohexane ring was employed to facilitate transfer of the GABA moiety into the central nervous system. Gabapentin is freely soluble in water *(64)*.

2.6.2. Pharmacology

Despite the fact that gabapentin was synthesized to serve as a GABA agonist in the CNS, this compound does not mimic the effects of GABA in experimental models *(65)*. Gabapentin appears to stimulate nonvesicular release of GABA through an unknown mechanism. Although it binds to a protein similar to the L-type voltage-sensitive Ca^{++} channels, gabapentin has no effect on calcium currents in root ganglion cells. Further, gabapentin does not effectively reduce sustained repetitive firing of action potentials as is seen with some other AEDs.

2.6.3. Pharmacokinetics

2.6.3.1. Absorption

Gabapentin is primarily absorbed in the small intestine. The L-amino acid carrier protein is responsible for absorption from the gut and distribution into the CNS. As a result of a saturable carrier-mediated absorption mechanism, bioavailability of gabapentin is dose-dependent *(66)*.

2. Antiepileptic Drugs

Oral bioavailability is reported as being 60%. In one multidose study of 1600 mg three times daily, bioavailability was reduced to approximately 35%. Maximal plasma concentrations are reached within 2 to 3 h of oral administration *(66)*.

2.6.3.2. DISTRIBUTION

Gabapentin is not appreciably bound to plasma proteins and exhibits an apparent volume of distribution of 0.65–1.04 L/kg. CSF concentrations of gabapentin range from 10 to 20% of plasma concentrations and distribution is limited by active transport through the L-amino acid carrier protein *(66)*. Optimal concentrations for therapeutic response to gabapentin have not been established.

2.6.3.3. METABOLISM

Gabapentin is not metabolized nor has it been found to interfere with the metabolism of other AEDs.

2.6.3.4. EXCRETION

Gabapentin is excreted exclusively in the urine. The reported half-life of gabapentin is 5–7 h but this may be significantly prolonged in patients with renal dysfunction *(67)*. Renal elimination of gabapentin is closely related to creatinine clearance and glomerular filtration rate. For this reason, dosage adjustments may be necessary for patients with renal disease.

2.6.4. Adverse Reactions

CNS side effects of gabapentin are the most common, tend to occur with initiation of therapy, and subside with continued use (Table 1). The most common of these effects are somnolence, dizziness, and fatigue. Ataxia has also been reported. Other rare CNS effects include nystagmus, tremor, and diplopia *(68)*.

Neuropsychiatric reactions including emotional lability, hostility, and thought disorders have been reported and may be more common among children and mentally retarded patients *(66)*. Weight gain is becoming more widely recognized as a long-term side effect of gabapentin use.

2.6.5. Contraindications and Precautions

Elderly patients or patients with impaired renal function should be monitored closely for the development of side effects secondary to reduced clearance and accumulation of gabapentin.

2.6.6. Drug Interactions

As previously mentioned, gabapentin is not appreciably metabolized by the cytochrome P450 system, nor does it alter the function of those enzymes. Cimetidine can decrease the renal clearance of gabapentin by 10% and aluminum-based antacids can decrease the bioavailability of gabapentin by as much as 20% (Table 3; *66*).

2.7. Topiramate

2.7.1. Chemistry

Topiramate is chemically unique from the more traditional AEDs in that it is a sulfamate-substituted monosaccharide. Topiramate is freely soluble in acetone, chloroform, dimethylsulfoxide, and ethanol. It is most soluble in aqueous environments with an alkaline pH *(69)*.

2.7.2. Pharmacology

Topiramate appears to have several mechanisms by which it exerts its antiseizure effects. First, topiramate reduces currents through voltage-gated Na^+ channels and may act on the inactivated state of these channels similarly to phenytoin, thus reducing the frequency of repetitive firing action potentials. In addition, topiramate increases postsynaptic GABA currents while also enhancing Cl^- channel activity. Further, topiramate decreases the activity of AMPA-kainate subtypes of glutamate receptors. Lastly, topiramate has been shown to function as a weak carbonic anhydrase inhibitor *(70,71)*.

2.7.3. Pharmacokinetics

2.7.3.1. ABSORPTION

Topiramate is readily absorbed with an estimated bioavailability of 80%. Food may delay absorption but does not alter bioavailability. Time to peak concentration ranges from 1.5 to 4 h after an oral dose *(72)*.

2.7.3.2. DISTRIBUTION

Topiramate is minimally bound to plasma proteins but does bind to erythrocytes. This unique phenomenon may lead to nonlinear changes in serum concentration until red cell binding sites have become saturated. The apparent volume of distribution is 0.6–0.8 L/kg *(72)*.

Topiramate dosage adjustments should be based upon therapeutic response as no defined therapeutic range has been established.

2.7.3.3. METABOLISM

Topiramate metabolism accounts for the disposition of less than 50% of an administered dose. Hepatic metabolism involves several pathways including hydroxylation, hydrolysis, and glucuronidation. Administration of enzyme-inducing drugs such as CBZ can increase the apparent hepatic clearance of topiramate by 50–100% with a corresponding decrease in the fraction excreted in the urine *(73)*.

2.7.3.4. EXCRETION

Greater than 50% of an administered dose of topiramate is eliminated unchanged in the urine. The elimination half-life ranges from 15 to 24 h. Clearance of topiramate may be reduced in patients with renal failure *(70)*.

2.7.4. Adverse Reactions

Primary side effects of topiramate are usually related to either the CNS or carbonic anhydrase inhibition (Table 1). CNS side effects are common and patients may become tolerant to them with continued use. These include fatigue, somnolence, dizziness, ataxia, confusion, psychomotor retardation, and difficulty concentrating. Visual disturbances such as diplopia and blurred vision and acute closed-angle glaucoma have also been reported *(74)*.

2. Antiepileptic Drugs

Side effects related to carbonic anhydrase inhibition include paresthesias and nephrolithiasis. Paresthesias are generally mild and transient. Renal stones were reported to occur in 1.5% of patients in premarketing studies but have been less frequent in postmarketing analyses *(70)*.

Two unique side effects have been attributed to topiramate. In contrast to other AEDs, long-term use of topiramate is associated with a decrease in body weight from 1 to 6 kg. This weight loss typically begins within the first 3 mo of therapy and peaks between 12 and 18 mo of use. Higher degrees of weight loss tend to occur in patients with higher pretreatment weight *(70)*.

Lastly, some users of topiramate report difficulty with word finding while talking. This has been attributed to the effects on psychomotor function and is not a specific effect on language or speech *(74)*.

No significant metabolic, hematologic, or hepatic effects have been attributed to the use of topiramate.

2.7.5. Contraindications and Precautions

Topiramate has demonstrated various teratogenic effects in animal models. Postmarketing surveillance has identified select cases of hypospadias in infants born to women taking topiramate alone or in combination with other AEDs during pregnancy. Topiramate is classified in the FDA Pregnancy Category C *(69)*.

Patients with impaired renal function may be at risk of toxicity due to accumulation of topiramate and should be monitored appropriately.

2.7.6. Drug Interactions

Topiramate does not appear to alter the metabolism or elimination of other AEDs. CBZ induces the metabolism of topiramate thus necessitating adjustment of the dosage of topiramate when used concomitantly (Table 2). Other potent enzyme inducing drugs such as phenytoin or phenobarbital may exhibit similar effects. It should also be noted that dose adjustments would be necessary upon discontinuation of an enzyme-inducing drug while continuing the topiramate *(75)*.

2.8. Tiagabine

2.8.1. Chemistry

Tiagabine is a nipecotic acid derivative synthesized by linking nipecotic acid to a lipophilic anchor compound. The addition of this anchor compound facilitates transfer of the nipecotic acid moiety across the blood–brain barrier. Tiagabine is sparingly soluble in water and practically insoluble in most organic solvents. However, it does remain soluble in ethanol *(76)*.

2.8.2. Pharmacology

Tiagabine reduces GABA uptake into presynaptic neurons by inhibiting the GABA transport protein, GAT-1. Inhibiting the reuptake of GABA results in increased extracellular concentrations of GABA and a prolongation of the inhibitory effect of GABA on neurons *(77)*.

2.8.3. Pharmacokinetics

2.8.3.1. ABSORPTION

Tiagabine is readily absorbed with oral bioavailability approaching 90%. Absorption is linear with maximum plasma concentrations occurring between 45 and 90 min after administration in the fasting state and after a mean of 2.6 h when taken with food. Though food may delay the absorption of tiagabine, the extent of absorption is unaffected. It is recommended by the manufacturer that tiagabine be administered with food to avoid side effects associated with high plasma concentrations *(78,79)*.

2.8.3.2. DISTRIBUTION

Tiagabine is highly bound to plasma proteins (96%) and is widely distributed throughout the body. The apparent volume of distribution is 1 L/kg *(78,79)*.

Though no therapeutic range for tiagabine has been established, because of the risk of drug interactions the manufacturer suggests that monitoring concentrations of tiagabine before and after the addition or discontinuation of interacting drugs may be useful *(76)*.

2.8.3.3. METABOLISM

Tiagabine is extensively metabolized in the liver via the CYP3A isozyme system with less than 2% of an administered dose excreted unchanged. The half-life of tiagabine ranges from 5 to 8 hours in patients receiving monotherapy but may be reduced to 2–3 h in patients taking enzyme-inducing medications *(80)*.

2.8.3.4. EXCRETION

Approximately 25% of an administered dose of tiagabine is eliminated in the urine with 40–65% of a dose eliminated in the feces within 3–5 d. This extended elimination may be due to enterohepatic recycling of tiagabine metabolites *(80)*.

2.8.4. Adverse Reactions

Side effects that occur more commonly with tiagabine than placebo include dizziness, asthenia, nervousness, tremor, diarrhea, and depression (Table 1). These side effects are usually mild and transient *(81)*.

More severe side effects such as ataxia, confusion, and itching or rash have been reported although rarely and should resolve upon discontinuation of tiagabine *(81)*.

2.8.5. Contraindications and Precautions

Animal teratogenicity studies demonstrate increased risks of embryo-fetal development abnormalities but no evidence of teratogenicity in humans has been seen. Tiagabine is classified as FDA Pregnancy Category C.

2.8.6. Drug Interactions

Many drugs are known to inhibit or induce the 3A isozyme family of the cytochrome system. The use of drugs that alter metabolism through these isozymes should be expected to alter the metabolism of tiagabine. Plasma concentrations of tiagabine will decrease with the addition of enzyme-inducing drugs such as CBZ and phenytoin whereas concentrations will increase with the addition of enzyme-inhibiting drugs such as cimetidine (Tables 2 and 3; *77*).

Although tiagabine is highly protein bound, plasma concentrations are low enough that significant displacement interactions do not occur.

2.9. Felbamate

2.9.1. Chemistry

Felbamate is a dicarbamate AED with a chemical structure similar to that of meprobamate. Whereas meprobamate incorporates an aliphatic chain at the 2-carbon position, felbamate includes a phenyl group at that position. Felbamate is a lipophilic compound that is only very slightly soluble in water and increasingly soluble in ethanol, methanol, and dimethyl sulfoxide *(82)*.

2.9.2. Pharmacology

Felbamate has a dual mechanism of action, inhibiting excitatory neurotransmission and potentiating inhibitory effects. Felbamate inhibits NMDA-evoked responses in rat hippocampal neurons. In addition, felbamate potentiates the effects of GABA in the same cell line *(83)*. By decreasing the spread of seizures to other neurons and increasing the seizure threshold, felbamate exhibits broad effects on various seizure types.

2.9.3. Pharmacokinetics

2.9.3.1. Absorption

Felbamate is readily absorbed from the gastrointestinal tract. Neither the rate nor the extent of absorption is altered by the presence of food. Greater than 90% of an orally administered dose of felbamate or its metabolites can be recovered in the urine or feces *(82)*.

2.9.3.2. Distribution

Felbamate is approximately 20–25% bound to plasma proteins and this is independent of total concentration. It readily crosses the blood–brain barrier with CSF concentrations nearly equal to plasma concentrations in animal models. No significant displacement of other compounds from protein-binding sites occurs with the use of felbamate *(84)*. The apparent volume of distribution of felbamate is 0.7–1 L/kg.

Though no therapeutic range has been defined for felbamate, it is suggested that concentrations of phenytoin, CBZ, be monitored when used concurrently with felbamate *(85)*.

2.9.3.3. Metabolism

Approximately 50% of an administered dose of felbamate is metabolized in the liver by hydroxylation and conjugation. One metabolite, atropaldehyde, has been implicated in the development of aplastic anemia associated with the use of felbamate. Atropaldehyde has been shown to alkylate proteins, which produces antigens that can generate a dangerous immune response in some individuals. Variations in the metabolism of felbamate as well as detoxification of atropaldehyde make it very difficult to predict which patients may be subject to this dangerous effect *(82)*.

2.9.3.4. Excretion

Urinary excretion of unchanged felbamate accounts for the disposition of 30–50% of an administered dose. This fraction can decrease to 9–22% in patients with renal dysfunction. The apparent half-life of felbamate has been reported to be between 16 and 22 h. This half-life may increase in patients with decreasing renal function *(85)*.

2.9.4. Adverse Reactions

Gastrointestinal upset, headache, anorexia, and weight loss have been reported to occur commonly among patients using felbamate (Table 1). Though most adverse effects will subside over time, anorexia and insomnia are more likely to persist with continued use.

Less common side effects such as diplopia, dizziness, and ataxia have been reported. However, these side effects occur more commonly with polytherapy than monotherapy and may be related to the other medications used, particularly CBZ *(86)*.

Postmarketing surveillance identified an increased risk of the development of aplastic anemia and hepatic failure among users of felbamate. Emerging risk factors for the development of these reactions are history of cytopenia, AED allergy or significant toxicity, viral infection, and/or immunologic problems *(82)*.

2.9.5. Contraindications and Precautions

Cross-sensitivity between felbamate and other carbamate drugs has been demonstrated. Caution is advised when treating a patient with carbamate hypersensitivity with felbamate.

Two known animal carcinogens, ethyl carbamate (urethane) and methyl carbamate, are found in felbamate tablets as a consequence of the manufacturing process. Quantities of these substances have been shown to be inadequate to stimulate tumor development in rats and mice. The implications of this in humans remains unknown *(82,87)*.

Teratogenicity studies in rats and mice revealed decreased rat pup weight and increased mortality during lactation but no effects on fetal development were identified. Felbamate is classified as FDA Pregnancy Category C.

Patients suffering from blood dyscrasias characterized by abnormalities in blood counts, platelet count, or serum iron concentrations should not receive felbamate without close evaluation of the risks and benefits of its use. Similarly, patients with a history of or current bone marrow suppression should not receive felbamate. This would also apply to patients receiving chemotherapy with agents known to cause bone marrow suppression *(82,88)*.

Because of the synthesis of atropaldehyde during felbamate metabolism and subsequent potential for immunologic response, patients with hepatic disease may be at increased risk for exacerbation of their condition *(82)*.

Caution should be exercised when patients with a history of myelosuppression or hematologic toxicity to any medication are prescribed felbamate as these patients may be at increased risk of felbamate-induced hematologic toxicity.

2.9.6. Drug Interactions

Felbamate has been reported to inhibit the metabolism of both phenytoin and valproic acid (Table 2). As felbamate increases the metabolism of CBZ serum concentra-

2. Antiepileptic Drugs

tions decrease whereas epoxide metabolite concentrations increase. Doses of phenytoin, CBZ, and VPA should be decreased by approximately 30% when felbamate is coadministered *(86,89)*.

Enzyme inducers like phenytoin and CBZ can increase the metabolism of felbamate. Felbamate has also been shown to decrease the metabolism of phenobarbital and warfarin (Table 3; *86,89*).

2.10. Vigabatrin

2.10.1. Chemistry

Vigabatrin, γ-vinyl GABA, is a structural analog of GABA. Vigabatrin is a racemic mixture of $R(-)$ and $S(+)$ isomers in equal proportions with no evident optical rotational activity. Although this compound is highly soluble in water, it is only slightly soluble in ethanol or methanol and remains insoluble in hexane or toluene *(90)*.

2.10.2. Pharmacology

Vigabatrin has been shown to effectively increase CNS concentrations of GABA in both animal models and humans with epilepsy in a dose-dependent fashion. Increased concentrations of other markers of GABA concentration (homocarnosine) have also been reported to occur in patients taking vigabatrin. The proposed mechanism by which vigabatrin facilitates these increases is through the inhibition of GABA transaminase, the primary enzyme involved in GABA metabolism. This inhibition occurs in an irreversible manner *(90)*. Therefore, despite a relatively short half-life, vigabatrin can be administered on a once-daily basis.

2.10.3. Pharmacokinetics

2.10.3.1. Absorption

Vigabatrin is readily absorbed from the gastrointestinal tract. Peak concentrations occur within 2 h of oral administration. Oral bioavailability is reported to be approximately 60%. Food has no effect on either the rate or extent of absorption of vigabatrin *(91)*.

2.10.3.2. Distribution

Vigabatrin has an apparent volume of distribution of 0.8 L/kg. There is virtually no binding to plasma proteins. CSF concentrations of vigabatrin are approximately 10% of concentrations in plasma samples. Uniquely, vigabatrin distributes into red blood cells with subsequent red blood cell concentrations approximating 30 to 80% of plasma concentrations *(90,91)*.

2.10.3.3. Metabolism

No human metabolites of vigabatrin have been identified and no therapeutic range has been established *(90,91)*.

2.10.3.4. Excretion

The manufacturer reports that up to 82% of an orally administered dose is recovered unchanged in the urine. The terminal half-life of vigabatrin is approximately 7 h, which can be significantly prolonged in patients with renal dysfunction. Although it has been suggested that doses of vigabatrin be reduced in patients with renal dysfunction, no guidelines in this regard have been published *(90,91)*.

2.10.4. Adverse Reactions

Vigabatrin is well tolerated with sedation and fatigue being the primary adverse effects associated with its use (Table 1). It has been shown to have no effect on cognitive abilities *(90,92)*.

Psychiatric and behavioral effects of vigabatrin have been reported. Agitation, irritability, depression, or psychosis have been reported in up to 5% of patients taking the drug with no prior history of psychosis *(90)*.

The development of visual-field defects has occurred in patients taking vigabatrin. These visual field defects are commonly asymptomatic and appear to be irreversible. The time course of the onset, relationship with dose, influence of other AEDs, and progression of visual-field deficits are unknown. It is suggested that patients treated with vigabatrin undergo visual-field testing regularly during therapy *(90)*.

2.10.5. Contraindications and Precautions

No evidence of carcinogenicity has been demonstrated in animal studies. Serious fetal neurotoxicity has been shown to occur in animal studies and vigabatrin is *not* recommended to be used during pregnancy *(90)*. Vigabatrin is classified as FDA Pregnancy Category D.

Vigabatrin should be used with caution in patients with aggressive tendencies or evidence of psychosis as these patients may be at higher risk for these types of episodes while using vigabatrin *(90,92)*.

Because the risk of accumulation, patients with impaired renal function or a creatinine clearance less than 60 mL/min should be monitored closely for the development of adverse effects *(92)*.

2.10.6. Drug Interactions

Few clinically significant drug interactions have been identified with vigabatrin. Vigabatrin use can increase serum concentrations of phenytoin by as much as 30% although the mechanism of this interaction is unknown (Table 2; *92*).

2.11. Levetiracetam

2.11.1. Chemistry

Levetiracetam is a unique AED that is chemically unrelated to any of the other currently available AEDs. This single *S*-enantiomer pyrrolidine compound is very soluble in water and decreasingly less soluble in chloroform or methanol, ethanol, and acetonitrile, and practically insoluble in n-hexane *(93)*.

2.11.2. Pharmacology

The mechanism of action of levetiracetam is distinct and unrelated to the effects of other AEDs. No evidence supports any effect on voltage-gated Na^+ channels or on GABA or benzodiazepine receptors. Levetiracetam has been shown to bind in a stereo-specific, saturable, and reversible manner to unknown binding sites in the CNS. These binding sites do appear to be confined to synaptic membranes in the CNS and not the

2. Antiepileptic Drugs

peripheral nervous system. Phenylenetetrazole and piracetam can effectively displace levetiracetam from these binding sites whereas there is no effect on binding caused by other antiepileptic drugs, picrotoxin, or bicuculline. Midazolam, a benzodiazepine receptor agonist, has no discernible effect on binding of levetiracetam to synaptic membranes *(94)*.

2.11.3. Pharmacokinetics

2.11.3.1. ABSORPTION

Levetiracetam is readily and completely absorbed after oral administration. Peak concentrations occur within 20–120 min of administration. Clinical studies have shown that although food does not decrease the extent of absorption, it can cause a delay in time to peak concentration by up to 1.5 h and decrease the peak concentration by as much as 20% *(94)*.

2.11.3.2. DISTRIBUTION

The apparent volume of distribution of levetiracetam is 0.7 L/kg. This drug and its metabolites are less than 10% bound to plasma proteins and protein displacement drug interactions are unlikely to occur. There has been no therapeutic range established for levetiracetam *(93,94)*.

2.11.3.3. METABOLISM

Levetiracetam is minimally metabolized in humans via a hydrolysis reaction. This metabolism does not involve hepatic microsomal enzymes and therefore is unlikely to be involved in metabolic drug interactions *(95)*.

2.11.3.4. EXCRETION

Renal excretion of parent drug accounts for 66% of the disposition of an orally administered dose of levetiracetam with an additional 25% of administered dose eliminated renally as metabolites. The elimination half-life is 6–8 h and may be prolonged as much as 2.5 h in elderly subjects due to changes in renal function. In addition, half-life is prolonged in patients with documented renal disease *(95)*.

2.11.4. Adverse Reactions

Common adverse effects of levetiracetam include somnolence, dizziness, asthenia, and fatigue (Table 1). Somnolence has been reported in up to 45% of patients receiving the drug. Coordination difficulties including ataxia, abnormal gait, and incoordination are also more common with levetiracetam than placebo. Behavioral symptoms have also been reported and include reactions such as psychosis, agitation, anxiety, hostility, emotional lability, depression, and others. These adverse effects typically appear early in therapy and may resolve with dose reduction *(93)*.

Little information is available regarding idiosynchratic reactions on hematologic and hepatic systems.

2.11.5. Contraindications and Precautions

Animal studies show that levetiracetam can cause developmental abnormalities at doses near that used in humans (93). Levetiracetam is classified as FDA Pregnancy Category C.

Levetiracetam dose should be reduced in patients with evidence of renal function impairment.

2.11.6. Drug Interactions

Pharmacokinetic studies of levetiracetam indicate that no clinically significant interactions of this sort occur. Levetiracetam neither induces nor inhibits cytochrome P450 isozymes nor does it alter UDP-glucuronidation *(95)*.

2.12. Zonisamide

2.12.1. Chemistry

Zonisamide is a unique AED with a sulfonamide structure. This compound is only moderately soluble in water and 0.1 N HCl *(96)*.

2.12.2. Pharmacology

Zonisamide exhibits antiseizure effects similar to other AEDs. It has been shown to inhibit T-type calcium currents as well as prolonging the inactivation of voltage-gated Na^+ channels, thus inhibiting sustained repetitive firing of neurons. These mechanisms are similar to those of phenytoin and CBZ. In addition, zonisamide may have some minimal carbonic anhydrase inhibitory activity *(94,96)*.

2.12.3. Pharmacokinetics

2.12.3.1. Absorption

Peak serum concentrations occur within 2–6 h of administration of an oral dose of zonisamide. Food may prolong the time to peak concentration (4–6 h) but has no effect on the extent of absorption *(94,96)*.

2.12.3.2. Distribution

Studies indicate that zonisamide is 40 to 50% protein bound. In addition, zonisamide is extensively bound to erythrocytes with erythrocyte concentrations eight times higher than serum concentrations. This binding to erythrocytes is saturable and may result in disproportionate increases in serum concentration with a given change in dose at higher doses. The volume of distribution is reported to be 1.4 L/kg. No therapeutic range has been established *(94,97)*.

2.12.3.3. Metabolism

The primary route of metabolism of zonisamide is reduction to 2-sulfamoylacetyl phenol (SMAP) by the CYP3A4 isozyme system. A minor metabolic route involves hydroxylation and acetylation to 5-N-acetylzonisamide. Zonisamide does not induce its own metabolism *(94,97)*.

2.12.3.4. Excretion

Renal elimination is the primary route for clearance of zonisamide. Thirty-five percent of an administered dose is recovered unchanged whereas the remaining 65% is eliminated in the urine as metabolites. The terminal half-life of zonisamide is 63 h, which may be prolonged in patients with renal or hepatic dysfunction *(94,97)*.

2.12.4. Adverse Reactions

Adverse effects most common with the use of zonisamide include somnolence, dizziness, ataxia, anorexia, headache, nausea, and anger/irritability (Table 1). Other CNS effects include psychomotor slowing, difficulty concentrating, and word-finding difficulties *(94,98)*.

Severe reactions including Stevens-Johnson syndrome, toxic epidermal necrosis, hepatic failure, aplastic anemia, agranulocytosis, and other blood dyscrasias have been reported in patients taking sulfonamides and should be considered potential side effects of zonisamide *(94,98)*.

Oligohydrosis and hyperthermia have been reported to occur in 13 pediatric patients during the first 11 yr of marketing of zonisamide in Japan. Although zonisamide is not approved for pediatric use in the United States, it is important to recognize that oligohydrosis and hyperthermia are potential adverse effects associated with the use of zonisamide *(98)*.

2.12.5. Contraindications and Precautions

Studies in rats and mice have shown teratogenic effects when zonisamide is administered during organogenesis in pregnancy. Embryo lethality has been demonstrated during the treatment of cynomolgus monkeys. Strong caution is advised against the use of zonisamide during pregnancy. Zonisamide is categorized as FDA Pregnancy Category C *(96)*.

Oligohydrosis and hyperthermia were reported to occur in Japanese children treated with zonisamide but has not occurred in Caucasians.

Decreases in clearance will occur in patients with impaired renal function and zonisamide should only be used under close supervision in patients with a glomerular filtration rate of <50 mL/min. In addition, metabolism of zonisamide may be decreased in patients with hepatic dysfunction.

2.12.6. Drug Interactions

Although zonisamide is metabolized via the CYP3A4 isozyme system, it has not been shown to alter the pharmacokinetics of other drugs metabolized through that isozyme. In contrast, CBZ, phenytoin, fosphenytoin, and phenobarbital have been shown to increase the clearance of zonisamide (Table 2). The clinical impact of these interactions are unknown as no therapeutic level for zonisamide has been determined *(94,97)*.

2.13. Conclusion

Epilepsy is a common neurologic condition that affects patients of all ages, although the incidence is higher among the youngest and oldest segments of the population. Historically, antiepileptic drug use has been fraught with complications, some of which are attributable to the many pharmacokinetic drug interactions encountered with this group of medications. In addition to the pharmacokinetic interactions that occur with antiepileptic drugs, clinicians must remain well informed and aware of the possibility of pharmacodynamic interactions that can occur with other medications known to have similar pharmacologic and toxicologic actions.

The close of the 20th century brought several new drugs to market for the treatment of epilepsy. Though each of these new drugs brings promise to the generations of patients that suffer from epilepsy, none is without risk.

REFERENCES

1. Hauser WA. Seizure disorders: the changes with age. Epilepsia 33(Suppl 4):S6–S14 (1992).
2. Hauser WA. The prevalence and incidence of convulsive disorders in children. Epilepsia 35(Suppl 2):S1–S6 (1994).
3. Leppik IE. Contemporary diagnosis and management of the patient with epilepsy, 1st ed. Newtown, PA: Handbooks in Health Care, 1993.
4. Dichter MA. Emerging insights into mechanisms of epilepsy: implications for new antiepileptic drug development. Epilepsia 35(Suppl 4):S51–S57 (1994).
5. Garnett WR. Antiepileptics. In: Schumacher GE, ed. Therapeutic drug monitoring. Norwalk, CT: Appleton & Lange, 1995:345–395.
6. Schmidt D and Haenel F. Therapeutic plasma levels of phenytoin, phenobarbital, and carbamazepine: individual variation in relation to seizure frequency and type. Neurology 34:1252–1255 (1984).
7. Schmidt D, Einicke I, and Haenel F. The influence of seizure type on the efficacy of plasma concentrations of phenytoin, phenobarbital, and carbamazepine. Arch Neurol 43:263–265 (1986).
8. Juul-Jensen P. Frequency of recurrence after discontinuance of anticonvulsant therapy in patients with epileptic seizures: a new follow-up study after 5 years. Epilepsia 9:11–16 (1968).
9. Camfield P and Camfield C. Acute and chronic toxicity of antiepileptic medications: a selective review. Can J Neurol Sci 21:S7–S11 (1994).
10. Bowden CL. Role of newer medications for bipolar disorder. J Clin Psychopharmacol 16: 48S–55S (1996).
11. McNamara JO. Drugs effective in the therapy of the epilepsies. In: Goodman LS, Gilman A, Hardman JG, Limbird LE, and Gilman AG, eds. Goodman & Gilman's the pharmacological basis of therapeutics, 10th ed. New York: McGraw-Hill, 2001:xxvii, 2148.
12. Browne T and LeDuc B. Phenytoin: chemistry and biotransformation. In: Levy RH, Mattson RH, and Meldrum BS, eds. Antiepileptic drugs, 4th ed. New York: Raven Press, 1995: 283–300.
13. Browne TR, Kugler AR, and Eldon MA. Pharmacology and pharmacokinetics of fosphenytoin. Neurology 46:S3–S7 (1996).
14. McLean MJ and Macdonald RL. Multiple actions of phenytoin on mouse spinal cord neurons in cell culture. J Pharmacol Exp Ther 227:779–789 (1983).
15. Treiman D and Woodbury D. Phenytoin: absorption, distribution, and excretion. In: Levy RH, Mattson RH, and Meldrum BS, eds. Antiepileptic drugs, 4th ed. New York: Raven Press, 1995:301–314.
16. Kostenbauder HB, Rapp RP, McGovren JP, Foster TS, Perrier DG, Blacker HM, et al. Bioavailability and single-dose pharmacokinetics of intramuscular phenytoin. Clin Pharmacol Ther 18:449–456 (1975).
17. Vajda F, Williams FM, Davidson S, Falconer MA, and Breckenridge A. Human brain, cerebrospinal fluid, and plasma concentrations of diphenylhydantoin and phenobarbital. Clin Pharmacol Ther 15:597–603 (1974).
18. Wallace S and Brodie MJ. Decreased drug binding in serum from patients with chronic hepatic disease. Eur J Clin Pharmacol 9:429–432 (1976).

2. Antiepileptic Drugs

19. Spielberg SP, Gordon GB, Blake DA, Mellits ED, and Bross DS. Anticonvulsant toxicity in vitro: possible role of arene oxides. J Pharmacol Exp Ther 217:386–389 (1981).
20. Tozer TN and Winter ME. Phenytoin. In: Evans WE, Schentag JJ, and Jusko WJ, eds. Applied pharmacokinetics: principles of therapeutic drug monitoring, 3rd ed. Vancouver, WA: Applied Therapeutics, 1992:25.1–25.44.
21. Kaneko S, Battino D, Andermann E, Wada K, Kan R, Takeda A, et al. Congenital malformations due to antiepileptic drugs. Epilepsy Res 33:145–158 (1999).
22. Mattson RH. Parenteral antiepileptic/anticonvulsant drugs. Neurology 46:S8–S13 (1996).
23. Liponi DF, Winter ME, and Tozer TN. Renal function and therapeutic concentrations of phenytoin. Neurology 34:395–397 (1984).
24. Olsen KM, Hiller FC, Ackerman BH, and McCabe BJ. Effect of enteral feedings on oral phenytoin absorption. Nutr Clin Pract 4:176–178 (1989).
25. Berg MJ, Fincham RW, Ebert BE, and Schottelius DD. Decrease of serum folates in healthy male volunteers taking phenytoin. Epilepsia 29:67–73 (1988).
26. Kutt H. Carbamazepine: chemistry and methods of determination. Adv Neurol 11:249–261 (1975).
27. Grant SM and Faulds D. Oxcarbazepine. A review of its pharmacology and therapeutic potential in epilepsy, trigeminal neuralgia and affective disorders. Drugs 43:873–888 (1992).
28. MacDonald R. Carbamazepine. Mechanisms of action. In: Levy RH, Mattson RH, and Meldrum BS, eds. Antiepileptic drugs, 3rd ed. New York: Raven Press, 1989:447–455.
29. Waldmeier PC, Baumann PA, Wicki P, Feldtrauer JJ, Stierlin C, and Schmutz M. Similar potency of carbamazepine, oxcarbazepine, and lamotrigine in inhibiting the release of glutamate and other neurotransmitters. Neurology 45:1907–1913 (1995).
30. McLean MJ, Schmutz M, Wamil AW, Olpe HR, Portet C, and Feldmann KF. Oxcarbazepine: mechanisms of action. Epilepsia 35(Suppl 3):S5–S9 (1994).
31. Schmutz M, Brugger F, Gentsch C, McLean MJ, and Olpe HR. Oxcarbazepine: preclinical anticonvulsant profile and putative mechanisms of action. [see comments.]. Epilepsia 35 (Suppl 5):S47–S50 (1994).
32. Morselli P. Carbamazepine: absorption, distribution, and excretion. In: Levy RH, ed. Antiepileptic drugs, 3rd ed. New York: Raven Press, 1989:473–490.
33. Meinardi H. CBZ. In: Woodbury DM, Penry JK, and Schmidt RP, eds. Antiepileptic drugs. New York: Raven Press, 1972:487–496.
34. Bell WL, Crawford IL, and Shiu GK. Reduced bioavailability of moisture-exposed carbamazepine resulting in status epilepticus. Epilepsia 34:1102–1104 (1993).
35. Riad LE, Chan KK, Wagner WE Jr, and Sawchuk RJ. Simultaneous first- and zero-order absorption of carbamazepine tablets in humans. J Pharm Sci 75:897–900 (1986).
36. Morselli PL and Frigerio A. Metabolism and pharmacokinetics of carbamazepine. Drug Metab Rev 4:97–113 (1975).
37. Morselli PL, Baruzzi A, Gerna M, Bossi L, and Porta M. Carbamazepine and carbamazepine-10, 11-epoxide concentrations in human brain. Br J Clin Pharmacol 4:535–540 (1977).
38. Wisner KL and Perel JM. Serum levels of valproate and carbamazepine in breastfeeding mother–infant pairs. J Clin Psychopharmacol 18:167–169 (1998).
39. Kerr B and Levy R. Carbamazepine: carbamazepine and carbamazepine-epoxide. In: Levy RH, ed. Antiepileptic drugs, 3rd ed. New York: Raven Press, 1989:505–520.
40. Hundt HK, Aucamp AK, Muller FO, and Potgieter MA. Carbamazepine and its major metabolites in plasma: a summary of eight years of therapeutic drug monitoring. Ther Drug Monit 5:427–435 (1983).
41. Lloyd P, Flesch G, and Dieterle W. Clinical pharmacology and pharmacokinetics of oxcarbazepine. Epilepsia 35(Suppl 3):S10–S13 (1994).

42. Zakrzewska JM and Patsalos PN. Oxcarbazepine: a new drug in the management of intractable trigeminal neuralgia. J Neurol Neurosurg Psychiatry 52:472–476 (1989).
43. Bertilsson L and Tomson T. Clinical pharmacokinetics and pharmacological effects of carbamazepine and carbamazepine-10,11-epoxide. An update. Clin Pharmacokinet 11:177–198 (1986).
44. Bertilsson L, Hojer B, Tybring G, Osterloh J, and Rane A. Autoinduction of carbamazepine metabolism in children examined by a stable isotope technique. Clin Pharmacol Ther 27:83–88 (1980).
45. Bertilsson L, Tomson T, and Tybring G. Pharmacokinetics: time-dependent changes—autoinduction of carbamazepine epoxidation. J Clin Pharmacol 26:459–462 (1986).
46. Konishi T, Naganuma Y, Hongo K, Murakami M, Yamatani M, and Okada T. Carbamazepine-induced skin rash in children with epilepsy. Eur J Pediatr 152:605–608 (1993).
47. Van Amelsvoort T, Bakshi R, Devaux CB, and Schwabe S. Hyponatremia associated with carbamazepine and oxcarbazepine therapy: a review. Epilepsia 35:181–188 (1994).
48. Lander CM and Eadie MJ. Antiepileptic drug intake during pregnancy and malformed offspring. Epilepsy Res 7:77–82 (1990).
49. Messenheimer JA. Lamotrigine. Epilepsia 36(Suppl 2):S87–S94 (1995).
50. Goa KL, Ross SR, and Chrisp P. Lamotrigine. A review of its pharmacological properties and clinical efficacy in epilepsy. Drugs 46:152–176 (1993).
51. Rambeck B and Wolf P. Lamotrigine clinical pharmacokinetics. Clin Pharmacokinet 25:433–443 (1993).
52. Richens A. Safety of lamotrigine. Epilepsia 35(Suppl 5):S37–S40 (1994).
53. Messenheimer J, Mullens EL, Giorgi L, and Young F. Safety review of adult clinical trial experience with lamotrigine. Drug Saf 18:281–296 (1998).
54. Davis R, Peters DH, and McTavish D. Valproic acid. A reappraisal of its pharmacological properties and clinical efficacy in epilepsy. Drugs 47:332–372 (1994).
55. Dreifuss FE, Santilli N, Langer DH, Sweeney KP, Moline KA, and Menander KB. Valproic acid hepatic fatalities: a retrospective review. Neurology 37:379–385 (1987).
56. May RB and Sunder TR. Hematologic manifestations of long-term valproate therapy. Epilepsia 34:1098–1101 (1993).
57. Bjerkedal T, Czeizel A, Goujard J, Kallen B, Mastroiacova P, Nevin N, et al. Valproic acid and spina bifida. Lancet 2:1096 (1982).
58. Pisani F, Narbone M, and Trunfio C. Ethosuximide: chemistry and biotransformation. In: Levy RH, Mattson RH, and Meldrum BS, eds. Antiepileptic drugs, 4th ed. New York: Raven Press, 1995:655–658.
59. Glauser T. Ethosuximide. In: Wyllie E, ed. The treatment of epilepsy: principles and practice, 3rd ed. Baltimore: Williams & Wilkins, 2001:881–891.
60. Horning MG, Brown L, Nowlin J, Lertratanangkoon K, Kellaway P, and Zion TE. Use of saliva in therapeutic drug monitoring. Clin Chem 23:157–164 (1977).
61. Yamamoto T, Pipo JR, Akaboshi S, and Narai S. Forced normalization induced by ethosuximide therapy in a patient with intractable myoclonic epilepsy. Brain Dev 23:62–64 (2001).
62. Gibaldi M. Adverse drug effect-reactive metabolites and idiosyncratic drug reactions: part I. Ann Pharmacother 26:416–421 (1992).
63. Dreifuss F. Ethosuximide: toxicity. In: Levy RH, Mattson RH, and Meldrum BS, eds. Antiepileptic drugs, 4th ed. New York: Raven Press, 1995:675–679.
64. Schmidt B. Potential new antiepileptic drugs: gabapentin. In: Levy RH, Mattson RH, and Meldrum BS, eds. Antiepileptic drugs, 3rd ed. New York: Raven Press, 1989:925–935.
65. Taylor CP, Gee NS, Su TZ, Kocsis JD, Welty DF, Brown JP, et al. A summary of mechanistic hypotheses of gabapentin pharmacology. Epilepsy Res 29:233–249 (1998).

66. McLean MJ. Gabapentin. In: Wyllie E, ed. The treatment of epilepsy: principles and practice, 3rd ed. Philadelphia: Lippincott Williams & Wilkins, 2001:915–932.
67. Wong MO, Eldon MA, Keane WF, Turck D, Bockbrader HN, Underwood BA, et al. Disposition of gabapentin in anuric subjects on hemodialysis. J Clin Pharmacol 35:622–626 (1995).
68. Goa KL and Sorkin EM. Gabapentin. A review of its pharmacological properties and clinical potential in epilepsy. Drugs 46:409–427 (1993).
69. (March 1998). Package insert: topamax. Ortho-McNeil Pharmaceuticals, Raritan, NJ.
70. Privitera M, Ficker D, and Welty T. Topiramate. In: Wyllie E, ed. The treatment of epilepsy: principles and practice, 3rd ed. Philadelphia: Lippincott Williams & Wilkins, 2001:939–945.
71. DeLorenzo RJ, Sombati S, and Coulter D. Effects of topiramate on sustained repetitive firing and spontaneous recurrent seizure discharges in cultured hippocampal neurons. Epilepsia 41(Suppl 1):S40–S44 (2000).
72. Doose DR, Walker SA, Gisclon LG, and Nayak RK. Single-dose pharmacokinetics and effect of food on the bioavailability of topiramate, a novel antiepileptic drug. J Clin Pharmacol 36:884–891 (1996).
73. Sachdeo RC, Sachdeo SK, Walker SA, Kramer LD, Nayak RK, and Doose DR. Steady-state pharmacokinetics of topiramate and carbamazepine in patients with epilepsy during monotherapy and concomitant therapy. Epilepsia 37:774–780 (1996).
74. Walker MC and Sander JW. Topiramate: a new antiepileptic drug for refractory epilepsy. Seizure 5:199–203 (1996).
75. Bourgeois BF. Drug interaction profile of topiramate. Epilepsia 37(Suppl 2):S14–S17 (1996).
76. Schachter S. Tiagabine. In: Wyllie E, ed. The treatment of epilepsy: principles and practice, 3rd ed. Philadelphia: Lippincott Williams & Wilkins, 2001: 930–938.
77. Schachter SC. A review of the antiepileptic drug tiagabine. Clin Neuropharmacol 22:312–317 (1999).
78. Mengel H. Tiagabine. Epilepsia 35(Suppl 5):S81–S84 (1994).
79. Gustavson LE and Mengel HB. Pharmacokinetics of tiagabine, a gamma-aminobutyric acid-uptake inhibitor, in healthy subjects after single and multiple doses. Epilepsia 36: 605–611 (1995).
80. Gustavson LE, Mengel HB. Pharmacokinetics of tiagabine, a gamma-aminobutyric acid-uptake inhibitor, in healthy subjects after single and m ultiple doses. Epilepsia 36(6):605–611 (1995).
81. Leppik IE. Tiagabine: the safety landscape. Epilepsia 36(Suppl 6):S10–S13 (1995).
82. Faught E. Felbamate. In: Wyllie E, ed. The treatment of epilepsy: principles and practice, 3rd ed. Philadelphia: Lippincott Williams & Wilkins, 2001:953–960, 1188.
83. White HS, Wolf HH, Swinyard EA, Skeen GA, and Sofia RD. A neuropharmacological evaluation of felbamate as a novel anticonvulsant. Epilepsia 33:564–572 (1992).
84. Adusumalli VE, Wichmann JK, Kucharczyk N, Kamin M, Sofia RD, French J, et al. Drug concentrations in human brain tissue samples from epileptic patients treated with felbamate. Drug Metab Disp 22:168–170 (1994).
85. Wilensky AJ, Friel PN, Ojemann LM, Kupferberg HJ, and Levy RH. Pharmacokinetics of W-554 (ADD 03055) in epileptic patients. Epilepsia 26:602–606 (1985).
86. Graves NM. Felbamate. Ann Pharmacother 27:1073–1081 (1993).
87. McGee JH, Butler WH, Erikson DJ, and Sofia RD. Oncogenic studies with felbamate (2-phenyl-1,3-propanediol dicarbamate). Toxicol Sci 45:146–151 (1998).
88. Kaufman DW, Kelly JP, Anderson T, Harmon DC, and Shapiro S. Evaluation of case reports of aplastic anemia among patients treated with felbamate. [see comments.]. Epilepsia 38: 1265–1269 (1997).
89. Wagner ML, Remmel RP, Graves NM, and Leppik IE. Effect of felbamate on carbamazepine and its major metabolites. Clin Pharmacol Ther 53:536–543 (1993).

90. Ben-Menachem E. Vigabatrin. In: Wyllie E, ed. The treatment of epilepsy: principles and practice, 3rd ed. Philadelphia: Lippincott Williams & Wilkins, 2001:961–968.
91. Durham SL, Hoke JF, and Chen TM. Pharmacokinetics and metabolism of vigabatrin following a single oral dose of [14C]vigabatrin in healthy male volunteers. Drug Metab Dispos 21:480–484 (1993).
92. Grant SM and Heel RC. Vigabatrin. A review of its pharmacodynamic and pharmacokinetic properties, and therapeutic potential in epilepsy and disorders of motor control. [erratum appears in Drugs 1991 Aug;42(2):330.]. Drugs 41:889–926 (1991).
93. (March 2000). Package insert: keppra. UCB Pharma, Smyrna, GA.
94. Delanty N and French J. Newer antiepileptic drugs. In: Wyllie E, ed. The treatment of epilepsy: principles and practice, 3rd ed. Philadelphia: Lippincott Williams & Wilkins, 2001: 977–983.
95. Patsalos PN. Pharmacokinetic profile of levetiracetam: toward ideal characteristics. Pharmacol Ther 85:77–85 (2000).
96. (May 2000). Package insert: zonegran. Elan pharmaceuticals, San Francisco, CA.
97. Perucca E and Bialer M. The clinical pharmacokinetics of the newer antiepileptic drugs. Focus on topiramate, zonisamide and tiagabine. Clin Pharmacokinet 31:29–46 (1996).
98. Mimaki T. Clinical pharmacology and therapeutic drug monitoring of zonisamide. Ther Drug Monit 20:593–597 (1998).
99. Gidal BE, Garnett WR, and Graves NM. Epilepsy. In: DiPiro JT, ed. Pharmacotherapy: a pathophysiologic approach, 5th ed. New York: McGraw-Hill, 1999:1031–1060.

Chapter 3

Opioids and Opiates

Seyed-Adel Moallem, PharmD, PhD, Kia Balali-Mood, PhD, and Mahdi Balali-Mood, MD, PhD

1. INTRODUCTION

The term opioid applies to any substance, whether endogenous or synthetic, that produces morphine-like effects. Opiates are restricted to synthetic morphine-like drugs with nonpeptidic structure. Opium is an extract of the juice of the poppy *Papaver somniferum*, which has been used socially and medicinally as early as 400 to 300 BC. In the early 1800s, morphine was isolated and in the 1900s its chemical structure was determined. Opium contains many alkaloids related to morphine. Many semisynthetic and fully synthetic compounds have been made and studied. The main groups of drugs include morphine analogs such as oxymorphone, codeine, oxycodone, hydrocodone, heroin (diamorphine), and nalorphine; and the synthetic derivatives such as meperidine, fentanyl, methadone, propoxyphene, butorphanol, pentazocine, and loperamide *(1)*.

2. PHARMACOKINETICS

Some of the pharmacokinetic parameters for opioids are summarized in Table 1 *(1,2)*. Most opioids are readily absorbed from the gastrointestinal tract; they are also absorbed from the nasal mucosa, the lung, and after subcutaneous or intramuscular injection. With most opioids and due to significant but variable first-pass effect, the effect of a given dose is more after parenteral than after oral administration. The enzyme activity responsible for opioid metabolism in the liver varies considerably in different individuals. Thus, the effective oral dose in a particular patient may be difficult to predict.

All opioids bind to plasma proteins with varying affinity. However, the drugs rapidly leave the blood and localize in highest concentrations in tissues that are highly perfused. Brain concentrations of opioids are usually relatively low in comparison to most other organs. In neonates the blood–brain barrier for opioids is effectively lacking.

From: *Handbook of Drug Interactions: A Clinical and Forensic Guide*
A. Mozayani and L. P. Raymon, eds. © Humana Press Inc., Totowa, NJ

Table 1
Pharmacokinetic Parameters and Receptor Subtypes Activity of Some Opioids

Generic Name	Brand Name	Dose (mg)	Administration	Duration of Analgesia (hours)	Addiction/ Abuse Potential	μ	δ	κ
Buprenorphine	Buprenex	0.3	im, iv, sc	4–8	Low	P		—
Butorphanol	Stadol	2	im, iv, Nasal Spray	3–4	Low	P		+++
Codeine		30–60	Oral, sc	3–4	Medium	+	+	
Fentanyl	Sublimaze	0.1	im, iv, Transdermal	1–2	High	+++		
Hydromorphone	Dilaudid	1.5	Oral, sc	4–5	High	+++		+
Mepridine	Demerol	50–100	Oral, im	1–3	High	++		
Methadone	Dolphine	10	Oral, sc	3–5	High	+++		
Morphine	Statex, Kadian	10	Oral, im, iv, sc	4–5	High	+++		+
Naloxone	Narcan	0.4	im, iv	—	—	—	—	—
Oxycodone	Percodan	5	Oral	3–5	Medium	+	+	
Oxymorphone	Numorphan	1–2	im, iv, sc	3–5	High	+++		+
Pentazocine	Talwin	25–50	Oral, im	3–4	Low	P		++
Propoxyphene	Darvon	60–120	Oral	2–4	Low	++		
Tramadol	Ultram	50–100	Oral, im	1–6	Low	+		

+, agonist; —, antagonist; P, partial agonist. Data compiled from various sources.

3. Opioids and Opiates

Because of this, easy transport of opioids through the placenta, and the low conjugating capacity in neonates, opioids used in obstetrics analgesia have a much longer duration of action and can easily cause respiratory depression in neonates *(3)*.

Hepatic metabolism is the main mode of inactivation, usually by conjugation with glucuronide. Esters (e.g., heroin) are rapidly hydrolyzed by common tissue esterases. Heroin is hydrolyzed to monoacetylmorphine and finally to morphine, which is then conjugated with glucuronic acid. These metabolites were originally thought to be inactive, but it is now believed that morphine-6-glucuronide is more active as analgesic than morphine. Accumulation of these active metabolites may occur in patients in renal failure and may lead to prolonged and more profound analgesia even though central nervous system (CNS) entry is limited *(2)*.

Some opioids are also N-demethylated by CYP3A and O-demethylated by CYP2D6 in the liver but these are minor pathways. Codeine, oxycodone, and hydrocodone are converted to metabolites of increased activity by CYP2D6. Genetic variability of CYP2D6 and other CYP isozymes may have clinical consequences in patients taking these compounds. Accumulation of a demethylated metabolite of meperidine, normeperidine, may occur in patients with decreased renal function or those receiving multiple high doses of the drug. In sufficiently high concentrations, the metabolite may cause seizures, especially in children. However, these are exceptions, and opioid metabolism usually results in compounds with little or no pharmacologic activity *(2)*.

Hepatic oxidative metabolism, mainly N-dealkylation by CYP3A4, is the primary route of degradation of the phenylpiperidine opioids (e.g., fentanyl) and eventually leaves only small quantities of the parent compound unchanged for excretion *(2)*.

3. PHARMACODYNAMICS

Morphine and most other opioids elicit a mixture of stimulatory and inhibitory effects, with the major sites of action being the brain and the gastrointestinal tract. Areas of the brain receiving input from the ascending spinal pain-transmitting pathways are rich in opioid receptors.

3.1. Opioid Receptors

Three major classes of opioid receptors have been identified in various nervous system sites and in other tissues. They are mu (μ), delta (δ), and kappa (κ). The newly discovered N/OFQ receptor, initially called the opioid-receptor-like 1 (ORL-1) receptor or "orphan" opioid receptor has added a new dimension to the study of opioids. Each major opioid receptor has a unique anatomical distribution in brain, spinal cord, and the periphery. These distinctive patterns of localization suggest specific possible functions. There is little agreement regarding the exact classification of opioid receptor subtypes. Pharmacological studies have suggested the existence of multiple subtypes of each receptor. Behavioral and pharmacological studies suggested the presence of μ_1 and μ_2 subtypes. The μ_1 site is proposed to be a very high affinity receptor with little discrimination between μ and δ ligands. The data supporting the existing of δ-opioid receptor subtypes are derived mainly from behavioral studies. In the case of κ receptor, numerous reports indicate the presence at least one additional subtype *(3)*.

Table 2
Classification of Opioid Receptors and Their Effects

Functional Effects	μ	δ	κ
Analgesia			
Supraspinal	++	+	+
Spinal	++	++	+
Respiratory depression	+++	+	–
Reduced GI motility	++	+	++
Pupil constriction	+	–	+
Euphoria	+++	–	–
Sedation	++	–	++
Physical dependence	+++	–	–

Opioids show different activities at these receptors (Table 1). Most of the clinically used opioids are relatively selective for μ receptors. It is crucial to note that opioids that are relatively selective at standard doses will interact with additional receptor subtypes when given at sufficiently high doses, leading to possible changes in their pharmacological profile. Classification of opioid receptor subtypes and actions is shown in Table 2 *(2,3)*. Opioid receptors have been cloned and belong to the G protein-coupled family of receptor proteins *(4)*.

3.2. Endorphins

Opioid alkaloids (e.g., morphine) produce analgesia through actions at regions in the brain that contain peptides that have opioid-like pharmacologic properties. The general term currently used for these endogenous substances is *endogenous opioid peptides,* which replaces the other term *endorphin.* There are three families of endogenous opioid peptides. The best-characterized of the opioid peptides possessing analgesic activity are the pentapeptides methionine-enkephalin (met-enkephalin) and leucine-enkephalin (leu-enkephalin), which were the first opioid peptides to be isolated and purified. Leu- and met-enkephalin have slightly higher affinity for the δ than for the μ opioid receptor. Two recently discovered peptides, endomorphin I and endomorphin II, have very high μ receptor selectivity *(2,3)*.

These endogenous peptides are derived by proteolysis from much larger precursor proteins. The principal precursor proteins are prepro-opiomelanocortin (POMC), preproenkephalin (proenkephalin A), and preprodynorphin (proenkephalin B). POMC contains the met-enkephalin sequence, β-endorphin, and several nonopioid peptides, including ACTH, β-lipotropin, and melanocyte-stimulating hormone. Preproenkephalin contains six copies of met-enkephalin and one copy of leu-enkephalin. Preprodynorphin yields several active opioid peptides that contain the leu-enkephalin sequence. These are dynorphin A, dynorphin B, and alpha and beta neoendorphins *(2,3)*.

The endogenous opioid precursor molecules are present at brain sites that have been implicated in pain modulation. Evidence suggests that they can be released during stress such as pain or the anticipation of pain. The precursor peptides are also found in the adrenal medulla and neural plexuses of the gut. Recent studies indicate that several phenanthrene opioids (morphine, codeine) may also be found as endogenous substances

3. Opioids and Opiates 127

at very low (picomolar) concentrations in mammalian tissues; their role at such sites has not been established *(2,3)*.

3.3. Mechanism of Action

Activation of opioids receptors has a number of cellular consequences, including inhibition of adenyl cyclase activity, leading to a reduction in intracellular cAMP concentration. This fall in neuronal cAMP is believed to account mostly for the analgesic effect of opioids.

Opioids vary not only in their receptor specificity, but also in their efficacy at different types of receptors. Some agents act as agonists on one type of receptor and antagonists or partial agonists at another, producing a very complicated pharmacological picture. Most opioids are pure agonists, pentazocine and nalorphine are partial agonists, and naloxone and naltrexone act as antagonists (Table 1).

The opioids have two well-established direct actions on neurons. They either close a voltage-gated Ca^{2+} channel on presynaptic nerve terminals and thereby reduce transmitter release, or they hyperpolarize and thus inhibit postsynaptic neurons by opening K^+ channels *(2–4)*. The presynaptic action (depressed transmitter release) has been demonstrated for release of a large number of neurotransmitters, including acetylcholine, norepinephrine, glutamate, serotonin, and substance P *(2)*.

All three major receptors are present in high concentrations in the dorsal horn of the spinal cord. Receptors are present both on spinal cord pain transmission neurons and on the primary afferents that relay the pain message to them. Opioid agonists inhibit the release of excitatory transmitters from these primary afferents, and they directly inhibit the dorsal horn pain transmission neuron. Thus, opioids exert a powerful analgesic effect directly upon the spinal cord. This spinal action has been exploited clinically by direct application of opioid agonists to the spinal cord, which provides a regional analgesic effect while minimizing the unwanted respiratory depression, nausea and vomiting, and sedation that may occur from the supraspinal actions of systematically administered drugs *(2)*. Different combinations of opioid receptors are found in supraspinal regions implicated in pain transmission and modulation. Of particular importance are opioid-binding sites in pain-modulating descending pathways, including the rostral ventral medulla, the locus ceruleus, and the midbrain periaqueductal gray area. At these sites as at others, opioids directly inhibit neurons, yet neurons that send processes to the spinal cord and inhibit pain transmission neurons are activated by the drugs. In addition, part of the pain-relieving action of exogenous opioids involves the release of endogenous opioid peptides *(2)*.

Clinical use of opioid analgesics consists primarily in balancing the analgesia against adverse side effects. Their depressive effect on neuronal activity, increase in pain threshold, and sedation is often accompanied by euphoria. A summary of opioid pharmacological effects is shown in Table 3 *(1,2)*.

4. OPIOID USE AND ABUSE

4.1. Introduction: The Size of the Problem

Man has used drugs for recreational purposes as long as history itself. Arabic traders smoked opium in the third century BC. In the last 30 yr the number of people

Table 3
Pharmacodynamic Properties of Opioids

Central Nervous System Effects
Suppression of pain; analgesia
Drowsiness and decreased mental alertness; sedation
Respiratory function depression (at the same dose that produce analgesia)
Euphoria
Psychotomimetic effects (nightmares, hallucinations)
Suppression of cough; codeine is used primarily as antitussive
Miosis, mediated by parasympathetic pathways
Nausea and vomiting, by activating the brain stem chemoreceptor trigger zone
Antimuscarinic effects by meperedine

Peripheral Effects
Increased intracranial pressure
Hypotension, if cardiovascular system is stressed
Bradycardia
Decreased peristalsis; constipation
Decreased gastric acid secretion
Inhibition of fluid and electrolyte accumulation in intestinal lumen
Increased tone of intestinal smooth muscle
Increased tone of sphincter of Oddi; increased biliary pressure
Increased tone of detrusor muscle and vesical sphincter
Decreased uterine tone
Stimulation of the release of antidiuretic, prolactine, and somatotropine hormones
Inhibition of luteinizing hormone release
Skin flushing and warming; sweating; itching
Immune system modulation

using recreational drugs, particularly opioids, appears to have increased. By 1997, 25% of the population reported using illicit drugs at some point in their lives and 10% within the last year. In 1999, there were 179,000 treatment admissions for primary-injection drug abuse and 34,000 admissions for secondary-injection drug abuse in the United States. Opiates accounted for 83% of substance abuse treatment admissions for injection drug abuse, followed by methamphetamine/amphetamines (11%) and cocaine (5%). Injection drug admissions of young people aged 15–25 yr old increased between 1992 and 1999. Injection drug users tended to use drugs for many years before entering the substance abuse treatment system. Heroin treatment admission rates between 1993 and 1999 increased by 200% or more in 6 states and by 100–199% in another 11 states. The West and Northeast had the highest heroin treatment admission rates between 1993 and 1999 (Website of National Institute of Drug Abuse, 2001).

There are numerous medical consequences to recreational drug use. Follow-up studies of heroin addicts indicate an annual mortality of 4%. Thus, physicians should consider substance abuse in any unexplained illness. Recent evidence suggests that more than 40% of young people in the UK have tried illicit drugs at some time *(5)*. It is estimated that 9.5% of total mortality in Australians aged 15–39 years can be attrib-

3. *Opioids and Opiates*

uted to regular use of illicit opiates. Australian mortality data for 1992 indicate that approximately 401 male deaths and 161 female deaths occurred as a result of opiate use. This represents some 15,429 and 6261 person-years of life lost to age 70, for males and females, respectively *(6)*. In the UK in 1991, 44 heroin deaths out of 113,620 yields a mortality of 1 in 2582 and 74 methadone deaths of 9880 gives a mortality of 1 in 134. Thus, methadone would appear to be 19 times more toxic than heroin, similar to previous findings in New York. Yet methadone is a manufactured pharmaceutical product, whereas heroin is usually adulterated from the street *(7)*. Although methadone has been used as a maintenance therapy for opiate addicts, several reports on the fatal methadone overdose have been published *(8,9)*. Serious side effects of some opioids such as hydrocodone have been reported. This powerful and potentially addictive painkiller used by millions of Americans is causing rapid hearing loss and even deafness *(10)*. In another report, sublingual buprenorphine caused 20 fatalities in France over a 6-mo period in five urban areas. Buprenorphine and its metabolites were found in postmortem fluids and viscera *(11)*.

4.2. Pathophysiology of Opiate Use

The physiologic effects of opioids are actually the result of interaction between the individual agent and multiple receptors. These interactions exert their primary effects on the central nervous system (CNS) and the respiratory system; however, the other organs particularly the cardiovascular system and the gastrointestinal system may also be affected *(3)*.

4.2.1. Central Nervous System

The CNS effects include analgesia, via altered pain tolerance, sedation, euphoria, and dysphoria. Morphine-like drugs produce analgesia, drowsiness, changes in mood, and mental clouding. A significant feature of the analgesia is that it occurs without loss of consciousness, although drowsiness commonly occurs. Nausea and vomiting are secondary to stimulating the chemoreceptor trigger zone in the medulla. As the dose is increased, the subjective analgesic and toxic effects, including respiratory depression become more pronounced. Morphine does not possess anticonvulsant activity and usually does not cause slurred speech *(12)*.

4.2.2. Respiratory System

Respiratory depression occurs by direct effect on the medullary/respiratory center. The diminished sensitivity at this region results in an elevation of pCO_2 with resultant cerebral vasodilation, increased cerebral perfusion pressure and increased intracranial pressure. Hypoxic stimulation of the chemoreceptors still may be effective when opioids have decreased the responsiveness to CO_2, and the inhalation of O_2 may thus produce apnea *(3)*. In human beings, death from morphine poisoning is nearly always due to respiratory arrest. Therapeutic doses of morphine depress all phases of respiratory activity (rate, minute volume, and tidal exchange) and may also produce irregular and periodic breathing. The diminished respiratory volume is due primarily to a slower rate of breathing *(13)*. Toxic doses may pronounce the aforementioned effects and the respiratory rate may fall even to less than three or four breaths per minute. Although respiratory effects can be documented readily with standard doses of morphine, respiratory depression is rarely a problem clinically in the absence of underlying pulmonary dysfunction. However, the combination of opiates with other medications such as general anesthetics, alcohol, or sedative-hypnotics may present a greater risk of respiratory depression resulting from the synergic effects of these drugs on the respiratory center.

Morphine and related opioids also depress the cough reflex at least in part by a direct effect on a cough center in the medulla. There is no positive relationship between depression of respiration and depression of coughing. Effective antitussive agents such as dextrometorphan do not depress respiration. Suppression of cough by such agents appears to involve the medulla that are less sensitive to naloxone than to the other opioid analgesics *(3)*.

4.2.3. Cardiovascular System

Cardiovascular effects are trivial at therapeutic doses. However, peripheral vasodilation resulting in orthostatic hypertension may occur. Histamine release may contribute to the haemodynamic changes as well as dermal pruritus. Transient bradycardia and hypotension secondary to occasional vasovagal episodes may accompany nausea and vomiting. In supine patients, therapeutic doses of morphine-like opioids have no major effect on blood pressure and cardiac rate and rhythm. Such doses do produce peripheral vasodilation, reduced peripheral resistance, and inhibition of baroreceptor reflexes. When supine patients assume the head-up position, orthostatic hypotension and fainting may occur. The peripheral, arteriolar, and venous dilatation produced by morphine involves several mechanisms. It provokes release of histamine, which sometimes plays a central role in hypotension. However, vasodilation is usually only partially blocked by H_1 antagonists, but is effectively reversed by naloxone. Morphine also attenuates the reflex vasoconstriction caused by increased PCO_2 *(3)*. Myocardial damage and rhabdomyolisis associated with prolonged hypoxic coma, following opiate overdose, has been reported *(14)*.

4.2.4. Gastrointestinal System

Gastrointestinal effects result in gastric motility. Increased antral and proximal duodenal muscle tone results in delayed gastric emptying. This may also contribute to the observed nausea and vomiting. Increased segmental tone and decreased longitudinal peristaltic contractions in the small intestine and colon may result in the common side effect of constipation. Spasm of the Oddi sphincter may also occur with certain narcotics, resulting in symptoms that are characteristic of biliary colic. Morphine and other μ agonists usually decrease the secretion of HCl, although stimulation is sometimes evident. It also diminishes biliary, pancreatic, and intestinal secretions *(15)*. Morphine delays ingestion of food in the small intestine. The upper part of the small intestine, particularly the duodenum, is more affected than the ileum.

4.3. Tolerance and Physical Dependence

Tolerance and dependence are physiological responses seen in all patients and are not predictors of abuse. For example, cancer pain often requires prolonged treatment with high doses of opioids leading to tolerance and dependence, although abuse in this setting is very unusual. Neither the presence of tolerance and dependence nor the

3. Opioids and Opiates

fear that it may develop should interfere with the appropriate use of opioids. Opioids can be discontinued in dependent patients without subjecting them to withdrawal. Suppression of withdrawal requires only minimal doses. Clinically, the dose can be decreased by 50% every several days and eventually stopped, without severe signs and symptoms of withdrawal. However, decreases in dosage may lead to reduction of the degree of pain control. Blockade of glutamate actions by noncompetitive and competitive NMDA antagonists (N-methyl, D-aspartic acid) receptors inhibits morphine tolerance *(16)*. Although the role of the NMDA receptor in the development and expression of opiate tolerance, dependence, and withdrawal is well established in adults, different mechanisms may exist in infants *(17)*.

Nitric oxide production has also been implicated in morphine tolerance, as inhibition of nitric oxide synthesis also blocks morphine tolerance *(18)*. These studies indicate that several important aspects of tolerance and dependence are involved. First, the selective actions of drugs on tolerance and dependence demonstrate that analgesia can be dissociated from these two unwanted actions. Second, the reversal of preexisting tolerance by NMDA antagonists and nitric oxide synthetase inhibitors indicates that tolerance is a balance between activation of processes and reversal of those processes.

The clinical importance of these observations is speculative, but they suggest that in the future, tolerance and dependence in the clinical management of pain can be minimized.

4.4. Clinical Presentations of Opioid Overdose

Opioid overdose may occur in children as accidental or in adults as intentional and rarely as a criminal act. The body packers who present with the leakage of drugs from the packets that are being transported with the gastrointestinal tract, may also be encountered. Opium body packing is a health problem in Iran *(19)*. Overdoses in addicts generally occur in two ways. The first is the user who unknowingly uses a more potent grade of opioid. The second is the uninitiated or abstaining user who had administered a dose beyond his or her perceived tolerance. In both ways, excessive opioid effects are observed and excessive respiratory depression may result. The patient is typically found or presents in an obtused state with worrying degrees of respiratory depression. Diagnosis is usually aided by the presence of miosis and track mark (scarring from prior iv administration) or evidence of skin popping (scarring from prior subcutaneous administration). Positive rapid response to the administration of naloxone is usually confirmatory.

Pediatric patients often present with overdose resulting from access to pain medication or methadone from a family member or other individual in the household. Interpretation of clinical manifestations in this situation is very important as the available history may be very limited or nonexistent, particularly in cases which illicit drugs are involved.

The suicidal patient may present with a mixed picture, resulting from polysubstance ingestion, frequently accompanied by the coingestion of alcohol. History may be more helpful than in the prior scenarios. The patient is frequently accompanied by family members or friends, who confirm the use of medication by the patient or may simply have found pill bottles. Toxic doses of opioids may be difficult to assess in this situation, as tolerance, underlying medical conditions, and the other substances abused play a role in the severity of poisoning. Patients with mild overdose present with slight depression in mental status, miosis, and minimal respiratory depression. Severe overdoses result in the triad of CNS depression, miosis, and respiratory depression. Effects on respiration usually begin with a decrease in respiratory rate whereas the tidal volume is maintained. In more severe overdoses, respiratory arrest may occur. Hypoxia due to respiratory depression is the main cause of most deaths of opioid drugs.

Certain opiates, particularly heroin, can cause a fulminant but rapidly reversible pulmonary edema. Noncardiogenic pulmonary edema (NCPE) has been described as the most frequent complication of heroin overdose, observed in up to 48% of the patients *(20)*. In contrast, a later study reported that NCPE was diagnosed in only 2.4% of patients presenting to the emergency departments *(21)*. The wide range may be reflective of numerous factors including changes in heroin purity and methods of administration. Pneumonia, the next leading of complication of heroin overdose (up to 30%), may also play a role in this discrepancy *(22)*.

The etiology of heroin-induced NCPE in heroin overdose remains unclear but may include a hypersensitivity reaction, an acute hypoxemia-induced capillary vasoconstriction resulting in increased hydrostatic pressure or capillary injury, secondary to the drug, or adultery *(23)*. NCPE is characterized by tachypnea, tachycardia, hypoxia, and rales on auscultation. Pulmonary capillary wedged pressure is typically normal. Laboratory abnormalities include respiratory acidosis and hypoxia. Radiographic evaluation usually demonstrates bilateral patchy infiltrates. Onset may occur from minutes to several hours after heroin use. Prior review indicates that onset maybe delayed as much as 24 h after heroin administration *(24)*, whereas a further study reported a much earlier onset *(20)*. Methadone and other opiates have also been linked to NCPE, although its occurrence is uncommon *(25,26)*.

Other complications from opioid overdose include seizures most often attributed to propoxifen *(27,28)*, or meperidine overdose *(29)*. Heroin also appears to be a potential causative agent *(30)*. The mechanism for opioid-induced seizures is not totally clear. However, two distinct causes have been postulated based on therapy with opioid antagonists. Although seizures from heroin, morphine, and propoxifen overdoses have been treated successfully with naloxone, animal studies indicate that naloxone will lower seizure threshold in meperidine overdoses. The toxic metabolite normeperidine has been implicated in cases involving meperidine *(31,32)*.

Cardiac conduction disturbances have also been reported and are primarily attributed to propoxifen and its metabolites *(33,34)*.

4.5. Diagnosis of Opioid Overdose

Diagnosis of opioid overdose should be based initially on history and clinical presentation. Additional laboratory analyses are useful particularly in the iv drug users who may have additional underlying conditions or complications. Drug screens of mixed utility depend on the information being obtained and the time frame in which results will be available to guide the clinical management of the patient. In patients with specific signs such as miosis, CNS and respiratory depression, particularly in severe poisoning with coma and respiratory insufficiency, iv administration of naloxone is a good diagnostic tool.

3. *Opioids and Opiates*   133

Situations involving poly substance usage maybe less straightforward, but clinical judgment and supportive measures are usually employed before receiving results of a toxic screen. However, in complicated cases opioid screens as well as other CNS depressants screening could be beneficial. Screening techniques must be able to detect parent compounds and their active metabolites in serum or urine. Urine drug screens can provide a qualitative method to detect many opioids, including propoxyphene, codeine, methadone, meperidine, and morphine. Screens for fentanyl and its derivatives are usually negative. Quantitative results on opiates from serum are not helpful in the routine management of overdoses. The serum drug screen maybe helpful in detecting the presence of agent other than opiates, such as acetaminophen that may require its specific antidote (N-acetyl cystein) therapy.

4.6. Management of Opioid Overdose

Management of opioid overdoses focuses on stabilization. Initial assessment and establishment of effective ventilation and oxygenation followed by ensuring adequate homodynamic support are followed. Initial support with a bag-valve-mask (BVM) is appropriate along with 100% oxygen supplementation. Oral or nasal airway placement may be required and in fact is vital in comatose patients. However, caution is advised with their use, to prevent vomiting and or aspiration. Suction apparatus should be available for immediate use at the patient's bedside. Ventilatory support can usually be provided with a BVM device while awaiting the reversal of respiratory depression by an opioid antagonist.

Endotracheal intubation is indicated in severely compromised patients in whom there is a real risk in aspiration or in patients who do not respond satisfactory to opioid antagonists. Treatment of NCPE will require 100% oxygen therapy with positive end expiratory pressure (PEEP), if necessary, to reverse hypoxia. Diuretics and digoxin have no role in treatment of NCPE. The options for opioid antagonists include naloxone, naltrexone, and the longer acting antagonist nalmefene *(35,36)*. This pure opiate antagonist with great affinity to μ receptors should be titrated according to the severity of poisoning.

Naloxone remains the drug of choice as the initial reversal agent in suspected opioid overdose, given its short half-life and ability to titrate for the effect. The need for immediate results (usually in the form of increased ventilation) is balanced by the potential unpleasant of inducing withdrawal symptoms in the chronic abuser. In the patient who presents with respiratory arrest, precipitation of some acute withdrawal symptoms may be unavoidable. To minimize this risk, naloxone should be given in small increments, titrated to the response. Naloxone can be administered iv, im, sc, endotracheally, or intralingually *(37–39)*.

Naloxone dose is based on the severity of poisoning. It generally ranges from 0.4 to 2.0 mg iv in the adult patient. For respiratory depression or arrest, 2 mg iv is suggested initially, to be repeated 2–5 min (or sooner if the patient is indeed in respiratory arrest) up to 10 mg. If no response is observed after 10 mg of naloxone, it is unlikely that opioids by themselves are playing a significant role in the patient's clinical status. Certain opiate overdoses such as codeine, propoxifen, pentazocine, methadone, and diphenoxylate may require repetitive or continuous administration. In cases of leaked opium body packing, repetitive or continuous naloxone administration is needed.

Nalmefene may provide an alternative to naloxone infusion, given its longer half-life (4–8 h) compared to (1 h) with naloxone *(36)*. Initial dose of 0.5 mg nalmefene iv reverses respiratory depression in the adult patients. A repeat dose of 1.0 mg can be given 2–5 min later if necessary.

The current recommendation for pediatric dosing of naloxone is 0.1 mg/kg given iv *(40)*. Continuous iv injection of naloxone (0.4–0.5 mg/h for 2.5–4 d) in two patients (aged 3 d to 1 yr) was also applied *(41)*.

Decontamination is generally reserved for opioid agents taken orally. Opiates cause decreased gastric emptying and pylorospasm. This decrease in gastrointestinal motility suggests that there may be some benefit to gastrointestinal emptying several hours after ingestion. Gastric aspiration and lavage is affected in debulking large amounts of ingestant; it may also be beneficial with smaller amounts of ingestant due to delayed gastric motility in the obtuse patient. Endotracheal intubation should be performed prior to the placement of orogastric or nasogastric tubes, to protect against aspiration in comatose patients. Activated charcoal and cathartics (magnesium citrate or sorbitol) should be administered after gastric emptying if bowel sounds are present. The initial dose of activated charcoal is 1.0 g/kg by mouth or per nasogastric tube. Repetitive dosing of activated charcoal may be beneficial in cases in which large amounts of ingestant such as body packers are suspected.

Muscle rigidity, though possible after all narcotics, appears to be more common after administration of bolus doses of fentanyl or its congeners. Rigidity can be treated with depolarizing or nondepolarizing neuromuscular blocking agents while controlling the patient's ventilation *(3)*.

Since the half-life of naloxone is short but the half-life of most opioids is long, the patients must not be discharged after recovery unless no signs of intoxication particularly CNS depression are found 24 h after cessation of naloxone therapy.

5. Drug Interactions

Opiates and opioids have a wide range of pharmacological and toxicological interactions with many classes of drugs. The pharmacological interactions can be divided into pharmacokinetics and pharmacodynamics.

5.1. Pharmacokinetic Interactions

5.1.1. Food

Oral morphine in sustained-release form (Oramorph SR) and morphine sulfate in a continuous preparation (MST continus) taken by 24 healthy male volunteers in a four-way crossover study revealed significant higher C_{max}, T_{max}, and AUC_{0-24} following high-fat breakfast than the fasting subjects *(42)*. In a randomized crossover study in 22 normal male and female subjects, it was revealed that oxycodone in sustained-release form had no significant interactions with food intake. However, both bioavailability and C_{max} were significantly altered by high-fat meal after taking immediate-release form of oxycodone *(43)*. It was shown that food has no effect on the pharmacokinetics of morphine following doses of immediate-release solution and the modified-release preparations. However, the lack of bioequivalence between some of the formulations sug-

3. Opioids and Opiates

gests that care should be taken by physicians in changes of modified-release formulations *(44)*. For morphine sulfate and dextrometorphan combination (MorphiDex) in a single-dose double-blind study in patients suffered from postoperation pain, food reduced C_{max}, but not the extent of absorption *(45)*. In another study with a new sustained-release form of tramadol in 24 healthy volunteers, food had no significant effects on the pharmacokinetics of the drug *(46)*.

5.1.2. Drug Absorption and Bioavailability

5.1.2.1. MORPHINE AND METOCLOPRAMIDE

Metoclopramide increases the rate of absorption of oral morphine and exacerbates its sedative effects. Ten mg of metoclopramide markedly increased the extent and speed of sedation due to a 20-mg oral dose of morphine over a period of 3–4 h in 20 patients undergoing surgery. Peak serum morphine concentrations and the total absorption remained unaltered. Metoclopramide increases the rate of gastric emptying so that the rate of morphine absorption from the small intestine is increased. An alternative idea is that both drugs act additively on opiate receptors to increase sedation *(47)*.

5.1.2.2. CODEINE AND SALICYLATE-CONTAINING HERBS

It has been suggested by some authorities that since salicylate-containing herbs can selectively precipitate some alkaloids, high doses of these herbs may impair the absorption of codeine *(48)*.

5.1.2.3. MORPHINE AND TRICYCLIC ANTIDEPRESSANTS

The bioavailability and the degree of analgesia of oral morphine are increased by the concurrent use of clomipramine, desipramine, and possibly amitriptyline. Clomipramine or amitriptyline in daily doses of 20–50 mg increased the area under the curve (AUC) of oral morphine by amounts ranging from 28 to 111% in 24 patients being treated for cancer pain. The half-life of morphine was also prolonged *(49)*. A previous study *(50)* found that desipramine but not amitriptyline increased and prolonged morphine analgesia and a later study by the same group *(51)* confirmed the value of desipramine. The reasons are not understood. The increased analgesia may be a result of not only the increase of serum/morphine concentrations but possibly also some alterations in the morphine receptors. Acute administration of clomipramine potentiates morphine analgesia in mice whereas chronic administration attenuates them *(52)*.

5.1.2.4. MORPHINE AND TROVAFLOXACIN

Coadministration of trovafloxacin and morphine in 19 healthy volunteers reduced the bioavailability and C_{max} of trovafloxacin but the effects were not significant *(53)*.

5.1.2.5. CODEINE AND IBUPROFEN

Relative bioavailabilities of ibuprofen and codeine in 24 healthy volunteers revealed no significant interactions *(54)*.

5.1.2.6. METHADONE AND ANTI-HIV DRUGS

Interactions between methadone and some HIV-related medications are known to occur, yet their characteristics cannot reliably be predicted based on current understandings of metabolic enzyme induction and inhibition, or through in vitro studies *(55)*.

Nevertheless, it has been shown that methadone elevates Zidovudine's serum concentration, increasing the risk of side effects *(56)*. In 17 study subjects using drugs for HIV and stable methadone therapy, methadone reduced the AUC of didanosine by 63%, suggesting larger doses of didanosine are required for these patients *(57)*.

5.1.2.7. METHADONE AND ANTICONVULSANTS

Classic anticonvulsant drugs, such as phenytoin, carbamazepine, and phenobarbital, produce dramatic decreases in methadone levels, which may precipitate a withdrawal syndrome; valproic acid and the new anticonvulsant drugs do not have these effects *(58,59)*.

5.1.3. Metabolism

Opioid interaction on drug metabolism that reported are mostly in vitro or in experimental studies. The interactions may occur by induction or inhibition of drug metabolism.

5.1.3.1. MORPHINE AND ALCOHOL

The respiratory depressant effect of morphine is significantly increased by alcohol. The use of morphine in patients who are intoxicated with alcohol is especially dangerous and even small doses can be fatal when there is a high concentration in the blood *(15)*. Loss of tolerance and concomitant use of alcohol and other CNS depressants, particularly morphine and its derivatives, clearly play a major role in fatality. However, age, gender, and other risk factors do not account for the strong age and gender patterns observed among victims of overdose. There is evidence that systemic diseases particularly pulmonary and hepatic disorders may be more prevalent in users who are at greater risk of overdose. There is no effective role for opiate mediation in ethanol intake as well as any ethanol sweet-fluid intake interactions *(60)*. Both ethanol and opioids are metabolized in part by the hepatic mixed enzyme oxidative system. When both drugs are used together, slower disposal rates and possibly higher toxicity may arise. Ethanol may affect some opiate receptors and possibly change the brain tissue endogenous opiate peptide levels in some loci. Mixed alcohol and opiate abusers did poorly in standard alcohol abstinence treatment compared to matched alcoholics without opiate abuse histories *(61)*.

5.1.3.2. MORPHINE AND RIFAMPIN

Rifampin significantly reduced the peak plasma morphine concentration and AUC and the analgesic effect of morphine in 10 healthy volunteers on a double-blind placebo-controlled study. It has been found that rifampin was found to reduce morphine's analgesic effects, probably due to the induction of its metabolism *(62)*.

5.1.3.3. MORPHINE AND CIMETIDINE

Respiratory depression, potentially fatal, occurred in patients receiving cimetidine with morphine or opium and methadone *(63)*. Decreased metabolism of morphine is the probable mechanism.

5.1.3.4. METHADONE AND ANTIDEPRESSANTS

Important pharmacokinetic interactions may occur between methadone and antidepressant drugs. Desipramine plasma levels are increased by methadone. Furthermore, fluvoxamine (and fluoxetine to a less extent) may cause an important increase in serum methadone concentrations *(64)*. In patients unable to maintain effective methadone blood level throughout the dosing interval, fluvoxamine can help increase the methadone blood level and alleviate opiate withdrawal symptoms *(65)*. The inhibition of different clusters of the cytochrome P450 system is involved in these interactions.

5.1.3.5. CODEINE AND QUINIDINE

Patients who lack CYP2D6 or whose CYP2D6 is inhibited by quinidine will not benefit from codeine *(66)*. Quinidine-induced inhibition of codeine O-demethylation is ethnically dependent with the reduction being greater in Caucasians *(67)*.

5.1.3.6. METHADONE AND CIPROFLOXACIN

Recent reports suggest a significant drug interaction between ciprofloxacin and methadone. Ciprofloxacin may inhibit cytochrome P450 3A4 up to 65%, thus elevating methadone levels significantly *(68)*.

5.1.3.7. PROPOXYPHENE AND CARBAMAZEPINE

Since propoxyphene inhibits hepatic metabolism of carbamazepine, decreased clearance of carbamazepine may result in its increased serum concentration and toxicity *(69)*.

5.1.4. Elimination

5.1.4.1. MORPHINE AND ORAL CONTRACEPTIVES

Clearance of morphine is approximately doubled by the concurrent use of oral contraceptives. The clearance of intravenous morphine (1 mg) was increased by 75%, oral morphine (10 mg) by 120% in six young women taking an oral contraceptive *(70)*. This implies that the dosage of morphine will need to be virtually doubled to achieve the same degree of analgesia. Urinary morphine concentration will then be greater in patients taking oral contraceptives.

5.1.4.2. MEPERIDINE AND PHENYTOIN

Meperidine systemic clearance rose from 1017 ± 225 mL/min to 1280 ± 130 mL/min during phenytoin dosing ($p < 0.01$) *(71)*.

5.1.4.3. MORPHINE AND 5-FLUROURACIL

The plasma clearance rate of 5-fluoro uracil (5FU) in mice is significantly reduced by concomitant use of morphine. The effects of morphine are due to reduced hepatic elimination of 5FU rather than to a decrease in its renal excretion *(72)*.

5.1.4.4. MORPHINE AND GENTAMICIN

Morphine administration significantly reduced the dose of infused gentamicin needed to achieve the critical lethal plasma level *(73)*.

5.1.4.5. METHADONE AND URINARY ACIDIFIERS

Several studies have shown that patients with a high clearance rate of methadone also have a low urine pH (1–3). In a study, the administration of ammonium chloride and sodium carbonate over 3 d each resulted in a mean methadone elimination half-life of 19.5 h, compared with 42.1 h following sodium carbonate *(74)*. This is because of increased methadone ionization and thus clearance.

5.1.4.6. Fentanyl (or Alfentanil) and Propofol

Although clinically the hypnotic effect of propofol is enhanced by analgesic concentrations of µ-agonist opioids (e.g., fentanyl), the bispectral index does not show this increased hypnotic effect *(75)*. It was shown that haemodynamic changes induced by propofol may have an important influence on the pharmacokinetics of alfentanil *(76)*.

5.2. Pharmacodynamic Interaction

5.2.1. Sedative-Hypnotics-Antipsychotics

5.2.1.1. Morphine and Barbiturates

Secobarbital increases the respiratory depressant effects of morphine, whereas diazepam appears not to interact in this way. In 30 normal subjects, it was found that quinalbarbitone and morphine depressed ventilation when given alone. However, a combination of quinalbarbitone and morphine resulted in a much greater and more prolonged depression. Other respiratory depressant drugs such as narcotics, opiates, and analgesics can also have additive effects *(77)*. In one study, it was found that fentanyl and alfentanil pretreatment have also reduced the dose of thiopental required for anesthesia induction *(78)*.

5.2.1.2. Morphine and Phenothiazines

Phenothiazines potentiate the depressant effects of morphine on the CNS, particularly with respect to respiration. Also, the simultaneous administration of morphine and phenothiazines can result in significant hypotension *(15)*.

5.2.1.3. Morphine and Benzodiazepines

The depressant effects of morphine on respiration are significantly greater if the patient is simultaneously taking benzodiazepines *(15)*. Alprazolam mediated analgesic effects, most probably via a µ opiate mechanism of action *(79)*.

5.2.1.4. Methadone and Psychoactive Agents

Psychoactive medication is frequently used in methadone maintenance treatment programs (MMP) to treat comorbid mental disorders (depression, anxiety, schizophrenia) in opiate addicts. Thus, several pharmacological interactions are possible. This problem becomes more relevant with the introduction of new CNS drugs like SSRI (serotonin selective reuptake inhibitor), atypical antipsychotics, or new anticonvulsants. For instance, sertaline increases the plasma methadone concentration significantly in depressed patients on methadone *(80)*. The most common interactions seen in practice are pharmacodynamic in nature, most often due to the cumulative effects of different drugs on the CNS (e.g., neuroleptics or benzodiazepine interactions). Several lines of evidence suggest that benzodiazepines and methadone may have synergistic interactions and that opiate sedation or respiratory depression could be increased. This is a serious problem, given the widespread use of benzodiazepines among MMP patients. Experimental but not clinical data support methadone and lithium interactions.

3. Opioids and Opiates

Accordingly, caution is advised in the clinical use of methadone when other CNS drugs are administered.

5.2.1.5. MEPERIDINE AND PHENOTHIAZINES

Although uncontrolled observations have supported concurrent administration of these agents to minimize narcotic dosage and control nausea and vomiting, serious side effects may outweigh the benefits. In a study, meperidine and chlorpromazine compared to meperidine and placebo resulted in significantly increased lethargy and hypotension *(81)*.

5.2.2. CNS Stimulants

Dexamphetamine and methylphenidate increase the analgesic effects of morphine and reduce some of its side effects such as respiratory depression and sedation. It seems there would be advantages in using two drugs in combination. D-amphetamine potentiates the effects of di-acetyl morphine (heroin). Opiate abusers use amphetamines to increase the effects obtained from poor quality heroin *(82)*.

5.2.3. Hallucinating Agents

5.2.3.1. OPIOIDS AND CANNABINOIDS

Cannabinoids and opioids share the same pharmacological properties and to a lesser extent in drug reinforcement. Braida and coworkers demonstrated that cannabinoids produce reward in conditioned place preference tests and interconnection of opioid and cannabinoid systems *(83)*. Functional interaction between opiate and cannabinoid system exists at immune level that differs form the interaction present in the CNS *(84)*. SR141716A, a CB1 receptor antagonist, significantly reduced the intensity of naloxone-induced opiate withdrawal in tolerant rats. SR141716A could be of some interest in ameliorating opiate withdrawal syndrome *(85)*. Maternal exposure to delta-p tetra hydro cannabinol (THC) has the potential effects of motivational properties in female adult rats, as measured by an intravenous opiate self-administration paradigm *(86)*.

5.2.3.2. OPIOIDS AND COCAINE

Enadolin, a selective and high efficacy κ agonist, and butorphanol, a mixed agonist with intermediate efficacy at both μ and κ receptors, failed to modify cocaine self-administration in humans *(87)*.

5.2.3.3. NALOXONE AND LYSERGIC ACID DIETHYLAMINE (LSD)

Naloxone attenuated haloucigenic effects of LSD and may subserve the development of tolerance to morphine-like drugs *(88)*.

5.2.4. Endocrine Drugs

Thyrotropin-releasing hormone (TRH) and related compounds appear to (a) antagonize hypothermia, respiratory depression, locomotor depression, and catalepsy but not the analgesia induced by opiates, (b) inhibit the development of tolerance to the analgesic effects but not to the hypothermic effects of opiate, (c) inhibit the development of physical dependence of opiates as evidenced by the inhibition of development of certain withdrawal syndromes, and (d) suppress the abstinence syndrome in opiate dependent rodents. TRH does not interact with the opiate receptors in the brain.

Potential therapeutic application of TRH and its synthetic analogs can be used in counteracting some of the undesirable effects of opiates *(89)*. Possible common mode of action of adrenocorticotropic hormone (ACTH) interaction with opiate agonist and antagonists that are dependent on time of the day and stress intensity have been reviewed *(90)*.

5.2.5. Muscle Relaxants

Patients recovering from relaxant anaesthesia are especially vulnerable to the respiratory depressant effects of morphine. Respiratory acidosis, secondary to acute hypercapnia, can result in reactivation of the long-acting relaxant on the completion of anesthesia, resulting in further depression of respiration. The combination of muscle relaxant and morphine could result in a rapidly progressing respiratory crisis *(15)*. Morphine and $GABA_B$ agonists (e.g., baclofen) shared the same mechanism of action and thus in combination with morphine tend to induce higher analgesic response in mice *(91)*.

5.2.6. Adrenergic Drugs

Agmatin (an endogenous polyamine metabolite formed by the carboxylation of L-arginine) potentiates antinociception of morphine via an $alpha_2$ adrenergic receptor-mediated mechanism. This combination may be an effective therapeutic strategy for the medical treatment of pain *(92)*. Yohimbine (an $alpha_2$ antagonist) tends to limit opiate antinociception and the additive potential of µ and delta opioid agonists *(93)*.

Clonidine (4 and 10 µg/kg) in cats had a differential degree of inhibition in the order of analgesia, much greater than hypotension, greater than bradycardia. Naloxone (0.4 and 1.0 mg/kg) failed essentially to antagonize these effects, suggesting the lack of involvement of the opiate receptors of endogenous opioids in these processes. Furthermore, pain suppression of clonidine appeared to be independent of vasodepression and cardio inhibition *(94)*. Clonidine did not affect the pain when administered with iv placebo. When administered with pentazocine, clonidine caused a statistically significant increase in pentazocine analgesia *(95)*. Clonidine induced dose- and time-dependent suprasensitivity to norepinephrine, similar to that produced by morphine. Thus, clonidine and morphine possess comparable properties on the antagonism of chronic morphine tolerance; and this maybe the therapeutic basis for clonidine's clinical application in the treatment of opiate addicts *(96)*.

5.2.7. Heroin and Alcohol

There have been numerous reports of the enhancement of acute toxicity and fatal outcome of overdose of heroin by ethanol. Losses of tolerance and concomitant use of alcohol and other CNS depressants clearly play a major role in fatality; however, such risk factors do not account for the strong age and gender patterns observed consistently among victims of overdose. There is evidence that systemic disease may be more prevalent in users at greatest risk of overdose. It is suggested that pulmonary and hepatic dysfunction resulting from such disease may increase susceptibility to both fatal and nonfatal overdose *(97)*. In one study, at all ranges of free-morphine concentrations, there was a greater percentage of heroin deaths when ethanol was present *(98)*. Toxicological evidence of infrequent heroin use was more common in decedents with blood ethanol concentration greater than 1 µg/mL than in those with lower concentrations *(99)*.

3. Opioids and Opiates

**Table 4
Drug Interactions of Some Opioids**

Object Drug(s)	Precipitant Drug(s)	Interaction	Ref.
Morphine	MAO Inhibitors	Increased effects of Morphine; anxiety, confusion, respiratory depression, coma	15
Morphine, Loperamide	Quinidine	Increased toxicity of opiates	104,105
Morphine, Methadone	Hexoses	Reduction in potency ratio of objects drugs	106
Morphine	Fluoxetine	Fluoxetine attenuated morphine analgesia but not pentazocine	107
Narcotics	Maternal tobacco smoking	Fatal intrauterine growth retardation	108
Morphine	Ginseng	Ginseng inhibited the analgesic activity, tolerance to and dependence on morphine	109
Buprenorphine	Naloxone	Low abuse potential; opiate withdrawal symptoms	110,111
Morphine, Cocaine	Buprenorphine	Buprenorphine significantly reduced both opiate and cocaine abuse	112
Yohimbine	Naltrexone	Altered sensitivity to yohimbine	113
Pentazocine	Amitriptyline	respiratory depression may be increased by their concomitant use	114
Codeine	Glutethimide	Specific concentrations of each drug in most cases were in the high therapeutic range, suggesting a possible toxic synergistic effect	115
Meperidine	Isoniazid	Isoniazid inhibits monoamine oxidase causing hypotensive episode or CNS depression	116

5.2.8. Genotoxic Damage and Immunosuppression

Opiate addicts have higher chromosome damage and sister chromatid exchange frequencies. Opiates diminish DNA repair and reduce immunoresponsivness as measured by T-cell E-rosetting and other assays. These interactions of opiates with T lymphocytes may regulate metabolism and could thereby be responsible for the sensitivity of cells from opiate addicts to both genotoxic damage and immunological effects *(100)*.

More drug interactions of some opioids are presented in Table 4.

6. POSTMORTEM EXAMINATIONS

The diagnosis of death due to opiates or opioids is based on the following:

1. Examination of the scene where the body is found.
2. Investigation of the circumstances.
3. History obtained from friends and relations.
4. Autopsy examination.
5. Toxicological evidence.

Before attributing death due to narcotism purely on the basis of circumstantial evidence, it is essential to exclude other natural or unnatural causes of death such as spontaneous intracranial hemorrhage, occult subdural hemorrhage, or evidence of non-narcotic drugs.

6.1. Postmortem Appearances

The appearances could be divided into external and internal:

1. External: the smell of opium may be present. The face is deeply cyanosed, almost black. The fingernails are blue. The veins are engorged and distended in the neck. The postmortem lividity is intense, almost black, and is better seen in a fair-skinned body. The pupils may be contracted or dilated. There is froth at the mouth and nose, but neither so fine nor as copious as in drowning.
2. Internal: the stomach may show the presence of small, soft, brownish lumps of opium and the smell of drug may be perceived. It disappears with the onset of putrefaction. The internal organs, especially the trachea, bronchi, lungs, and brain, exhibit a marked degree of venous congestion. In addition, the trachea and bronchi are covered with froth and the lungs are edematous. The blood is usually dark and fluid.

Associated with edema of the lungs, the intense lividity of the face almost approaching to blackness should make one suspicious of opium poisoning as the cause of death. Such intense lividity is seldom seen in any other condition *(101)*.

At autopsy of an individual who has died of an overdose of heroin, the lungs are heavy and show congestion, though the classic pulmonary edema mentioned in some of the other textbooks is not always present. Microscopic examination of the lungs commonly reveals foreign-body granulomas with talc crystals and cotton fibers. Samples of the venous blood, urine, stomach and contents, liver, and in some circumstances, additional samples such as bile, cerebrospinal fluid and vitreous humor, kidney, and brain, may be taken. When the drug has been injected, an ellipse of skin around the injection mark extending down through the subcutaneous tissue to the muscle should be excised, along with control area of skin from another noninjected site *(102)*.

6.2. Toxicological Analyses

Various analytical methods for the estimation of morphine and its derivatives have been reported. The most reliable methods are gas chromatography–mass spectrometry and radioimmunoassay. Blood and urine as well as the other samples such as gastric contents and the organ tissue extracts may be analyzed. In order to identify a certain opiate or opioid, a highly specific method should be used to determine the parent drug as well as the metabolites. For instance, if both morphine and monoacetylmorphine are detected in the blood, then, the individual took heroin.

Plasma concentrations of some opiates such as methadone correlated well with the intake doses. Plasma methadone concentration appears to increase by 263 ng/mL for every mg of methadone consumed per kilogram of body weight *(103)*.

6.3. Interpretation of the Results

Interpretation of the results of toxicological analyses is very important in both clinical and forensic toxicology. History of drug use and abuse, overdose, and clinical and postmortem findings should be considered for the evaluation and interpretation of the results.

As with all deaths from toxic substances, the interpretation of analytical results may present considerable difficulties. There might be a long delay between the intake of a drug and death, during which time the blood, urine, and even tissue levels may decline, or even disappear. Many drugs break down rapidly in the body and their metabolites may be the only recognizable products of their administration. In some cases, data on lethal blood levels may be imperfectly known and great variations in personal susceptibility may make the range of concentrations found in a series of deaths so wide as to be rather unhelpful.

If a person dies rapidly after the first episode of taking a normal dose of a drug, because of some ill-understood personal idiosyncrasy, the quantitative analysis may not assist.

Where habituation and tolerance has developed, drug users may have concentrations in their body fluids and tissues far higher than lethal levels published for nondependence. In general, the great usefulness of toxicological analysis is both qualitative and quantitative. The qualitative tests will show what drugs have been taken in the recent past; the length of time that drugs or their metabolites persist in different fluids and tissues varies widely.

The quantitative analysis can be useful, especially when the results reveal high levels—into the toxic or lethal ranges. These ranges are usually obtained anecdotally from surveys of large number of deaths but, as stated, can differ in terms of minimum and maximum values from different laboratories. Interaction of other drugs and alcohol or both, delayed death, and abnormal sensitivity are other problems that should be considered. Thus, the analysis is not the final arbiter of the cause of death, although it is a highly important component of the whole range of investigations *(102)*.

REFERENCES

1. Herz A. Handbook of experimental pharmacology vol. 104: Opioids. Berlin: Springer-Verlag, 1993.
2. Way WL, Fields HL, and Schumacher MA. Opioid analgesics & antagonists. In: Katzung BG, ed. Basic and clinical pharmacology. New York: McGraw-Hill, 2001:512–531.
3. Gutstein HB and Akil H. Opioid analgesics. In: Hardman JG and Limbird LE, eds. Goodman & Gilman's the pharmacological basis of therapeutics. New York: McGraw-Hill, 2001: 569–619.
4. Akil H, Owens C, Gutstein H, Taylon L, Curran E, and Watson S. Endogenous opioids: overview and current issues. Drug Alcohol Depend 51:127–140 (1998).
5. Crowe AV, Howse M, Bell GM, and Henry JA. Substance abuse and the kidney. Q J Med 93:147–152 (2000).
6. Hulse GK, English DR, Milne E, and Holman CD. The quantification of mortality resulting from the regular use of illicit opiates. Addiction 94:221–229 (1999).
7. Marks J. Deaths from methadone and heroin. Lancet 343:976 (1994).
8. Hendra TJ, Gerrish SP, and Forrest ARW. Fatal methadone overdose. Br Med J 313:481–482 (1996).
9. Nanji AA and Filipenko JD. Rhabdomyolisis and acute myoglobinuric renal failure associated with methadone intoxication. J Toxicol Clin Toxicol 20:353–360 (1983).
10. Friedman RA, House JW, Luxford WM, Gherini S, and Mills D. Profound hearing loss associated with hydrocodone/acetaminophen abuse. Am J Otol 21:188–191 (2000).

11. Tracqui A, Kintz P, and Ludes B. Buprenorphine-related deaths among drug addicts in France: a report on 20 fatalities. J Anal Toxicol 22:430–434 (1998).
12. Yaksh TL. CNS mechanisms of pain and analgesia. Cancer Surv 7:55–67 (1988).
13. Martin WR. Pharmacology of opioids. Pharmacol Rev 35:283–323 (1983).
14. Melandri R, Re G, Lanzarini C, Rapezzi C, Leone O, Zele I, and Rocchi G. Myocardial damage and rhabdomyolisis associated with prolonged hypoxic coma, following opiate overdose. J Toxicol Clin Toxicol 34:199–203 (1996).
15. Dollery C. Therapeutic drugs. Edinburgh: Churchill Livingston, 1999:231–233.
16. Elliott K, Minami N, Kolesnikov YA, Pasternak GW, and Inturrisi CE. The NMDA receptor antagonists, LY274614 and MK801, and the nitric oxide synthase inhibitor, NG-nitro-L-arginine, attenuate analgesic tolerance to the μ-opioid morphine but not to kappa opioids. Pain 56:69–75 (1994).
17. Zhu H and Barr GA. Opiate withdrawal during development: are NMDA receptors indispensable? Trends Pharmacol Sci 22:404–408 (2001).
18. Kolesnikov YA, Pick CG, Ciszewska G, and Pasternak GW. Blockade of tolerance to morphine but not kappa opioids by a nitric oxide synthase inhibitor. Proc Natl Acad Sci USA 90:5162–5166 (1993).
19. Balali-Mood M. Opium body packing in Mashhad, Iran. J Toxicol Clin Toxicol 38:177–178 (2000).
20. Duberstein JL and Kaufman DM. A clinical study of an epidemic of heroin intoxication and heroin induced pulmonary edema. Am J Med 51:704–714 (1971).
21. Smith DA, Leake L, Loflin JR, and Yealy DM. Is admission after intravenous heroin dose necessary? Ann Emerg Med 21:1326–1330 (1992).
22. Maurer PM and Bartkowski RR. Drug interactions of clinical significance with opioid analgesics. Drug Saf 8:30–48 (1993).
23. Wang ML, Lin JL, Liaw SJ, and Bullard MJ. Heroin lung: report of two cases. J Formos Med Assoc 93:170–172 (1994).
24. Steinberg AD and Karliner J. The clinical spectrum of heroin pulmonary edema. Arch Intern Med 122:122–127 (1968).
25. Kjeldgaard JM, Hahn GW, Heckenlively JR, and Genton E. Methadone-induced pulmonary edema. JAMA 218:882–883 (1971).
26. Persky VW and Goldfrank LR. Methadone overdoses in a New York City hospital. J Am Coll Emerg Phys 65:111–113 (1976).
27. Lovejoy FH, Mitchell AA, and Goldman PG. The management of propoxyphene poisoning. Pediatr 85:98–100 (1974).
28. Carson DJL and Carson ED. Fatal dextropropoxyphene poisoning in Northern Ireland. Lancet 1:894–897 (1977).
29. Clark RF, Wei EM, and Anderson PO. Meperidine: therapeutic use and toxicity. J Emerg Med 13:797–802 (1995).
30. Ng SK, Brust JC, Hauser WA, and Susser M. Illicit drug use and the risk of new-onset seizures. Am J Epidemiol 132:47–57 (1990).
31. Mauro VF, Bonfiglio MF, and Spunt AL. Meperidine-induced seizures in a patient without renal dysfunction or sickle cell anemia. Clin Pharmacol 5:837–839 (1986).
32. Bonfiglio MF and Mauro VF. Naloxone in the treatment of meperidine induced seizures. Drug Intell Clin Pharmacother 2:174–175 (1987).
33. Nickander R, Smits SE, and Steinberg MI. Propoxyphene and norpropoxyphene: pharmacologic and toxic effects in animals. J Pharmacol Exp Ther 200:245–253 (1977).
34. Holland DR and Steinberg MI. Electrophysiologic properties of propoxyphene and norpropoxyphene in canine conductive tissue in vitro and in vivo. J Pharmacol Exp Ther 47:123–133 (1979).

35. Kaplan JL and Marx JA. Effectiveness and safety of intravenous nalmefene for emergency department patients with suspected narcotic overdose: a pilot study. Ann Emerg Med 22: 187–190 (1993).
36. Glass PS, Jhaveri RM, and Smith LR. Comparison of potency and duration of action nalmefene and naloxone. Anesth Analg 78:536–541 (1994).
37. Martin WR. Naloxone. Ann Intern Med 85:765–768 (1976).
38. Greenberg MI. The use of endotracheal medication in cardiac emergencies. Resuscitation 12:155–165 (1984).
39. Maio RF, Gaukel B, and Freeman B. Intralingual naloxone injection for narcotic-induced respiratory depression. Ann Emerg Med 16:572–573 (1987).
40. Kauffman RE, Banner W Jr, and Blumer JL. Naloxone dosage and route of administration for infants and children. Pediatr 86:484–485 (1990).
41. Tenenbein M. Continous naloxone infusion for opiate poisoning in infancy. J Pediatr 105: 645–648 (1984).
42. Drake J, Kirkpatrick CT, Aliyar CA, Crawford FE, Gibson P, and Horth CE. Effect of food on the comparative pharmacokinetics of modified-release morphine tablet formulations: Oramorph SR and MST Continus. Br J Clin Pharmacol 41:417–420 (1996).
43. Benziger DP, Kaiko RF, Miotto JB, Fitzmartin RD, Reder RF, and Chasin M. Differential effects of food on the bioavailability of controlled-release oxycodone tablets and immediate-release oxycodone solution. J Pharm Sci 85:407–410 (1996).
44. Gourlay GK. Sustained relief of chronic pain. Pharmacokinetics of sustained release morphine. Clin Pharmacokinet 35:173–190 (1998).
45. Caruso FS. MorphiDex pharmacokinetic studies and single-dose analgesic efficacy studies in patients with postoperative pain. J Pain Symptom Manage 19:S31–S36 (2000).
46. Raber M, Schulz HU, Schurer M, Bias-Imhoff U, and Momberger H. Pharmacokinetic properties of tramadol sustained release capsules. 2nd communication: investigation of relative bioavailability and food interaction. Arzneimittelforschung 49:588–593 (1999).
47. Manara AR, Shelley MP, Quinn K, and Park GR. The effect of metoclopramide on the absorption of oral controlled release morphine. Br J Clin Pharmacol 25:518–521 (1988).
48. Brinker F. Interactions of pharmaceutical and botanical medicines. J Naturopathic Med 7: 14–20 (1997).
49. Ventafridda V, Ripamonti C, De Conno F, Bianchi M, Pazzuconi F, and Panerai AE. Antidepressants increase bioavailability of morphine in cancer patients. Lancet 1:1204 (1987).
50. Levine JD, Gordon NC, Smith R, and McBryde R. Desipramine enhances opiate postoperative analgesia. Pain 27:45–49 (1986).
51. Gordon NC, Heller PH, Gear RW, and Levine JD. Temporal factors in the enhancement of morphine analgesia by desipramine. Pain 53:273–276 (1993).
52. Fialip J, Marty H, Makambila MC, Civiale MA, and Eschalier A. Pharmacokinetic patterns of repeated administration of antidepressants in animals. II. Their relevance in a study of the influence of clomipramine on morphine analgesia in mice. J Pharmacol Exp Ther 248: 747–751 (1989).
53. Vincent J, Hunt T, Teng R, Robarge L, Willavize SA, and Friedman HL. The pharmacokinetic effects of coadministration of morphine and trovafloxacin in healthy subjects. Am J Surg 176:32S–38S (1988).
54. Laneury JP, Duchene P, and Hirt P. Comparative bioavailability study of codeine and ibuprofen after administration of the two products alone or in association to 24 healthy volunteers. Eur J Drug Metab Pharmacokinet 23:185–189 (1998).
55. Gourepitch MN and Friedland GH. Interactions between methadone and medications used to treat HIV infection: a review. Mt Sinai J Med 67:429–436 (2000).

56. Schwartz EL, Brechbuhl AB, Kahl P, Miller MA, Selwyn PA, and Friedland GH. Pharmacokinetic interactions of zidovudine and methadone in intravenous drug-using patients with HIV infection. J Acquir Immune Defic Syndr 5:619–626 (1992).
57. Rainey PM, Friedland G, and McCance-Katz EF. Interaction of methadone with didanosine and stavudine. J Acquir Immune Defic Syndr 24:241–248 (2000).
58. Tong TG, Rond SM, Kreek MJ, Jaffery NF, and Benowitz NL. Phenytoin-induced methadone withdrawal. Ann Int Med 94:349–351 (1981).
59. Bell J, Seres V, Bowron P, Lewis J, and Batey R. The use of serum methadone levels in patients receiving methadone maintenance. Clin Pharmacol Ther 43:623–629 (1988).
60. Goodwin FL, Campisi M, Babinska I, and Amit Z. Effects of naltrexone on the intake of ethanol and flavored solutions in rats. Alcohol 25:9–19 (2001).
61. Cushman P Jr. Alcohol and opioids: possible interactions of clinical importance. Adv Alcohol Subst Abuse 6:33–46 (1987).
62. Fromm MF, Eckhardt K, and Li S. Loss of analgesic effect of morphine due to coadministration of rifampin. Pain 72:261–267 (1997).
63. Sorkin EM and Darvey DL. Review of cimetidine drug interactions. Drug Intell Clin Pharm 17:110–120 (1983).
64. Bertschy G, Baumann P, Eap CB, and Baettig D. Probable metabolic interaction between methadone and fluvoxamine in addict patients. Ther Drug Monit 16:42–45 (1994).
65. De Maria PA and Serota RD. A therapeutic use of methadone fluvoxamine drug interaction. J Addict Dis 18:5–12 (1999).
66. Caraco Y, Sheller J, and Wood AJ. Pharmacogenetic determination of the effects of codeine and prediction of drug interactions. J Pharmacol Exp Ther 278:1165–1174 (1996).
67. Caraco Y, Sheller J, and Wood AJ. Impact of ethnic origin and quinidine coadministration on codeine's disposition and pharmacodynamic effects. J Pharmacol Exp Ther 290: 413–422 (1999).
68. Herr K, Segerdahi M, Gustafsson LL, and Kalso E. Methadone, ciprofloxacine and adverse drug reactions. Lancet 356:2069–2070 (2000).
69. Oles KS, Mirza W, and Penry JK. Catastrophic neurologic signs due to drug interaction: Tegretol and Darvon. Surg Neurol 32:144–151 (1989).
70. Watson KJR, Ghabrial H, Mashford ML, Harman PJ, Breen KJ, and Desmond PV. The oral contraceptive pill increases morphine clearance but does not increase hepatic blood flow. Gastroenterol 90:1779 (1986).
71. Pond SM and Kretschzmar KM. Effect of phenytoin on meperidine clearance and normeperidine formation. Clin Pharmacol Ther 30:680–686 (1981).
72. Li Y, Looney GA, Kimler BF, and Hurwitz A. Opiate effects on 5-fluorouracil disposition in mice. Cancer Chemother Pharmacol 39:273–277 (1997).
73. Hurwitz A, Garty M, and Ben Zvi Z. Morphine effects on gentamicin disposition and toxicity in mice. Toxicol Appl Pharmacol 93:413–420 (1988).
74. Nilsson MI, Widerlov E, Meresaar U, and Anggard E. Effect of urinary pH on the disposition of methadone in man. Eur J Clin Pharmacol 22:337–342 (1982).
75. Lysakowski C, Dumont L, Pellegrini M, Clergue F, and Tassonyi E. Effects of fentanyl, alfentanil, remifentanil and sufentanil on loss of consciousness and bispectral index during propofol induction of anaesthesia. Br J Anaesth 86:523–527 (2001).
76. Mertens MJ, Vuyk J, Olofsen E, Bovill JG, and Burm AG. Propofol alters the pharmacokinetics of alfentanil in healthy male volunteers. Anesthesiology 94:949–957 (2001).
77. Zsigmond EK and Flynn K. Effect of secobarbital and morphine on aterial blood gases in healthy human volunteers. J Clin Pharmacol 33:453–457 (1993).

78. Dundee JW, Halliday NJ, McMurray TJ, and Harper KW. Pretreatment with opioids. The effect on thiopentone induction requirements and on the onset of action of midazolam. Anaesthesia 41:159–161 (1986).
79. Pick CG. Antinociceptive interaction between alprazolam and opioids. Brain Res Bull 42: 239–243 (1997).
80. Hamilton SP, Nunes EV, Janal M, and Weber L. The effect of sertraline on methadone plasma levels in methadone-maintenance patients. Am J Addict 9:63–69 (2000).
81. Stambaugh JE Jr and Wainer IW. Drug interaction: meperidine and chlorpromazine, a toxic combination. J Clin Pharmacol 21:140–146 (1981).
82. Gaiardi M, Bartoletti M, Gubellini C, Bacchi A, and Babbini M. Modulation of the stimulus effects of morphine by d-amphetamine. Pharmacol Biochem Behav 59:249–253 (1998).
83. Braida D, Pozzi M, Cavallini R, and Sala M. Conditioned place preference induced by the cannabinoid agonist CP 55,940: interaction with the opioid system. Neuroscience 104: 923–926 (2001).
84. Massi P, Vaccani A, Romorini S, and Parolaro D. Comparative characterization in the rat of the interaction between cannabinoids and opiates for their immunosuppressive and analgesic effects. J Neuroimmunol 117:116–124 (2001).
85. Rubino T, Massi P, Vigano D, Fuzio D, and Parolaro D. Long-term treatment with SR141716A, the CB1 receptor antagonist, influences morphine withdrawal syndrome. Life Sci 66:2213–2219 (2000).
86. Ambrosio E, Martin S, Garcia-Lecumberri C, and Crespo JA. The neurobiology of cannabinoid dependence: sex differences and potential interactions between cannabinoid and opioid systems. Life Sci 65:687–694 (1999).
87. Walsh SL, Geter-Douglas B, Strain EC, and Bigelow GE. Enadoline and butorphanol: evaluation of kappa-agonists on cocaine pharmacodynamics and cocaine self-administration in humans. J Pharmacol Exp Ther 299:147–158 (2001).
88. Hadorn DC, Anistranski JA, and Connor JD. Influence of naloxone on the effects of LSD in monkeys. Neuroharmacol 23:1297–1300 (1984).
89. Bhargava HN, Yousif DJ, and Matwyshyn GA. Interactions of thyrotropin releasing hormone, its metabolites and analogues with endogenous and exogenous opiates. Gen Pharmacol 14:565–570 (1983).
90. Galina ZH and Amit Z. Interactions between ACTH, morphine, and naloxone and their effects on locomotor behavior. Prog Neuropsychopharmacol Biol Psych 9:691–695 (1985).
91. Zarrindast MR and Mahmoudi M. GABA mechanisms and antinociception in mice with ligated sciatic nerve. Pharmacol Toxicol 89:79–84 (2001).
92. Yesilyurt O and Uzbay IT. Agmatine potentiates the analgesic effect of morphine by an alpha(2)-adrenoceptor-mediated mechanism in mice. Neuropsychopharmacol 25:98–103 (2001).
93. Morales L, Perez-Garcia C, and Alguacil LF. Effects of yohimbine on the antinociceptive and place conditioning effects of opioid agonists in rodents. Br J Pharmacol 133:172–178 (2001).
94. Chan SH. Differential effects of clonidine on pain, arterial blood pressure, and heart rate in the cat: lack of interactions with naloxone. Exp Neurol 84:338–346 (1984).
95. Gordon NC, Heller PH, and Levine JD. Enhancement of pentazocine analgesia by clonidine. Pain 48:167–169 (1992).
96. Ramaswamy S, Pillai NP, Gopalakrishnan V, and Ghosh MN. Effect of clonidine on the chronic morphine tolerance and on the sensitivity of the smooth muscles in mice. Life Sci 33:1167–1172 (1983).

97. Warner-Smith M, Darke S, Lynskey M, and Hall W. Heroin overdose: causes and consequences. Addiction 96:1113–1125 (2001).
98. Levine B, Green D, and Smialek JE. The role of ethanol in heroin deaths. J Forensic Sci 40:808–810 (1995).
99. Ruttenber AJ, Kalter HD, and Santinga P. The role of ethanol abuse in the etiology of heroin-related death. J Forensic Sci 35:891–900 (1990).
100. Shafer DA, Falek A, Donahoe RM, and Madden JJ. Biogenetic effects of opiates. Int J Addict 25:1–18 (1990).
101. Parkin S. Somniferous poisons. In: Parkin S, ed. Parkin's textbook of medical jurisprodence and toxicology. Edinburgh: Livingstone, 1990:834–846.
102. Knight B. Deaths from narcotic and hallucinogenic drugs. In: Knight B, ed. Forensic Pathology. London: Arnold, 1996:568–570.
103. Schonwald S. Opiates. In: Schonwald S, ed. Medical toxicology—A synopsis and study guides. London: Williams and Wilkins, 2001:201–230.
104. Thompson SJ, Koszdin K, and Bernards CM. Opiate-induced analgesia is increased and prolonged in mice lacking P-glycoprotein. Anesthesiology 92:1392–1399 (2000).
105. Sadeque AJ, Wandel C, He H, Shah S, and Wood AJ. Increased drug delivery to the brain by P-glycoprotein inhibition. Clin Pharmacol Ther 68:231–237 (2000).
106. Brase DA, Ward CR, Bey PS, and Dewey WL. Antagonism of the morphine-induced locomotor activation of mice by fructose: comparison with other opiates and sugars, and sugar effects on brain morphine. Life Sci 49:723–734 (1991).
107. Gordon NC, Heller PH, Gear RW, and Levine JD. Interactions between fluoxetine and opiate analgesia for postoperative dental pain. Pain 58:85–88 (1994).
108. Sastry BV. Placental toxicology: tobacco smoke, abused drugs, multiple chemical interactions, and placental function. Reprod Fertil Dev 3:355–372 (1991).
109. Takahashi M and Tokuyama S. Pharmacological and physiological effects of ginseng on actions induced by opioids and psychostimulants. Methods Find Exp Clin Pharmacol 20:77–84 (1998).
110. Mendelson J, Jones RT, Fernandez I, Welm S, Melby AK, and Bagott MJ. Buprenorphine and naloxone interactions in opiate-dependent volunteers. Clin Pharmacol Ther 60:105–114 (1996).
111. Mendelson J, Jones RT, Welm S, Brow J, and Batki SL. Buprenorphine and naloxone interactions in methadone maintenance patients. Biol Psychiatry 4:1095–1101 (1997).
112. Mello NK, Mendelson JH, Lukas SE, Gastfriend DR, Teoh SK, and Holman BL. Buprenorphine treatment of opiate and cocaine abuse: clinical and preclinical studies. Harv Rev Psychiatry 1:168–183 (1993).
113. Rosen MI, Kosten TR, and Kreek MJ. The effects of naltroxone maintenance on the responses to yohimbine in healthy volunteers. Biol Psychiatry 45:1636–1645 (1999).
114. Savarialho-Kerc U, Mattila MJ, and Seppala T. Parenteral pentazocine: effects on psychomotor skills and respirations with amitryptiline. Eur J Clin Pharmacol 35:483–489 (1988).
115. Havier RG and Lin R. Deaths as a result of a combination of codeine and glutethimide. J Forensic Sci 30:563–566 (1985).
116. Gannon R, Pearsall W, and Rowley R. Isoniazid, meperidine, and hypotension. Ann Intern Med 99:415 (1983).

Chapter 4

Monoamine Oxidase Inhibitors and Tricyclic Antidepressants

Terry J. Danielson, PhD

1. INTRODUCTION

Depression is a disorder consisting, in varying degrees, of low mood, pessimism, lethargy, and loss of interest in former pleasures. Treatment of this disability frequently involves the use of drugs such as monoamine oxidase inhibitors (MAOIs), tricyclic antidepressants (TCAs), and, more recently, selective serotonin reuptake inhibitors (SSRIs). These drugs have multiple pharmacological and toxicological properties and are capable of producing severe effects independent of the antidepressant response.

In recent years the SSRIs have become a frequent choice in the pharmacological management of depressive illness because of the comparative infrequency and mildness of side effects during their use. For many years, the TCAs were the drugs of common choice, along with the MAOIs, in treatment of depressive illness and have long established their clinical efficacy, and a population does exist among well-managed, long-term patients or individuals unresponsive to other drugs for whom the TCAs or MAOIs remain the drugs of choice. Practitioners may also prefer these substances because of familiarity with their use and pharmacological actions *(1–3)*. The MAOIs and TCAs remain in use for treatment of refractive patients and the TCAs, in particular, remain frequent visitors to the toxicology laboratory.

This chapter will focus on the toxicological properties of the MAOIs and the TCAs. SSRIs are discussed only to the extent of their effects on the metabolism of the TCAs and their involvement in the "serotonin syndrome" associated with their combined administration with the MAOIs or certain of the TCAs. A more detailed discussion of the toxicological properties and drug interactions of the SSRIs is presented in an accompanying chapter.

From: *Handbook of Drug Interactions: A Clinical and Forensic Guide*
A. Mozayani and L. P. Raymon, eds. © Humana Press Inc., Totowa, NJ

2. Monoamine Oxidase Inhibitors

MAOI drugs evolved from the observation that patients treated with the antitubercular substance, iproniazid, often experienced elevated moods. Although the occurrence of hepatotoxicity reduced the clinical application of iproniazid, other MAOIs such as tranylcypromine (2-phenylcyclopropylamine, Parnate) and phenelzine (2-phenylethylhydrazine, Nardil), and more recently moclobemide are not hepatotoxic and have been widely applied in the treatment of depressive illness. In general, the MAOIs were seen to be less hazardous than the TCAs, particularly in patients with suicidal ideation.

As their name implies, the MAOIs reduce the activity of monoamine oxidase enzymes A and B, which degrade monoamine substrates such as dopamine, noradrenalin, and serotonin. Reduced degradation of monoamines after treatment with an MAOI is thought to increase the amount of available transmitter and thereby alter mood. In addition, tranylcypromine and phenelzine have been shown to increase transmitter release and to inhibit reuptake (4)

Deaths as a result of acute overdose with an MAOI are uncommon and amounts in blood in these instances are generally very much higher than the normal clinical range (5–7). The more commonly observed toxicological dangers associated with the MAOIs are, in many respects, extensions of the mechanism by which they produce their antidepressant effect. The two forms of MAO are distributed unequally throughout the tissues of the body. MAO-A is more prevalent in the central nervous system (CNS) and inhibition of this enzyme has been associated with the antidepressant response. MAO-B, on the other hand, is not associated with the antidepressant response and is more common in hepatic and intestinal tissue where it serves as a barrier to dietary sympathomimetic amines, such as tyramine, phenylethylamine, and tryptamine. On entry into the body, these simple amines promote release of noradrenalin in the peripheral nervous system and are capable of causing severe hypertensive crisis. Deactivation of intestinal and hepatic MAO-B enzymes effectively eliminates the barrier to these amines and places the patient at risk.

Food interactions with the nonselective MAOI are therefore common and life threatening and patients treated with MAOI drugs, such as tranylcypromine or phenelzine, must avoid amine-rich foods, such as chocolate, red wines, lager beers, and fermented cheeses and soy products (8,9).

Modern MAOI drugs have been developed to take advantage of the different distributions and substrate specificities of the MAO enzymes. Moclobemide is one example of an effective antidepressant that is highly selective toward MAO-A enzymes and, because of this selectivity, differs very significantly in its toxicological profile from the nonselective inhibitors (10–12). Therefore, due to inhibition of intestinal and hepatic MAO-B enzymes, nonselective inhibitors such as tranylcypromine and phenelzine increase the pressor response to oral tyramine more than do selective MAO-A inhibitors (13). Moclobemide is also considered reversible and regeneration of MAO-A activity occurs within days after withdrawal, in comparison to the several weeks required after tranylcypromine or phenelzine. Selective MAO-A inhibitors, like moclobemide, are therefore felt to be less prone to enhancement of the pressor response to sympathomimetic amines found in food. These comparisons also illustrate the fact that MAO inhibition by the traditional, nonselective MAOI is long term and dietary restrictions can apply for weeks after stopping the medication. Clinicians and patients need to be aware of the serious interactions that can occur during the interval between discontinuance of the drug and the return of MAO activity.

Interactions have also been reported with other amines, such as ephedrine. This amine is not a substrate for MAO enzymes and both moclobemide and nonselective inhibitors will enhance its pressor response *(14)*. In another instance *(15)*, 24 h after discontinuing phenelzine, a patient ingested a tablet containing ephedrine, caffeine, and theophylline. Eight hours later, she developed encephalopathy, neuromuscular irritability, hypotension, sinus tachycardia, rhabdomylosis and hyperthermia.

Combinations of MAOI, TCA, and/or SSRI have been employed in treatment of unresponsive depressed patients *(16–18)*. In most instances combined treatment is uneventful and very often is successful. However, combinations of an MAOI with an SSRI, or with a TCA having serotonin reuptake blocking activity, may result in a "serotonin syndrome" with a severe or fatal outcome *(19–23)*. Features of this syndrome might not develop until 6–12 h after overdose and include hyperpyrexia, disseminated intravascular coagulation, convulsions, coma, and muscle rigidity *(19)*. It bears reemphasis that the critical issue of this interaction is that it occurs between agents that act in concert to increase the amount of free serotonin. Therefore, because of the potential for severe toxicity, patients must follow a well-defined dosing regimen, be carefully monitored, and be informed of the immediate need for medical intervention should side effects occur. The serotonin syndrome has been observed subsequent to combined exposures to an MAOI plus a neuroleptic *(24)*, an SSRI *(25,26)*, or a TCA *(27,28)*.

Concurrent administration of MAOIs and narcotic analgesics has also been a cause of concern *(21)*. This phenomenon has been reviewed by Stack et al. *(29)* and Browne et al. *(30)*, who concluded that the most frequent and most serious interaction was between a nonselective, irreversible MAOI, such as phenelzine and meperidine. They also noted that the interaction with meperidine is of two distinct forms, excitatory and depressive. Meperidine has been demonstrated to inhibit the neuronal reuptake of serotonin and, like the SSRIs, can provoke an excitatory serotonin syndrome response when coadministered with an MAOI. Meperidine is the only commonly used narcotic analgesic reported to have elicited this excitatory response, which occurs in approximately 20% of patients treated with this drug combination.

There is evidence also that MAO-A and MAO-B must both be inhibited to increase meperidine toxicity *(31)* although a serotonin syndrome–like response has been observed on a single occasion between meperidine and the selective MAO-A inhibitor moclobemide *(32)*.

Serotonin syndrome has not been reported with any opiate, other than meperidine, when used in combination with an MAOI and a number of successful strategies have been developed for administration of anesthetics or analgesics without interrupting antidepressant therapy *(33–38)*.

The depressive form of the MAOI/narcotic analgesic interaction is characterized by respiratory depression, hypotension, and coma, and reflects accumulation of free narcotic due to inhibition of liver enzymes by the MAOI *(29,30)*. This latter interaction can occur with any analgesic and results in symptoms characteristic of analgesic overdose. If recognized beforehand the interaction can be avoided by adjustment of the narcotic analgesic dosage. A similar interaction with the MAOI has been reported with dextromethorphan, which, like meperidine, also blocks reuptake of serotonin *(39)*.

Analogies can also be drawn between the MAOI and the antitubercular agent, isoniazid. The use of isoniazid has increased recently largely as a result of treatment of human immunodeficiency virus infections. Interactions between isoniazid and the TCA drugs have in the past been attributed to the weak MAO-inhibiting properties of isoniazid *(40,41)*. More recently, evidence suggests that, at clinically relevant concentrations, isoniazid inhibits the enzymes critically involved in metabolism of the TCA *(42,43)*. Inhibition of TCA metabolism, and accumulation of the TCA, might therefore contribute to the interactions observed between isoniazid and a TCA.

3. Tricyclic Antidepressants

The term tricyclic antidepressant (TCA) refers to a group of medicinal substances useful in treatment of depression and bearing a common structure relationship to a tricyclic, dibenzocycloheptane ring system. The most prominent members of the group are amitriptyline, imipramine, doxepin, dothiepin, and clomipramine. Their chemical structures are shown in Fig. 1.

Even with the dramatically increased clinical use of less toxic SSRIs, the TCAs remain a drug class frequently encountered in emergency rooms and postmortem toxicology *(44,45)*. Clinical evidence suggests that suicidal ideation is not uncommon during a depressive illness *(46–48)* and that acting upon such impulses might lead to use of any available drug for improper, dangerous purposes. Suicidal ideation contributes but is not the sole explanation for the high incidence of TCA encounters in emergency wards or forensic laboratories. The TCA drugs, as a class, are characterized by a combination of low therapeutic indices *(49)* and less than ideal pharmacokinetic properties. Tissue concentrations at intoxication may be only low multiples of the therapeutic level. Also, since their primary route of elimination involves metabolic conversion to more easily eliminated, water-soluble molecules, introduction of any other substance that reduces the capacity for metabolic transformation might also promote accumulation of dangerously high levels of the TCAs. Recent surveys conducted around the world suggest that approximately 5–10% of fatal intoxications involve antidepressants, with TCAs accounting for near 80% of that number *(48,50–59)*.

The TCAs exhibit two main pharmacological properties: they alter the reuptake and deactivation of neurotransmitters released during neurotransmission and they are competitive antagonists at muscarinic acetylcholine receptors. It is believed that the antidepressant effects of the TCAs are related to effects on amine reuptake within the CNS. Symptoms such as sedation, blurred vision, dry mouth, and urinary retention appear to be related to the antimuscarinic actions. Hypotension after the TCA is also closely related to antimuscarinic properties and changes in cardiac output and also to alpha-adrenergic antagonism.

Intoxication with the TCAs is therefore manifest by hypotension, cardiac arrhythmias, and/or CNS symptoms such as seizures *(45,60)*. In a group of 64 patients, treated for TCA overdose, 22 (34%) had systolic blood pressure less than 95 mm Hg on first presentation *(45)*. The authors observed a relationship among the presentations of hypo-

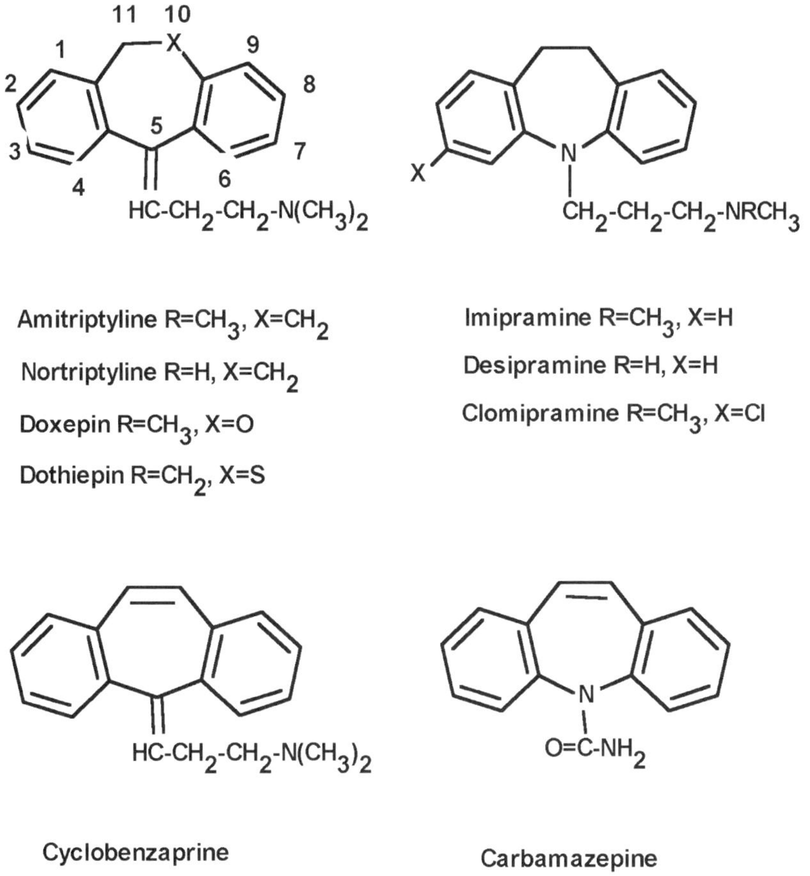

4. MAOIs and Tricyclic Antidepressants

Fig. 1. Chemical structures of common tricyclic antidepressants and two related drugs.

tension, cardiac arrhythmias, and pulmonary edema. Seizures were independent of these signs. Other studies also indicate that CNS symptoms can occur as the sole manifestation of TCA overdose (61). In a small number of cases, involvement of other organs has also been observed (62).

Notably, and of very great toxicological significance, the TCAs, through antimuscarinic mechanisms, lower the threshold for ventricular fibrillation and predispose to sudden death (63). Electrocardiographic monitoring therefore plays a major role in diagnosis of TCA overdose (64,65).

Regardless of presentation, overdose with the TCAs represents a serious medical crisis and even under intensive-care conditions 2–3% of patients die. The seriousness of TCA overdose is further magnified by the fact that the majority of self-poisonings occur while alone and at home, without the benefit of supportive intervention (59,66).

In this section we will discuss the common TCA drugs and review the chemical features important to their pharmacological properties. A major portion of the discussion will deal with the metabolism of the TCAs and the drug interactions that can contribute to accumulation of a TCA and the occurrence of TCA intoxication.

3.1. Chemistry and Pharmacology of the TCAs

The chemical structures of five common TCAs, plus cyclobenzaprine and carbamazepine, have been indicated in Fig. 1. These later compounds are shown to emphasis the structural features of the TCAs that are important to retention of the major pharmacological properties of the drug class.

The TCAs are chemically based on a dibenzocycloheptane ring system with a three-carbon chain separating the methylene bridgehead carbon (C-5) from a mono- or dimethyl-amino group (Fig. 1). Amitriptyline and imipramine are the most intensely studied of the TCA group and represent the parent molecules on which the remainder is based. Chemically, imipramine differs from amitriptyline only by replacement of the C-5 exocyclic double bond by a nitrogen atom. Antidepressant and anticholinergic activities are retained after insertion of oxygen or sulfur heteroatoms at C-10 of the ethylene bridge (cf. amitriptyline, doxepin, and dothiepin) or substitution of halogen at C-3 on the aromatic ring (cf. imipramine and clomipramine).

It is also important to note that the C-5 double bond in amitriptyline introduces a plane of symmetry that passes through C-5 and the C-10, C-11 bond of the molecule. Analogs or metabolites of amitriptyline can therefore be separated into isomers, differing only by introduction of substituents into the half of the molecule on the same (cis or Z) or opposite side of the double bond (trans or E) as the ethylamino aliphatic chain. This type of isomerism exists with amitriptyline, doxepin, and dothiepin but is absent for imipramine and clomipramine because of the ready inversion of the bridgehead nitrogen atom.

Metabolic studies in rats and humans have demonstrated that this form of E/Z geometric isomerism is important to the clinical and metabolic properties of the TCAs. Doxepin, for example, is marketed as an irrational 85:15, E:Z mixture and the less active E-isomer of N-desmethyldoxepin is metabolized more quickly than Z-N-desmethyldoxepin *(67,68)*.

Other changes in the dibenzocycloheptane ring system can dramatically alter the pharmacological properties of a TCA analog. Useful antidepressant activity is lost after dehydrogenation of the two-carbon ethylene bridge (C-10, C-11) and cyclobenzaprine is employed clinically as a centrally acting muscle relaxant. Some conflict as to the overdose risk of cyclobenzaprine is present in the literature. Some data suggest that cyclobenzaprine is an overdose risk in its own right *(69,70)*. However, in a 5-yr multicenter study of over 400 cyclobenzaprine overdoses, no deaths occurred. Arrhythmias were infrequent and cyclobenzaprine did not appear to be life threatening after doses up to 1 g *(71)*. Finally, carbamazepine differing by C-10, C-11 unsaturation, plus modification of the side chain at C-5, lacks both antidepressant and anticholinergic actions. Levels of carbamazepine required in blood for expression of toxic signs are severalfold higher than those of either the TCA or cyclobenzaprine *(69)*.

3.2. Metabolism of the TCAs

The TCAs are extensively metabolized and less than 1% of an administered dose of any of the five model TCAs is recovered in the urine as unchanged drug *(72–76)*. In addition, it is a long-standing general observation that, during TCA therapy, responses vary considerably between patients treated with similar dosages. Although differences

4. MAOIs and Tricyclic Antidepressants

in clinical response may reflect the psychological characteristics of individual effective disorders, differing abilities among individuals to maintain clinically effective concentrations in plasma, has also been realized as an important contributor toward overall clinical outcome *(77)*.

The extensive metabolism of the TCAs, their narrow therapeutic index, and the tendency for high interpatient response variability make the TCAs ideal candidates for plasma drug monitoring. The rationale in support of drug monitoring has been summarized for clomipramine *(78)*. Clinical evidence suggests that, during treatment with amitriptyline, efficacy is greatest when combined levels in serum of amitriptyline and its N-desmethyl metabolite, nortriptyline, are in a range between approximately 100 and 200 ng/mL *(79,80)*. Other studies suggest levels of imipramine in blood greater than a threshold level near 180 ng/mL *(81)* or in a range of 200–300 ng/mL were consistent with a good clinical response *(82,83)*. In comparison, combined levels of parent TCAs plus their major active metabolites greater than 500 ng/mL have been associated with clinical signs of overdose and toxicity *(45,84)* and combined levels near 1000 ng/mL have been associated with severe toxicity *(85–88)*. This suggests only a three- to fourfold difference between therapeutic and toxic amounts in blood.

A review of the literature suggests that genetic variations between individuals can determine abilities to metabolize the TCA and that inhibition of metabolism by some coadministered drugs, can cause the amounts of active antidepressant in blood to vary beyond the concentration range associated with the clinical antidepressant response.

Figure 2 illustrates the common metabolic transformations undergone by amitriptyline. Similar reactions are observed with each of the other TCAs *(69)*. As a group, the TCA undergo hydroxylation reactions and N-demethylation to the mono-N-desmethyl homologues (Fig. 2). These demethylated homologues accumulate in plasma and tissues and retain the pharmacological properties of the parent drug. They are felt to contribute to the overall clinical and toxicological response to the TCAs. In fact, the mono-N-demethylated metabolites of amitriptyline and imipramine, nortriptyline and desipramine respectively, are marketed in their own right as antidepressant drugs *(70)* and are toxic at levels in blood similar to their N,N-dimethyl- homologs *(69)*.

Hydroxylation (Fig. 2) followed by conjugation represents the principal metabolic route for elimination of the TCAs. In addition, the 2- and 10-hydroxy metabolites of the TCAs, and of their N-demethylated homologues, appear able to contribute to the pharmacological and potentially to the toxicological properties of the TCA. For example, clinical observations suggest the presence of an antidepressant response among patients treated with E-10-hydroxynortriptyline *(89)* and a superior clinical outcome was measured in patients favoring higher plasma levels of amitriptyline and Z-10-hydroxymetabolites in comparison to patients favoring formation of nortriptyline and E-10-hydroxy metabolites *(90)*.

The potential role played by hydroxylated metabolites in the cardiac toxicity of the TCA has also been studied after administration of the authentic compounds to animals. In these experiments 2-hydroxyimipramine produced a significantly greater incidence of life-threatening arrhythmias than did its parent, imipramine *(91)*. In comparison, E-10-hydroxynortriptyline produced fewer cardiac arrhythmias than did nortriptyline or Z-10-hydroxynortriptyline *(92)*. However, even though the hydroxylated metabolites of the TCA do appear to possess toxicological properties, they also undergo conju-

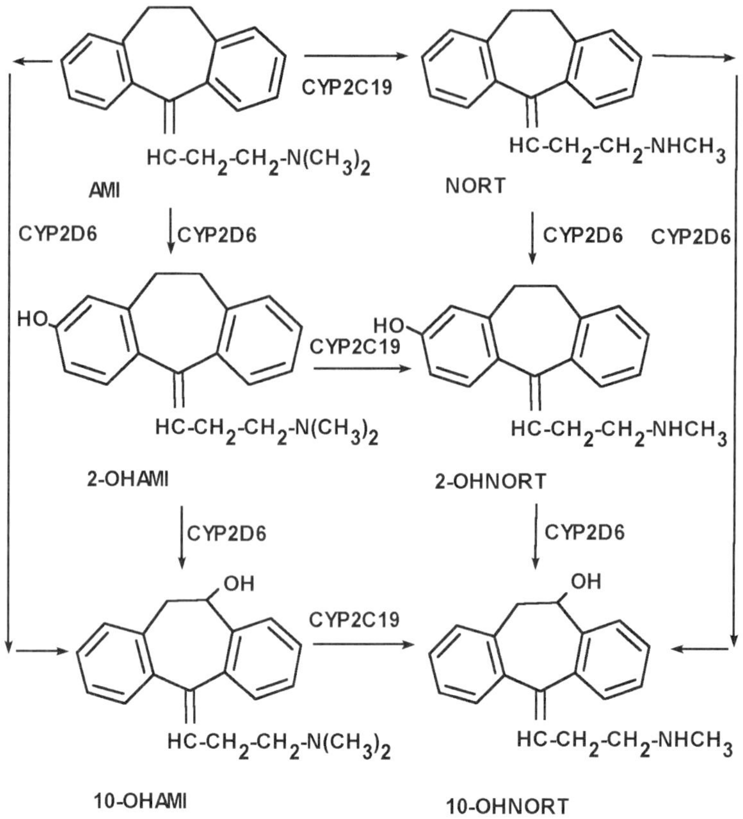

Fig. 2. Major metabolic transformations of common tricyclic antidepressants (AMI = amitriptyline, 2-OHAMI = 2-hydroxyamitriptyline, 10-OHAMI = 10-hydroxyamitriptyline, Nort = nortrityline, 2-OHNORT = 2-hydroxynortiptyline, 10-OHNORT = 10-hydroxynortiptyline).

gation reactions and are eliminated from the body more rapidly than the nonhydroxylated TCA *(93)*. No evidence for accumulation of hydroxylated metabolites into blood or tissue has been reported and their overall contribution to toxicity may be minor.

In contrast to the hydroxylated metabolites, the N-demethylated metabolites do accumulate into blood and tissue and have biological half-lives and pharmacological properties similar to their precursor TCAs. These differences from the hydroxylated metabolites has resulted in extensive research to determine the genetic variations among patients and drug interactions that reduce the rate of hydroxylation and, as a result, increase the levels and persistence of the TCAs and their N-desmethyl-metabolites.

3.3. Genetic Polymorphism and Metabolism of the TCA

In the middle 1980s Mellstrom et al. *(94)* demonstrated a relationship between debrisoquin hydroxylation and amitriptyline/nortriptyline metabolism. This cytochrome P450 enzyme has since come to be known as CYP2D6 and has been confirmed as a common mediator of TCA hydroxylation *(95,96)*. In addition, individuals less capable of CYP2D6-catalyzed metabolism have been shown to be more susceptible to TCA

4. MAOIs and Tricyclic Antidepressants

overdose and toxicity *(97,98)*. This unambiguous demonstration of the involvement of a CYP450 enzyme in the metabolism of the TCAs sparked an understanding of the potential for drug interactions and the influence of genetic differences on the responses to the TCAs.

Since the observation that a relationship existed in human subjects between debrisoquin hydroxylation and TCA metabolism *(94)*, at least five CYP450 enzymes have been demonstrated to participate, in varying degrees, to the N-demethylation and 2- or 10-hydroxylation of the TCAs. These CYP450 enzymes are CYP1A2, CYP2C9, CYP2C19, CYP2D6, and CYP3A4 *(99–107)*. However, because of different affinities toward the TCAs, or differing degrees of expression, not all of these enzymes are significantly involved in TCA metabolism at clinically relevant TCA concentrations. In vitro studies have confirmed that the enzymes involved in TCA metabolism differ between low and high concentrations of the TCAs.

Ghahramani et al. *(100)* studied amitriptyline N-demethylation in human liver microsomes and heterologously expressed human enzymes over a concentration range from 1 to 500 µM (250 to 12,500 ng/mL) and showed that N-demethylation of amitriptyline involved CYP3A4, CYP2C9, and CYP2D6. However, when experiments were conducted at a more clinically significant level of imipramine, near 500 ng/mL, CYP2C19 was shown to have major involvement in N-demethylation. CYP2D6, with a minor contribution from CYP2C19, was the major catalyst of 2-hydroxylation *(101)*.

In combination these studies *(99–108)* have contributed to an interpretation that although at least five CYP450 enzymes contribute to metabolism of the TCAs over a broad range of concentrations, CYP2D6 and CYP2C19 are of predominant importance at clinically relevant concentrations.

Genetically-determined differences in the distribution of CYP2C19 and CYP2D6 also play important roles in determining the ability of individuals to metabolize the TCAs, and ultimately their susceptibility to accumulation of toxic concentrations of the TCAs.

Polymorphic distribution of CYP2D6 was first demonstrated approximately 20 yr ago *(109,110)*. Currently, close to 50 CYP2D6 alleles are known, but fewer than 10 exceed the 1% frequency requirement *(111)* to be considered significant. Several of these alleles encode for functionally defective CYP2D6 enzymes with reduced, or without metabolic capability. Depending on genetic complement, an individual may be an extensive (EM), intermediate (IM) or a poor metabolizer (PM). In addition, the CYP2D6 gene may be duplicated, or multiduplicated, resulting in ultrafast metabolizers (UM) *(112,113)*. That is, although most individuals metabolize CYP2D6 substrates at rates expected of the normal population (EM plus IM), some individuals are unable to metabolize (PM) whereas others are extraordinarily capable (UM). For example, in a group of unrelated German volunteers, Sachse et al. *(114)* reported three main alleles, CYP2D6*1 (EM), CYP2D6*2 (IM), and CYP2D6*4 (PM). Frequencies of these alleles were 0.36, 0.32, and 0.21, respectively. Approximately 7% of the population were in the PM genotype, whereas 0.5% had multiple copies of the CYP2D6*1 allele (UM).

As one might expect of a genetically determined polymorphism, PM frequency follows strong ethnic lines *(115–117)*. This distribution can be seen with the CYP2D6 PM phenotype. Whereas 5.5% of Dutch volunteers were PMs *(118)* only 1–2% of subjects tested in Turkey and East and South Africa were of the PM phenotype *(119,120)*.

Less than 1% of a group of 216 black Tanzanians were PM but fully 9% exhibited allele duplication consistent with UM status *(121)*. Asian populations also have a low CYP2D6 PM frequency but, because of a high incidence of defective alleles of intermediate efficiency, the CYP2D6 metabolic capability of the Asian EM phenotype is somewhat lower than in other parts of the world.

These various observations suggest a Northern European bias toward the CYP2D6 PM phenotype and this bias has been observed to influence the metabolism of TCA drugs in patients. For example, 8% of a group of Swedish Caucasians were found to have reduced abilities to hydroxylate the CYP2D6 probe, debrisoquin, and also to 2-hydroxylate desipramine *(122)*. In the Danish population the PM frequency is also about 7% and in one reported instance a Danish woman, of the PM phenotype, developed toxic serum levels after successive treatments with 100 mg/d of nortriptyline. After adjusting the dosage to 25 mg/d the woman's depression disappeared without any side effects of note *(97)*.

At therapeutically relevant concentrations, N-demethylation of the tertiary amine TCA is catalyzed by CYP2C19 *(101,123,124)*. As is the case with CYP2D6, there is a marked interethnic difference in the incidence of the PM phenotype. Approximately 3–6% of Caucasians and 13–23% of Asians are slow metabolizers *(125,126)*.

The effects of CYP2D6 and CYP2C19 phenotype on TCA metabolism have been examined in several clinical studies. These studies often involve Chinese or Japanese subjects because of the higher frequency of the CYP2D6*10 allele and, of the CYP2C19 PM phenotype in general, among the Asian population. The CP2D6*10 (IM) allele occurs in approximately 34% of the Asian population. This allele encodes for an enzyme with reduced metabolic activity but is included in the EM phenotype and contributes to the general lowering of rate of derisoquin hydroxylation observed in the Asian EM phenotype. In one study the pharmacokinetics of nortriptyline and 10-hydroxynortriptyline were compared among subjects homozygous for CYP2D6*1, homozygous for CYP2D6*10, or heterozygous for these two alleles (CYP2D6*1*10) *(127)*. The study showed that the CYP2D6*10*10 subjects had impaired metabolism of nortriptyline, the plasma half-life of nortriptyline was prolonged, and the area under the plasma concentration time curve was greater in this group than in either of the other two groups. Two additional studies have examined the impact of CYP2D6 genotype on nortriptyline and desipramine metabolism *(128,129)*. These again showed that the rate of hydroxylation was reduced in subjects with either one or two defective alleles and that, in subjects with two defective CYP2D6 alleles, amounts of nortriptyline or desipramine in blood were more than twofold greater than in individuals in the EM phenotype.

Examination of the effects of CYP2C19 PM status on the metabolism of the TCAs are less common. However, in three studies subjects homozygous for defective CYP2C19 alleles again had approximately double the plasma concentrations of imipramine or clomipramine as did the members of the homozygous EM phenotype *(122–124)*.

3.4. Drug Interactions with Metabolism of the TCA

Patient phenotype has been seen to play an important role in determining the pharmacokinetic impact of interactions between the TCAs and drugs interfering with CYP450-catalyzed metabolism. For example, in 1992, Crewe et al. *(130)* reported that several of the SSRI antidepressant drugs inhibited CYP2D6-catalyzed metabolism. They observed that paroxetine had the greatest inhibitory effect and fluvoxamine, the least. Fluoxetine and sertraline had intermediate activities. They also observed that, whereas the N-desmethyl- metabolite of fluoxetine was a potent inhibitor, metabolites of paroxetine caused negligible inhibition. In general, this rank order of CYP2D6-inhibitor activity has stood the test of time and reexamination *(108,131)*. However, because the N-desmethylated metabolite of fluoxetine is more persistent in blood and tissues and is a potent inhibitor of CYP2D6 in its own right, inhibition of TCA hydroxylation in clinical settings may be more significant after fluoxetine than after any of the other SSRIs.

In human patients, treated with amitriptyline (50 mg/d) and fluoxetine (20 mg/d) for long durations, the steady-state concentration of amitriptyline in blood was increased approximately twofold, and that of nortryptyline ninefold, relative to patients treated only with amitriptyline *(132)*. In comparison, paroxetine, 20 mg/d for 2 wk, increased amitriptyline and imipramine by approximately 50% and doubled the concentrations at steady state of nortryptyline and desipramine *(133)*. Some of the apparent difference between these inhibitors might be due to the fact that patients were treated with fluoxetine/TCA combinations for longer periods than were the paroxetine/TCA group. Such being the case, the clinical observations suggest inhibitory effects due to fluoxetine or paroxetine and that the effects of metabolic inhibition on the concentrations of the TCA in blood may increase in a manner related to the duration of combined exposure. In both experiments, also, the effect of the inhibitor was approximately four times greater toward the accumulation of desmethylated metabolites than toward accumulation of the parent TCA. This difference is consistent with an interaction at the level of CYP2D6, which catalyzes the second, and apparently rate-determining, hydroxylation step of TCA metabolism.

The effects of the SSRIs on the pharmacokinetics of the demethylated TCA, desipramine and nortriptyline, have also been examined in clinical settings. These experiments very clearly confirm the rank order of the SSRI interactions with the TCAs.

For example, fluoxetine (20 mg/d) or sertraline (50 mg/d) were coadministered with desipramine (50 mg/d) *(134)*. After 3 wk of combined treatment, fluoxetine increased the Cmax levels of desipramine and area under the plasma concentration vs time curve (AUC0-24) by 400 and 480%, respectively. In this same experiment, sertraline increased Cmax and AUC0-24 by only 31 and 23%, respectively. Fluoxetine had a greater pharmacokinetic interaction with desipramine than did sertraline. Inhibitory effects of paroxetine and sertraline on desipramine pharmacokinetics have also been compared *(135)*. In these experiments, 24 healthy, CYP2D6 EM phenotype, males received desipramine, 50 mg/d for 7 d and then were cotreated with either paroxetine, 20 mg/d, or sertraline, 50 mg/d. After 10 d of cotreatment, desipramine concentrations in plasma increased greater than fourfold, from 38 to 173 ng/mL, in the paroxetine/desipramine group but only by approximately half, from 36 to 52 ng/mL, in the sertraline/desipramine group. The experiments were consistent with a greater pharmacokinetic interaction by paroxetine than by sertraline. A similar small effect by sertraline on nortriptyline accumulation has also been reported *(136)*.

Each of these reports again supports the original assignment of relative inhibitory actions decreasing in the order fluoxetine/paroxetine/sertraline. Citalopram and venlafaxine either do not appear to inhibit CYP450 metabolism or have only very modest clinical impacts *(137,138)*.

The results of these mixed antidepressant studies and previously noted phenotype studies are consistent with the presence of two alternative pathways, demethylation and hydroxylation, that are available for TCA metabolism. Olesen and Linnet *(102)* have estimated that 90% of the metabolism of nortriptyline is dependent on hydroxylation by CYP2D6 and the effect of a coadministered SSRI on the pharmacokinetics of the TCAs can be explained as an interaction, by the higher affinity SSRI, at the level of the CYP2D6 enzyme. Since hydroxylation of the TCAs by CYP2D6 behaves as the rate-determining step in the overall elimination process, inhibition of hydroxylation by the SSRIs results in accumulation of the parent TCA and also the N-desmethylated metabolite.

The interaction between the TCAs and SSRIs is greatest in individuals from the UM and EM phenotypes and metabolism of the TCAs by patients from the PM phenotype is largely uneffected *(139)*. The lack of inhibitory effect in PM subjects is due to lack of CYP2D6 enzyme and illustrates that these PM subjects metabolize the TCAs by alternate enzymes. There are no reports of inhibition of TCA metabolism in the PM phenotype by an SSRI and the SSRI would not be expected to further reduce the already slowed TCA metabolism in this phenotype.

A clinical application has been proposed for the interaction between the TCAs and SSRIs *(140)*. Clinical experience has shown that, because of very rapid metabolism, patients in the CYP2D6 UM phenotype may require larger doses of a TCA to maintain therapeutically useful concentrations in plasma. Simultaneous treatment with low doses of paroxetine, 10 mg/d, reduced the rate of debrisoquine hydroxylation and produced an apparent conversion from UM to EM status. After conversion, four of the five subjects achieved therapeutic levels of nortriptyline. After a higher dose of paroxetine, 20 mg/d, two subjects converted to PM status. Conversion to PM status in part of the patient population illustrates the variability in responses to inhibitors such as paroxetine and further supports the implementation of TCA-monitoring procedures.

The interaction between TCAs and the predominant demethylating enzyme, CYP2C19, is less studied because highly potent and selective inhibitors are not currently available. However, the SSRI drug fluvoxamine is a potent inhibitor of CYP1A2, and also a moderately potent inhibitor of CYP2C19, and has been demonstrated to effectively inhibit CYP2C19-catalyzed metabolism of the antimalarial drug, proquanil, in vivo *(102)*. Since the contribution of CYP1A2 to desipramine metabolism at clinically relevant concentrations is slight, fluvoxamine may act as a relatively specific inhibitor of metabolism by CYP2C19 enzyme. In one report, prior treatments with fluvoxamine (100 mg/d, 10 d) prolonged the elimination half-life of imipramine from 23 to 40 h and reduced apparent oral clearance *(141)*. No effect on desipramine pharmacokinetics was observed. In another instance, fluvoxamine, administered at a dose of 100 mg/d for 14 d, increased the elimination half-life of imipramine from 23 to 39 h, reduced the apparent oral clearance from 1.3 to 0.6 L/h/kg, and doubled the maximum concentration of imipramine in plasma. The maximum concentration of desipramine was halved, in a manner consistent with inhibition of imipramine N-demethylation *(142)*. Finally, in a single UM patient treated with clomipramine (150–225 mg/d), fluvoxamine (100 mg/d) increased the amount of clomipramine in plasma from 53 to 223 ng/mL and reduced the amount of N-desmethylclomiprimine from 87 to 49 ng/mL *(143)*.

An important difference between the effects of inhibition of CYP2D6 (hydroxylation) and CYP2C19 (N-demethylation) can be seen. The predominant effect of inhibition of CYP2D6 catalyzed hydroxylation by an SSRI is to increase the amount of the N-desmethylated TCA metabolites in blood by approximately four- to ninefold *(131–134,144)*. Effects on the parent N,N-dimethylated TCA are less dramatic. In comparison, inhibition of CYP2C19 primarily results in an approximately twofold increase in the amount of unmetabolized, tertiary amine, parent TCA *(141–144)*. Amounts of the N-desmethylated TCA tend to decrease because only demethylation, and not hydroxylation, has been inhibited.

3.5. Other Drug Effects on Metabolism of the TCA

The incidence of effects of other prescription drugs on the metabolism of amitriptyline and nortriptyline has been assessed through analysis of drug-level data collected on several thousand patients *(145)*. These data indicate that amounts of the TCAs in blood were decreased by carbamazepine, due to enzyme induction, and increased by dextropropoxyphene and neuroleptics, particularly thioridazine. The thioridazine effect on TCA metabolism exhibited a complex dose dependency and was greatest after low doses of the TCA and high doses of the neuroleptic. Treatments with thioridazine have been shown to convert CYP2D6 EM phenotype patients to the PM phenotype *(146,147)* and in one instance, involving a pediatric patient, coadministration of thioridazine was seen to increase amounts of imipramine in blood into a toxic range *(148)*.

Effects by amitriptyline on thioridazine metabolism may be more significant, both pharmacokinetically and clinically. Recent studies support the common belief that cardiovascular mortality is greater among psychiatric patients receiving neuroleptics than in the general population *(149,150)*. Other evidence suggests that the risk cardiotoxicity may be greater with thioridazine than other neuroleptics *(151)* and that cardiac effects such as delayed ventricular repolarization are dose related and due predominantly to unmetabolized thioridazine *(152)*. In a rodent model, treatment with imipramine or amitriptyline increased the blood plasma levels of thioridazine and its metabolites 20- and 30-fold, respectively *(153)*. These authors noted that the TCA/thioridazine concentration ratio was important in determining the final result of the TCA: neuroleptic interaction. This observation is consistent with the observations in psychiatric patients that the effect of thioridazine on amitriptyline metabolism varied with the antidepressant/neuroleptic:dose ratio *(153)*. When the ratio favored amitriptyline, thioridazine metabolism was inhibited. When the ratio favored thioridazine, amitriptyline metabolism was inhibited.

An example of a pharmaceutical agent with a potential to interact in the metabolism of the TCA is ticlopidine. Ticlopidine is employed clinically as an inhibitor of platelet aggregation and is also a potent inhibitor of CYP2D6 and CYP2C19 *(154–157)*, the enzymes critically involved in the hydroxylation and N-demethylation of the TCA. Examples of an interaction between ticlopidine and a TCA have not been reported. However, known interactions between ticlopidine and the anticonvulsant, dilantin, might serve as examples *(154–155)*. Dilantin is metabolized predominantly by CYP2C9 and

CYP2C19 isoforms and combined therapy with ticlopidine has been seen to dangerously elevate blood levels of dilantin. In addition, since inhibition by ticolidine may be mechanism based, which by definition permanently inactivates the metabolizing enzyme, inhibition may be long term *(156–157)*.

Carbamazepine and ethyl alcohol have also been shown to influence the response to the TCA. Carbamazepine is a structural analog of imipramine with anticonvulsant properties (Fig. 1), and has been combined with a TCA in the treatment of refractory, treatment-resistant depression *(158)*. The improved clinical response is, however, in direct contrast with the effect of carbamazepine on TCA metabolism. Therapeutic drug-level reviews and clinical studies have shown that patients also treated with carbamazepine have amounts of parent and demethylated TCA in blood reduced by as much as 60%, in comparison with patients treated with a comparable dose of TCA alone *(145, 159–161)*. These effects by carbamazepine on TCA metabolism appear to be mediated through induction of CYP1A2 and CYP3A4 enzymes *(106,162)*. By most standards, the amounts of TCA plus demethylated metabolites in blood from these patients might be seen as subtherapeutic, even though the clinical response may be increased. These contradictory observations of low levels in blood and increased clinical efficacy appear relayed to changes in the amount of drug available for pharmacological action. Under normal circumstances, greater than 95% of a TCA is bound to plasma protein and the pharmacological response is related to the smaller (5%) unbound fraction. Some evidence suggests that carbamazepine acts to reduce binding of the TCA to plasma protein and thereby increase the amount of free drug available for pharmacological effect *(162)*. Attempts to adjust the TCA dosage to obtain amounts in blood within a "therapeutic window" may not be necessary.

Ethanol may also have a clinically important interaction with the TCA. Dorian et al. *(163)* have demonstrated that ethanol ingested together with amitriptyline, increased the amount of the TCA which reached the systemic circulation, possibly because of reduced hepatic clearance during absorption. They also noted that postural sway and short-term memory impairments were increased by the combination. The effects of the combined exposure to ethanol and amitriptyline on skills such as driving have been reviewed *(164)*.

4. CLINICAL SIGNIFICANCE OF POLYMORPHISM AND DRUG INTERACTIONS

Are genetic polymorphisms, and CYP 450 interactions with the SSRIs or other drugs, significant factors in the toxicology of the TCAs? Clinically effective levels of the TCAs plus the N-desmethylated metabolites have been proposed to lie between approximately 100 and 300 ng/mL *(79–83)*. In comparison, clinical toxicity has been observed at concentrations over 500 ng/mL *(45,84)* and severe toxicity at levels over 1000 ng/mL *(85–88,165)* although in one nonfatal intoxication, amounts of clomipramine and N-desmethylclomipramine in plasma exceeded 2000 ng/mL *(166)*. Clinically toxic, nonfatal, levels of nortriptyline, near 600 mg/mL have been reported in a CYP2D6 PM *(97)*. Postmortem concentrations of imipramine and desipramine of 3000 and 9600 ng/mL were determined in blood from an individual treated with a paroxetine/imipramine combination *(167)*.

Druid et al. *(168)* determined CYP2D6 phenotype in 22 postmortem cases where amounts of a parent drug were disproportionately higher than levels of metabolite in femoral blood. They concluded that the incidence of the PM phenotype within this group was not different from the general population. Similarly, Spigset et al. *(169)* also reported that CYP2D6 or CYP2C19 genotype were not associated with the incidence of seizures or myoclonus during antidepressant treatment. Vandel et al. *(170)* have reviewed the available literature and have also added their own observations regarding TCA plasma levels after combined therapy with fluoxetine. They observed that, even though amounts of clomipramine in plasma increased to as much as 965 ng/mL, and imipramine to 785 ng/mL, no signs of toxicity were observed in their patients. Similarly, Bonin et al. *(171)* studied 10 patients treated simultaneously with a TCA and fluoxetine. In three of these patients, amounts of TCA plus the N-desmethylated metabolite in blood exceeded 500 ng/mL. In the short term, clinical tolerance to the treatment was "very good." Combined treatments with a TCA and fluoxetine have also been examined for beneficial effects in depressed patients previously unresponsive to either drug alone. In these cases, individuals who responded favorably to the combination, experienced blood levels that averaged greater than 750 ng/mL *(172)*. Nevertheless, fatalities have been associated with combined fluoxetine/amitriptyline and paroxetine/imipramine therapy *(167,173)*.

One factor that may contribute to a lack of recognition of SSRI or phenotype interactions with the TCAs is that, because of their long elimination half-life, increases in blood content may occur gradually, and go unrecognized because of slow development of symptoms. It is also clear that individual patients are more, or less, responsive to either the beneficial or toxic effects of the TCA. Amounts of the TCA in plasma from living patients cover a rather broad range and this range in the total of patients is greater than the clinical to toxic range in any individual patient.

Another factor is the observation that, in postmortem cases, amounts of a TCA in blood occur in a broad range and are often several times higher than normally seen in living, even severely intoxicated, persons *(174–176)*. Pounder and Jones studied this phenomenon of postmortem redistribution and observed diffusion of drugs, along a concentration gradient, out of solid organs and into the blood *(177)*. Highest levels were seen in pulmonary arteries and veins and lowest in peripheral vessels. They reported that amounts of doxepin or clomipramine in postmortem blood collected from different sites ranged from 3.6 to 12.5 mg/L and from 4.0 to 21.5 mg/L, respectively. Other investigators have since confirmed the phenomenon *(178–181)*. The consequence of postmortem redistribution is that reference data are rendered less useful unless a record of the site of collection is available. It is therefore a common practice to assay the TCAs in blood collected from different peripheral vascular sites, and in tissues such as liver, in order to increase the probability of a correct interpretation.

5. Conclusions

Depression, and its allied disorders, is common in modern society and drug intervention will continue to be a major mechanism in its control. Beneficial clinical responses after the MAOIs or TCAs are not less than those observed after treatment with the SSRIs and many thousands of people have benefited from these antidepressant drugs. Their use is not without risk of severe drug interactions and toxicities.

In this chapter the common toxicology of the MAOIs and TCAs has been presented. Some of the interactions may appear small in comparison to a broad range of therapeutic concentrations, but effects in a single patient can be dramatic. It has therefore been the objective of this chapter to describe these interactions, and to provide a basis on which they can be applied toward interpretation of a toxic response by a single patient.

REFERENCES

1. Paykel ES and Priest RG. Recognition and management of depression in general practice: consensus statement. Br Med J 305:1198–1202 (1992).
2. Owens D. New or old antidepressants: benefits of new drugs are exaggerated. Br Med J 309: 1281–1822 (1994).
3. Barbui C and Hotopf M. Amitriptyline v. the rest: still the leading antidepressant after 40 years of randomized controlled trials. Br J Psychiatry 178:129–144 (2001).
4. Baker GB, Coutts RT, McKenna KF, and Sherry-McKenna RL. Insights into the mechanisms of action of the MAO inhibitors phenelzine and tranylcypromine: a review. J Psychiatry Neurosci 17:206–214 (1992).
5. Linden CH, Rumack BH, and Strehlke C. Monoamine oxidase inhibitor overdose. Ann Emerg Med 13:1137–1144 (1984).
6. Lichtenwalner MR, Tully RG, Cohn RD, and Pinder RD. Two fatalities involving phenelzine. J Anal Toxicol 19:265–266 (1995).
7. Boniface PJ. Two cases of fatal intoxication due to tranylcypromine overdose. J Anal Toxicol 15:38–40 (1991).
8. Gardner DM, Shulman KI, Walker SE, and Tailor SA. The making of a user friendly MAOI diet. J Clin Psychiatry 57:99–104 (1996).
9. Shulman KI, Tailor SA, Walker SE, and Gardner DM. Tap (draft) beer and monoamine oxidase inhibitor dietary restrictions. Can J Psychiatry 42:310–312 (1997).
10. Norman TR and Burrows GD. A risk-benefit assessment of moclobemide in the treatment of depressive disorders. Drug Saf 12:46–54 (1995).
11. Antal EJ, Hendershot PE, Batts DH, Sheu WP, Hopkins NK, and Donaldson KM. Linezolid, a novel oxazolidinone antibiotic: assessment of monoamine oxidase inhibition using pressor response to oral tyramine. J Clin Pharmacol 41:552–562 (2001).
12. Callingham BA. Drug interactions with reversible monoamine oxidase-A inhibitors. Clin Neuropharmacol 16(Suppl 2):S42–S50 (1993).
13. Zimmer R. Relationship between tyramine potentiation and monoamine oxidase (MAO) inhibition comparison between moclobemide and other MAO inhbitors. Acta Psychiatr Scand Suppl 360:81–83 (1990).
14. Dingemanse, J, Guentert T, Gieschke R, and Stabl M. Modification of the cardiovascular effects of ephedrine by the reversible monoamine oxidase A-inhibitor moclobemide. J Cardiovasc Pharmacol 28:856–861 (1996).
15. Dawson JK, Earnshaw SM, and Graham CS. Dangerous monoamine oxidase inhibitor interactions are still occurring in the 1990s. J Accid Emerg Med 12:49–51 (1995).
16. Ponto LB, Perry PJ, Liskow BI, and Seaba HH. Drug therapy reviews: tricyclic antidepressant and monoamine oxidase inhibitor combination therapy. Am J Hosp Pharm 34:954–961 (1977).

17. Schmauss M, Kapfhammer HP, Meyr P, and Hoff P. Combined MAO-inhibitor and tri- (tetra) cyclic antdepressant treatment in therapy resistant depression. Prog Neuropsychopharmacol Biol Psychiatry 12:523–532 (1988).
18. Berlanga C and Ortega-Soto HA. A 3-year follow up of a group of treatment-resistant depressed patients with a MAOI/tricyclic combination. J Affect Disord 34:187–193 (1995).
19. Sporer KA. The serotonergic syndrome. Implicated drugs, pathophysiology and management. Drug Saf 13:94–104 (1995).
20. Brubacher JR, Hoffman RS, and Lurin MJ. Serotonin syndrome from venlafaxine-tranylcypromine interaction. Vet Hum Toxicol 38:358–361 (1996).
21. Meyer D and Halfin V. Toxicity secondary to meperidine in patients on monoamine oxidase inhibitors: a case report and critical review. J Clin Psychopharmacol 1:319–321 (1981).
22. Nielson K. Hyperpyrexia following poisoning with a monoamine oxidase inhibitor. Ugeskr Laeger 151:774–775 (1989).
23. Verrilli MR, Sanglanger VD, Kozachuck WE, and Bennetts M. Phenelzine toxicity responsive to dantroline. Neurology 37:865–867 (1987).
24. Lannas PA and Pachar JV. A fatal case of neuroleptic malignant syndrome. Med Sci Law 33:86–88 (1993).
25. Hodgman MJ, Martin TG, and Krenzelok EP. Serotonin syndrome due to venlafaxine and maintenance tranylcypromine therapy. Hum Exp Toxicol 16:14–17 (1997).
26. Brubacher JR, Hoffman RS, and Lurin MJ. Serotonin syndrome from venlafaxine-tranylcypromine interaction. Vet Hum Toxicol 38:358–361 (1996).
27. Cagliesi Cingolani R and Benici A. 2 fatal cases of reaction to the combination of MAO inhibitors and tricyclic antidepressants. Medico-legal aspects. Riv Patol Nerv Ment 103: 21–31 (1982).
28. White K. Tricyclic overdose in a patient given combined tricyclic-MAOI treatment. Am J Psychiatry 135:1411 (1978).
29. Stack CG, Rogers P, and Linter SPK. Monoamine oxidase inhibitors and anaesthesia. A review. Br J Anaesth 60:222–227 (1988).
30. Browne B and Linter S. Monoamine oxidase inhibitors and narcotic analgesics. A critical review of the implications for treatment. Br J Psychiatry 151:210–212 (1987).
31. Boden R, Botting R, Coulson P, and Spanswick G. Effect of nonselective and selective inhibitors of monoamine oxidases A and B on pethidine toxicity in mice. Br J Pharmacol 82:151–154 (1984).
32. Gillman PK. Possible serotonin syndrome with moclobemide and pethidine. Med J Aust 162:554 (1995).
33. Zimmer R, Gieschke R, Fischbach R, and Gasic S. Interaction studies with moclobemide. Acta Psychiatr Scand Suppl 360:84–86 (1990).
34. Sedgwick JV, Lewis IH, and Linter SP. Anesthesia and mental illness. Int J Psychiatry Med 20:209–225 (1990).
35. Blom-Peters L and Lamy M. Monoamine oxidase inhibitors and anesthesia: an updated literature review. Acta Anaesthesiol Belg 44:57–60 (1993).
36. Pavy TJ, Kliffer AP, and Douglas MJ. Anaesthetic management of labour and delivery in a woman taking long-term MAOI. Can J Anaesth 42:618–620 (1995).
37. Fischer SP, Mantin R, and Brocke-Utne JG. Ketorolac and propofol anaesthesia in a patient taking chronic monoamine oxidase inhibitors. J Clin Anesth 8:245–247 (1996).
38. Ure DS, Gillies MA, and James KS. Safe use of remifentanil in a patient treated with the monoamine oxidase inhibitor phenelzine. Br J Anaesth 84:414–416 (2000).
39. Rivers N and Horner B. Possible lethal reaction between nardil and dextromethorphan. Can Med Assoc J 103:85 (1970).

40. Judd FK, Mijch AM, Cockram A, and Norman TR. Isoniazid and antidepressants: is there cause for concern. Int Clin Psychpharmacol 9:123–125 (1994).
41. DiMartini A. Isoniazid, tricyclics and the "Cheeze Reaction." Psychopharmacol 10:197–198 (1995).
42. Desta Z, Soukhova NV, and Flockhart DA. Inhibition of cytochrome P450 (CYP450) by isoniazid: potent inhibition of CYP2C19 and CYP3A. Antimicrob Agents Chemother 45: 382–392 (2001).
43. Wen X, Wang JZ, Neuvonen PJ, and Backman JT. Isoniazid is a mechanism-based inhibitor of cytochrome P450 1A2, 2A6, 2C19 and 3A4 isoforms in human liver microsomes. Eur J Clin Pharmacol 57:799–804 (2002).
44. Amann B, Grunze H, Hoffmann J, Schafer M, and Kuss HJ. Non-fatal effect of highly toxic amitriptyline level after suicide attempt. A case report. Nervenarzt 72:52–55 (2001).
45. Shannon M, Merola J, and Lovejoy FH. Hypotension in severe tricyclic antidepressant overdose. Am J Emerg Med 6:439–442 (1988).
46. Montgomery SA. Suicide and antidepressants. Ann NY Acad Sci 836:329–338 (1997).
47. Goodwin FK. Anticonvulsant therapy and suicide risk in affective disorders. J Clin Psychiatry 60:89–93 (1999).
48. Muller-Oerlinghaussen B. Arguments for the specificity of the antisuicidal effect of lithium. Eur Arch Psychiatry Clin Neurosci 251(Suppl 2):II72–II75 (2001).
49. Ostapowicz A, Zejmo M, Wrzesniewska J, Bialecka M, Gornik W, and Gawronska-Szklarz B. Effect of therapeutic drug monitoring of amitriptyline and genotyping on efficacy and safety of depression therapy. Psychiatr Pol 34:595–605 (2000).
50. Ohberg A, Vuori E, Klaukka T, and Lonnqvist J. Antidepressants and suicide mortality. J Affect Disord 50:225–233 (1998).
51. Schreinzer FR, Stimpfl T, Vycudilik W, Berzlanovich A, and Kasper S. Suicide by antidepressant intoxication identified at autopsy in Vienna from 1991–1997: the favourable consequences of the increasing use of SSRIs. Eur Neuropsychopharmacol 10:133–142 (2000).
52. Isacsson G, Holmgren P, Druid H, and Bergman U. The utilization of antidepressants—a key issue in the prevention of suicide: an analysis of 5281 suicides in Sweden during the period 1992–1994. Acta Psychiatr Scand 96:94–100 (1997).
53. Henry JA. Epidemiology and relative toxicity of antidepressant drugs in overdose. Drug Saf 16:374–390 (1997).
54. Battersby MW, O'Mahoney JJ, Beckwith AR, and Hunt JL. Antidepressant deaths by overdose. Aust N Z J Psychiatr 30:223–228 (1996).
55. Ghazi-Khansari M and Oreizi S. A prospective study of fatal outcome of poisonings in Tehran. Vet Hum Toxicol 37:449–452 (1995).
56. Jick SS, Dean AD, and Jick H. Antidepressants and suicide. BMJ 310:215–218 (1995).
57. Obafunwa JO and Busuttil A. Deaths from substance overdose in the Lothian and Borders region of Scotland (1983–1991). Hum Exp Toxicol 13:401–406 (1994).
58. Shah R, Uren Z, Baker A, and Majeed A. Deaths from antidepressants in England and Wales 1993–1997: analysis of a new national database. Psychol Med 31:1203–1210 (2001).
59. Buckley NA, Whyte IM, Dawson AH, McManus PR, and Ferguson NW. Self-poisoning in Newcastle, 1987–1992. Med J Austr 162:190–193 (1995).
60. Kerr GW, McGuffie AC, and Wilkie S. Tricyclic antidepressant overdose: a review. Emerg Med J 18:236–241 (2001).
61. Roberge RJ and Krenzelok EP. Prolonged coma and loss of brainstem reflexes following amitriptyline overdose. Vet Hum Toxicol 43:42–44 (2001).
62. Pezzilli R, Melandri R, Barakat B, Broccoli BL, and Miglio F. Pancreatic involvement associated with tricyclic overdose. Ital J Gastroenterol Hepatol 30:418–420 (1998).

63. Tobis JM, Aronow WS. Effect of amitriptyline antidotes on repetitive extrasystole threshold. Clin Pharmacol Ther 27:602–606 (1980).
64. Singh N, Singh HK, and Fahn IA. Serial electrocardiographic changes as a predictor of cardiovascular toxicity in acute tricyclic antidepressant overdose. Am J Ther 9:75–79 (2002).
65. Harrigan RA and Brady WJ. ECG abnormalities in tricyclic antidepressant ingestion. Am J Emerg Med 17:387–393 (1999).
66. Jonasson B, Johnasson U, and Saldeen T. Among fatal poisonings dextropropoxyphene predominates in younger people, antidepressants in the middle aged and sedatives in the elderly. J Forensic Sci 45:7–10 (2000).
67. Shu YZ, Hubbard JW, Cooper JK, McKay G, Korchinsky ED, Kumar R, and Midha KK. The identification of urinary metabolites of doxepin in patients. Drug Metab Dispos 18: 735–741 (1990).
68. Yan JH, Hubbard JW, McKay G, and Midha KK. Stereoselective in vivo and in vitro studies on the metabolism of doxepin and N-desmethyldoxepin. Xenobiotica 27:1245–1257 (1997).
69. Baselt RC and Cravey RH. Disposition of toxic drugs and chemicals in man, 4th ed. Foster City, CA: Chemical Technology Institute, 1995.
70. Parfitt K, ed. Martindale. The complete drug reference, 32nd ed. Parfitt K, ed. London: Pharmaceutical Press, 1999.
71. Spiller HA, Winter ML, Mann KV, Borys DJ, Muir S, and Krenzelok EP. Five year retrospective review of cyclobenzaprine toxicity. J Emerg Med 13:781–785 (1995).
72. Diamond S. Human metabolism of amitriptyline tagged with carbon 14. Curr Ther Res 7: 170–175 (1965).
73. Crammer JL, Scott B, and Rolfe B. Metabolism of ^{14}C-imipramine: II, Urinary metabolites in man. Pschopharmacology 15:207–225 (1969).
74. Kawahara K, Awajji T, Uda K, Sakai Y, and Hashimoto Y. Urinary excretion of conjugates of dothiepin and northiepin (mono-N-demethyl-dothiepin) after an oral dose of dothiepin to humans. Eur J Drug Met Pharmacokin 11:29–32 (1986).
75. Dusci LJ and Hackett LP. Gas chromatographic determination of doxepin in human urine following therapeutic doses. J Chrom 61:231–236 (1971).
76. Dubois J, Kung W, Theobald W, and Wirz B. Measurement of clomipramine, N-desmethylclomipramine, imipramine and dehydroimipramine in biological fluids by selective ion monitoring, and pharmacokinetics of clomipramine. Clin Chem 22:892–897 (1976)
77. Mellstrom B and von Bahr C. Demethylation and hydroxylation of amitriptyline, nortriptyline and 10-hydroxyamitriptyline in human liver microsomes. Drug Metab Dispos 9: 565–568 (1981).
78. Balant-Gorgia AE, Gex-Fabry M, and Balant LP. Clinical pharmacokinetics of clomipramine. Clin Pharmacokinet 20:447–462 (1991).
79. Ulrich S, Northoff G, Wurthman C, Partscht G, Pester U, Herscu H, and Meyer FP. Serum levels of amitriptyline and therapeutic effect in non-delusional moderately to severely depressed in-patients: a therapeutic window relationship. Pharmacopsyhiatry 34:33–40 (2001).
80. Breyer-Pfaff U, Geidke H, Gaertner HJ, and Nill K. Validation of a therapeutic plasma level in amitriptylene in treatment of depression. J Clin Psychopharmacol 9:116–121 (1989).
81. Perel JM, Mendlewicz J, Shostak M, Kantor SJ, and Glassman AH. Plasma levels of imipramine in depression. Environmental and genetic factors. Neuropsychobiology 2:193–202 (1976).
82. Preskorn SH, Burke MJ, and Fast GA. Therapeutic drug monitoring. Principles and practice. Psychiatr Clin North Am 16:611–645 (1993).
83. Eilers R. Therapeutic drug monitoring for the treatment of psychiatric disorders. Clinical use and cost effectiveness. Clin Pharmacokinet 29:442–450 (1995).

84. Preskorn SH and Fast GA. Tricyclic antidepressant-induced seizures and plasma drug concentrations. J Clin Psychiatry 53:160–162 (1992).
85. Biggs JT, Spiker DG, Petit JM, and Ziegler VE. Tricyclic antidepressant overdose: incidence of symptoms. JAMA 238:135–138 (1977).
86. Spiker DG, Weiss AN, Chang SS, Rutwitch JF, and Biggs JT. Tricyclic antidepressant overdose: clinical presentation and plasma levels. Clin Pharmacol Ther 18:539–546 (1975).
87. Caravati EM and Bossart PJ. Demographic and electrocardiographic factors associated with severe tricyclic antidepressant toxicity. J Toxicol Clin Toxicol 29:31–34 (1991).
88. Haddard LM. Managing tricyclic antidepressant overdose. Am Fam Physician 46:153–159 (1992).
89. Nordin C, Bertilsson L, Dahl ML, Resul B, Toresson G, and Sjoqvist F. Treatment of depression with E-10-hydroxynortriptyline—a pilot study on biochemical effects and pharmacokinetics. Psychopharmacology 103:287–290 (1991).
90. Shimoda K, Yasuda S, Morita S, Shibasaki M, Someya T, Bertilsson L, and Takahashi S. Psychiatry Clin Neurosci 51:35–41 (1997).
91. Pollock BG and Perel JM. Imipramine and 2-hydroxyimipramine: comparative cardiotoxicity and pharmacokinetics in swine. Psychopharmacology 109:57–62 (1992).
92. Pollock BG, Everett G, and Perel JM. Comparative cardiotoxicity of nortryptyline and its isomeric 10-hydroxymetabolites. Neuropsychopharmacology 6:1–10 (1992).
93. Dahl-Puustinen ML, Perry TJ Jr, Dumont E, von Bahr C, Nordin C, and Bertilsson L. Stereospecific disposition of racemic E-10-hydroxynortriptyline in human beings. Clin Pharmacol Ther 45:650–656 (1989).
94. Melstrom B, Sawe J, Bertilsson L, and Sjoqvist F. Amitriptyline metabolism: association with debrisoquin hydroxylation in nonsmokers. Clin Pharmacol Ther 39:369–371 (1986).
95. Brosen K, Zeugin T, and Meyer UA. Role of P450IID6, the target of sparteine-debrisoquin oxidation polymorphism, in the metabolism of imipramine. Clin Pharmacol Ther 49:609–617 (1991).
96. Breyer-Pfaff U, Pfandl B, Nill K, Nusser E, Monney C, Jonzier-Perey M, et al. Enantioselective amitriptyline metabolism in patients phenotyped for two cytochropme P450 isozymes. Clin Pharmacol Ther 52:350–358 (1992).
97. Petersen P and Brosen K. Severe nortriptyline poisoning in poor metabolisers of the sparteine type. Ugeskr Laeger 153:443–444 (1991).
98. Dahl ML, Bertilsson L, and Nordin C. Steady-state plasma levels of nortriptyline and its 10-hydroxymetabolite: relationship to the CYP2D6 genotype. Psycopharmacology (Berl) 123:315–319 (1996).
99. Lemoine A, Gautier JC, Azoulay D, Kiffel L, Belloc C, Guengerich FP, et al. Major pathway of imipramine metabolism is catalyzed by cytochromes P-450 1A2 and P-450 3A2 in human liver. Mol Pharmacol 43:827–832 (1993).
100. Ghahramani P, Ellis SW, Lennard MS, Ramsay LE, and Tucker GT. Cytochromes P450 mediating the demethylation of amitriptyline. Br J Clin Pharmacol 43:137–144 (1997).
101. Koyama E, Chiba K, Tani M, and Ishizaki T. Reappraisal of human CYP isoforms involved in imipramine N-demethylation and 2-hydroxylation: a study using microsomes obtained from putative extensive and poor metabolizers of S-mephenytoin and eleven recombinant human CYPs. J Pharmacol Exp Ther 281:1199–1210 (1997).
102. Olsen OV and Linnet K. Hydroxylation and demethylation of the tricyclic antidepressant nortriptyline by cDNA-expressed human cytochrome P-450 isoenzymes. Drug Metab Dispos 25:740–744 (1997).
103. Venkatakrishnan K, Greenblatt DJ, von Moltke LL, Schmider J, Harmatz JS, and Shader RI. Five distinct human cytochromes mediate amitriptyline N-demethylation in vitro: dominance of CYP 2C19 and 3A4. J Clin Pharmacol 38:112–121 (1998).

104. Venkatakrishnan K, Schmider J, Harmatz JS, Ehrenberg BL, von Moltke LL, Graf JA, et al. Relative contribution of CYP3A to amitriptyline clearance in humans: *in vitro* and *in vivo* studies. J Clin Pharmacol 41:1043–1054 (2001).
105. Coutts RT, Bach MV, and Baker GB. Metabolism of amitriptyline with CYP2D6 expressed in a human cell line. Xenobiotica 27:33–47 (1997).
106. Venkatakrishnan K, von Moltke LL, and Greenblatt DJ. Nortriptyline E-10-hydroxylation in vitro is mediated by human CYP2D6 (high affinity) and CYP3A4 (low affinity): implications for interactions with enzyme inducing drugs. J Clin Pharmacol 39:567–577 (1999).
107. Haritos VS, Ghabrial H, Ahokas JT, and Ching MS. Role of cytochrome P450 2D6 (CYP2D6) in the stereospecific metabolism of E- and Z-doxepin. Pharmacogenetics 10:591–603 (2000).
108. Ereshefsky AJ, Zarycranski W, Taylor K, Albano D, and Klockowski PM. Effect of venlafaxine vrs fluoxetine on metabolism of dextromethorphan, a CYP2D6 probe. J Clin Pharmacol 41:443–451 (2001).
109. Pelkonen O, Raunio H, Rautio A, and Lang M. Xenobiotic-metabolizing enzymes and cancer risk: correspondence between genotype and phenotype. In: Vineis P, ed. Metabolic polymorphisms and susceptibility to cancer: Lyon: International Agency for Cancer Research. 1999:77–88.
110. Mahgoub A, Idle JR, Dring LG, Lancaster R, and Smith RL. Polymorphic hydroxylation of debrisoquine in man. Lancet 2:584–586 (1997).
111. Eichelbaum M, Spanbrucker N, Steincke B, and Dengler HG. Defective N-oxidation of sparteine in man: a new pharmacogenetic defect. Eur J Clin Pharmacol 16:183–187 (1979).
112. Daly AK, Armstrong M, Monkman SC, Idle ME, and Idle JR. Genetic and metabolic criteria for the assignment of debrisoquine 4-hydroxylation (cytochrome P4502D6) phenotypes. Pharmacogenetics 1:33–41 (1991).
113. Kroemer HK and Eichelbaum M. Molecular basis and clinical consequences of genetic cytochrome P450 2D6 polymorphism. Life Sci 56:2285–2298 (1995).
114. Sachse C, Brockmoller J, Bauer S, and Roots I. Cytochrome P450 2D6 variants in a Caucasian population: allele frequencies and phenotypic consequences. Am J Hum Genet 60: 284–295 (1997).
115. Mayer UA and Zanger UM. Molecular mechanisms of genetic polymorphisms of drug metabolism. Annu Rev Pharmacol Toxicol 37:269–296 (1997).
116. Nebert DW. Pharmacogenetics: 65 candles on the cake. Pharmacogenetics 7:435–440 (1997).
117. Ingelman-Sundberg M, Oscarson M, and McLellan RA. Polymorphic human cytochrome P450 enzymes: an opportunity for individualized drug treatment. Trends in Pharmacological Sciences 20:342–349 (1999).
118. Tamminga WJ, Wemer J, Oosterhuis B, de Zeeuw RA, de Leij L, and Jonkman JH. The prevalence of CYP2D6 and CYP2C19 genotypes in a population of healthy Dutch volunteers. Eur J Clin Pharmacol 57:717–722 (2001).
119. Aynacioglu AS, Sachse C, Bozkurt A, Kortunay S, Nacak M, Schroder T, et al. Low frequency of defective alleles of cytochrome P450 enzymes 2C16 and 2C19 in the Turkish population. Clin Pharmacol Ther 66:185–192 (1999).
120. Dandara C, Masimirembwa CM, Magimba A, Sayi J, Kaaya S, Sommers DK, et al. Genetic polymorphism of CYP2D6 and CYP2C19 in east- and southern African populations including psychiatric patients. Eur J Clin Pharmacol 57:11–17 (2001).
121. Bathum L, Skejelbo E, Mutabingwa TK, Madsen H, Horder M, and Brosen K. Phenotypes and genotypes for CYP2D6 and CYP2C19 in a black Tanzanian population. Br J Clin Pharmacol 48:395–401 (1999).
122. Yue QY, Zhong ZH, Tybring G, Dalen P, Dahl ML, Bertilsson L, and Sjoqvist F. Pharmacokinetics of nortriptyline and its 10-hydroxy metabolite in Chinese subjects of different CYP2D6 genotypes. Clin Pharmacol Ther 64:384–390 (1998).

123. Dahl ML, Iselius L, Alm C, Svensson JO, Lee D, Johansson I, and Ingelman-Sundberg M. Polymorphic 2-hydroxylation of desipramine. A population and family study. Eur J Clin Pharmacol 44:445–450 (1993).
124. Skjelbo E, Brosen K, Hallas J, and Gram LF. The mephentoin oxidation polymorphism is partially responsible for the N-demethylation of imipramine. Clin Pharmacol Ther 49: 18–23 (1991).
125. Koyama E, Sohn D-R, Shin S-G, Chiba K, Shin J-G, Kim Y-H, et al. Metabolic distribution of imipramine in oriental subjects: relation to motoprolol α-hydroxylation and S-mephenytoin-4-hydroxylation phenotypes. J Pharmacol Exp Ther 271:860–867 (1994).
126. Nakamura K, Goto F, Ray WA, McAllister CB, Jacqz E, Wilkinson GR, and Branch RA. Interethnic differences in genetic polymorphism of debrisoquin and mephenytoin hydroxylation between Japanese and Caucasian populations. Clin Pharmacol Ther 38:402–408 (1985).
127. Horai Y, Nakano M, Ishizaki T, Ishikawa K, Zhou H-H, Zhou B-J, et al. Metoprolol and mephenytoin oxidation polymorphisms in Far Eastern oriental subjects: Japanese versus mainland Chinese. Clin Pharmacol Ther 46:198–207 (1989).
128. Morita S, Shimoda K, Someya T, Yoshimura Y, Kamijima K, and Kato N. Steady-state plasma levels of nortriptyline and its hydroxylated metabolites in Japanese patients: impact of CYP2D6 genotype on the hydroxylation of nortriptyline. J Clin Psychopharmacol 20: 141–149 (2000).
129. Shimoda K, Morita S, Hirokane G, Yokono A, Someya T, and Takahashi S. Metabolism of desipramine in Japanese psychiatric patients: the impact of CYP2D6 genotype on the hydroxylation of desipramine. Pharmacol Toxicol 86:245–249 (2000).
130. Crewe HK, Lennard MS, Tucker GT, Woods FR, and Haddock RE. The effect of selective serotonin re-uptake inhibitors on cytochrome P4502D6 (CYP2D6) activity in human liver microsomes. Brit J Clin Pharmacol 34:262–265 (1992).
131. Alfaro CL, Lam YW, Simpson J, and Ereshefsky L. J Clin Pharmacol 40:58–66 (2000).
132. el-Yazigi A, Chaleby K, Gad A, and Raines DA. Steady-state kinetics of fluoxetine and amitriptyline in patients treated with a combination of these drugs as compared to those treated with amitriptyline alone. J Clin Pharmacol 35:17–21 (1995)
133. Leuch S, Hackl HJ, Steimer W, Angersbach D, and Zimmer R. Effect of adjunctive paroxetine on serum levels and side effects of tricyclic antidepressants in depressive inpatients. Psychopharmacology 147:378–383 (2000).
134. Preskorn SH, Alderman J, Chung M, Harrison W, Messig M, and Harris S. Pharmacokinetics of desipramine coadministered with sertraline or fluoxetine. J Clin Psychopharmacol 14:90–98 (1994).
135. Alderman J, Preskorn SH, Greenblatt J, Harrison W, Penenberg D, Allison J, and Chung M. Desipramine pharmacokinetics when coadministered with paroxetine or sertraline in extensive metabolizers. J Clin Psychopharmacol 17:284–291 (1997).
136. Solai LK, Mulsant BH, Pollock BG, Sweet RA, Rosen J, Yu K, and Reynolds CF 3rd. Effects of sertraline on plasma nortriptyline levels in depressed elderly. J Clin Psychiatry 58:440–443 (1997).
137. Brosen K and Naranjo CA. Review of pharmacokinetic and pharmacodynamic studies with citalopram. Eur Neuropsychopharmacol 11:275–283 (2001).
138. Albers LJ, Reist C, Vu RL, Fujimoto K, Ozdemir V, Helmeste D, et al. Effect of venlafaxine on imipramine metabolism. Psychiatry Res 96:235–243 (2000).
139. Brozen K, Hansen JG, Nielsen KK, Sindrup SH, and Gram LF. Inhibition by paroxetine of desipramine metabolism in extensive but not in poor metabolizers of sparteine. Eur J Clin Pharmacol 44:349–355 (1993).

140. Laine K, Tybring G, Harrter S, Andersson K, Svensson JO, Widen J, and Bertilsson L. Inhibition of cytochrome P4502D6 activity with paroxetine normalizes the ultrarapid metabolizer phenotype as measured by nortriptyline pharmacokinetics and the debrisoquine test. Clin Pharmacol Ther 70:327–335 (2001).
141. Rasmussen BB, Nielsen TL, and Brosen K. Fluvoxamine inhibits the CYP2C19-catalyzed metabolism of proquanil in vitro. Eur J Clin Pharmacol 54:735–740 (1998).
142. Spina F, Pollicino AM, Avenoso A, Campo GM, Perruca E, and Caputi AP. Effect of fluvoxamine on the pharmacokinetics of imipramine and desipramine in healthy subjects. Ther Drug Monit 15:243–246 (1993).
143. Xu ZH, Huang SL, and Shou HH. Inhibition of imipramine N-demethylation by fluvoxamine in chinese young men. Zhongguo Yao Li Xue Bao 17:399–402 (1996).
144. Conus P, Bondolfi G, Eap CB, Macciardi F, and Baumann P. Pharmacokinetic fluvoxamine-clomipramine interaction with favorable therapeutic consequences in therapy-resistant depressive patient. Pharmacopsychiatry 29:108–110 (1996).
145. Jerling M, Bertilsson L, and Sjoqvist F. The use of therapeutic drug monitoring data to document kinetic drug interactions: an example with amitriptyline and nortriptyline. Ther Drug Monit 16:1–12 (1994).
146. Baumann P, Meyer JW, Amey M, Baettig D, Bryois C, Jonzier-Perey M, et al. Dextromethorphan and mephenytoin phenotyping of patients treated with thioridazine or amitriptyline. Ther Drug Monit 14:1–8 (1992).
147. Llerena A, Berecz R, de la Rubia A, Fernandez-Salguero P, and Dorado P. Effect of thioridazine dosage on the debrisoquine hydroxylation phenotype in psychiatric patients with different CYP2D6 genotypes. Ther Drug Monit 23:616–620 (2001).
148. Maynard GL and Soni P. Thioridazine interferences with imipramine metabolism and measurement. Ther Drug Monit 18:729–731 (1996).
149. Gury C, Canceil O, and Iaria P. Antipsychotic drugs and cardiovascular safety: current studies of prolonged QT interval and risk of ventricular arrhythmia. Encephale 26:62–72 (2000).
150. Ray WA, Meredith S, Thapa PB, Meador KG, Hall K, and Murray KT. Antipsychotics and the risk of sudden cardiac death. Arch Gen Psychiatry 58:1161–1167 (2001).
151. Buckley NA, Whyte IM, and Dawson AH. Cardiotoxicity more common in thioridazine overdose than with other neuroleptics. J Toxicol Clin Toxicol 33:199–204 (1995).
152. Hartigan-Go K, Bateman DN, Nyberg G, Martensson E, and Thomas SH. Concentration related pharmacodynamic effects of thioridazine and its metabolites in humans. Clin Pharmacol Ther 60:543–553 (1996).
153. Daniel WA, Syrek M, Haduch A, and Wojcikowski J. Pharmacokinetics and metabolism of thioridazine during coadministration of tricyclic antidepressants. Br J Pharmacol 131:287–295 (2000).
154. Donahue SR, Flockhart DA, Abernethy DR, and Ko JW. Ticlopidine inhibition of phenytoin metabolism mediated by potent inhibition of CYP2C19. Clin Pharmacol Ther 62:572–577 (1997).
155. Lopez-Aritzegui N, Ochoa M, Sanchez-Migallon MJ, Nevado C, and Martin M. Acute phenytoin poisoning secondary to and interaction with ticlopidine. Rev Neurol 26:1017–1018 (1998).
156. Ko JW, Desta Z, Soukhova NV, Tracy T, and Flockhart DA. In vitro inhibition of the cytochrome P450 (CYP450) system by the antiplatelet drug ticlopidine: potent effect on CYP2C19 and CYP2D6. Br J Clin Pharmacol 49:343–351 (2000).
157. Ha-Duong NT, Dijols S, Macherey AC, Goldstein JA, Dansette PM, and Mansuy D. Ticlopidine as a selective mechanism-based inhibitor of human cytochrome P450 2C19. Biochemistry 40:12112–12122 (2001).

158. Dietrich DE and Emrich HM. The use of anticonvulsants to augment antidepressant medication. J Clin Psychiatry 59(Suppl 5):57–58 (1998).
159. Leinonen E, Lillsunde P, Laukkanen V, and Ylitali P. Effects of carbamazepine on serum antidepressant concentrations in psychiatric patients. J Clin Psychopharmacol 11:313–318 (1991).
160. Spina E, Pisani F, and Perucca E. Clinically significant pharmacokinetic drug interactions with carbamazepine. An update. Clin Pharmacokinet 31:198–214 (1996).
161. Szymura-Oleksiak J, Wyska E, and Wasieczko A. Pharmacokinetic interaction between imipramine and carbamazepine in patients with major depression. Psychpharmacology 154: 38–42 (2001).
162. Parker AC, Pritchard P, Preston T, and Choonara I. Induction of CYP1A2 activity by carbamazepine in children using the caffeine breath test. Brit J Clin Pharmacol 45:176–178 (1998).
163. Dorian P, Sellers EM, Reed KL, Warsh JJ, Hamilton C, Kaplan HL, and Fan T. Amitriptyline and ethanol: pharmacokinetic and pharmacodynamic interaction. Eur J Clin Pharmacol 25:325–331 (1983).
164. Basalt RC. Amitriptyline. In: Drug Effects on Psychomotor Performance. Foster City, CA: Biomedical Publications, 2001.
165. Power BM, Hackett LP, Dusci LJ, and Ilett KF. Antidepressant toxicity and the need for identification and concentration monitoring in overdose. Clin Pharmacokinet 29:154–171 (1995).
166. Stolk LML and Geest S van der. Plasma concentrations after a clomipramine intoxication. J Anal Toxicol 22:612–613 (1998).
167. Vermeulen T. Distribution of paroxetine in three postmortem cases. J Anal Toxicol 22: 541–544 (1998).
168. Druid H, Holmgren P, Carlsson B, and Ahlner J. Cytochrome P450 2D6 (CYP2D6) genotyping on postmortem blood as a supplementary tool of forensic toxicological results. Forensic Sci Int 99:25–34 (1999).
169. Spigset O, Hedenmalm K, Dahl ML, Wilholm BE, and Dahlqvist R. Seizures and myoclonus associated with antidepressant treatment: assessment of potential risk factors, including CYP2D6 and CYP2C19 polymorphisms, and treatment with CYP2D6 inhibitors. Acta Psychiatr Scand 96:379–384 (1997).
170. Vandel S, Bertschy G, Bonin B, Nezelof S, Fransois TH, Vandel B, et al. Tricyclic antidepressant plasma levels after fluoxetine addition. Neuropsychobiology 25:202–207 (1992).
171. Bonin B, Bertschy G, Baumann P, Francois T, Vandel P, Vandel S, et al. Fluoxetine and tricyclic antidepressants: clinical tolerance in short-term combined administration. Encephale 22:221–227 (1996).
172. Levitt AJ, Joffe RT, Kamil R, and McIntyre R. Do depressed subjects who have failed fluoxetine and a tricyclic antidepressant respond to the combination? J Clin Psychiatry 60: 613–616 (1999).
173. Preskorn SH and Baker B. Fatality associated with combined fluoxetine-amitriptyline therapy. JAMA 277:1682 (1997).
174. Chaturvedi AK, Hidding JT, Rao JT, Smith JT 2nd, and Bredehoeft SJ. Two tricyclic antidepressant poisonings: levels of amitriptyline, nortriptyline and desipramine in postmortem blood. Forensic Sci Int 33:93–101 (1987).
175. September 11September 11ns. J Anal Toxicol 13:303–304 (1989).
176. Musshoff F, Grellner W, and Madea B. Toxicological findings in suicide with doxepin and paroxetine. Arch Kriminol 204:28–32 (1999).
177. Pounder DJ and Jones GR. Post-mortem drug redistribution—a toxicological nightmare. Forensic Sci Int 45:253–263 (1990).

178. Pounder DJ, Hartley AK, and Watmough PJ. Postmortem redistribution and degradation of dothiepin. Human case studies and an animal model. Am J Forensic Med Pathol 15:231–235 (1994).
179. Hilberg T, Morland J, and Bjroneboe A. Postmortem release of amitriptyline from the lungs; a mechanism of post-mortem drug redistribution. Forensic Sci Int 64:47–55 (1994).
180. Hilberg T, Rogde S, and Morland J. Post-mortem drug redistribution—human cases related to results in experimental animals. J Forensic Sci 44:3–9 (1999).
181. Pounder DJ, Owen V, and Quigley C. Postmortem changes in blood amitriptyline concentration. Am J Forensic Med Pathol 15:224–230 (1994).

Chapter 5

Selective Serotonin Reuptake Inhibitors

Mojdeh Mozayani, PharmD
and Ashraf Mozayani, PharmD, PhD

1. INTRODUCTION

Selective serotonin reuptake inhibitors (SSRIs) are one of the newer classes of antidepressants. Since their introduction in the United States, they have been greatly used and accepted in the psychiatric field *(1)*. SSRIs presently available in the United States include fluoxetine, paroxetine, sertraline, fluvoxamine, and citalopram. SSRIs act by inhibiting neuronal uptake of serotonin (5HT). SSRIs are generally shown to be as effective and overall better tolerated than tricyclic antidepressants (TCAs) in treatment of depression *(2,3)*. SSRIs are also used in treating other psychiatric disorders such as panic disorder *(4,13)*, obsessive compulsive disorder, and social anxiety disorder *(5–7)*.

Depression is among the most common illnesses in the United States *(8)*. However, it is underdiagnosed and undertreated in this country *(9)*. In recent years, there has been a significant increase in the number of patients who received outpatient treatment for depression *(7,8)*. SSRIs are widely used in the treatment of psychiatric disorders *(5–7,10)*; therefore, understanding drug interactions involving this class of agents is very important. In this chapter, SSRIs' mechanism of action, pharmacokinetics, drug and herbal interactions, and adverse reactions are described.

2. MECHANISM OF ACTION

SSRIs, as indicated by their name, block the central nervous system (CNS) neuronal uptake of serotonin (5HT), which is related to their antidepressant action *(11)*. SSRIs

From: *Handbook of Drug Interactions: A Clinical and Forensic Guide*
A. Mozayani and L. P. Raymon, eds. © Humana Press Inc., Totowa, NJ

Table 1
Pharmacokinetic Parameters of SSRIs

Drug (ref)	Vd (L/kg)	$t_{1/2}$ (hours)	Time to Steady State (days)
Fluoxetine (15)	20–45	24–72	30–660
Paroxetine (19,23)	20	7–37	7–14
Sertraline (12,22)	20	22–36	5–7
Citalopram (24,25)	12–15	25–35	6–15
Fluvoxamine (18)	5	8–28	10

selectively inhibit the reuptake of serotonin; however, they also have a different degree of effect on blocking the reuptake of norepinephrine and dopamine (11,12). Paroxetine is the most potent SSRI available; however, it has less selectivity for serotonin sites than do fluvoxamine and sertraline (12). Citalopram is the most selective SSRI on the market (12). Sertraline is both the second most potent and second most selective SSRI (12).

3. PHARMACOKINETICS

In order to better understand the drug interactions involving SSRIs, it is essential to understand their pharmacokinetic properties.

3.1. Absorption

SSRIs are in general well absorbed from the gastrointestinal tract, however they undergo hepatic first-pass metabolism to a varying degree. This reduces the amount of intact drug that reaches the systemic circulation (12).

Fluoxetine, fluvoxamine, paroxetine, sertraline, and citalopram are well absorbed (15–17,19). Food does not alter their absorption significantly (14). All SSRIs, with the exception of citalopram, undergo extensive hepatic first-pass metabolism (15–17,19).

3.2. Distribution

SSRIs have a relatively large volume of distribution (Vd) due to their lipophilic properties. These large Vds suggest extensive accumulation in tissues, particulary fatty tissues (15). Fluoxetine, paroxetine, and sertraline are highly protein bound, especially to α-1 acid glycoproteins (15). Citalopram and fluvoxamine do not bind as extensively to plasma proteins (15).

For drugs that exhibit single-compartment pharmacokinetic behavior, a steady-state plasma concentration is achieved in about four to five half-lives. Drugs that are extensively distributed throughout the deep-tissue reservoirs of the body (i.e., those drugs with large Vd) take a longer time to achieve a steady-state concentration because of the increased time and amount of drug required to attain equilibrium in these deep-tissue stores. SSRIs therefore require a significantly longer time to attain a steady-state concentration.

Table 2
Active Metabolites of SSRIs

SSRIs	Active Metabolites	Clinically Significant
Fluoxetine	Norfluoxetine	Yes
Fluvoxamine	—	—
Paroxetine	—	—
Sertraline	Desmethylsertraline	? No
Citalopram	Desmethylcitalopram, Didesmethylcitalopram	No

The Vd, $t_{1/2}$ (terminal elimination half-life), and time to steady state of these SSRIs are summarized in Table 1.

3.3. Metabolism and Elimination

Metabolism is the main route of elimination for all SSRIs *(12)*. SSRIs are mainly hepatically metabolized and renally excreted *(25)*. Fluoxetine is metabolized extensively by CYP2D6 to its active metabolite (norfluoxetine) and other metabolites *(28)*. It is reported that half-lives ($t_{1/2}$s) of fluoxetine and its metabolite norfluoxetine range from 1 to 5 d and 7 to 20 d, respectively *(20,21)*. Fluvoxamine is metabolized by CYP1A2 and CYP2D6 *(29)*. Its metabolites are inactive *(17)*. Fluvoxamine's $t_{1/2}$ is between 8 and 28 h *(18)*. Paroxetine is also metabolized to clinically inactive metabolites by CYP2D6 *(30)*. Its $t_{1/2}$ is variable depending on the subject, dosage, and duration of administration *(16)*. Its terminal half-life is about 1 d *(16,19)*. Metabolism is also the main route of elimination for sertraline. Its main active metabolite, desmethylsertraline, is obtained by demethylation of sertraline by CYP3A4 *(31)*. This metabolite has a half-life three times longer than sertraline (60–100 h) *(22,26)*. Sertraline has a longer $t_{1/2}$ in elderly and female volunteers (32.1–36.7 h) than in young male volunteers (22.4 h) *(22)*. Citalopram is metabolized by CYP2C19 and CYP3A4 to several metabolites, including two pharmacologically active metabolites: desmethylcitalopram and didesmethylcitalopram *(27,32)*. The half-life for citalopram ranges from 35 to 58.5 h depending on the study *(24,25)*. Although its active metabolites have two to three times longer half-lives, their activity, because of their low potency, is not clinically important *(12,24)*. Refer to Table 2 for a summary of active metabolites.

4. CYTOCHROME P450 SYSTEM

SSRIs are extensively metabolized as discussed previously. Cytochrome P-450 iso-enzymes play a major role in their metabolism and, hence, their interactions with other drugs *(15)*. Therefore, in order to better understand the drug interactions involving SSRIs, it is essential to understand this system. Cytochrome P-450 is composed of many enzymes; however, most drugs are metabolized by three families of enzymes in this system: CYP1A2, CYP2D6, and CYP3A4. SSRIs' inhibitory effects on these enzymes play a major role in most of their drug interactions *(33)*. Fluoxetine, its metabolite norfluoxetine, and paroxetine are potent inhibitors of CYP2D6 enzymes, and there-

Table 3
Metabolization and Inhibition of SSRIs by Cytochrome P-450

SSRIs	Metabolized by	CYP450 Enzyme Inhibited
Fluoxetine	CYP2D6	CYP2C19, CYP2D6***
Norfluoxetine	—	CYP2D6***
Fluvoxamine	CYP1A2, CYP2D6	CYP2C19, CYP1A2,*** CYP3A4*
Paroxetine	CYP2D6	CYP2D6,*** CYP2C19***
Sertraline	CYP3A4	CYP2D6**
Citalopram	CYP2C19, CYP3A4	CYP2D6*
Desmethylcitalopram	—	CYP2D6**

Degree of inhibition is indicated by: ***, Potent; **, Moderate; *, Weak.

fore inhibit the metabolism of many TCAs and antipsychotic drugs *(33,34,36)*. Fluoxetine and fluvoxamine also inhibit CYP2C19 to a lesser extent *(21,36)*. Fluvoxamine is a strong inhibitor of CYP1A2, therefore very likely to interact with other drugs *(17,33, 34,36)*. Sertraline has a moderate inhibitory effect on CYP2D6 *(34)*. Citalopram does not seem to have many pharmacokinetic drug interactions, since it is a weak inhibitor of CYP2D6 *(35,36)*. Table 3 summarizes the actions of these enzymes.

5. Drug–Drug Interactions

Drug interactions are classified into two major groups: pharmacodynamic interactions and pharmacokinetic interactions. Pharmacodynamic interactions are described as a change in the pharmacologic effect of the target drug produced by the activity of another drug at the same receptor or a different site (with the same activity or a different or opposite effect). In other words, the mechanism of action of one drug may amplify or diminish the mechanism of action of the other drug *(37)*. Pharmacokinetic interactions involve any alteration in absorption, distribution, metabolism, or elimination of the target drug caused by coadministration of another medication.

5.1. Pharmacodynamic Interactions

Serotonin syndrome is a major pharmacodynamic interaction that occurs when SSRIs are administered concomitantly with other drugs including monoamine oxidase inhibitors (MAOIs), lithium, other SSRIs, dextromethorphan, meperidine, L-tryptophan, sumatriptan, risperidone, and MDMA (known as ecstasy) *(37,39,40)*. However, other mechanisms such as defects in monoamine metabolism and hepatic and pulmonary insufficiency may contribute in developing this condition *(42)*.

Serotonin syndrome is described as serotonergic hyperstimulation. Any drug or drug combinations that increase serotonin neurotransmission can cause serotonin syndrome *(37)*. Serotonin syndrome is an acute condition that is characterized by changes in mental status, restlessness, dyskinesia, clonus and myoclonus, autonomic dysfunction such as mydriasis, hyperthermia, shivering, diaphoresis, and diarrhea *(37–39,41)*. Neuroleptic malignant syndrome is described as an idiosyncratic response of patients to mostly neuroleptic agents with high D2 potency *(37)*. Serotonin syndrome and neuroleptic malignant syndrome are very similar in signs and symptoms. It is difficult to differentiate between these two syndromes, but in general patients with neuroleptic malignant syndrome present with higher fever and more muscle rigidity; on the other hand, patients with serotonin syndrome have more gastrointestinal dysfunction and myoclonus *(43)*. Symptoms in neuroleptic malignant syndrome appear more gradual and resolve more slowly *(38)*. Both syndromes are treated by discontinuing the offending agent and supportive care *(38,43)*. Caution is advised if initiating drug therapy in these two syndromes. Some patients with serotonin syndrome may require drug therapy with antiserotonergic agents such as cyproheptadine, methysergide, and propranolol *(37)*. These agents may not be effective in treating neuroleptic malignant syndrome. Dopamine agonists that are used to treat neuroleptic malignant syndrome may exacerbate a serotonin syndrome *(38)*.

Serotonin syndrome is usually mild and resolves quickly when the serotonergic drugs are discontinued and supportive care is provided. However, there have been numerous cases of fatalities due to this syndrome. These are mostly caused by intentional drug overdosage and/or combining different serotonergic drugs *(44–48)*.

5.2. Pharmacokinetic Interactions

Oral absorption can be affected by the presence of certain drugs that can change gastrointestinal motility or pH. Food can also change drug absorption. SSRIs' interactions involving absorption are not clinically significant *(49)*.

Drug distribution is influenced by such factors as blood flow, drug lipophilicity, and its protein-binding ability. Only the unbound drug (free fraction) is able to act on the receptor site. Although SSRIs are highly protein bound, their interaction involving protein binding is clinically minor *(49)*.

Interactions involving metabolism and the enzymes that facilitate this process are the most studied. There is also individual variability in metabolizing drugs. For example, it is a well-established fact that there are individuals who do not synthesize the enzyme CYP2D6, leading to poor metabolism of the drugs metabolized by this enzyme. As indicated in Table 2, SSRIs inhibit some of the most important CYP450 enzymes involved in other drugs' metabolism, hence leading to increased levels of those drugs. There are a great number of drugs that are metabolized by these enzymes. A few examples are given in Table 4 *(50)*.

On the other hand, since SSRIs are metabolized by mostly the same enzymes, their metabolism can be affected by inhibitors and inducers of these enzymes. Drugs such as sulfonylureas, barbiturates, phenytoin, carbamazepine, rifampin, and primidone are CYP enzyme inducers that cause an increase in metabolism of the drugs including SSRIs, whose main route of metabolism is by CYP450 system enzymes. Enzyme inhibitors such as cimetidine, erythromycin, isoniazid, verapamil, and propoxyphene can lead to an increase in plasma levels of affected drugs. Table 5 summarizes a number of drug–drug interactions mediated by metabolic enzymes. It should be emphasized that this table does not include all the drug interactions involving SSRIs. However, it indicates the importance of understanding pharmacokinetic drug interactions involving this class of drugs.

Table 4
Drugs Metabolized by CYP450 Isoenzymes

Enzyme	Examples of Metabolized Drugs
CYP1A2	TCAs (amitriptyline, imipramine), clozapine, propranolol, theophylline, R-warfarin
CYP2C19	Citalopram, imipramine, barbiturates, propranolol
CYP2D6	Antiarrythmics (propafenone, flecainide), β-blockers (propranolol, metoprolol, timolol), opiates, SSRIs (fluoxetine, paroxetine), TCAs, venlafaxine
CYP3A3/4	Acetaminophen, codeine, dextromethorpahn
CYP2C9/10	Phenytoin, S-warfarin, tolbutamide

6. DRUG–NATURAL PRODUCT INTERACTION

There are not many clinical trials on the potential of SSRIs' interaction with herbal products. It is suggested that if a natural product has an effect on CYP450 isoenzymes it potentially can interact with drugs metabolized by these enzymes. However this is not a reliable predictor for drug–natural product interaction (67). Examples of known drug–natural product interaction are: fluvoxamine significantly increases melatonin (sleep aid) levels by reducing its metabolism due to inhibition of CYP1A2 and CYP2C9 (67). Ayahuasca is an Amazonian psychoactive beverage that contains potent monoamine oxidase–inhibiting alkaloids (harmalines). It may induce serotonin syndrome if given with SSRIs (68,69). St John's wort (*Hypericum perforatum*) is used for mild to moderate depression. It may cause mild serotonin syndrome when given with SSRIs (70).

7. ADVERSE REACTIONS

SSRIs are generally well tolerated (71,76). However, they are associated with a few adverse effects. The most commonly reported adverse reactions to SSRIs are nausea, anorexia, diarrhea, insomnia, nervousness, headache, anxiety, dry mouth, constipation, hypotension, and fatigue (72). Cases of hyponatremia caused by SSRIs have also been reported (11,73). Mydriasis has been reported with paroxetine and sertraline (74). SSRIs are also implicated in extrapyramidal side effects and akathisia (75). Although SSRIs are relatively safe in cases of overdose, they have been associated with seizures in overdose situations (77).

8. CONCLUSIONS

SSRIs have become the first line of therapy in treatment of depression. They are also used in other areas of psychiatry such as obsessive-compulsive disorder and panic disorder. In general, SSRIs are considered to be well tolerated and safe. Therapeutic drug monitoring (TDM) is not commonly done with SSRIs, because there is no clear relationship between drug plasma concentrations and clinical response (79). However TDM may be useful in patients with poor compliance. It is also suggested that TDM of SSRIs can be a factor in overall cost reduction (80). SSRIs are involved in many drug–drug interactions, because of their activities on CYP enzymes. Therefore, when deal-

Table 5
Drug Interactions of SSRIs

Drug Causing Effect	Drug Affected	Observed Effect
Paroxetine	Codeine	Loss of efficacy *(50)*
Paroxetine	Risperidone	Inc. plasma levels *(51)*
Fluoxetine	Phentermine	Inc. plasma levels *(52)*
Fluoxetine, norfluoxetine, fluvoxamine, paroxetine, sertraline	Phenytoin	Inc. plasma levels *(53,60)*
Fluvoxamine	Methadone	Inc. plasma levels *(54)*
Sertraline	Alprazolam	No effect *(55,66)*
Fluoxetine, fluvoxamine, paroxetine	Benzodiazepines	Inc. plasma levels *(50)*
SSRIs	TCAs	Inc. plasma levels *(56)*
Rifampin	Sertraline	Dec. plasma levels *(57)*
Fluoxetine, paroxetine, fluvoxamine	Propafenone	Inc. plasma levels *(58)*
Fluoxetine, fluvoxamine	Warfarin	Inc. risk of bleeding *(59)*
Citalopram	Carbamazepine	No effect *(61)*
Fluoxetine, fluvoxamine	Carbamazepine	Inc. plasma levels *(11)*
Fluoxetine	Methadone	Inc/dec. plasma levels *(54,62)*
Paroxetine	Lithium	No effect *(63,64)*
Paroxetine	Metoprolol	Inc. plasma levels *(65)*

ing with SSRIs, it is essential for the clinician to have a thorough knowledge of the drugs' activity on CYP enzymes, and their metabolism. Although these interactions are usually undesirable, there have been instances when clinicians have taken advantage of them to successfully treat resistant cases *(81)*.

REFERENCES

1. Leonard B and Tollfeson G. Focus on SSRIs: broadening the spectrum of clinical use. J Clin Psychiatry 55:459–466 (1994).
2. Menting JE, Honig A, Verhey FR, Hartmans M, Rozendaal N, de Vet HC, and van Praag HM. Selective serotonin reuptake inhibitors (SSRIs) in the treatment of elderly depressed patients: a qualitative analysis of the literature on their efficacy and side effects. Int Clin Psychopharmacol 11(3):165–175 (1996).
3. Anderson IM. Selective serotonin reuptake inhibitors versus tricyclic antidepressants: a meta-analysis of efficacy and tolerability. J Affect Disord 58(1):19–36 (2000).
4. Otto MW, Tuby KS, Gould RA, McLean RY, and Pollack MH. An effect-size analysis of the relative efficacy and tolerability of serotonin reuptake inhibitors for panic disorder. Am J Psychiatry 158(12):1989–1992 (2001).
5. Tollefson GD, Rampey AH Jr, Potvin JH, Jenike MA, Rush AJ, Kominguez RA, et al. A multicenter investigation of fixed dose fluoxetine in the treatment of obsessive compulsive disorder. Arch Gen Psychiatry 51(7):559–567 (1994).
6. Wagstaff AJ, Cheer SM, Matheson AJ, Ormond D, and Goa KL. Paroxetine: an update of its use in psychiatric disorder in adults. Drugs 62(4):655–703 (2002).
7. Montgomery SA, Kasper S, Stein DJ, Bang Hededgaard K, and Lemming OM. Citalopram 20 mg, 40 mg, and 60 mg are all effective and well tolerated compared with placebo in obsessive compulsive disorder. Int Clin Psychopharmacol 16(2):75–86 (2001).

8. Fichter MM, Narrow WE, Roper MT, Rehm J, Elton M, Rae DS, et al. Prevalence of mental illness in Germany and the United States: comparison of the Upper Bavarian Study and the Epidemiologic Catchment Area Program. J Nerv Ment Dis 184:598–606 (1996).
9. Hirschfeld RM, Keller MB, Panico S, et al. The National Depressive and Manic-Depressive Association consensus statement on the under treatment of depression. JAMA 277: 333–340 (1997).
10. Gregor KJ, Way K, Young CH, and James SP. Concomitant use of selective serotonin reuptake inhibitors with other cytochrome P450 2D6 or 3A4 metabolized medications: how often does it really happen? J Affect Disord 46(1):59–67 (1997).
11. Drug facts and comparison, Jan 2000.
12. Hiemke C and Hartter S. Pharmacokinetics of selective serotonin reuptake inhibitors. Pharmacol Ther 85(1):11–28 (2000).
13. Rapaport MH, Wolkow R, Rubin A, Hackett E, Pollack M, and Ota KY. Sertraline treatment of panic disorder: results of a long-term study. Acta Psychiatrica Scandinavica 104(4): 289–298 (2001).
14. DeVane CL. Pharmacokinetics of the newer antidepressants: clinical relevance. Am J Med 97(6A):13S–23S (1994).
15. Catterson M and Preskorn SH. Pharmacokinetics of selective serotonin reuptake inhibitors: clinical relevance. Pharmacol Toxicol 78(4):203–208 (1996).
16. Van Harten J. Clinical pharmacokinetics of selective serotonin reuptake inhibitors. Clin Pharmacokinet 24:203–220 (1993).
17. DeVane CL and Gill HS. Clinical pharmacokinetics of fluvoxamine: applications to dosage regimen design. J Clin Psychiatry 58(5):7–14 (1997).
18. DeVries MH, Raghoebar M, Mathlener IS, and van Harten J. Single and multiple oral dose fluvoxamine kinetics in young and elderly subjects. Therap Drug Monit 14:493–498 (1992).
19. Kaye CM, Haddock RE, Langley PF, Mellows G, Tasker TCG, Zussman BD, and Greb WH. A review of the metabolism of paroxetine in man. Acta Psychiatr Scand 80(350):60–75 (1989).
20. Gram LF. Fluoxetine. N Engl J Med 331:1354–1361 (1994).
21. Harvey AT and Preskorn SH. Fluoxetine pharmacokinetics and effect on CYP2C19 in young and elderly volunteers. J Clin Psychopharmacol 21(2):161–166 (2001).
22. Ronfeld RA, Tremaine LM, and Wilner KD. Pharmacokinetics of sertraline and N-demethyl-metabolite in elderly and young male and female volunteers. Clin Pharmacokinet 32(Suppl 1):22–30 (1997).
23. Lundmark J, Scheel Thomsen I, Fjord-Larsen T, Manniche PM, Mengel H, Moller-Nielsen EM, et al. Paroxetine: pharmacokinetic and antidepressant effect in the elderly. Acta Psychiatr Scand 350:76–80 (1989).
24. Kragh-Sorensen P, Overo KF, Peterson OL, Jensen K, and Parnas W. the kinetics of citalopram: single and multiple dose studies in man. Acta Pharmacol Toxicol 48(1):53–60 (1981).
25. Gutierrez M and Abramowitz W. Steady-state pharmacokinetics of citalopram in young and elderly subjects. Pharmacotherapy 20(12):1441–1447 (2000).
26. Murdoch D and McTavish D. Sertraline. A review of its pharmacodynamic and pharmacokinetic properties, and therapeutic potential in depression and obsessive-compulsive disorder. Drugs 44(4):604–624 (1992).
27. Milne RJ and Goa KL. Citalopram. A review of its pharmacodynamic and pharmacokinetic properties, and therapeutic potential in depressive illness. Drugs 41(3):450–477 (1991).
28. Fjordside L, Jeppsen U, Eap CB, Powell K, Baumann P, and Brosen K. The stereoselective metabolism of fluoxetine in poor and extensive metabolisers of sparteine. Pharmacogentics 9:55–60 (1999).

29. Carrillo JA, Dahl ML, Svensson JO, Alm C, Rodriguez I, and Bertillsson L. Disposition of fluvoxamine in humans is determined by the polymorphic CYP2D6 and also by the CYP1A2 activity. Clin Pharmacol Ther 60:183–190 (1996).
30. Bloomer JC, Woods FR, Haddock RE, Lennard MS, and Tucker GT. The role of cytochrome P-450D6 in the metabolism of paroxetine by human liver microsomes. Br J Clin Pharmacol 33:521–523 (1992).
31. Preskorn SH. Clinically relevant pharmacology of selective serotonin reuptake inhibitors. An overview with emphasis on pharmacokinetics and effects on oxidative drug metabolism. Clin Pharmacokinet 32(Suppl 1):1–21 (1997).
32. Rochat B, Amey M, Gillet M, Meyer UA, and Baumann P. Identification of three cytochrome P-450 isozymes involved in N-demethylation of citalopram enantiomers in human liver microsomes. Pharmacogentics 7:1–10 (1997).
33. Richelson E. Pharmacology of antidepressants. Mayo Clinic Proceedings 76(5):511–527 (2001).
34. Brosen K. The pharmacogenetics of the selective serotonin reuptake inhibitors. Clin Investig 71:1002–1009 (1993).
35. Gram LF, Hansen MG, Sindrup SH, Brosen K, Poulsen JH, Aaes-Jorgensen T, and Overo KF. Citalopram: interaction studies with levomepromazine, imipramine, and lithium. Ther Drug Monit 15:18–24 (1993).
36. Jeppesen U, Gram LF, Vistisen K, Loft S, Poulsen HE, and Brosen K. Dose-dependent inhibition of CYP1A2, CYP2C19 and CYP2D6 by citalopram, fluoxetine, fluvoxamine and paroxetine. Eur J Clin Pharmacol 51:73–78 (1996).
37. Lane R and Baldwin D. Selective serotonin reuptake inhibitor-induced serotonin syndrome: review. J Clin Psychopharmacol 17(3):208–221 (1997).
38. Mills KC. Serotonin syndrome. Am Fam Physician 52(5):1475–1482 (1995).
39. Hamilton S and Malone K. Serotonin syndrome during treatment with paroxetine and risperidone. J Clin Psychopharmacol 20(1):103–105 (2000).
40. Voirol P, Hodel PF, Zullino D, and Baumann P. Serotonin syndrome after small doses of citalopram or sertraline. J Clin Psychopharmacol 20(6):713–714 (2000).
41. Weitzel C and Jiwanlal S. The darker side of SSRIs. RN 64(8):43–48 (2001).
42. Brown TM, Skop BP, and Mareth TR. Pathophysiology and management of the serotonin syndrome. Ann Pharmacother 30:527–533 (1996).
43. Carbone JR. The neuroleptic malignant and serotonin syndromes. Emerg Med Clin North Am 18(2):317–325 (2000).
44. Dams R, Benijts TH, Lambert WE, Van Bocxlaer JF, Van Varenbergh D, Van Peteghem C, and De Leenheer AP. A fatal case of serotonin syndrome after combined moclobemide-citalopram intoxication. J Anal Toxicol 25(2):147–151 (2001).
45. Hernandez AF, Montero MN, Pla A, and Villanueva E. Fatal moclobemide overdose or death caused by serotonin syndrome? J Forensic Sci 40(1):128–130 (1995).
46. Rogde S, Hillberg T, and Teige B. Fatal combined intoxication with new antidepressants. Human cases and an experimental study of postmortem moclobemide redistribution. Forensic Sci Int 100(1–2):109–116 (1999).
47. Goeringer KE, Raymon L, Christian GD, and Logan BK. Postmortem forensic toxicology of selective serotonin reuptake inhibitors: a review of pharmacology and report of 168 cases. J Forensic Sci 45(3):633–648 (2000).
48. Keltner N and Harris CP. Serotonin syndrome: a case of fatal SSRI/MAOI interaction. Perspect Psychiatr Care 30(4):26–31 (1995).
49. DeVane CL and Nemroff CB. 2000 guide to psychtropic drug interactions. Primary Psych 7(10):40–68 (2000).

50. Preskorn SH. Clinical pharmacology of selective serotonin reuptake inhibitors, 1st ed. Caddo, OK: Professional Communications Inc., 1996.
51. Spina E, Avenoso A, Facciol G, Scordo M, Anciono M, and Madia A. Plasma concentrations of risperidone and 9-hydroxyrisperidone during combined treatment with paroxetine. Ther Drug Monit 23(3):223–227 (2001).
52. Bostwick J and Brown T. A toxic reaction from combining fluoxetine and phentermine. J Clin Psychopharmacol 16(2):189–190 (1996).
53. Mamiya K, Kojima K, Yukawa E, Higuchi S, Ieiri I, Ninomiya H, and Tashiro N. Phenytoin intoxication induced by fluvoxamine. Ther Drug Monit 23(1):75–77 (2001).
54. Eap C, Bertschy G, Powell K, and Baumann P. Fluvoxamine and fluoxetine do not interact in the same way with the metabolism of the enantiomers of methadone. J Clin Psychopharmacol 17(2):113–117 (1997).
55. Preskorn S, Greenblatt D, and Harvey A. Lack of effect of sertraline on the pharmacokinetics of alprazolam. J Clin Psychopharmacol 20(5):585–586 (2000).
56. Taylor D. Selective serotonin reuptake inhibitors and tricyclic antidepressants in combination. Interactions and therapeutic uses. Br J Psychiatry 167(5):575–580 (1995).
57. Markowitz J and DeVane CL. Rifampin induced selective serotonin reuptake inhibitor withdrawal syndrome in a patient treated with sertraline. J Clin Psychopharmacol 20(1):109–110 (2000).
58. Hemeryck A, De Vriendt C, and Belapaire FM. Effect of selective serotonin reuptake inhibitors on the oxidative metabolism of propafenone: in vitro studies using human liver microsomes. J Clin Psychopharmacol 20(4):428–434 (2000).
59. Sayal K, Duncan-McConnell DA, McConnell HW, and Taylor D. Psychotropic interactions with warfarin. Acta Psychiatr Scand 102(4):250–255 (2000).
60. Nelson MH, Birnbauma AK, and Remmel RP. Inhibition of phenytoin hydroxylation in human liver microsomes by several selective serotonin reuptake inhibitors. Epilepsy Res 44(1):71–82 (2001).
61. Moller SE, Larsen F, Khan A, and Rolan PE. Lack of effect of citalopram on the steady state pharmacokinetics of carbamazepine in healthy male subjects. J Clin Psychopharmacol 21(5):493–499 (2001).
62. Bertschy G, Eap CB, Powell K, and Baumann P. Fluoxetine addition to methadone in addicts: pharmacokinetic aspects. Ther Drug Monit 18(5):570–572 (1996).
63. Bauer M, Zaninelli R, Muller-Oerlinghausen B, and Meister W. Paroxetine and amitriptyline augmentation of lithium in the treatment of major depression: a double-blind study. J Clin Psychopharmacol 19(2):164–171 (1999).
64. Fagiolini A, Buysse DJ, Frank E, Houck P, Luther JF, and Kupfer DJ. Tolerability of combined treatment with lithium and paroxetine in patients with bipolar disorder and depression. J Clin Psychopharmacol 21(5):474–478 (2001).
65. Hemeryck A, Lefebvre R, De Vriendt CE, and Belpaire FM. Paroxetine affects metoprolol pharmacokinetics and pharmacodynamics in healthy volunteers. Clin Pharmacol Ther 67(3):283–291 (2000).
66. Hassan P, Sproule B, Naranjo C, and Hermann N. Dose-response evaluation of the interaction between sertraline and alprazolam in vivo. J Clin Psychopharmacol 20(2):150–158 (2000).
67. Scott GN and Elmer GW. Update on natural product-drug interactions. Am J Health Syst Pharm 59(4):339–347 (2002).
68. Callaway JC and Grob CS. Ayahuasca preparations and serotonin reuptake inhibitors: a potential combination for severe adverse interactions. J Psychoactive Drugs 30(4):367–369 (1998).

69. Callaway JC, McKenna DJ, Grof CS, Brito GS, Raymon LP, Poland RE, et al. Pharmacokinetics of Hoasca alkaloids in healthy humans. J Ethnopharm 65(3):243–246 (1999).
70. Izzo AA and Ernst E. Interactions between herbal medicines and prescribed drugs: a systemic review. Drugs 61(15):2163–2175 (2001).
71. Montgomery SA and Judge R. Treatment of depression with associated anxiety: comparisons of tricyclic and selective serotonin reuptake inhibitors. Acta Psychiatr Scand 101(403): 9–16 (2000).
72. Trindade E, Menon D, Topfer LA, and Coloma C. Adverse effects associated with selective serotonin reuptake inhibitors and tricyclic antidepressants: a meta-analysis. CMAJ 159: 1245–1252 (1998).
73. Corrington KA, Gatlin C, and Fields K. A case of SSRI-induced hyponatremia. J Am Board Fam Pract 15(1):63–65 (2002).
74. McKoy GK, ed., American Hospital Formulary Service Drug Information. Bethesda, MD: American Society of Health-System Pharmacists (1954 & 1966), 1999.
75. Lane RM. SSRI-induced extrapyramidal side-effects and akathisia: implications for treatment. J Psychopharmacol 12(2):192–214 (1998).
76. Emslie GJ, Walkup JT, Pliszka SR, and Ernst M. Nontricyclic antidepressants: current trends in children and adolescents. J Am Acad Child Adolesc Psychiatry 38(5):517–528 (1999).
77. Alldredge BK. Seizure risk associated with psychotropic drugs: clinical and pharmacokinetic considerations. Neurology 53(5):S68–S75 (1999).
78. Olfson M, Marcus SC, Druss B, Elinson L, Tanielian T, and Pincus HA. National trends in the outpatient treatment of depression. JAMA 287(2):203–209 (2002).
79. Rasmussen B and Brosen K. Is therapeutic drug monitoring a case for optimizing clinical outcome and avoiding interactions of the selective serotonin reuptake inhibitors? Ther Drug Monit 22(2):143–154 (2000).
80. Lundmark J, Bengtsson F, Nordin C, Reis M, and Walinder J. Therapeutic drug monitoring of selective serotonin reuptake inhibitors influences clinical dosing strategies and reduces drug costs in depressed elderly patients. Acta Psychiatr Scand 101(5):354–359 (2000).
81. Baumann P, Nil R, Souche A, Montaldi S, Baettig D, Lambert S, et al. A double blind, placebo-controlled study of citalopram with and without lithium in the treatment of therapy-resistant depressive patients: a clinical, pharmacokinetic, and pharmacogenetic investigation. J Clin Psychopharmacol 16(4):307–314 (1996).

Chapter 6

Antipsychotic Drugs and Interactions

Implications for Criminal and Civil Litigation

Michael Welner, MD

1. ANTIPSYCHOTICS AND DRUG INTERACTIONS

Antipsychotics include two general classes of drugs. *Traditional antipsychotics* are thought to act by exerting effects principally on the dopamine neurotransmitter system *(1)*. The traditional antipsychotics became known to many as neuroleptics based on their frequent effects of substantially slowing movement *(1)*. *Atypical antipsychotics*, designed in laboratories to provide psychotic symptom relief without movement problems, affect other neurotransmitter systems *(2)*, and present other potential concerns.

Table 1 lists available antipsychotic medicines, as well as their brand names.

Interactions involving antipsychotics (a) make side effects of the antipsychotics more pronounced, (b) render the antipsychotics less effective, and (c) affect the metabolism of other medicines, and prolong their effects and side effects

Both older and more recently developed varieties of antipsychotics are known for their manifold side effects on numerous organ systems. Interactions have forensic significance when efficacy and/or side effects are heightened by the coprescription of medicines that affect antipsychotic metabolism.

Drug interactions involving antipsychotics warrant particular scrutiny in the elderly, the brain-damaged, those on other psychotropics, and those with a history of special sensitivity to antipsychotics.

Given the severe conditions for which antipsychotic prescribing is reserved, interactions also have forensic relevance when an antipsychotic is no longer effective because of the medicines prescribed along with it. In these cases, the greatest forensic significance of the drug interaction is the relapse of the root illness, rather than drug side effects.

Table 1
Commonly Prescribed Antipsychotics

Name	Generic Name	Chemical Type	Atypical/Traditional
Clozaril	Clozapine	Dibenzodiazepines	Atypical
Haloperidol Decanoate	Haloperidol	Butyrophenones	Traditional
Loxitane	Loxapine	Dibenzoxazepine	Traditional
Moban	Molindone	Dihydroindole	Traditional
Geodon	Ziprasidone	Benzisothiazole	Atypical
Orap	Pimozide	Diphenylbutylpiperidine	Traditional
Risperdal	Risperidone	Benzisoxazole	Atypical
Seroquel	Quetiapine Fumarate	Dibenzothiazepine	Atypical
Navane	Thiothixene	Thioxanthene	Traditional
Zyprexa	Olanzapine	Thienobenzodiazepine	Atypical

Data from Physicians' Desk Reference, 57th ed. ©2003 Medical Economics Company, Inc. New Jersey.

Before we explore how these interactions manifest themselves in criminal and civil case scenarios, an appreciation for the neurochemistry involved is necessary.

2. KEY NEUROCHEMISTRY OF ANTIPSYCHOTICS

Antipsychotics are able to exert their effects by influencing how specific chemicals, known as neurotransmitters, move through the brain. Messages pass through the nervous system, from cell to cell, by these chemical neurotransmitters (3). Psychosis and other psychiatric maladies occur when the delicate equilibrium of each of these microscopic neurochemical transmitters is disrupted. The chemical imbalance causes chain reactions that result in the development of symptoms or outwardly visible behaviors.

Antipsychotics impact a number of neurotransmitters and regulatory systems in the body. Like other psychotropics, antipsychotics exert their effects on receptors of these neurotransmitters, receptors that normally catch and relay the transmitting neurochemical that has been released by the nerve cell nearby.

In addition to directly blocking dopamine transmission at D2 receptors, antipsychotics have antihistaminic and antiadrenergic effects (4). All traditional antipsychotics, particularly those that are classified as low potency, have anticholinergic effects focusing on the muscarinic class of receptors (5). The effects of such neurotransmitter blockade depend not only on the neurotransmitter, but where in the brain that neurotransmitter is active, and what role in human functioning it plays.

Atypical antipsychotic drugs earn their name, in part, because they do not cause effects on movement in the way traditional antipsychotic drugs do. Whereas each of the atypical antipsychotics impacts a distinct profile of neurotransmitters, all of the atypical class block dopamine D2 receptors, as well as serotonin 2A receptors (6).

2.1. Dopamine: Benefits and Movement Problems Caused by Its Blockade

Dopamine has been the foundation of antipsychotic treatment. Traditional antipsychotics' influence on the different centers of dopamine activity has directly and indirectly accounted for side effects of forensic significance.

6. Antipsychotic Drugs and Interactions

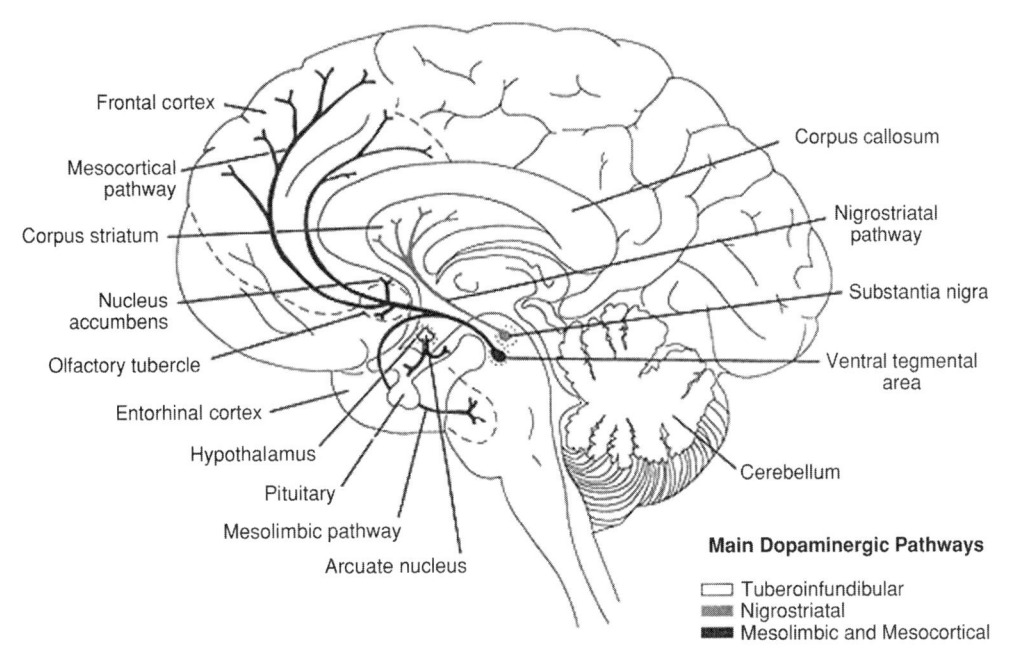

Fig. 1. Sagittal section of human brain showing the dopaminergic pathways involved in the actions of antipsychotic drugs.

Psychotic illnesses and certain drug intoxications, such as cocaine and amphetamines, arise from altered dopamine transmission. Traditional antipsychotics decrease or eliminate psychotic symptoms like hallucinations and delusions, and organize confused thinking, regardless of their origin. These medicines block dopamine transmission at D2 receptors in the mesolimbic nerve pathways that lead to the nucleus accumbens in the limbic system of the brain *(7)*.

Dopamine activity is associated with numerous vital human functions. Therefore, regrettably, dopamine blocking in other areas of the brain results in unwanted consequences as well.

Parkinsonism, dystonia, akathisia, tardive dyskinesia, and tardive dystonia stem, through a variety of mechanisms, from the capacity of antipsychotics to block dopamine transmission in the brain *(8)*. Dopamine activity in the brain substantia nigra is necessary for unrestricted movement. Potent blockade of dopamine transmission from the substantia nigra at D2 receptors is therefore associated with severely slowed movements, a resting tremor, loss of the ability to instinctively maintain upright posture (postural reflex), and trouble initiating movement *(8,9)*.

These symptoms mimic the movement disorders of Parkinson's disease, in which the degeneration of dopamine-transmitting nerve cells leads to symptoms *(10)*. Because the nerve cells of those receiving antipsychotic treatment are not deteriorating—it is merely the transmission of dopamine that is blocked—the symptoms of dopamine blocker-induced parkinsonian-type symptoms are reversible (*see* Fig. 1).

Parkinsonism may result in more dangerous consequences, particularly when problems with regulating postural reflexes manifest. A person so affected, when pushed, has trouble regaining footing; falls can result, and in the elderly or those with advanced osteoporosis, spills may cause hip fractures *(11)*. Compounding the significance of this risk is the greater sensitivity of the elderly to parkinsonian effects from traditional antipsychotics *(12)*.

Though one might assume, logically, that reversing these symptoms should be accomplished with a medicine that promotes dopamine transmission to overcome a dopamine blockade, remember that dopamine transmission in mesolimbic nerve pathways would aggravate the symptoms of psychosis that start this mess in the first place. Clinicians thus rely upon the important relationship between acetylcholine and dopamine to remedy some movement problems, specifically the parkinsonian symptoms.

Dopamine released in the substantia nigra blocks acetylcholine transmission *(13)*. Therefore, dopamine-blocking drugs prevent the suppression of acetylcholine. Anticholinergics such as benztropine and trihexyphenidyl reduce the dopamine-blocking effects on the substantia nigra without affecting dopamine blocking that treats psychosis *(14)*. Anticholinergics are also instrumental at providing an immediate reversal of symptoms of dystonia *(14)*.

Dystonia involves the relatively abrupt onset of severe and extended spasm of a muscle group. Typically, muscles of the back, neck, eyes, or tongue are involved *(15)*. But when muscles of the larynx spasm, a person can suffocate *(16)*. Fortunately, over 90% of dystonic reactions occur within 2 wk of starting treatment *(17)*. Furthermore, anticholinergics quickly reverse these effects *(18)*. However, a dystonic reaction in the wrong setting can still inspire fear, humiliation, and an unwillingness to continue with treatment.

Unlike Parkinsonian effects, dystonia has not been definitively localized as originating in the substantia nigra. However, its dramatic reversal by anticholinergics is further evidence of an elegant balance between dopamine blockage and the potency of acetylcholine transmission.

Dopamine blockade at D2 receptors in other movement centers in the brain is not so easily reversed by anticholinergics. Other dopamine-induced movement disorders are thought to result from phenomena that have less to do with acetylcholine, and more with other of the numerous effects of the traditional antipsychotics.

2.2. Antipsychotics and Akathisia

Akathisia, unlike dystonia and parkinsonism, begins to develop—often insidiously—weeks after antipsychotic treatment begins *(19)*. The subjective sense of restlessness, akathisia is exquisitely uncomfortable *(20)*. Visitors to psychiatric wards who encounter patients pacing the hallways are likely witnessing a person's response to akathisia.

Primarily high-potency traditional antipsychotics are associated with the development of akathisia. These include haloperidol, fluphenazine, triflulopenzine, and thiothixene *(21)*. Risperidone, an atypical antipsychotic, also causes akathisia in some of the patients taking that medicine. Pimozide is a high-potency traditional antipsychotic, but is typically prescribed at very low doses for its clinical effect.

Because atypical antipsychotics do not frequently cause akathisia, many presume that the dopamine-blocking qualities of traditional antipsychotics account for this movement disorder. However, drugs that promote dopamine transmission, or anticholinergics that reverse dopamine-blocking effects leading to parkinsonism, do not relieve akathisia.

The delay in onset of akathisia suggests that traditional antipsychotics' causative influence is indirect—namely, the antipsychotics initiate a chain reaction that, for some, culminates in akathisia.

Further shrouding the neurochemical understanding of akathisia is its treatment; beta-blockers and benzodiazepines, which improve akathisia, act in a general manner on both the central and peripheral nervous system *(22)*. Therefore, unlike the anticholinergics, for example, the mystery of why akathisia can be improved by broadly acting drugs conceals the neurochemical and neuroanatomic mechanisms responsible for akathisia in the first place.

Fluphenazine and haloperidol are especially relevant to consideration of akathisia and other high-potency side effects such as tardive dyskinesia. These two antipsychotics are often prescribed in oil-based depot forms that are injected into fatty areas of the buttocks or rear shoulder, and release themselves steadily into the bloodstream over a period of 2–4 wk *(23)*.

Since the onset of akathisia is more common weeks after a medicine has begun, and since those patients on depot medicines have the prospect of slowly metabolizing antipsychotics accumulating in their system, these patients are at higher risk for developing akathisia. Because patients taking depot haloperidol or fluphenazine are managed as outpatients, their akathisia may go undetected, relative to the discomfort of someone on a hospital ward who is under intermittent observation all day, every day.

An additional dilemma associated with akathisia is that patients often find it difficult to express the source of their discomfort or restlessness. Families or physicians may note a sense of increasing distress, and may mistakenly—and sometimes understandably—attribute that disquiet to psychosis, from *under*treatment or noncompliance with the antipsychotic. If the psychiatrist's reaction is to then increase the dose of the dopamine-blocking antipsychotic, the akathisia only gets worse. By the time the basis for the patient's discomfort is identified, the mounting discomfort may cause the patient to refuse further treatment—or worse.

2.3. Civil and Criminal Law and Implications of Akathisia

Those who experience akathisia feel a driven pressure to keep moving, and the effects are enough to have been occasionally associated with suicide *(24)*.

The clinician must distinguish akathisia's internal discomfort from the outward expression of discomfort, through hostility and assaultiveness. Theoretically, one might imagine a scenario in which someone is so uncomfortable from his akathisia that he might strike out at another. However, resolving this idea requires factoring in a person's inherent predisposition to assaulting others to begin with.

The notion of someone's violence arising exclusively from akathisia in a person who is not otherwise violent is unsubstantiated in the clinical literature. As such, this notion would likely not achieve *Daubert* standards for having been systematically studied and confirmed as a cause–effect relationship between akathisia and violence.

2.4. Tardive Dyskinesia

Tardive dyskinesia baffled clinicians for decades. This involuntary and disfiguring twisting movement of muscles of the face, tongue, hands, or feet *(25)* was found in people who had been treated with traditional antipsychotics, particularly those who had been treated with those drugs for an extended period *(26)*. Complicating tardive dyskinesia was its sometimes irreversible course *(27)*; many who stop traditional antipsychotics, hoping the tardive dyskinesia would somehow improve, note no change *(28)*. Some even experience a worsening of symptoms that improve only when their medicines are restored *(29)*.

Traditional antipsychotics have all been known to frequently cause tardive dyskinesia *(30)*, as often as 20% for those who have taken these medicines as long as four years *(31)*. Less commonly, the antipsychotics cause tardive dystonia, an involuntary tightening of muscle groups, usually of the head and neck *(32)*. The pronounced impact of irreversible tardive dyskinesia and dystonia on appearance and body image has civil-liability implications. Disfigurement can be as grievous surgical errors in the head and neck or other sensitive body areas.

The discovery, in recent years, of the benefits of megadoses of vitamin E in treating tardive dyskinesia *(33)* has not resolved the lingering mystery of what causes this condition. Furthermore, atypical antipsychotics of the newer generation are far less likely to cause tardive dyskinesia *(34)*. Of course, once these medicines have been in use for many years, we may learn otherwise. But now that traditional antipsychotics are less readily prescribed, there is less research initiative for resolving the origins of tardive dyskinesia.

Current neuropsychiatric perspective primarily endorses the idea that dopamine receptor hypersensitivity is responsible for tardive dyskinesia *(35)*. This idea, though otherwise completely consistent with our understanding of neurotransmitters and psychotropic drugs' impact on the sensitivity of neuroreceptors, does not successfully account for vitamin E's therapeutic effects.

2.5. Dopamine Blockade and Interactions

The parkinsonian side effects of traditional antipsychotics are enhanced by the coadministration of the mood stabilizer lithium *(36)*. Lithium added to traditional antipsychotics also increases the risk for tardive dyskinesia, and of akathisia *(36)*. Still, the combination of traditional antipsychotics with lithium is safe and essential for many individuals whose health would collapse otherwise from persistent psychosis.

The risk of parkinsonism, and of akathisia, is also heightened when fluphenazine is taken by those who chew betel nut. Betel nut, chewed as a recreational drug in many countries, is a mild stimulant, also known as *areca catechu (37)*.

2.6. Dopamine Blockade: Cognitive Side Effects of Note

The frontal cortex of the brain includes some of the most sophisticated intellectual and cognitive qualities that distinguish man as the most able of the animal kingdom. Dopamine transmission occurs in the frontal lobe as well *(38)*. Blockade of dopamine transmission through mesocortical nerve pathways to the frontal lobe is therefore accompanied by substantial intellectual impairment *(39)*. Closer study has specified these problems as attention, memory, planning, problem solving, and effortful cognitive processing *(40)*.

The dopamine-blocking effects of traditional antipsychotics on the frontal cortex may be difficult to readily detect, especially in diagnosis on the schizophrenia spectrum (schizophrenia, schizoaffective disorder, schizoid personality). Each of these conditions is associated with a baseline of low initiative, simple thinking, passivity, emotional withdrawal, anhedonia, lack of spontaneity, poor attention, and/or more impoverished expression, or negative symptoms *(41)*. Perhaps these qualities reflect that dopamine activity in the frontal lobe is diminished to begin with, even before the patient takes medicines *(42)*.

For this reason, medication side effects on the frontal lobe, particularly because they are subtle to begin with, commonly go unnoticed. Further complicating the aforementioned overlap is the resemblance of these symptoms to depression, and to a lack of stimulation resulting from the abandonment of many with this condition.

The standard for care in psychiatry has not achieved the attentiveness to schizophrenia that mandates neurocognitive testing of those being medicated with dopamine blockers in order to ensure that cognitive effects independent of the disease process can be accounted for. However, as our sensitivity to the functional rights of our patients improves, this seems to be an appropriate objective—certainly in line with informed consent.

2.7. Antipsychotics, Cognition, and Implications for Criminal Law

Impaired cognition can be especially relevant in the appraisal of a defendant's ability to render a knowing and intelligent confession. Cognitive impairment may impact a defendant's competency, or his or her criminal responsibility.

The limited cognitive flexibility of those with schizophrenia and the subduing qualities of dopamine blockade do not include a suspension of morality. Antipsychotic-induced cognitive changes, pertinent to the aforementioned issues, pale in importance to the cognitive processes of the underlying disease. It is not the dopamine blockade that impacts mental competency for specific tasks within the course of a criminal case, but the underlying condition may be relevant, especially if the legal issues are nuanced and the deficits are pronounced.

Cognitive problems associated with some traditional antipsychotics have been attributed to the anticholinergic properties of the given medicines, in addition to effects on dopamine transmission in the cortex *(43)*. Memory and mental clarity can be affected in this way *(44)*. Chlorpromazine, thioridazine, and mesoridazine each possess higher anticholinergic qualities, and are more sedating as well *(45)*. Higher doses of antipsychotics cause increased sedation, at which point all cognitive domains are affected *(45)*.

In the unusual circumstance of anticholinergic toxicity, confusion may be implicated in crime, particularly a disorganized event. An acute change in mental status, such as would be seen in a delirium associated with anticholinergic drug toxicity, would give reason to question competency to waive Miranda. The fast reversibility of this drug effect, however, renders this of unlikely consequence in cases of questioned trial or sentencing competency.

2.8. Antipsychotics, Cognition, and Implications for Civil Law

Impaired cognition associated with the effects of traditional antipsychotics may be responsible for motor-vehicle or heavy-equipment accidents that kill or injure the patient or someone else. In other instances, work proficiency may be affected, resulting in the loss of a job.

The cognitive deficits identified with traditional antipsychotics do not readily affect decision making for parenting, contracts, and other simple transactions. The cognitive effects of the underlying condition are of more likely pertinence to problems people experience in these matters. However, presuming parental, contract, and other incompetence on the basis of even an advanced presentation of schizophrenia—without a specific assessment relating to capacity—is unfair and professionally irresponsible.

Atypical antipsychotics may impact cognition as well; these effects are more directly related to the sedating qualities of the medicines, however, than anticholinergic properties *(46)*. Clearly, however, there are cognitive advantages to the atypical antipsychotics, which we will review and explain below.

2.9. Other Dopamine Blockade Side Effects of Note

Dopamine transmission from the hypothalamus to the anterior pituitary is also blocked by traditional antipsychotics *(47)*. This blockade causes an increase in circulating prolactin levels. Indirectly, therefore, dopamine blockade results, through this mechanism, in unexpected breast secretions, or galactorrhea, menstrual interruption, and amenorrhea *(47)*.

Sexual dysfunction occurs in a number of individuals taking dopamine-blocking antipsychotics *(48)*. Whether elevated prolactin levels—or direct effects of dopamine blockade on the sexual-arousal cycle—are responsible, has not yet been determined. Nevertheless, atypical antipsychotics that do not cause a rise in prolactin levels have and have not been shown to be associated with sexuality effects *(49)*.

Closer attention to the sexual-arousal cycle is necessary in order to sort out the potential troubles that both traditional and atypical antipsychotics can cause. After discussing neurotransmitters other than dopamine, we will focus on sexuality later in the chapter, as well as the civil forensic implications.

2.10. Acetylcholine Blockade Through Antimuscarinic Effects

In addition to the cognitive side effects noted previously, anticholinergic effects also include dry mouth, blurred vision, constipation, and urinary retention *(50)*.

Independent of cognitive effects, visual problems can affect work performance, or equipment and motor vehicle operation. Furthermore, visual impairment may result in misdiagnosis of other eye conditions, prompting unnecessary treatment.

Chlorpromazine, thioridazine, perphenazine, mesoridazine, and molindone are most frequently associated with causing blurred vision *(51)*. However, those who are especially sensitive to the anticholinergic properties of traditional antipsychotics may experience vision effects as well.

Older individuals, particularly men with benign prostatic hypertrophy, are going to be more sensitive to the urinary side effects of anticholinergics. Protracted effects can contribute to serious kidney problems, because urine is not passing through the excretory channels. Risk is heightened when the patient has only sporadic outpatient follow-up.

Though a desire to avoid the parkinsonian, dystonic, and akathisia effects associated with high-potency neuroleptics might favor low-potency antipsychotics, anticholinergic side effects offset any apparent advantage. Some patients simply are too affected

6. *Antipsychotic Drugs and Interactions* 195

by the anticholinergic and other effects of the low-potency drugs, which are far more pronounced than they are in high-potency antipsychotic drugs.

2.11. Antihistaminic Effects and Weight Gain

Traditional antipsychotics also have been associated with blocking histamine and adrenergic receptors. Antihistaminic effects are responsible for sedation and weight gain. The weight gain, unfortunately, may persist even with careful dieting and exercise.

All traditional and atypical antipsychotics have antihistaminic effects (with the reported exception of the atypical antipsychotic ziprasidone) and are associated with substantial weight gain *(52)*. This side effect has important implications for the management of heart disease, diabetes, and high blood pressure, as well as other conditions that are aggravated by obesity.

This is more than merely an "eating hot dogs causes cancer" point. If someone can trace the origin of weight gain or diabetes to prescription of an antipsychotic, then scrutiny of the basis for the physician's conceding those health risks must be warranted. This is part of the standard dialog of today's doctor–patient care, particularly because medication alternatives are available.

2.12. Sugar Metabolism

Traditional and atypical antipsychotics, especially clozapine, commonly impair glucose metabolism *(53)* (though risperidone has proven in the period of its use to be less associated with this side effect) *(54)*. For those with diabetes, or who develop Type 2 diabetes, the progression of this pernicious condition has a major impact on quality of life in many functional domains.

New-onset diabetes from atypical antipsychotics *(55)* does not merely introduce long-term risks of stroke, heart disease, and end-organ damage. A number of cases of sudden death from diabetic ketoacidosis have been attributed to atypical antipsychotics *(55)*.

Given the Achilles' heel of the advanced treatments, regularly monitoring sugar metabolic functions is therefore a responsibility of prescribing psychiatrists.

2.13. Atypical Antipsychotics: Different Areas of the Brain, Different Effects

Serotonin inhibits dopamine release. Blockade of serotonin 2A receptors, therefore, allows dopamine transmission to occur *(56)*. Atypical antipsychotics have serotonin- and D2-blocking properties *(56)*. With the potential for both dopamine stimulation as well as blockade, and the side effects of blockade, the answer to the riddle of atypical antipsychotics rests in the neuroanatomy.

In the nigrostriatal area, atypical antipsychotics block a far lower percentage of D2 receptors than traditional antipsychotics. The degree of blockade remains below the threshold to produce parkinsonian effects *(56)*.

Dopamine blockade causes prolactin release; serotonin blockade limits prolactin release *(56)*. Effects on prolactin levels differ between antipsychotics, suggesting other neurochemical or neuroanatomical forces are also pertinent.

In the mesolimbic pathway, where dopamine transmission influences psychotic symptoms, dopamine blockade predominates over the effects of serotonin 2A blockade

(56). Therefore, atypical antipsychotics are able to successfully exert their clinical effects without the baggage of dopamine blockade in untargeted areas of the brain.

As for the mesocortical pathway, serotonin 2A blockade activity predominates in the atypical antipsychotics, so dopamine transmission in the frontal lobes is ultimately enhanced *(56)*. This accounts for improvements in initiative, expression, interest, and a variety of other frontal-lobe functions in those with schizophrenia-spectrum disorders.

The availability of atypical antipsychotics, with their favorable effects on cognition, increases the viability of malpractice liability for the effects of traditional antipsychotics. No longer can the effects of traditional antipsychotics be readily explained away by the severity of the illness, and the "lesser of two evils" argument.

As social and occupational reintegration of the chronic mentally ill assumes greater importance in mental-health care, the expectations of the chronic mentally ill will be felt in liability demands and request for workplace and parental accommodations because of the cognitive enhancing potential of the atypical antipsychotics relative to the traditional antipsychotics.

2.14. α-Adrenergic Effects

Antiadrenergic effects, which act at $\alpha 1$ receptors, are implicated in sedation, as well as sudden drops of blood pressure upon rising from a lying or sitting position (orthostatic hypotension) *(57)*.

The traditional antipsychotics, particularly chlorpromazine, thioridazine, and mesoridazine, may cause precipitous drops in blood pressure through α-adrenergic blockade *(58)*. These medicines have been implicated as well in sudden death *(59)*. Effects on blood pressure, specifically in the case of chlorpromazine and thioridazine, may be amplified by the antihypertensives propranolol and pindolol; the latter α blockers have been shown to increase the blood levels of both of those antipsychotics *(60)*, and add to the hypotensive effects of the antipsychotics; however, so do other antihypertensives such as ACE (angiotensin-converting enzyme) inhibitors and clonidine, which have no effect on the amount of antipsychotic in the bloodstream *(61)*.

Though novel antipsychotics are otherwise appreciated for their less pronounced effects on blood pressure, clozapine, the atypical antipsychotic, has nevertheless been frequently associated with precipitous drop of blood pressure *(62)*. Clozapine has also been reported to cause inflammation of the heart muscle (myocarditis) and degeneration of the heart muscle (cardiomyopathy) *(63)*. Furthermore, alcohol and benzodiazepines increase orthostatic hypotension when taken along with olanzapine *(64)*.

Therefore, clinicians should regard advantages of newer antipsychotic medicines in less absolute terms, so as to avoid overlooking the need to monitor patients for dizziness and to educate them to recognize signs of such circulatory problems.

2.15. Sudden Death and Cardiac Conductance

Sudden death from antipsychotics does not result typically from hypotension, but from arrhythmias *(65)*. The effects at this writing appear to begin with antipsychotic-induced blockade of potassium channels, through which electrical signals flow through the heart to make it beat in an orderly manner *(66)*. The resulting disturbance, in the rare instances in which it progresses to ventricular arrhythmia, would cause sudden death.

Pharmaceutical marketing campaigns have highlighted the association of thioridazine, especially, with torsades de pointes, a disturbance featuring prolonged cardiac rhythm conduction *(67)*. Theoretically, torsades de pointes may be responsible for some sudden deaths attributed to antipsychotics, if heart rhythm conduction is slowed to a severe degree. However, because antipsychotics and diagnoses of torsades de pointes have no more than rarely been demonstrated in practice *(68)*, the current discussion in the medical literature may prove to be overestimated in its importance to later forensic questions.

Given that the rare phenomenon of sudden death is real, the need to minimize the risk of torsades de pointes is necessary. Attention to combinations of medicines and their relative risk is therefore essential. Antipsychotics that may introduce risk in patients who are on other medicines that affect cardiac conduction also include droperidol *(69)*. This medicine, used more frequently in perioperative settings, or in emergency rooms, has been assigned a special warning by the FDA, for reasons similar to the noticeably more risky thioridazine *(70)*.

2.16. Neuroleptic Malignant Syndrome

This very uncommon, but emergent condition may spontaneously arise in those who have been prescribed antipsychotics, particularly the traditional variety *(71)*. Neuroleptic malignant syndrome (NMS) is characterized by a collapse of the body's regulatory system—blood pressure, temperature, and pulse—followed by catastrophic muscle breakdown all over the body. If not treated, NMS results in death from respiratory failure (resulting from breakdown of muscles in the respiratory apparatus), or kidney failure (resulting from sludging of proteins from muscles being broken down) *(72)*.

It is not so simple to explain NMS as attributable to dopamine blockade. The primary treatment of NMS is a neuromuscular blocking agent. And, in more recent years, atypical antipsychotics have been implicated in cases of NMS, specifically olanzapine *(73)*, quetiapine *(74)*, clozapine *(75)*, and risperidone *(76)*.

The neurophysiologic causes of NMS have not been identified, and no way of preventing it has been found. Clinicians are thus forced to be vigilant for signs of early NMS, in order to immediately stop the antipsychotic medication or arrange for more supportive care, if necessary. NMS is clearly a condition where immediate recognition and aggressive response is necessary in order to prevent death. Unfortunately, in some cases, quick intervention is still too late.

2.17. Sexual Side Effects: Serotonin and Others

A number of neurochemicals affected by antipsychotics impact the sexual-response cycle. Stage one of the cycle, *libido*, is enhanced by dopamine *(77)* and diminished by prolactin *(77)*. Antipsychotics therefore can potentially diminish libido by dopamine blockade and/or enhancing prolactin release.

Stage two, *arousal*, involves erection in men and lubrication in women. Arousal is enhanced by acetylcholine, and more indirectly by dopamine. Serotonin indirectly may reduce arousal, but this effect has been identified only in patients taking antidepressants *(78)*. Arousal, therefore, can be inhibited by both traditional and atypical antipsychotics through two mechanisms, anticholinergic and dopamine-blocking activity.

Stage three, *orgasm*, is not affected by dopamine, acetylcholine, or other of the principal neurochemicals of antipsychotics. However, serotonin diminishes orgasm *(79)*, which may explain orgasm difficulties found in those prescribed atypical antipsychotics.

Thus, most traditional and atypical antipsychotics invariably affect the gonadotropic hormonal system. Ultimate effects on relationships and marriages, as well as procreation, can be profound.

Priapism is a rare side effect in which blood is trapped in the erect penis because of circulatory changes *(80)*. This rare effect is associated with those antipsychotics, chlorpromazine and thioridazine in particular, with the greatest α-adrenergic blockade *(80)*. Fortunately, this reaction is very rare, enough that it should not be affecting prescribing decisions unless it has happened. An informed patient can recognize that priapism is medicine related, and can seek treatment in an emergency room without panic.

The management of sexual side effects is, well, a touchy subject. Many of those who take antipsychotics have very guarded boundaries and have difficulty broaching issues of sexuality. Impotence and sexual disinterest is embarrassing for them, and often feeds into and off of a low self-esteem that becomes the major, chronic illness. This area is an example of the burden facing the psychiatrist to educate patients at the time of informed consent about sexual side effects, and to probe side effects beyond perfunctory general questions or questionnaires. However questionnaires may satisfy standards of care, they do not represent quality care.

2.18. Seizures

Traditional antipsychotics lower the threshold at which someone with a history of seizures will experience a seizure *(81)*. In practice, this risk is primarily pertinent to those with already diagnosed seizure disorders. The atypical antipsychotic clozapine may directly cause seizures at higher dose, even in patients with no previous history *(82)*. If there are no treatment alternatives, that drawback does not outweigh the benefits of continuing to prescribe the medicine.

However, seizures from medications can be reduced in frequency with antiseizure medicines added to the regimen. Other interactions must then be addressed, specifically those resulting from the tendency of many antiseizure medicines to lower blood concentrations of antipsychotics.

Poor physician management of antipsychotic drug treatment is often the reason for intolerable side effects. If patients discontinue treatment because of unacceptable experiences with antipsychotics when medicines might have been helpful had they been competently managed, injury relating to unmanaged illness may establish a viable malpractice claim.

2.19. Interactions and Drug Metabolism

Ingested and injected antipsychotics are eventually broken down in the liver, through the enzyme system known as cytochrome P450 (CYP). From there, a transformed product, as well as unchanged drug, enter the bloodstream to exert their effects *(83)*.

This CYP system involves many subsystems, or isoenzymes *(84)*. Research in recent years has increasingly delineated which of the isoenzymes systems is responsible for metabolizing which drugs, what drugs inhibit that metabolism, and what drugs

Table 2
Antipsychotics and the Cytochrome P450 System

Enzyme	Drugs Metabolized
CYP1A2	clozapine, chlorpromazine, mesoridazine, thioridazine, olanzapine, trifluoperazine, thiothixene
CYP2D6	clozapine, olanzapine, sertindole, thioridazine, risperidone, perphenazine, molindone, fluphenazine, mesoridazine, chlorpromazine, thiothixene
CYP3A	pimozide, quetiapine, ziprasidone, clozapine, chlorpromazine, mesoridazine, haloperidol, sertindole

stimulate that metabolism. Well over 30 isoenzymes in the CYP system have been identified to date. The known isoenzymes associated with antipsychotic metabolism are listed in Table 2.

Generally, antipsychotics are metabolized by multiple means; this may explain why the blood levels of antipsychotics, based on available research, tend to be less affected by medicines that activate or inhibit at the level of the CYP system *(85)*. Most combinations of medicines with antipsychotics have not yet been studied to the end point of clear impact of medicines on the metabolism of that specific drug, with a few exceptions.

Medicines that slow the metabolism of traditional antipsychotics do so by inhibiting those enzymes in the liver that would otherwise break down the antipsychotics. This causes the antipsychotics to accumulate, and for side effects, including cognitive effects, to be more pronounced *(86)*. A list of medicines that inhibit the breakdown of the above antipsychotics appears in Table 3.

Still other medicines add their own anticholinergic properties, and can heighten the cognitive impairing effects of traditional antipsychotics *(86)*. The antidepressants with the highest anticholinergic qualities are amitryptyline and imipramine.

Whereas these medicines are far less commonly prescribed for depression and anxiety compared to previous years, tricyclic antidepressants often are prescribed to help treat pain. Therefore, particularly when patients are seeing more than one specialist, communication between all clinicians is vital to minimize risks associated with prescribing a patient an overly anticholinergic regimen.

Those medicines that stimulate CYP enzymes in the liver to break down antipsychotics faster gain forensic significance when a subsequent drop in medication levels leads to a relapse of symptoms, and behaviors or consequences of the relapsed condition. The accompanying Table 4 lists medicines that lower the blood levels of circulating antipsychotics.

2.19.1. Other Agents Affecting Antipsychotic Blood Levels

The antidepressant nefazodone has been shown to decrease the clearance of haloperidol from the body by about 33%. Given haloperidol's association with parkinsonism, and that effect's increase in risk associated with falls, coadministration of these drugs should be performed with attentive care. On the other hand, another antidepressant, venlafaxine, has been shown to increase the clearance of a single dose of haloperidol *(87)*.

Table 3
Antipsychotics and Inhibition of P450 Enzymes

CYP System	Antipsychotic Whose Metabolism Inhibited	Inhibiting Medicine-Type or Use of Medicine	Degree of Inhibition, if Known
1A2	clozapine, chlorpromazine, mesoridazine, thioridazine, olanzapine, trifluoperazine, thiothixene	fluvoxamine—antidepressant	high
		cimetidine—gastric distress	
		ciprofloxacin—antibiotic	high
		norfloxacin—antibiotic	
		paroxetine—antidepressant	moderate
		moclobemide—antidepressant	
		tertiary tricyclic antidepressants	moderate
2D6	clozapine, olanzapine, sertindole, thioridazine, risperidone, perphenazine, fluphenazine, mesoridazine, chlorpromazine	ritonavir—anti-AIDS	moderate
		indinavir—anti-AIDS	low
		fluoxetine—antidepressant	high
		paroxetine—antidepressant	high
		sertraline—antidepressant	moderate
		fluvoxamine—antidepressant	low
		citalopram—antidepressant	low
		venlafaxine—antidepressant	low
		bupropion—antidepressant	low
		secondary tricyclic antidepressants	moderate
		moclobemide—antidepressant	low
		perphenazine—antipsychotic	low
		fluphenazine—antipsychotic	low
		mesoridazine—antipsychotic	low
		haloperidol—antipsychotic	low
		chlorpromazine—antipsychotic	low
		sertindole—antipsychotic	
		thioridazine—antipsychotic	
		cimetidine—gastric distress	
		cocaine	
		methadone	
		quinidine—anti-arrhythmic	
		amiodarone—anti-arrhythmic	

(continued)

Tricyclic antidepressants increase the blood levels of one or both drugs when administered together with antipsychotics *(87)*.

For some with psychotic illnesses, combination drug therapy with multiple antipsychotics is employed. This practice has been described as causing untoward and unusual side effects, from increasing the likelihood of parkinsonism to NMS *(88)*.

The antipsychotic thioridazine and the antiseizure medicine phenytoin have been shown to decrease circulating levels of quetiapine, however *(89)*. And, administration of the antipsychotic risperidone, or clozapine, with the antimanic valproate results in an inconsistent concentration of both drugs *(89)*. These interactions are clinically sig-

Table 3 (*continued*)

CYP System	Antipsychotic Whose Metabolism Inhibited	Inhibiting Medicine-Type or Use of Medicine	Degree of Inhibition, if Known
3A	pimozide, quetiapine, ziprasidone, clozapine, sertindole, chlorpromazine, mesoridazine, haloperidol	ritonavir—anti-AIDS	high
		indinavir—anti-AIDS	high
		amprenavir—anti-AIDS	
		nelfinavir—anti-AIDS	moderate
		saquinavir—anti-AIDS	high
		fluvoxamine—antidepressant	high
		fluoxetine—antidepressant	high
		sertraline—antidepressant	moderate
		paroxetine—antidepressant	moderate
		nefazadone—antidepressant	high
		tricyclic—antidepressants	moderate
		thioridazine—antipsychotic	
		sertindole—antipsychotic	
		haloperidol—antipsychotic	low
		erythromycin—antibiotic	high
		clarithromycin—antibiotic	high
		azithromycin—antibiotic	high
		troleandomycin—antibiotic	
		diltiazem—antihypertensive	high
		verapamil—antihypertensive	
		ketoconazole—antifungal	
		fluconazole—antifungal	
		omeprazole—antiulcer	
		itraconazole—antifungal	
		dexamethasone—steroid	low
		cimetidine—anti-gastric upset	high
		amiodarone—antiarrhythmic	
		mibefradil—antihypertensive	high

nificant because of the life morbidity associated with relapsing bipolar disorder and unstable schizophrenia-spectrum disorders, and the need to treat those conditions with strict compliance.

Clozapine, when administered together with a benzodiazepine, may result in confusion, excess sedation, or even rare respiratory collapse *(90)*. Caffeine increases blood levels of clozapine *(91)*; clinicians are wise to anticipate the scenario of a patient self-medicating for fatigue, with coffee, who initiates a cycle of more sedation and consequent self-medication with coffee.

Risperidone increases blood levels of clozapine *(92)*. A clinician who adds risperidone to clozapine, expecting synergistic antipsychotic effects, may get more synergy than he or she bargained for.

Clozapine continues to represent a fascinating quandary for clinicians. For those with difficult to treat psychotic disorders, many experience that drug as the most likely

Table 4
Antipsychotics and Inducing of P450 Systems

CYP System	Antipsychotic Whose Metabolism Activated	Activating Medicine-Type or Use of Medicine	Degree of Activation, if Known
1A2	clozapine, chlorpromazine, mesoridazine, thioridazine, olanzapine, trifluoperazine, thiothixene	ritonavir—anti-AIDS phenytoin—antiseizure carbamazepine—antiseizure/ mood stabilizer barbiturates—antiseizure/sedative marijuana cigarettes omeprazole—antiulcer	
2D6	clozapine, olanzapine, sertindole, thioridazine, risperidone, perphenazine, fluphenazine, mesoridazine, chlorpromazine		
3A4	pimozide, quetiapine, ziprasidone, clozapine, chlorpromazine, mesoridazine, haloperidol, sertindole	ritonavir—anti-AIDS rifampin—anti-TB efavirenz—anti-AIDS nevirapine—anti-AIDS rifabutin—antibiotic St. John's wort—antidepressant felbamate—antiseizure topiramate—antiseizure oxcarbazepine—antiseizure/ mood stabilizer carbamazepine—antiseizure/ mood stabilizer phenytoin—antiseizure barbiturates—antiseizure/ sedative dexamethasone-steroids troglitazone—antidiabetic	

antipsychotic to offer meaningful benefit. The drug has its loyalists who contend that it is the best antipsychotic psychiatry has to offer. However, clozapine's increased likelihood of problematic sedation, orthostatic hypotension, cardiomyopathy, myocarditis, weight gain, seizures, and effects on bone marrow pose civil medicolegal risks as well.

One study found that clozapine-treated patients were 3.6 times more likely to suffer sudden death compared to patients treated with other psychiatric agents. The same study, however, showed that those clozapine-treated patients were five times less likely to die of a condition related to their psychiatric disease *(93)*.

Ultimately, the more potentially toxic the antipsychotic, the more significant a clinician should appraise a potential interaction, since even a small effect on the metabolism of that antipsychotic may elicit side effects that are intolerable even in minor or less frequent form. Alternatively, the seemingly minor effect of a small lowering of the blood level of a medicine may result in a relapse of terribly psychotic symptoms such as hallucinations or delusions.

The effect of medicines on each other's metabolism must be remembered when discontinuing a treatment. Medications that inhibited antipsychotic metabolism, such as paroxetine or fluoxetine, when discontinued, may have unexpected effects. Levels of the antipsychotic, no longer inhibited in its metabolism, may drop—resulting in far worse control over psychotic symptoms. In this manner, a person may be totally compliant yet demonstrate a "surprise" clinical change with forensic ramifications.

Theoretically—and this point must be emphasized—the same point can be made about smoking. Cigarette smoking activates the metabolism of CYP1A2. Therefore, a person who stops smoking may have a corresponding increase in blood levels of an antipsychotic metabolized through this pathway—along with serious side effects associated with that change, especially if dramatic.

3. INTERACTIONS OF ANTIPSYCHOTICS WITH OTHER AGENTS

Antipsychotics are less appreciated for the significance of their influence on the metabolism of other medicines through the CYP system, although perphenazine and other antipsychotics' effects as a 2D6 inhibitor are particularly chronicled. This 2D6 inhibitor may become pertinent in reconstructive investigations involving drugs who are metabolized through that CYP isoenzyme—such as desipramine, nortryptyline, codeine, antiarrhythmics, and some β blockers. All of these 2D6 medicines can accumulate to a lethal degree in the bloodstream; any drug that inhibits their metabolism, therefore, is of forensic interest.

Many psychotropics have sedating qualities. Not surprisingly, the sedating qualities of antipsychotics are additive to the effects of other medicines *(94)*. This may have forensic significance, particularly if such oversedation results in an accident.

However, additive effects of antipsychotics cannot be presumed. Thioridazine, as noted above, actually decreases circulating blood levels of quetiapine *(95)*.

4. INDIVIDUALITY AND METABOLISM

Forensic examination that focuses on drug interactions must consider that 5–10% of the Caucasian population, genetically, has a poor capacity to metabolize drugs through the CYP isoenzyme 2D6 *(96)*. This point is especially important with antipsychotics, which are principally metabolized via this particular isoenzyme. If need be, a person's capacity to metabolize may be tested to resolve forensic questions.

Medicine appreciates the principle that metabolic potential worsens as a person advances into old age. Therefore, the elderly may be vulnerable to untoward effects of medicines dosed at prescriptions that may even be modest *(97)*.

Differences in metabolism are increasingly identified that link to gender and race. Poor 2D6 metabolizers, for example, have been found to be less frequent among Asians and African Americans, compared to Caucasian populations *(98)*. Though isoenzyme activity of CYP3A4 has been demonstrated to be 40% greater in younger women *(99)*, however, the distinctions relating to other isoenzymes are less pronounced. Furthermore, the distinctions noted in 3A4, and in 2D6 (lower activity during the luteal phase of the menstrual cycle) *(100)*, have not been linked by any research to findings that specifically relate to antipsychotic drug metabolism.

Still, this stage of understanding directs the forensic examiner to monitor the research in this rapidly evolving area, for research findings will increase the relevance of identifying ages and stages of culture- and gender-distinct metabolism.

5. IMPLICATIONS FOR CRIMINAL LAW

Drug interactions in criminal law are far less pertinent to cases than the conditions antipsychotics are prescribed for. For example, most defendants who are unable to render a knowing or intelligent confession have moderate to severe mental retardation or significant brain damage that exists independent of the medicine they are taking. With respect to the voluntariness of their confession, antipsychotics again have little bearing; even in higher or toxic doses, involuntary actions are not attributable to the medicines themselves.

Forensic scrutiny of competency to stand trial, or to represent one's self, should incorporate a consideration of the medication regimen. Subtle issues noted below are clearly related to drug interactions. As in other criminal matters, however, symptoms that compromise competency are more likely to result from the condition itself than the treatments for it.

Criminal responsibility may be alleged to relate to involuntary intoxication with medicines, or an untoward reaction from a combination of psychotropics. However, antipsychotics do not cause violence or criminality. In the particular case of clozapine, the medicines may be responsible for preventing violence *(101)*. Mitigated criminal responsibility—as a byproduct of antipsychotic use—would be theoretically more related to crimes clearly committed during a period of frank confusion, in the absence of sustained purposefulness. Though obscure, such a plausible scenario will be depicted below.

Far more likely an issue, for an individual prescribed antipsychotics, is the influence of the condition itself—or an untreated co-occurring condition—on criminal responsibility.

5.1. Questioning Considerations

How do drug interactions involving antipsychotics impact a knowing and intelligent confession? Let us consider the following example:

Jimmy Martin, a 25-year-old with a history of schizophrenia, has been admitted to the emergency room under arrest. He allegedly attacked his neighbor with a stick, after which the neighbor called the police, and Jimmy is psychotic.

Seen by the ER attending, Jimmy declares that he is "allergic to Haldol." He is given chlorpromazine 25 mg along with the benzodiazepine lorazepam. Thirty minutes later, he is seen with a stiff neck, and is diagnosed with dystonia. Given benztropine, Jimmy's dystonia lifts.

Once he is calmer, police interview Jimmy, a man of average intelligence. He tells police he attacked his neighbor.

Was his confession intelligent, and knowing? The forensic examiner needs to review the results of the examinations closest in time to the administration of his benztropine and chlorpromazine to appraise whether there were any signs of confusion or memory disturbance originating from anticholinergic effects.

Reviewing the confession statement, should it be taped or transcribed, enables the examiner to match details of the confession with the alleged crime. Inconsistent details, a changing story, and/or a confused pattern of relating may herald cognitive impairment originating from a drug interaction involving an anticholinergic antipsychotic.

Of course, should Jimmy be noted as difficult to rouse, due to the cumulative sedation of the lorazepam and chlorpromazine, the ER chart would indicate such a condition.

Adequate medical chart documentation of the mental-status exam of prisoners helps resolve questions of knowing and intelligent communications. Never should side effects be presumed. On the contrary, traditional charting practices note changes in the mental status; no news in an ER is more often no news (or not examined). A lack of documentation bespeaks an unmonitored patient, or a patient that did not call attention to her or himself through a deteriorating or obviously changed condition.

Irrespective of legal burdens, the medical chart defines events or nonevents. The burden is on a disagreeing party to prove documentation wrong. Future examiners should later raise suspicion of the role of drug interactions only when (a) a change in cognitive ability is documented and (b) that change coincides with the administration schedule of the medicine, as well as the expected times of their expression of effects and side effects.

5.2. Criminal Competencies

When one considers the abilities being assessed, there is truly no basis to contest competency to stand trial on the basis of theoretical drug interactions alone. Given that the trial is extended, any communication between the attorney, or the court, with a defendant should elicit evidence that a person has memory, concentration, or attention problems attributable to the medication regimen. Because these effects are easily reversible, typically within hours to days, a simple telephone call to a caregiving physician can remedy a problem rather than derailing the administration of justice by months simply to lower the dose of a drug.

Mac Brown, a 50-year-old bank employee charged with robbery, has asked the court if he can represent himself. Currently prescribed mesoridazine and trihexyphenidyl, he seemed a bit confused in court, though he is relatively intelligent and educated.

An examination of Mr. Brown reveals him to have a mild delirium. Alteration of his medicines results in a full resolution of the confusion within 18 hours.

Of course, in such cases, modifying the medication may provide only temporary improvement. In fact, lowering the medicines may prompt a relapse of dramatic symptoms of the underlying illness, which may affect competency far more vividly than mere drug interactions.

For this reason, delaying the proceedings an additional several days to monitor for mental deterioration of other origin makes good clinical and judicial sense. In the end, drug interactions leading to compromised competency to stand trial need not result in the kinds of delays associated with allowing the effects of acute illness to simmer down.

Competency to be executed is, of course, a standard that is so easy to achieve that a person who is quite mentally impaired may still satisfy criteria. Advanced illness is invariably the causal factor behind such pronounced incapacitation. However, the desperate culture—among both doctors opposed to capital punishment and patients determined to evade the death penalty—makes for interesting possibilities.

For instance, Barry Peterson, convicted of the sex murder of a child, is sentenced to death. Over the course of his stay on death row, and while receiving counseling, he is prescribed sedating antipsychotics to sleep. As his execution date approaches, he becomes progressively more confused. His attorney contests his competency to be executed.

The death row setting and the stress of impending execution are extreme enough to precipitate psychosis. But opposing counsel should still order a comprehensive drug screen, with quantification if necessary. Given the pills and drugs that circulate among prisoners and prison employees, the ease with which a prisoner can hoard and employ mind-altering medicines must be accounted for in any such forensic examination.

So, too, must the prescription decisions of physicians. A doctor may choose, for unconscious or conscious reasons, a prescription whose drug interactions render a death row patient exceptionally disoriented. Without careful accountability, this can be explained away in a medical chart as arising from illness.

Physicians are to be assumed to mean well. However, we must also remember that to many doctors, meaning well involves saving the life of a condemned person at all costs. Careful oversight into the prescribing history of the death row psychiatrist is therefore sensible diligence for the attorney presented with an inmate who has become less competent, perhaps incompetent, to be executed.

5.3. Medication Defenses

Antipsychotics do not directly disinhibit, and do not cause acute psychiatric illnesses. In unusual circumstances, interactions can result in crimes that reflect the product of untoward medication effects.

Sharon Perez was prescribed thiothixene and benztropine. Her psychiatrist felt she looked a bit stiff in her previous appointment, and increased the benztropine. Ms. Perez became increasingly confused, and later exited her apartment at approximately 10:00 PM after hanging up with her mother. Her mother was worried enough after the conversation to drive over to Sharon's house.

Too late. Sharon had already gone for a drive. She had driven aimlessly for about 2 miles, before pulling into a convenience store. In so doing, she ran over a customer walking to her car. Police personnel who arrived at the scene found Sharon, perplexed, surrounded by store customers. Asked to read her rights, Ms. Perez complained of blurry vision, though her answers were often irrational.

Notwithstanding the above bizarre example, a prescribed antipsychotic far more likely reflects diminished capacity through the suggestion that whatever the defendant was taking at the time of the crime, it may not have been enough.

Therefore, medicines that accelerate the metabolism of the antipsychotic may be pertinent to a criminal defense, especially if behavioral changes coincided with the time course of the regimen. If the patient followed a doctor's instructions, then the unexpected ineffectiveness of the medicine may be even further supportive to the defense *(102)*.

Jerry Kasner has been prescribed clozapine for a number of years. He is compliant with his appointments, sees his doctors every 2 weeks, and had blood levels taken of the drug that show him to be in the therapeutic range.

Recently, he takes up smoking. At some point, between appointments, his friends notice he becomes increasingly withdrawn, taking poor care of his hygiene. On one occasion, ambling out in a mall, he attacks a young lady, whose screams alert passersby to intervene.

Jerry is noted to be peculiar in his manner on arrest, but says very little. Follow-up blood testing reflects that clozapine is still in his system, but in a substantially lower blood concentration.

Typically, patients who consume intoxicants are judged as having become voluntarily intoxicated *(103)*. Laws may be more accommodating to the benefit of the defense if a defendant drank alcohol or took an illicit drug with the expectation of relief, especially if he were suffering from psychotic mental illness, and the existing antipsychotic regimen was ineffective *(104)*.

6. IMPLICATIONS FOR CIVIL CASES

Antipsychotics have traditionally been the heaviest artillery in the psychiatric drug armamentarium. Also known as "major tranquilizers," the traditional antipsychotics assumed forensic significance because of the significant side effects that could appear fairly dramatically with relatively small fluctuations in dose of the medicine.

With the revolution of psychopharmacology, and the release and widespread use of atypical antipsychotics, forensic civil implications have changed for these medicines. Because there are medicines now available that are not as associated with significant side effects, future civil forensics will relate more directly to the decision to choose traditional vs atypical antipsychotics.

7. DISABILITY, WORKPLACE, AND AMERICANS WITH DISABILITIES ACT

Adaptation to the workplace when taking traditional antipsychotics was long a major obstacle. As significant as the impairments from schizophrenia, schizoaffective disorder, bipolar disorder, and psychotic depression are, the impact of those illnesses on employability was worsened by the often-unavoidable side effects of traditional antipsychotics.

The effects of akathisia, driving a person to perpetual motion, would interfere with the essential functions of most work. The cognitive effects of other traditional antipsychotics also limit even compliant patients with major psychiatric disorders from fulfilling the core demands of intellectual dexterity of many positions.

Parkinsonism also impacts on one's ability to perform essential functions. The condition, which limits the ability to move quickly and spontaneously, may substantially curtail the efficiency with which one can do any task that requires movement. Furthermore, the masklike face of parkinsonism *(105)* calls attention to an employee as "medicated," and can further isolate someone who especially needs the support.

7.1. New Frontiers of Accommodation

With the release of clozapine, and later, olanzapine, and seroquel, treatments became available that do not affect movement, do not cause parkinsonism, and do not produce confusion. Employees can now engage in more intellectually competitive pursuits, even while taking atypical antipsychotics *(106)*.

The obstacles of traditional antipsychotics have been removed by the next generation. Now, employers can more easily anticipate reversible side effects, and more easily accommodate side effects of interactions such as increased sedation (a side effect of all of the atypical antipsychotics), or dizziness upon rapidly standing (clozapine) *(107)*.

Advances in antipsychotic technology are the most important development in the reintegration of employees under the Americans with Disabilities Act (ADA). They render many questions of insurmountable side effects obsolete.

Poor compliance with treatment has also had a major impact on accommodating employees with psychotic mental illness. Atypical antipsychotics have been demonstrated to have superior compliance *(108)*, which in turn promotes maintaining a symptom-free presentation and adherence to a plan worked out for an employee.

7.2. Tomorrow's Cases

Mark Frost, 28, has a history of bipolar disorder. He began psychiatric treatment for the first time last month. At the time of the onset of his illness, he was 6 months removed from law school and had no health insurance. Upon admission to a city hospital, he was given fluphenazine and lithium. His symptoms resolved relatively quickly.

After his discharge, Mark began a new position. While he remained without manic symptoms, he noticed a subjective sense of great restlessness. Others at his firm noticed that he was pacing about the office. After gentle input, a senior partner demanded a drug test, suspecting Mark of being on cocaine or amphetamines.

No cocaine was found in Mark's blood; however, when he demonstrated traces of fluphenazine, and his firm confronted him, Mark disclosed his condition. The employer contacted Mark's psychiatrist to advise him of the firm's concerns; the psychiatrist changed Mark's antipsychotic to olanzapine. Soon afterward, Mark spent noticeably more time at his own desk, without pacing about, and others noted him to be more creative as well.

However, Mark would appear somewhat sluggish in the early morning. A follow-up call to the psychiatrist resulted in the firm's agreement to shift his starting time at work to 10:00 AM. Mark settled into the firm and remains a key part of the firm's future.

As we become more acquainted with the atypical drugs, previously unrecognized interactions will be discovered. Case reports describe panic attacks arising, for example, in those treated with high-dose antipsychotics *(109)*. Modifying the regimen and early intervention, in such cases, quickly reverses the side effects without necessarily having to accommodate the condition by changing occupational responsibilities.

Unfortunately for some, even those who derive benefit from the atypical antipsychotics, residual symptoms of the condition may linger. If these symptoms interfere with the performance of essential functions, then even the most tolerable medicines will not salvage the employee's job or warrant accommodation by the employer.

Whenever an employee on an antipsychotic raises an ADA issue, the workplace should immediately establish channels of communication with the treating psychiatrist. Should an employee demonstrate a sudden mental or physical deterioration, any necessary changes relating to contributing drug interactions can be recommended, with quick response. Such structure also reinforces the need for continued compliance with treatment. Adherence to boundaries of confidentiality can still be easily respected.

8. MALPRACTICE AND OTHER TORT LITIGATION

Malpractice litigation relating to interactions of antipsychotics is evolving. In the past, physicians confronted liability based on the consequences of traditional antipsychotic side effects, heightened by interactions. In the future, malpractice suits will originate based upon the physician's decision to prescribe a traditional antipsychotic instead of an atypical antipsychotic.

Informed consent continues to be overlooked in malpractice litigation. However, informed consent requires disclosure of alternative forms of treatment. Atypical antipsychotics are drugs of choice; therefore, liability may be clear when a patient suffers from the side effects of a traditional antipsychotic when an atypical agent was available and this option was not presented to the patient or otherwise considered.

Since psychiatric malpractice originates most commonly after unwanted death, particular attention needs to be directed to medication regimens in cases of sudden death. Postmortem toxicology studies may rule out overdose, but medications may still be responsible. Chlorpromazine and thioridazine are two antipsychotics that can cause substantial drops in blood pressure *(110)*. This effect can be more pronounced in patients given tricyclic antidepressants and monoamine oxidase inhibitors *(110)*.

Significant hypotension has also been described with mesoridazine and clozapine *(110)*. Since so many other medication options are available to treat acute agitation, and psychosis, clinical practice warrants accounting for why these medicines are prescribed instead of medicines that do not represent any risk to the circulatory system—particularly in the medically vulnerable or in those at risk for suicide by overdose.

Unwanted lethality may rarely arise from the very rare side effect of agranulocytosis, or loss of ability to make white blood cells, attributed to clozapine. Risk of this side effect may be heightened by a number of anti-AIDS *(111)* or anticancer agents *(112)*, as well as with carbamazepine *(113)*. Again, accounting for this risk is sufficient, especially if clinical choices are more restricted.

Other interactions are not so easy to resolve in a cause–effect manner. Sometimes, polypharmacy can collectively worsen a condition. Sometimes the interactions of medicines prescribed for nonpsychiatric conditions can affect glucose metabolism, or worsen sexual function, or contribute to weight gain. These problems may lead to the development of diabetes, divorce, or cardiac problems, respectively. The prescribing physician has a duty to monitor for these difficulties, and to discuss and resolve the problems with his or her patient, regardless of the different possible causes.

Interactions with antipsychotics may impact tort liability if a patient's excessive sedation or confusion results in impaired operation of a motor vehicle or other lethal equipment. Interactions that increase blood levels of clozapine may be responsible for causing seizures *(114)*, which can create a highway catastrophe. In this regard, standard psychiatric practice has reinforced the responsibility for psychiatrists to advise patients of risks associated with operating such items when prescribed antipsychotics.

9. COMPETENCY TO INVEST, TESTAMENTARY CAPACITY

Legal questions, often posthumous, arise over decisions to invest or to earmark assets. Since trusts and wills often concern individuals with health problems, such decisions may be affected by the interactions of prescribed drugs. Cases involving such competencies therefore warrant close scrutiny of medical, prescription, and pharmacy records. Comparison of decisions made, with corresponding dates, yields vital detail about the relevance of drug interactions.

As agitation in the medically ill, and in the elderly, is often treated with antipsychotics, confusion and sedation may be attributable to the medicine—if not the underlying condition. Careful consideration of the clinical course will enable the distinction of whether a drug interaction was responsible.

The elderly, and those incapacitated who are making financial decisions, are particularly vulnerable to undue influence. Loving relatives with self-serving motives can position themselves opportunistically. For this reason, sedation, heightened by drug interactions, should also be tracked. If undue influence is suspected, and the agent had continuous proximity to an ill but wealthy patient, the deceased's blood should be tested to ensure that no medicines were administered, in combination, that would have perpetuated mental incapacity or hastened death.

The study of drug interactions is ongoing. New discoveries from clinical use of combinations of an ever-growing pharmacopoeia add to our appreciation of interactions. These findings will one day provide answers to some of the peculiar forensic scenarios that we now suspect are influenced by drug interactions, but cannot yet explain.

REFERENCES

1. Kaplan H, Sadock B, and Grebb J. Synopsis of psychiatry: behavioral sciences clinical psychology. Baltimore: Williams and Wilkins, 1994:940–960.
2. Stahl SM. "Hit-and-run" actions at dopamine receptors, part 1: mechanism of action of atypical antipsychotics. J Clin Psychiatry 62(9):670–671 (2001).
3. Stahl S. Essential psychopharmacology. Cambridge, England: Cambridge University Press, 2000:2.
4. Stahl S. Essential psychopharmacology. Cambridge, England: Cambridge University Press, 2000:411–414.
5. Kaplan H, Sadock B, and Grebb J. Synopsis of psychiatry: behavioral sciences clinical psychiatry. Baltimore: Williams & Wilkins, 1994:984.
6. Seeman P. Atypical antipsychotics: mechanism of action. Canadian J of Psychiatry 47(1): 27–38 (2000).
7. Stahl S. Essential psychopharmacology. Cambridge, England: Cambridge University Press, 2000:375.
8. Wirshing W. Movement disorders associated with neuroleptic treatment. J Clin Psychol 62(Suppl 21):15 (2001).
9. Sethi K. Movement disorders induced by dopamine blocking agents. Semin Neurol 21(1): 60 (2001).

10. Kaufman DM. Clinical neurology for psychiatrists, 3rd ed. Philadelphia: Saunders, 1990: 368.
11. Wallis LA. Textbook of women's health. Philadelphia: Lippincott-Raven, 1998.
12. Mamo D, Sweet R, Mulsant B, Rosen J, and Pollock BG. Neuroleptic-induced parkinsonism in Alzheimer's disease. Psychiatric Annals 32(4):249–252 (2002).
13. Stahl S. Essential psychopharmacology, Cambridge, England: Cambridge University Press, 2000:408.
14. Kaplan H, Sadock B, and Grebb J. Synopsis of psychiatry: behavioral sciences clinical psychiatry, 7th ed. Baltimore: Williams & Wilkins, 1994:896–897.
15. Kaufman DM. Clinical neurology for psychiatrists, 3rd ed. Philadelphia: Saunders, 1990: 379.
16. Kaplan H, Sadock B, and Grebb J. Synopsis of psychiatry: behavioral sciences clinical psychiatry, 7th ed. Baltimore: Williams & Wilkins, 1994:950.
17. Matsumoto RR and Pouw B. Correlation between neuroloeptic binding to singam(1) and sigma(2): receptors and acute dystonic reactions. Eur J Pharmacol 401(2):155–160 (2000).
18. Velickovic M, Benabou R, and Brin MF. Cervical dystonia pathophysiology and treatment options. Drugs 61(13):1921–1943 (2001).
19. Csernansky JG and Schuchart EK. Relapse and rehospitalisation rates in patients with schizophrenia: effects of second generation antipsychotics. CNS Drugs 16(7):473–484 (2002).
20. Gorman JM, ed. The essential guide to psychiatric drugs. New York: St. Martins Press, 1990:218.
21. Holloman LC and Marder SR. Management of acute extrapyramidal effects induced by antipsychotic drugs. Am J Health Syst Pharm 54(21):2461–2477 (1997).
22. Lima AR, Soares-Weiser K, Bacaltchuk J, and Barnes TRE. Benzodiazepines for neuroleptic-induced acute akathisia. Cochrane Database System Review (1):CD001950 (2002).
23. Bernstein JG. Clinical psychopharmacology, 2nd ed. Littleton, CO: Library of Congress, 1984:162.
24. Siris S. Suicide and schizophrenia. J Psychopharm 15(2):127–135 (2001).
25. Kaufman DM. Clinical neurology for psychiatrists, 3rd ed. Philadelphia: Saunders, 1990: 394.
26. Kaplan H, Sadock B, and Grebb J. Synopsis of psychiatry: behavioral sciences clinical psychiatry, 7th ed. Baltimore: Williams & Wilkins, 1994:885.
27. Sethi K. Movement disorders induced by dopamine blocking agents. Semin Neurol 21(1): 59–68 (2001).
28. Casey DE. Tardive dyskinesia and atypical antipsychotic drugs. Schizophr Res 35:S61–S66 (1999).
29. Kaplan H, Sadock B, and Grebb J. Synopsis of psychiatry: behavioral sciences clinical psychiatry, 7th ed. Baltimore: Williams & Wilkins, 1994:951.
30. Wirshing W. Movement disorders associated with neuroleptic treatment. J Clin Psychol 62(Suppl 21):15–18 (2001).
31. Stahl S. Essential psychopharmacology. Cambridge, England: Cambridge University Press, 2000:406.
32. Sethi K. Movement disorders induced by dopamine blocking agents. Semin Neurol 21(1): 61 (2001).
33. Soares KV and McGrath JJ. Vitamin E for neuroleptic-induced tardive dyskinesia. Cochrane Database System Review (2):CD000209 (2000).
34. Llorca PM, Chereau I, Bayle FJ, et al. Tardive dyskinesias and antipsychotics: a review. Eur Psychiatry 17(3):129–138 (2002).
35. Stahl S. Essential psychopharmacology. Cambridge, England: Cambridge University Press, 2000:406.

36. Ghadirian AM, Annable L, Belanger MC, and Chouinard G. A cross-sectional study of parkinsonism and tardive dyskinesia in lithium-treated affective disordered patients. J Clin Psychiatry 57(1):22–28 (1996).
37. Ayd F. Evaluating the interactions between herbal and psychoactive medications. Psychiatric Times December: 45–46 (2000).
38. Goldberg E, ed. The executive brain. New York: Oxford University Press, 2001:94.
39. Physicians' desk reference, 57th ed. Montvale, NJ: Medical Economics Company, Inc., 2003:1787.
40. Asarnow RF. Neurocognitive impairments in schizophrenia: a piece of the epigenetic puzzle. Eur Child Adolesc Psychiatry 8(Suppl 1):15–18 (1999).
41. Diagnostic and statistical manual of mental disorders, 4th ed., text revision. Washington, DC: American Psychiatric Association, 2000:301.
42. Stahl S. Essential psychopharmacology. Cambridge, England: Cambridge University Press, 2000:370.
43. Kaplan H and Sadock B. Synopsis of psychiatry: behavioral sciences clinical psychology, 7th ed. Baltimore: Williams and Wilkins, 1994.
44. Knegtering H, Eijck M, and Hijsman A. Effects of antidepressants on cognitive functioning of elderly patients. Drugs Aging 5(3):192–199 (1994).
45. Bernstein JB. Clinical psychopharmocology, 2nd ed. Boston: John Wright, 1984.
46. Kaplan H and Sadock B. Synopsis of psychiatry: behavioral sciences clinical psychology, 7th ed. Baltimore: Williams and Wilkins, 1994:945.
47. Stahl S. Essential psychopharmacology. Cambridge, England: Cambridge University Press, 2000:378.
48. Physicians' desk reference, 57th ed. Montvale, NJ: Medical Economics Company, Inc., 2003:1789.
49. Turrone P, Kapur S, Seeman MV, and Flint AJ. Elevation of prolactin levels by atypical antipsychotics. Am J Psychiatry 159(1):133–135.
50. Kaplan H, Sadock B, and Grebb J. Synopsis of psychiatry: behavioral sciences clinical psychiatry, 7th ed. Baltimore: Williams & Wilkins, 1994:948.
51. Physicians' desk reference, 57th ed. Montvale, NJ: Medical Economics Company, Inc., 2003:1053, 1299, 1417, 1651–1652.
52. Allison DB, Mentore JL, and Heo M. Antipsychotic-induced weight gain: a comprehensive research synthesis. Am J Psychiatry 156:1686–1696 (1999).
53. McIntyre R. Psychotropic drugs and adverse events in the treatment of bipolar disorders revisited. J Clin Psychol 63(3):15–20 (2002).
54. Haupt D and Newcomer J. Hyperglycemia and antipsycotic medications. J Clin Psychol 62(27):15–26 (2001).
55. Jin H, Meyer JM, and Jeste DV. Phenomenology of and risk factors for new-onset diabetes mellitus and diabetic ketoacidosis associated with atypical antipsychotics: an analysis of 45 published cases. Ann Clin Psychiatry 14(1):59–64 (2002).
56. Stahl S. Essential psychopharmacology, Cambridge, England: Cambridge University Press, 2000:415–421.
57. Kaplan H, Sadock B, and Grebb J. Synopsis of psychiatry: behavioral sciences clinical psychiatry, 7th ed. Baltimore: Williams & Wilkins, 1994:947.
58. Jusic N and Lader M. Post-mortem antipsychotic drug concentrations and unexplained deaths. Br J Psychiatry 165:787–791 (1994).
59. Ray W. Arch Gen Psychiatry 58(11):1168–1170 (2001).
60. Markowitz JS, Wells BG, and Carson WH. Interactions between antipsychotic and antihypertensive drugs. Ann Pharmacother 29:603–609 (1995).

6. Antipsychotic Drugs and Interactions

61. Devane C and Markowitz J. Avoiding psychotropic drug interactions in the cardiac patient. TEN 3(5):67–71 (2001).
62. Grohman R, Ruther E, Sassim N, et al. Adverse effects of clozapine. Psychopharmacology (Berl) 99:101–104 (1989).
63. Killian JG, Kerr K, Lawrence C, and Celermajer DS, et al. Myocarditis and cardiomyopathy associated with clozapine. Lancet 354:1841–1845 (1999).
64. DeVane CL and Nemeroff CB. Drug interactions in psychiatry. Primary Psychiatry 7(10): 67 (2000).
65. Haddad PM and Anderson IM. Antipsychotic-related QTc prolongation, torsade de pointes and sudden death. Drugs 62(11):1649–1671 (2002).
66. Menkes DB and Knight JC. Cardiotoxicity and prescription of thioridazine in New Zealand. Aust N Z J Psychiatry 36(4):492–498 (2002).
67. FDA Psychopharmacological Drugs Advisory Committee. Briefing document for ziprasidone hydrochloride. July 19, 2000.
68. Glassman AH and Bigger JT. Antipsychotic drugs: prolonged QTc interval, torsades de pointes and sudden death. Am J Psychiatry 158(11):1774–1782 (2001).
69. Young D. Black-box warning for droperidol surprises pharmacists. Am J Health Syst Pharm 59(6):494, 497, 502–504 (2002).
70. Glassman AH and Bigger JT. Antipsychotic drugs: prolonged QTc interval, torsades de pointes and sudden death. Am J Psychiatry 158(11):1774–1782 (2001).
71. Smego RA and Durack DT. The neuroleptic malignant syndrome. Arch Intern Med 142: 1183–1185 (1982).
72. Friedman JH. Recognition and treatment of the neuroleptic malignant syndrome. Curr Opin Neurol 1:310–311 (1988).
73. Reeves RR, Torres RA, Liberto V, and Hart RH. Atypical neuroleptic malignant syndrome associated with olanzapine. Pharmacotherapy 22(5):641–644 (2002).
74. Sing KJ, Ramaekers GM, and Van Harten PN. Neuroleptic malignant syndrome and quetiapine. Am J Psychiatry 159(1):149–150 (2002).
75. Blum MW, Siegel AM, Meier R, et al. Neuroleptic malignant-like syndrome and acute hepatitis during tolcapone and clozapine medication. Eur Neurol 46(3):158–160 (2001).
76. Aboraya A, Schumacher J, Abdalla E, LePage J, et al. Neuroleptic malignant syndrome associated with risperidone and olanzapine in first-episode schizophrenia. W V Med J 98(2):63–65 (2002).
77. Stahl S. Essential psychopharmacology. Cambridge, England: Cambridge University Press, 2000:540.
78. Clayton AH. Reconstruction and assessment of sexual dysfunction associated with depression. J Clin Psychiatry 62(Suppl 3):5–9 (2001).
79. Stahl S. Essential psychopharmacology. Cambridge, England: Cambridge University Press, 2000:542.
80. Compton MT and Miller AH. Priapism associated with conventional and atypical antipsychotic medications: a review. J Clin Psychiatry 62(5):362–366 (2001).
81. Bernstein JB. Clinical psychopharmocology, 2nd ed. Boston: John Wright, 1984.
82. Pacia SV and Devinsky O. Clozapine-related seizures: experience with 5,629 patients neurology. Neurology 44(12):2247–2249 (1994).
83. Stahl S. Essential psychopharmacology. Cambridge, England: Cambridge University Press, 2000:207.
84. DeVane CL and Nemeroff C. Primary Psychiatry. 7(10):(2000).
85. Jibson M and Tandon R. An overview of antischizophrenic medications. CNS News Special Edition, December: 49–54 (2001).

86. Kaplan H and Sadock B. Synopsis of psychiatry: behavioral sciences clinical psychology, 7th ed. Baltimore: Williams and Wilkins, 1994:940–960.
87. Weber S. Drug interactions with antidepressants. CNS News February: 27–34 (2002).
88. Kontaxakis VP, Havaki-Kontaxaki BJ, Stamouli SS, and Christodoulou GN. Toxic interaction between risperidone and clozapine: A case report. Prog Neuropsychopharm Biol Psychiatry 26(2):407–409 (2002).
89. Mental fitness physician resource series. Primary Psychiatry November: 36–37 (2000).
90. Grohman R, Ruther E, Sassim N, et al. Adverse effects of clozapine. Psychopharmacology 99:101–104 (1989).
91. Mental fitness physician resource series. Primary Psychiatry November: 36 (2000).
92. DeVane CL and Nemeroff CB. Drug Interactions in psychiatry. Primary Psychiatry 7(10): 66 (2000).
93. Modai I, Hirschmann S, and Rava A. Sudden death in patients receiving clozapine treatment: a preliminary investigation. J Clin Psychopharmacol 20(3):525–327 (2000).
94. Kaplan H and Sadock B. Synopsis of psychiatry: behavioral sciences clinical psychology, 7th ed. Baltimore: Williams and Wilkins, 1994.
95. DeVane CL and Nemeroff CB. Quetiapine drug interactions. Primary Psychiatry 7(10): (2000).
96. Greenblatt D. Symposium, American Association for Geriatric Psychiatry, 2001 annual meeting, San Francisco, CA.
97. Pies R. Geriatric psychopharmacology. Am Fam Physician 28(4):171–176 (1983).
98. Pollock BG. Recent developments in drug metabolism of interest to psychiatrists. Harv Rev Psychiatry 2(4):204–213 (1994).
99. Tsunoda SM, Harris RZ, Mroczkowski PJ, and Benet LZ. Preliminary evaluation of progestins as inducers of cytochrome 3A4 activity in post-menopausal women. J Clin Pharmacology 38:1137–1143 (1998).
100. Tamminga WJ, Werner J, Oostehuis B, Wieling J, Wilffert B, de Liej LFMH, de Zeeuw RA, and Jonkman JHG. CYP2D6 and CYP2C19activity in a large population of Dutch healthy volunteers: indications for oral contraceptive-related gender differences. Euro J Clin Pharmacol 55(3):177–184 (1999).
101. Volavka J. The effects of clozapine on aggression and substance abuse in schizophrenic patients. J Clin Psychol 60(Supp 12):43–46 (1999).
102. Perkins v United States 228 F 408 (1915).
103. Lexsee 73 ALR 3d 195; 2001, West Group.
104. *Teeters v Commonwealth* 310 Ky 546, 221 SW2d 85 (1949).
105. Wyngaarden JB, Smith LH, and Bennett JC. Cecil textbook of medicine. Philadelphia: Saunders, 1992.
106. Meyer PS, Bond GR, and Tunis SL. Comparison between the effects of atypical and traditional antipsychotics on work status for clients in a psychiatric rehabilitation program. J Clin Psychiatry 63(2):108–116 (2002).
107. Grohman R. Adverse effects of clozapine. Psychopharmacology 99(Suppl):S101–S104 (1989).
108. Rosenheck R, Chang S, Choe Y, Cramer J, Xu W, Thomas J, Henderson W, and Charney D. Medication continuation and compliance: a comparison of patients treated with clozapine and haloperidol. J Clin Psychiatry 61(5):382–386 (2000).
109. Higuchi H, Kamata M, Yoshimoto M, Shimisu T, and Hishikawa Y. Panic attacks in patients with chronic schizophrenia: a complication of long-term neuroleptic treatment. *Psychiatry Clin Neurosci* 53(1):91–94 (1999).

110. Physicians' desk reference, 57th ed. Montvale, NJ: Medical Economics Company, Inc., 2003:1651–1652.
111. Gillenwater D and McDaniel J. Rational psychopharmacology for patients with HIV infection and AIDS. Psychiatric Annals 31(1):28–32 (2001).
112. Safdar A and Armstrong D. Infectious morbidity in critically ill patients with cancer. Crit Care Clin 17(3):531–570 (2001).
113. Kaplan H and Sadock B. Synopsis of psychiatry: behavioral sciences clinical psychology, 7th ed. Baltimore: Williams and Wilkins, 1994:934.
114. Welch J, Manschreck T, and Redmond D. Clozapine-induced seizures and EEG changes. J Neuropsychiatry Clin Neurosci 6(3):250–256 (1994).

PART II
Cardiovascular Drugs

Chapter 7

Cardiovascular Drugs

Johann Auer, MD

1. ANTIARRHYTHMICS

1.1. Drug Classification (see Fig. 1)

According to the Vaughan Williams classification *(1)*, class I drugs block the fast sodium channel. They, in turn, may be divided into three subgroups:

1. Class IA. Drugs that reduce Vmax and prolong action potential duration: quinidine, procainamide, disopyramide; kinetics of onset and offset in blocking the Na^+ channel are of intermediate rapidity (<5 s).
2. Class IB. Drugs that do not reduce Vmax and that shorten action potential duration: mexiletine, phenytoin, and lidocaine; fast onset and offset kinetics (<500 ms).
3. Class IC. Drugs that reduce Vmax, primarily slow conduction, and can prolong refractoriness minimally: flecainide, propafenone, and probably moricizine; slow onset and offset kinetics (10–20 s).
4. Class II drugs block beta-adrenergic receptors and include propranolol, timolol, metoprolol, and others.
5. Class III drugs block potassium channels and prolong repolarization. They include sotalol, amiodarone, bretylium, and ibutilide.
6. Class IV drugs block the slow calcium channel and include verapamil, diltiazem.

A more realistic view of antiarrhythmic agents is provided by the "Sicilian gambit *(2)*." This approach to drug classification is an attempt to identify the mechanisms of a particular arrhythmia, determine the vulnerable parameter of the arrhythmia most susceptible to modification, define the target most likely to affect the vulnerable parameter, and then select a drug that will modify the target.

Use of antiarrhythmic agents requires particular care because of the narrow therapeutic index of these drugs. Fortunately, we have reliable clinical end points for assessing efficacy and toxicity with a number of these agents *(3)*. Unfortunately, however,

From: *Handbook of Drug Interactions: A Clinical and Forensic Guide*
A. Mozayani and L. P. Raymon, eds. © Humana Press Inc., Totowa, NJ

Class Ia drugs (quinidine, procainamide, disopyramide)

Class Ib drugs (mexiletine, phenytoin, and lidocaine)

Class Ic drugs (flecainide, propafenone, and moricizine)

Class III drugs (sotalol, amiodarone, bretylium, ibutilide)

Class III drugs (verapamil, diltiazem)

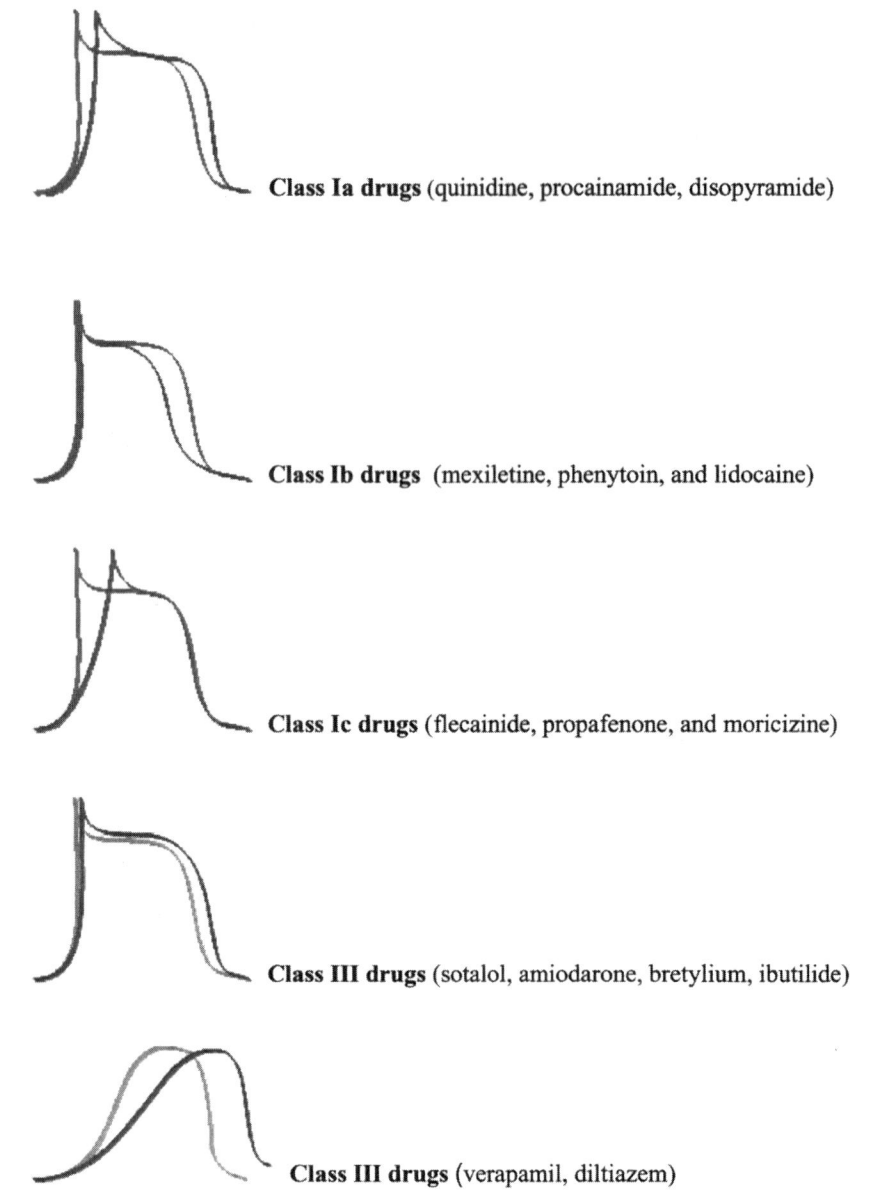

Fig. 1. Action potential and antiarrhythmic drug class (darker = drug effect on action potential).

toxicity can manifest as the very same arrhythmias for which these drugs are instituted. As a consequence, the clinician can make the potentially fatal error of misdiagnosing toxicity as lack of efficacy and responding in a manner antithetical to that required.

This phenomenon is of particular concern for the class I agents (as with quinidine and flecainide, e.g.). These agents are usually used to treat ventricular tachyarrhythmias, but their own inherent cardiotoxicity may be the same arrhythmia. It is important to emphasize that the pharmacologic effects of these drugs can often be quantified by measuring the cardiac-output (QT) interval, corrected for heart rate, and the duration

7. Cardiovascular Drugs

of the QRS (quick release system) complex. If a patient manifests ventricular tachyarrhythmias with prolongation of the QT interval or widening of the QRS complex, one should suspect a toxic etiology for these arrhythmias rather than lack of efficacy of the drugs. If such toxicity is misdiagnosed and treatment is continued or higher doses are instituted, the consequences could be disastrous.

1.2. Side Effects

Antiarrhythmic drugs produce one group of side effects that relate to excessive dosage and plasma concentrations, resulting in both noncardiac (e.g., neurological defects) and cardiac (e.g., heart failure, some arrhythmias) toxicity, and another group of side effects unrelated to plasma concentrations, termed idiopathic. Examples of the latter include procainamide-induced lupus syndrome, amiodarone-induced pulmonary toxicity (although a recent publication relates maintenance dose to this side effect), and some arrhythmias such as quinidine-induced torsades de pointes.

Drug-induced or drug-aggravated cardiac arrhythmias (*proarrhythmia*) are a major clinical problem. Electrophysiological mechanisms probably relate to prolongation of repolarization, the development of early afterdepolarizations to cause torsades de pointes, and alterations in reentry pathways to initiate or sustain ventricular tachyarrhythmias. Proarrhythmic events can occur in as many as 5–10% of patients. Heart failure increases proarrhythmic risk. Patients with atrial fibrillation treated with antiarrhythmic agents had a 4.7 relative risk of cardiac death if they had a history of heart failure compared with patients not so treated who had a 3.7 relative risk of arrhythmic death. Patients without a history of congestive heart failure had no increased risk of cardiac mortality during antiarrhythmic drug treatment. Reduced left ventricular function, treatment with digitalis and diuretics, and longer pretreatment QT interval characterize patients who develop drug-induced ventricular fibrillation. The more commonly known proarrhythmic events occur within several days of beginning drug therapy or changing dosage and are represented by such developments as incessant ventricular tachycardia, long QT syndrome, and torsades de pointes. However, in the Cardiac Arrhythmia Suppression Trial (CAST) *(4)*, encainide and flecainide reduced spontaneous ventricular arrhythmias but were associated with a total mortality of 7.7 vs 3.0% in the group receiving placebo. Deaths were equally distributed throughout the treatment period, raising the important consideration that another kind of proarrhythmic response can occur some time after the beginning of drug therapy. Such late proarrhythmic effects may relate to drug-induced exacerbation of regional myocardial conduction delay due to ischemia and heterogeneous drug concentrations that may promote reentry. Moricizine also increased mortality, leading to termination of CAST II *(5)*.

1.2.1. Quinidine (Class IA)

The most common adverse effects of chronic oral quinidine therapy are gastrointestinal (GI), including nausea, vomiting, diarrhea, abdominal pain, and anorexia. GI side effects may be milder with the gluconate form. Central nervous system (CNS) toxicity includes tinnitus, hearing loss, visual disturbances, confusion, delirium, and psychosis. Cinchonism is the term usually applied to these side effects. Allergic reactions may be manifested as rash, fever, immune-mediated thrombocytopenia, hemolytic anemia, and rarely, anaphylaxis. Thrombocytopenia is due to the presence of antibodies to quinidine-platelet complexes, causing platelets to agglutinate and lyse. In patients receiving oral anticoagulants, quinidine may cause bleeding. Side effects may preclude long-term administration of quinidine in 30–40% of patients. Quinidine can slow cardiac conduction, sometimes to the point of block, manifested as prolongation of the QRS duration or sinoatrial (SA) or arterovenous (AV) nodal conduction disturbances. Quinidine-induced cardiac toxicity can be treated with molar sodium lactate. Quinidine can prolong the QT interval and cause torsades de pointes in 1–3% of patients. Quinidine may produce syncope in 0.5–2.0% of patients, most often the result of a self-terminating episode of torsades de pointes. Torsades de pointes may be due to the development of early afterdepolarizations, as noted. Quinidine prolongs the QT interval in most patients, whether or not ventricular arrhythmias occur, but significant QT prolongation (QT interval of 500–600 ms) is often a characteristic of quinidine syncope. Many of these patients are also receiving digitalis or diuretics. Syncope is unrelated to plasma concentrations of quinidine or duration of therapy. Hypokalemia often is a prominent feature. Therapy for quinidine syncope requires immediate discontinuation of the drug and avoidance of other drugs that have similar pharmacological effects, such as disopyramide, since cross-sensitivity exists in some patients. Magnesium given intravenously (2 gm over 1–2 min, followed by an infusion of 3–20 mg/min) is probably the initial drug treatment of choice. Atrial or ventricular pacing can be used to suppress the ventricular tachyarrhythmia and may act by suppressing afterdepolarizations. For some patients, drugs that do not prolong the QT interval, such as lidocaine or phenytoin, can be tried. When pacing is not available, isoproterenol can be given with caution.

Drugs that induce hepatic enzyme production, such as phenobarbital and phenytoin, can shorten the duration of quinidine's action by increasing its rate of elimination. Quinidine may elevate serum digoxin and digitoxin concentrations by decreasing total-body clearance of digitoxin and by decreasing the clearance, volume of distribution, and affinity of tissue receptors for digoxin.

1.2.2. Procainamide (Class IA)

Multiple adverse noncardiac effects have been reported with procainamide administration and include skin rashes, myalgias, digital vasculitis, and Raynaud's phenomenon. Fever and agranulocytosis may be due to hypersensitivity reactions, and white blood cell and differential blood counts should be performed at regular intervals. GI side effects are less frequent than with quinidine, and adverse CNS side effects are less frequent than with lidocaine. Procainamide can cause giddiness, psychosis, hallucinations, and depression. Toxic concentrations of procainamide can diminish myocardial performance and promote hypotension. A variety of conduction disturbances or ventricular tachyarrhythmias can occur similar to those produced by quinidine, including prolonged QT syndrome and polymorphous ventricular tachycardia. *N*-Acetylprocainamide (NAPA) also can induce QT prolongation and torsades de pointes. In the absence of sinus node disease, procainamide does not adversely affect sinus node function. In patients with sinus dysfunction, procainamide tends to prolong corrected sinus node recovery time and can worsen symptoms in some patients who have the bradycardia-tachycardia syndrome. Procainamide does not increase the serum digoxin concentration. Arthralgia, fever, pleuropericarditis, hepatomegaly, and hemorrhagic pericardial effusion with tamponade have been described in a systemic lupus erythematosus (SLE)-like syndrome. The syndrome can occur more frequently and earlier in patients who are "slow acetylators" of procainamide and is influenced by genetic factors. The aromatic amino group on procainamide appears important for induction of SLE syndrome, since acetylating this amino group to form NAPA appears to block the SLE-inducing effect. Sixty to 70% of patients who receive procainamide on a chronic basis develop antinuclear antibodies, with clinical symptoms in 20–30%, but this is reversible when procainamide is stopped. When symptoms occur, SLE cell preparations are often positive. Positive serological tests are not necessarily a reason to discontinue drug therapy; however, the development of symptoms or a positive anti-DNA antibody is, except for patients whose life-threatening arrhythmia is controlled only by procainamide. Steroid administration in these patients may eliminate the symptoms. In contrast to naturally occurring SLE, the brain and kidney are spared, and there is no predilection for females.

1.2.3. Disopyramide (Class IA)

Three categories of adverse effects follow disopyramide administration. The most common relates to the drug's potent parasympatholytic properties and includes urinary hesitancy or retention, constipation, blurred vision, closed-angle glaucoma, and dry mouth. Symptoms may be minimized by concomitant administration of pyridostigmine. Second, disopyramide can produce ventricular tachyarrhythmias that are commonly associated with QT prolongation and torsades de pointes. Some patients can have "cross-sensitivity" to both quinidine and disopyramide and develop torsades de pointes while receiving either drug. When drug-induced torsades de pointes occurs, agents that prolong the QT interval should be used very cautiously or not at all. Finally, disopyramide can reduce contractility of the normal ventricle, but the depression of ventricular function is much more pronounced in patients with preexisting ventricular failure. Occasionally, cardiovascular collapse can result.

1.2.4. Lidocaine (Class IB)

The most commonly reported adverse effects of lidocaine are dose-related manifestations of CNS toxicity: dizziness, paresthesias, confusion, delirium, stupor, coma, and seizures. Occasional sinus node depression and His-Purkinje block have been reported. In patients with atrial tachyarrhythmias, ventricular rate acceleration has been noted. Rarely, lidocaine can cause malignant hyperthermia. Both lidocaine and procainamide can elevate defibrillation thresholds.

1.2.5. Mexiletine and Tocainide (Class IB)

These drugs, with a lidocaine-like spectrum of activity but active after oral administration, are both weak bases that demonstrate increased excretion with acidification of the urine. This phenomenon is unlikely to be clinically important, for the urine pH is normally acidic, and the amount of drug excreted in the urine unchanged is less than 10 and 30–50%, respectively. However, there remains the potential for patients with disorders of urinary acidification to accumulate either of these drugs to toxic levels. It does not appear that decreased renal function per se importantly influences the kinetics of either of these agents.

1.2.6. Flecainide (Class IC)

Proarrhythmic effects are one of the most important adverse effects of flecainide. Its marked slowing of conduction precludes its use in patients with second-degree AV block without a pacemaker and warrants cautious administration in patients with intraventricular conduction disorders. Aggravation of existing ventricular arrhythmias or onset of new ventricular arrhythmias can occur in 5–30% of patients, the increased percentage in patients with preexisting sustained ventricular tachycardia, cardiac decompensation, and higher doses of the drug. Failure of the flecainide-related arrhythmia to respond to therapy, including electrical cardioversiondefibrillation, may result in a mortality as high as 10% in patients who develop proarrhythmic events. Negative inotropic effects can cause or worsen heart failure. Patients with sinus node dysfunction may experience sinus arrest, and those with pacemakers may develop an increase in pacing threshold. In the CAST, patients treated with flecainide had 5.1% mortality or nonfatal cardiac arrest compared with 2.3% in the placebo group over 10 mo. Mortality was highest in those with non-Q-wave infarction, frequent premature ventricular complexes, and faster heart rates, raising the possibility of drug interaction with ischemia and electrical instability. Exercise can amplify the conduction slowing in the ventricle produced by flecainide and in some cases can precipitate a proarrhythmic response. Therefore, exercise testing has been recommended to screen for proarrhythmia. CNS complaints, including confusion and irritability, represent the most frequent noncardiac adverse effect.

1.2.7. Propafenone (Class IC)

Minor noncardiac effects occur in about 15% of patients, with dizziness, disturbances in taste, and blurred vision the most common and gastrointestinal side effects next. Exacerbation of bronchospastic lung disease can occur. Cardiovascular side effects occur in 10–15% of patients, including conduction abnormalities such as AV block, sinus node depression, and worsening of heart failure. Proarrhythmic responses, more often in patients with a history of sustained ventricular tachycardia and decreased ejection fractions, appear less commonly than with flecainide and may be in the range of 5%. The applicability of data from the CAST about flecainide to propafenone is not clear, but limiting propafenone's application in a manner similar to other IC drugs seems prudent at present until more information is available. Its beta-blocking actions may make it different, however.

1.2.8. Moricizine (Class IC)

Usually the drug is well tolerated. Noncardiac adverse effects primarily involve the nervous system and include tremor, mood changes, headache, vertigo, nystagmus, and dizziness. GI side effects include nausea, vomiting, and diarrhea. Worsening of congestive heart failure is uncommon but can happen. Proarrhythmic effects have been reported in about 3–15% of patients and appear to be more common in patients with severe ventricular arrhythmias. Advancing age increases the susceptibility to adverse effects.

1.2.9. β-Blockers (Class II)

Adverse cardiovascular effects from propranolol include unacceptable hypotension, bradycardia, and congestive heart failure. The bradycardia may be due to sinus

7. Cardiovascular Drugs

bradycardia or AV block. Sudden withdrawal of propranolol in patients with angina pectoris can precipitate or worsen angina and cardiac arrhythmias and cause an acute myocardial infarction, possibly owing to heightened sensitivity to β-agonists caused by previous β-blockade (upregulation). Heightened sensitivity may begin several days after cessation of propranolol therapy and may last 5 or 6 d. Other adverse effects of propranolol include worsening of asthma or chronic obstructive pulmonary disease, intermittent claudication, Raynaud's phenomenon, mental depression, increased risk of hypoglycemia among insulin-dependent diabetic patients, easy fatigability, disturbingly vivid dreams or insomnia, and impaired sexual function.

1.2.10. Amiodarone (6,7) (Class III)

Adverse effects are reported by about 75% of patients treated with amiodarone for 5 yr but compel stopping the drug in 18–37%. The most frequent side effects requiring drug discontinuation involve pulmonary and GI complaints. Most adverse effects are reversible with dose reduction or cessation of treatment. Adverse effects become more frequent when therapy is continued long term. Of the noncardiac adverse reactions, pulmonary toxicity is the most serious; in one study it occurred between 6 d and 60 mo of treatment in 33 of 573 patients, with three deaths. The mechanism is unclear but may relate to a hypersensitivity reaction and/or widespread phospholipidosis. Dyspnea, nonproductive cough, and fever are common symptoms, with rales, hypoxia, a positive gallium scan, reduced diffusion capacity, and radiographic evidence of pulmonary infiltrates noted. Amiodarone must be discontinued if such pulmonary inflammatory changes occur. Steroids can be tried, but no controlled studies have been done to support their use. A 10% mortality in patients with pulmonary inflammatory changes results, often in patients with unrecognized pulmonary involvement that is allowed to progress. Chest roentgenograms at 3-mo intervals for the first year and then twice a year for several years have been recommended. At maintenance doses less than 300 mg daily, pulmonary toxicity is uncommon. Advanced age, high drug maintenance dose, and reduced predrug diffusion capacity (DLco) are risk factors for developing pulmonary toxicity. An unchanged DLco volume may be a negative predictor of pulmonary toxicity. Although asymptomatic elevations of liver enzymes are found in most patients, the drug is not stopped unless values exceed two or three times normal in a patient with initially abnormal values. Cirrhosis occurs uncommonly but may be fatal. Neurological dysfunction, photosensitivity (perhaps minimized by sunscreens), bluish skin discoloration, corneal microdeposits (in almost 100% of adults receiving the drug more than 6 mo), gastroenterological disturbances, and hyperthyroidism (1–2%) or hypothyroidism (2–4%) can occur. Amiodarone appears to inhibit the peripheral conversion of T4 to T3 so that chemical changes result, characterized by a slight increase in T4, reverse T3 and thyroid-stimulating hormone (TSH), and a slight decrease in T3. Reverse T3 concentration has been used as an index of drug efficacy. During hypothyroidism, TSH increases greatly whereas T3 increases in hyperthyroidism. Cardiac side effects include symptomatic bradycardias in about 2%, aggravation of ventricular tachyarrhythmias (with occasional development of torsades de pointes) in 1–2%, possibly higher in women, and worsening of congestive heart failure in 2%. Possibly due to interactions with anesthetics, complications after open-heart surgery have been noted by some, but not all, investigators, including pulmonary dysfunction, hypotension, hepatic dysfunction, and low cardiac output. Important interactions with other drugs occur, and when given concomitantly with amiodarone, the dose of warfarin, digoxin, and other antiarrhythmic drugs should be reduced by one-third to one-half and the patient watched closely. Drugs with synergistic actions, such as beta-blockers or calcium channel blockers, must be given cautiously.

1.2.11. Bretylium (Class III)

This drug, which is used for refractory ventricular tachyarrhythmias, may present particular problems in patients with renal dysfunction because its kinetics appear complex and have not been defined for this group of patients. Therapy with this drug in patients with renal disease should be extremely conservative.

1.2.12. Sotalol (Class III)

Proarrhythmia is the most serious adverse effect *(8)*. Overall, new or worsened ventricular tachyarrhythmias occur in about 4%, and this response is due to torsades de pointes in about 2.5%. The incidence of torsades de pointes increases to 4% in patients with a history of sustained ventricular tachycardia and is dose related, reportedly only 1.6% at 320 mg/d but 4.4% at 480 mg/d. Other adverse effects commonly seen with other beta-blockers also apply to sotalol. Sotalol should be used with caution or not at all in combination with other drugs that prolong the QT interval. However, such combinations have been used successfully.

1.2.13. Adenosine

Transient side effects occur in almost 40% of patients with supraventricular tachycardia given adenosine and are most commonly flushing, dyspnea, and chest pressure. These symptoms are fleeting, generally less than 1 min, and are well tolerated. Premature ventricular complexes, transient sinus bradycardia, sinus arrest, and AV block are common when a supraventricular tachycardia abruptly terminates. Induction of atrial fibrillation can be problematic in patients with the Wolff-Parkinson-White syndrome or rapid AV conduction.

1.3. Drug Interactions (Selection; Amiodarone Preferred)

Drug interactions associated with amiodarone are pharmacodynamic and/or pharmacokinetic in nature. The pharmacodynamic interactions associated with amiodarone occur primarily with other antiarrhythmics and are a consequence of additive or synergistic electrophysiologic effects. As the pharmacologic effects of amiodarone are delayed by several days even with adequate loading doses, concomitant use of another antiarrhythmic is often necessary. Should this be the case, the dose of the secondary antiarrhythmic should, in general, be decreased by 30–50% after the first few days of initiating amiodarone therapy. Discontinuation of the second antiarrhythmic agent should be attempted as soon as the therapeutic effects of amiodarone are observed. Conversely, in patients requiring combination therapy, the dose of the second antiarrhythmic should, in general, be decreased by 50% until amiodarone eliminated from the body. Proarrhythmia, including torsade de pointes (Table 1) and monomorphic ventricular tachycardia can and has occurred when amiodarone was administered in combination with any num-

7. Cardiovascular Drugs 227

Table 1
List of Drugs That May Induce Torsades de Pointes

Antiarrhythmic drugs	
Class I	quinidine, disopyramide, procainamide
Class III	sotalol, amiodarone
Non-antiarrhythmic drugs	
Antibiotic	erythromycin, bactrim
Antifungal	ketoconazole, itraconazole
Antihistamine	terfenadine, astermizole
Psychiatric drugs	tricyclic antidepressants, phenothiazines, haloperidol
Cholinergic antagonists	cisapride, organophophates
Other drugs	cocaine, arsenic

ber of antiarrhythmic compounds including Class IA agents, mexilitine and propafenone. Caution should be exercised when amiodarone is administered with any drug with electrophysiologic effects.

Amiodarone inhibits the activity of two cytochrome P450 enzymes, CYP2D6 and CYP2C9. As a consequence, it has been reported to reduce the metabolism of certain drugs. Of these drugs, the most significant interactions are reported with anticoagulants, antiarrhythmics, phenytoin, and cyclosporin. The anticoagulant effects of warfarin and nicoumalone are significantly increased when amiodarone is added.

Concurrent use of amiodarone with cyclosporin need not be avoided but cyclosporin serum levels can be increased and must be monitored. Cyclosporin dosage reductions are usually required. Amiodarone also increases serum digoxin concentrations.

Flecainide concentrations increase by an average of 60% with concomitant amiodarone therapy. Although the exact mechanism of the interaction is unknown, it is postulated that the hepatic metabolism and/or renal clearance of flecainide may be decreased. Careful clinical observation of the patient as well as close monitoring of the electrocardiogram (EKG) and plasma flecainde concentrations is essential with adjustment of the flecainide dosing regimen performed as necessary to avoid enhanced toxicity or pharmacodynamic effects. An empiric reduction of the flecainide dose by 50% is suggested 2–3 d following initiation of amiodarone therapy.

Quinidine serum concentrations generally increase by about 33% in patients receiving concomitant amiodarone therapy. Although the mechanism is unclear, it appears that hepatic and/or renal clearance may be diminished and quinidine may also be displaced from tissue- and protein-binding sites. Prolongation of the QT interval is well documented with quinidine, and the addition of amiodarone may dramatically increase this effect, placing the patient at an increased risk for the development of torsade de pointes. Careful clinical observation of the patient as well as close monitoring of the EKG and serum quinidine concentrations is essential with adjustment of the quinidine dosing regimen performed as necessary to avoid enhanced toxicity or pharmacodynamic effects. An empiric reduction of the quinidine dose by 50% is suggested within 2 d following initiation of amiodarone therapy with consideration given to immediately discontinuing quinidine once amiodarone therapy is begun.

Procainamide and N-acetylprocainamide or NAPA (a pharmacologically active metabolite) concentrations increase by approximately 55 and 33%, respectively, during the first 7 d of concomitant amiodarone therapy. The precise pharmacokinetic mechanism of this interaction has not been elucidated, although a reduction in the renal clearance of both parent and metabolite, as well as a reduction in hepatic metabolism seem likely. Additive electrophysiologic activity occurs with combination therapy and prolonged QT and QRS intervals or acceleration of preexisting ventricular tachycardia may result. Careful clinical observation of the patient as well as close monitoring of the EKG and serum procainamide and NAPA concentrations is essential with adjustment of the procainamide dosing regimen performed as necessary to avoid enhanced toxicity or pharmacodynamic effects. In general, it is recommended to discontinue completely or reduce the procainamide daily dose by 25% during the first week of initiating amiodarone therapy.

Concomitant administration of β-blockers, or calcium-channel blockers with amiodarone may result in additive electrophysiologic effects including bradycardia, sinus arrest, and atrioventricular block. This is particularly likely in patients with preexisting sinus node dysfunction. In general these drugs should only be continued in patients at risk of significant bradycardia if a permanent artificial pacemaker is in place. In addition, amiodarone can decrease the clearance of drugs eliminated by hepatic metabolism. Severe cardiovascular reactions were observed when amiodarone was coadministered with metoprolol and propranolol.

Amiodarone increases serum levels of digoxin when given concomitantly, and an empiric 50% dosage reduction is advised upon initiation of amiodarone therapy. The degree to which digoxin serum concentrations will increase is not predictable and reassessment of the need for both drugs is prudent. As always, careful clinical observation of the patient, and close monitoring of the ECG and serum digoxin concentrations is essential to ensure efficacy and to avoid enhanced toxicity with adjustment of the digoxin dose performed as necessary. The mechanism of the increase in digoxin serum concentration is complex and not well understood, but is thought to result from an amiodarone-induced displacement of digoxin from tissue-binding sites, an increase in bioavailability, and/or a decrease in renal or nonrenal clearance. Furthermore, amiodarone may induce changes in thyroid function and alter sensitivity to cardiac glycosides, and thyroid function should be monitored closely in patients receiving both drugs simultaneously.

Concurrent administration of amiodarone with coumarin or indandione anticoagulants (warfarin) results in at least a doubling of prothrombin time (PT), significantly increasing the international normalized ratio (INR) in virtually all patients receiving this drug combination and can cause serious or potentially fatal hemorrhagic complications. This effect can occur as early as 4–6 d following the initial administration of the drugs in combination but can be delayed for weeks in some cases. Given the extremely long half-life of amiodarone, the interaction may persist for weeks or even months after discontinuance of amiodarone. A 50% reduction in the dosage of warfarin is recommended if amiodarone therapy is initiated with intensive clinical observation and frequent determination of PT and INR values to evaluate the extent of the interaction and guide further adjustments in therapy.

7. Cardiovascular Drugs

Concomitant administration of amiodarone and phenytoin may result in phenytoin toxicity, secondary to a two- or threefold increase in total, steady-state serum phenytoin concentrations likely due to a amiodarone-induced decrease in phenytoin metabolism. Close monitoring for symptoms of phenytoin toxicity including nystagmus, lethargy, and ataxia; and evaluation of serum phenytoin concentrations with appropriate dosage reduction as necessary, is essential in patients receiving these medications.

Amiodarone may enhance cardiovascular adverse effects such as hypotension and atropine-resistant bradycardia in patients receiving inhalation anesthetics, possibly due to a drug interaction.

Concomitant use of amiodarone with tricyclic antidepressants, phenothiazines, or any drug with the potential to prolong the QT interval may cause additive prolongation of the QT interval, and, rarely, torsades de pointes.

Although limited data exist, anecdotal reports have demonstrated a cholestyramine-induced reduction in amiodarone elimination half-life and subsequently serum concentrations. This interaction may be of benefit in temporally reducing the serum amiodarone, and presumably desethylamiodarone (DEA) concentrations prior to surgery in an attempt to limit the cardiac depressant effects of the drug in the immediate postsurgical period.

Two protease inhibitors, ritonavir and nelfinavir, are potent P450 enzyme inhibitors. Theoretically, they would both be expected to produce a large increase in amiodarone concentrations, due to the inhibition of its metabolism. However, there are no published reports of this interaction to date but it is suggested that there may be an increased risk of ventricular arrhythmias, so concurrent use should still be avoided.

Possible pharmacodynamic interactions can occur between levomethadyl and potentially arrhythmogenic agents such as amitriptyline, calcium channel blockers, class I antiarrhythmics, class III antiarrhythmics, monoamine oxidase inhibitors, citalopram, fluoxetine, nortriptyline, sertraline, and terfenadine, among others that prolong the QT interval. Levomethadyl is contraindicated in patients being treated with any of these agents.

Paroxetine impairs metabolism of the CYP2D6 (cytochrome P450 isoenzyme 2D6) pathway at therapeutic doses. Paroxetine should be used cautiously in patients receiving type 1C antiarrhythmics (such as propafenone, flecainide, or encainide) and quinidine. Competition for hepatic CYP2D6 (cytochrome P450 isoenzyme 2D6) by paroxetine may potentiate the toxicity of these antiarrhythmics.

Drug interaction between antifungal drugs and macrolide antibiotics, e.g., ketoconazole and erythromycin, which are metabolized by the same cytochrome P450 3A4 hepatic isoenzyme, can cause LQT-syndrome and torsades de pointes.

2. SYMPATHOPLEGICS

2.1. α-2-Agonists and Other Centrally Acting Drugs

2.1.1. Clonidine and Other Centrally Acting Drugs (9,10)

Current use of these drugs is relatively limited, particularly as first-line therapy, due to a relatively high incidence of side effects such as dry mouth, sedation, and/or sexual dysfunction. In addition, there is a risk of rebound hypertension following sudden discontinuation of therapy, particularly with the shorter-acting clonidine.

The centrally acting sympatholytic agents, like methyldopa, clonidine, guanabenz, and guanfacine, are a class of effective antihypertensive agents that do not have adverse effects on lipid and carbohydrate metabolism. They act by stimulating the α-2a adrenergic receptors in the CNS, leading to a reduction in central sympathetic outflow. In comparison, the α-2b receptors are responsible for causing vasoconstriction in vascular smooth muscle.

Clonidine and other α-2-receptor agonists (methyldopa, guanabenz) should be used with caution in asthmatics. Oral doses of these agents do not change baseline air flow in asthmatics, but they do increase bronchial reactivity to inhaled histamine. Prazosin (an α-1-receptor antagonist) may lead to a subjective increase in wheezing in patients with asthma, but there was no measurable change in pulmonary function.

The bioavailability of clonidine is 75–95%. A skin patch is available that provides stable serum concentrations for 1 wk. Clonidine is excreted unchanged by about 40–70% and protein binding is 20–30%. This does not change in renal disease. Half-life of clonidine is 7–18 h, and in end-stage renal disease 30–40 h. Dose adjustment according to creatinine clearance is required: (a) >50 mL/min: normal dose; (b) 20–50 mL/min: one-half normal dose, (c) <20 mL/min: one-third to one-half normal dose; (d) hemodialysis: no additional dose adjustment necessary. Dosing with the conventional formulation is twice a day. Patch application is once per week.

A variety of drugs, including hydralazine and methyldopa, have been identified as being causes of lupus.

Several drugs are known dopamine receptor antagonists, and raise serum prolactin by that mechanism. These include neuroleptic drugs, but also such antihypertensive drugs as methyldopa and reserpine, neither of which is commonly used now. Methyldopa inhibits dopamine synthesis, whereas reserpine inhibits dopamine storage.

2.2. α-Blockers

These drugs are effective in acutely lowering blood pressure, but their effects are offset by an accompanying increase in cardiac output, and side effects are frequent and bothersome. Their limited efficacy may reflect their blockade of presynaptic α-adrenergic receptors, which interferes with the feedback inhibition of norepinephrine release. Increased catecholamine release would then blunt the action of postsynaptic α-adrenergic receptor blockade. Their use has largely been limited to the treatment of patients with pheochromocytomas.

The selective α-1-blockers, such as prazosin, terazosin, and doxazosin (which is the longest acting), are the only class of antihypertensive agents that may have the combined effect of lowering low-density lipoprotein (LDL)-cholesterol, raising high-density lipoprotein (HDL)-cholesterol levels, and improving insulin sensitivity *(11–13)*. The α-blockers, however, are associated with relatively bothersome side effects, including dizziness (rarely inducing syncope), headache, and weakness. As an example, a prospective trial in which six different antihypertensive drugs were compared found the highest incidence of adverse drug effects with prazosin. These problems appear to be minimized with long-acting doxazosin, which was as effective and as well tolerated as other antihypertensive drugs in the Treatment of Mild Hypertension Study.

Dizziness is most prominent with the first dose or with an increase in dose, particularly in patients who are volume depleted (usually due to diuretic therapy) or who are taking other antihypertensive drugs. The incidence can be diminished by beginning with a low dose of a long-acting agent such as 1 mg of doxazosin.

An interim analysis of the Antihypertensive and Lipid-Lowering Treatment to Prevent Heart Attack Trial (ALLHAT) *(14,15)* found that doxazosin increases the risk of congestive heart failure compared to that associated with the administration of a diuretic, chlorthalidone. ALLHAT is a randomized prospective study of nearly 25,000 patients with hypertension and one additional risk factor for coronary heart disease designed to evaluate whether the incidence of a primary (e.g., fatal coronary heart disease and nonfatal myocardial infarction) or secondary outcome (e.g., all-cause mortality, stroke, and combined cardiovascular disease events [including congestive heart failure]) differed among those randomized to chlorthalidone vs one of three other antihypertensive drugs: amlodipine, lisinopril, or doxazosin. The doxazosin arm was prematurely terminated because of the finding of a markedly increased risk of congestive heart failure (8.13 vs 4.45% for chlorthalidone at 4 yr, $p < 0.001$). Both drugs had equivalent risks of death from coronary heart disease and nonfatal myocardial infarction.

Why doxazosin was associated with an increased incidence of congestive heart failure is unclear; however, it was not felt to be due to the 2- to 3-mmHg difference in mean systolic blood pressure observed between the two groups.

The net effect is that the α-1-blockers should not be used as first-line treatment of hypertension. One possible exception is older men who also have symptomatic benign prostatic hyperplasia in whom an α-1-blocker may lead to symptomatic improvement.

2.2.1. Indications and Usage

2.2.1.1. BENIGN PROSTATIC HYPERPLASIA (BPH)

Doxazosin mesylate is indicated for the treatment of both the urinary outflow obstruction and obstructive and irritative symptoms associated with BPH: obstructive symptoms (hesitation, intermittency, dribbling, weak urinary stream, incomplete emptying of the bladder) and irritative symptoms (nocturia, daytime frequency, urgency, burning). Doxazosin mesylate may be used in all BPH patients whether hypertensive or normotensive. In patients with hypertension and BPH, both conditions were effectively treated with doxazosin mesylate monotherapy. Doxazosin mesylate provides rapid improvement in symptoms and urinary flow rate in 66–71% of patients. Sustained improvements with doxazosin mesylate were seen in patients treated for up to 14 wk in double-blind studies and up to 2 yr in open-label studies.

2.2.1.2. HYPERTENSION

Doxazosin mesylate is also indicated for the treatment of hypertension. Doxazosin mesylate may be used alone or in combination with diuretics, β-adrenergic blocking agents, calcium channel blockers, or angiotensin-converting enzyme (ACE) inhibitors *(16–18)*.

2.2.2. Contraindications

Doxazosin mesylate is contraindicated in patients with a known sensitivity to quinazolines (e.g., prazosin, terazosin).

2.2.3. Warnings

2.2.3.1. SYNCOPE AND FIRST-DOSE EFFECT

Doxazosin, like other α-adrenergic blocking agents, can cause marked hypotension, especially in the upright position, with syncope and other postural symptoms such as dizziness. Marked orthostatic effects are most common with the first dose but can also occur when there is a dosage increase, or if therapy is interrupted for more than a few days. To decrease the likelihood of excessive hypotension and syncope, it is essential that treatment be initiated with the 1-mg dose. The 2-, 4-, and 8-mg tablets are not for initial therapy. Dosage should then be adjusted slowly with evaluations and increases in dose every 2 wk to the recommended dose. Additional antihypertensive agents should be added with caution. Patients being titrated with doxazosin should be cautioned to avoid situations where injury could result should syncope occur, during both the day and night.

In an early investigational study of the safety and tolerance of increasing daily doses of doxazosin in normotensives beginning at 1 mg/d, only two of six subjects could tolerate more than 2 mg/d without experiencing symptomatic postural hypotension. In another study of 24 healthy normotensive male subjects receiving initial doses of 2 mg/d of doxazosin, seven (29%) of the subjects experienced symptomatic postural hypotension between 0.5 and 6 h after the first dose necessitating termination of the study. In this study, two of the normotensive subjects experienced syncope. Subsequent trials in hypertensive patients always began doxazosin dosing at 1 mg/d resulting in a 4% incidence of postural side effects at 1 mg/d with no cases of syncope.

In multiple-dose clinical trials in hypertension involving over 1500 hypertensive patients with dose titration every 1–2 wk, syncope was reported in 0.7% of patients. None of these events occurred at the starting dose of 1 mg and 1.2% (8/664) occurred at 16 mg/d.

In placebo-controlled, clinical trials in BPH, 3 out of 665 patients (0.5%) taking doxazosin reported syncope. Two of the patients were taking 1 mg doxazosin, whereas one patient was taking 2 mg doxazosin when syncope occurred. In the open-label, long-term extension follow-up of approximately 450 BPH patients, there were three reports of syncope (0.7%). One patient was taking 2 mg, one patient was taking 8 mg, and one patient was taking 12 mg when syncope occurred. In a clinical pharmacology study, one subject receiving 2 mg experienced syncope.

If syncope occurs, the patient should be placed in a recumbent position and treated supportively as necessary.

2.2.3.2. PRIAPISM

Rarely (probably less frequently than once in every several thousand patients), α-1 antagonists such as doxazosin have been associated with priapism (painful penile erection, sustained for hours and unrelieved by sexual intercourse or masturbation). Because this condition can lead to permanent impotence if not promptly treated, patients must be advised about the seriousness of the condition.

2.2.4. Drug Interactions

Most (98%) of plasma doxazosin is protein bound. In vitro data in human plasma indicate that doxazosin mesylate has no effect on protein binding of digoxin, warfarin, phenytoin, or indomethacin. There is no available data on the effect of other highly plasma protein-bound drugs on doxazosin. Doxazosin mesylate has been administered without any adverse drug interaction to patients receiving thiazide diuretics, β-blocking agents, and nonsteroidal antiinflammatory drugs (NSAIDs). In a placebo-controlled clinical trial, concomitant administration of a single 1-mg dose of doxazosin mesylate and cimetidine (at the dose of 400 mg twice daily) resulted in a 10% increase in mean AUC of a single dose of doxazosin (p = 0.006), and a slight but not statistically significant increase in mean C_{max} and mean half-life of doxazosin. The clinical significance of this increase in doxazosin AUC is unknown. In clinical trials, doxazosin mesylate tablets have been administered to patients on a variety of concomitant medications; though no formal interaction studies have been conducted, no interactions were observed. Doxazosin mesylate tablets have been used with the following drugs or drug classes:

1. Analgesic/antiinflammatory (e.g., acetaminophen, aspirin, codeine and codeine combinations, ibuprofen, indomethacin).
2. Antibiotics (e.g., erythromycin, trimethoprim and sulfamethoxazole, amoxicillin).
3. Antihistamines (e.g., chlorpheniramine).
4. Cardiovascular agents (e.g., atenolol, hydrochlorothiazide, propranolol).
5. Corticosteroids.
6. Gastrointestinal agents (e.g., antacids).
7. Hypoglycemics and endocrine drugs.
8. Sedatives and tranquilizers (e.g., diazepam).
9. Cold and flu remedies.

In a study (n = 24) where terazosin and verapamil were administered concomitantly, terazosin's mean AUC_{0-24} increased 11% after the first verapamil dose and after 3 wk of verapamil treatment it increased by 24% with associated increases in C_{max} (25%) and C_{min} (32%) means. Terazosin mean T_{max} decreased from 1.3 h to 0.8 h after 3 wk of verapamil treatment. Statistically significant differences were not found in the verapamil level with and without terazosin. In a study (n = 6) where terazosin and captopril were administered concomitantly, plasma disposition of captopril was not influenced by concomitant administration of terazosin and terazosin maximum plasma concentrations increased linearly with dose at steady state after administration of terazosin plus captopril.

Combined use with other antihypertensive drugs (e.g., β-blockers, calcium channel blockers, diuretics, ACE inhibitors) can cause additive blood pressure lowering effects with severe symptomatic hypotension.

Prazosin has enhanced hypotensive effects with alcohol and antipsychotic drugs.

2.3. β-Blocking Agents (Table 2)

β-Adrenergic antagonists *(19,20)* are identified by their affinity for binding to β-adrenergic receptors, which is sufficiently high to antagonize the binding of endogenous agonists like norepinephrine and epinephrine at blood and tissue concentrations that do not cause other undesirable effects. Historically, these agents have been classified according to their:

- relative selectivity for the β1- or β2-adrenergic receptors,
- their ability to bind other adrenergic receptors, usually α receptors,

Table 2
Beta-Blockers: Overview

Class	Drug name	Starting dose	Maximal dose
nonselective	Propranolol	40 mg bid	120 mg bid
cardioselective	Metoprolol	25 mg bid	100 mg bid
cardioselective	Atenolol	25 mg qd	100 mg qd
nonselective	Nadolol	25 mg qd	240 mg qd
ISA[a]	Pindolol	5 mg bid	30 mg bid
α-Blocker	Labetalol	100 mg bid	600 mg bid
α-Blocker + antioxidative properties	Carvedilol	12.5 mg bid	25 mg bid
Cardioselective	Bisoprolol	2.5 mg qd	10 mg qd

[a]ISA = intrinsic activity

- and their interactions with other molecular targets at clinically relevant doses, for example the K^+ channel antagonist activity of the [+]enantiomer of sotalol *(21)*.
- Many β-adrenergic antagonists are characterized by their ability not only to prevent the binding of endogenous catecholamines but also to act as partial agonists (so-called intrinsic sympathomimetic activity [ISA]),
- and also by chemical characteristics of the compound itself (e.g., lipophilicity) that determine the tissue distribution, oral bioavailability, and clearance mechanisms of each compound.

β-Blockers are in widespread use for the treatment of a variety of cardiovascular diseases: these include stable and unstable angina pectoris, hypertension, acute myocardial infarction, congestive heart failure *(22)* due to systolic or diastolic dysfunction, and the therapy and prevention of some arrhythmias *(23)*. There are many β-blockers available and although they all have the same mechanism of action, i.e., blockade of the β-adrenoreceptor, there are various characteristics that differ among these agents; these characteristics primarily impact upon drug metabolism and the side-effect profile but not efficacy *(24)*.

β-Blockers are competitive inhibitors of catecholamines at beta-adrenoreceptor sites. They act to reduce the effect of the catecholamine agonist on sensitive tissues. Most β-blockers exist as pairs of optical isomers and are marketed as racemic mixtures. Almost all of the β-blocking activity is found in the negative levorotatory L-stereoisomer, which can be up to 100 times more active than the positive dextrorotatory D-isomer. The D-isomers of β-blocking drugs have no apparent clinical value except for D-sotalol, which has type III antiarrhythmic properties; that is, it blocks the potassium channel and prolongs membrane repolarization, thereby increasing the QT interval. D-Propranolol has type I (quinidine-like) membrane-stabilizing activity that is manifested only when very high doses of racemic propranolol are administered.

Although the β-blockers have similar pharmacotherapeutic effects, their pharmacokinetic properties differ significantly in ways that may influence their clinical usefulness and side effects. Among individual drugs, there are differences in completeness of GI absorption, amount of first-pass hepatic metabolism, lipid solubility, protein binding, extent of distribution in the body, penetration into the brain, concentration in the

7. Cardiovascular Drugs

heart, rate of hepatic biotransformation, pharmacologic activity of metabolites, and renal clearance of the drug and its metabolites.

On the basis of their pharmacokinetic properties, the β-blockers can be classified into two broad categories: those eliminated by hepatic metabolism, and those excreted unchanged by the kidney. Drugs in the first group (such as propranolol and metoprolol) are lipid soluble, almost completely absorbed by the small intestine, and largely metabolized by the liver. They enter the CNS in high concentrations, possibly resulting in an increased incidence of CNS side effects. They tend to have highly variable bioavailability and relatively short plasma half-lives. In contrast, drugs in the second category (such as atenolol and sotalol) are more water soluble, incompletely absorbed through the gut, eliminated unchanged by the kidney, and do not as readily enter the CNS. They show less variance in bioavailability and have longer plasma half-lives. Ultra-short-acting β-blockers (such as esmolol) with a half-life of no more than 10 min offer advantages in some patients. They can be given for the treatment of supraventricular arrhythmias and, as a test dose, to a patient who has a questionable history of congestive heart failure. The short half-life of esmolol is due to its rapid metabolism by blood tissue and hepatic esterases.

β-Blockers are generally well tolerated but have a well-recognized set of potential side effects that can limit their use. Summarized briefly, the following are the major concerns with β-blocker therapy *(25,26)*:

1. Decreases in heart rate, contractility, and AV node conduction can lead to severe sinus bradycardia, sinus arrest, heart failure, and AV block.
2. Bronchoconstriction, due to β2-receptor blockade, can be induced by nonselective agents and high doses of cardioselective agents. Nonselective agents are generally contraindicated in patients with asthma and most patients with chronic obstructive lung disease; cardioselective agents or those with ISA must be used very cautiously in these settings.
3. Nonselective β-blockers can cause worsening of symptoms of severe peripheral vascular disease or Raynaud's phenomenon but usually not milder disease with mild to moderate intermittent claudication. Cardioselective β-blockers are probably preferable in such patients.
4. Fatigue may be due to the reduction in cardiac output or to direct effects on the CNS. Other central side effects that can occur include depression, nightmares, insomnia, and hallucinations. Impotence can also be a problem.
5. Nonselective β-blockers (including labetalol) can mask the early, sympathetically mediated symptoms of hypoglycemia in patients with insulin-dependent diabetes mellitus; they can also delay the rate of recovery of the blood glucose concentration.
6. Perturbations of lipoprotein metabolism accompany the use of β-blockers. Nonselective agents cause greater rises in triglycerides and falls in cardioprotective high-density lipoprotein-cholesterol levels, whereas ISA agents cause less or no effect and some agents such as celiprolol may raise HDL cholesterol levels. Patients with renal failure may take β-blockers without additional hazard, although modest falls in renal blood flow and glomerular filtration rate have been measured, presumably from renal vasoconstriction. Caution is advised in the use of β-blockers in patients suspected of harboring a pheochromocytoma, because unopposed α-adrenergic agonist action may precipitate a serious hypertensive crisis if this disease is present. Morover, caution is advised in the use of β-blockers in patients suspected of harboring Prinzmetal angina

Table 3
Major Drug Interactions with β-Blockers

Drug	Possible Effects	Precautions
Absorption		
Aluminium	Decreased β-blocker adsorption and therapeutic effect	Avoid β-blocker-aluminium hydroxide combination
cholestyramine colestipol	Decreased β-blocker adsorption	Avoid β-blocker-cholestyramine-combination
Metabolism		
Cimetidine	Prolongs half-life of propranolol	Combination should be used with caution
Aminophylline	Mutual inhibition	Observe patient's response
Lidocaine	Propranolol pretreatment increases Lidocaine levels with potential toxicity	Combination should be used with caution; use lower doses of lidocaine
Rifampin	Increased metabolism of β-blockers	Observe patient's response
Smoking	Increased metabolism of β-blockers	Observe patient's response
Pharmacodynamic Interactions		
AV-node		
Calcium channel Inhibitors (verapamil, diltiazem)	Potentiation of bradycardia, myodepression and hypotension	Avoid use, although few patients show ill effects
Amiodarone	May induce cardiac arrest	Combination should be used with caution
Digitalis glycosides	Potentiation of bradycardia	Observe patient's response; Interactions may benefit Angina patients with Abnormal ventricular Function

(continued)

and Mb. Raynaud, because use of β-adrenergic anatagonists in such patients may cause or enhance vasospasm. The use of β-blockers during pregnancy has been clouded by scattered case reports of various fetal problems. Moreover, prospective studies have found that the use of β-blockers during pregnancy may lead to fetal growth retardation.

When a β-blocker is discontinued, angina pectoris and myocardial infarction may occur. Therefore, patients with ischemic heart disease must be warned not to rapidly discontinue treatment, since this can lead to a withdrawal syndrome characterized by accelerated angina, myocardial infarction, and even death. These findings, which can occur even in patients without previously known coronary disease, probably result from upregulation of the beta receptors following chronic β-blockade.

2.3.1. *Major Drug Interactions with β-Blockers (27)*
(see also *Table 3*)

2.3.1.1. Decreased Absorption

Propranolol absorption is decreased by antacids and by cholestyramine and probably colestipol *(28)*. Taking propranolol 1 h before these medications will eliminate this interaction.

7. Cardiovascular Drugs

Table 3 (*continued*)

Drug	Possible Effects	Precautions
Conduction/Ventricular Function		
Phenytoin	Additive cardiac depressant effects	Administer IV phenytoin with great caution
Quinidine	Additive cardiac depressant effects	Observe patient's response; few patient show ill effects
Tricyclic antidepressants	Inhibits negative inotropic and chronotropic effects of β-blockers	Observe patient's response
Hypertension/Hypotension		
Clonidine	Hypertension during clonidine withdrawal	Monitor for hypertensive response; withdraw β-blocker before withdrawing clonidine
Levodopa	Antagonism of levodopa's hypotensive and positive inotropic effects	Monitor for altered response; interaction may have favorable results
Methyldopa	Hypertension during stress	Monitor for hypertensive episodes
Phenyllpropranolamine	Severe hypertensive reaction	β-Blocker may be safer doses of phenothiazines
Indomethacin	Inhibition of antihypertensive response to β-blockade	Observe patient's response
Reserpine	Excessive sympathetic blockade	Observe patient's response
Isoproterenol	Mutual inhibition	Avoid concurrent use or Choose cardiac-selective β-blocker
Phenothazines	Additive hypotensive effects	Monitor for altered response, especially with high
Halofenate	Reduced β-blocking activity; induction of propranolol withdrawal rebound	Observe for impaired response to β-blockade
Vasoconsriction		
Ergot alkaloids	Excessive vasoconstriction	Observe patient's response; Few patients show ill effects
Glucose Metabolism		
Glucagon	Inhibition of hyperglycemic effect	Monitor for reduced response
Antidiabetic agents	Enhanced hypoglycemia; hypertension	Monitor for altered diabetic response
Others		
MAO inhibitors	Uncertain, theoretical	Manufacturer of propanolol considers concurrent use contraindicated
Tubocurarine	Enhanced neuromuscular blockade	Observe response in surgical patients', especially after high doses of propranolol

2.3.1.2. Altered Metabolism (29–40)

Cimetidine can inhibit hepatic cytochrome P450IID6. This will decrease both the first-pass and systemic elimination of propranolol, causing plasma concentrations to increase as much as fourfold. Thus, cautious dosing of propranolol is required in this setting. Other drugs are also potent inhibitors of this cytochrome isoenzyme and decrease the metabolism of propranolol, including quinidine, propafenone, chlorpromazine, flecainide, fluoxetine (and its metabolite norfluoxetine), paroxetine, fluvoxamine, and tricyclic antidepressants. On the other hand, propranolol can inhibit the hepatic metabolism and raise the plasma levels of certain drugs by decreasing hepatic blood flow rather than enzyme activity. Among the drugs that can be affected are flecainide, lidocaine, nifedipine, and nisoldipine. Other β-blockers will probably have a similar effect.

3. DIRECT-ACTING VASODIALATATORS

3.1. NO-Drugs

3.1.1. Nitroprusside

Nitroprusside *(41,42)* is an arteriolar and venous dilator, given as an intravenous infusion. Initial dose is 0.25–0.5 µg/kg per min; maximum dose is 8–10 µg/kg per min. Nitroprusside acts within seconds and has a duration of action of only 2–5 min. Its effects are evident within 60–90 s after initiation of the infusion and should an adverse effect such as symptomatic hypotension occur, the vasodilating properties usually abate within 20–30 min after discontinuation. Thus, hypotension can be easily reversed by temporarily discontinuing the infusion. However, the potential for cyanide toxicity limits its prolonged use *(43,44)*.

Nitroprusside is metabolized to cyanide *(45)*, which rarely causes toxicity because it is converted to thiocyanate by the enzyme rhodonase, which is a thiosulfate-cyanide transferase. The thiosulfate is substrate limiting. If it is depleted, cyanide accumulates sufficiently to cause toxicity. Conversely, such an event can be treated by administering thiosulfate. Once thiocyanate is formed, it is excreted by the kidney. If it accumulates, it causes adverse CNS effects. The half-life of thiocyanate is 2–7 d, and in end-stage renal disease 9 d. Thiocyanate can accumulate, and its levels should be monitored in patients with decreased renal function.

Nitroprusside is a powerful vasodilator with potent afterload-reducing properties. It is the agent most frequently used early in the treatment of acute heart failure, particularly when a rapid and substantial reduction in systemic vascular resistance is necessary. Common clinical conditions would include complications of myocardial infarction such as acute mitral regurgitation secondary to papillary muscle dysfunction or rupture, ventricular septal defect, and acute aortic regurgitation. Nitroprusside relaxes arterial and venous smooth muscle via the production of nitric oxide and nitrosothiols leading to an increase in cyclic guanosine monophosphate and smooth muscle relaxation. Similar to nitroglycerin, nitroprusside causes preload reduction by diminishing heightened venous tone and increasing venous capacitance with a concomitant shift in central blood volume to the periphery. This causes a reduction in right ventricular pressure and volume. Unique to nitroprusside is its rapid and powerful effect on afterload. This agent reduces the major components of aortic impedance (mean and hydraulic vascular load) resulting in an improved and often dramatic increase in forward stroke volume and cardiac output with reductions in left ventricular filling pressure, volume, and valvular regurgitation. In most patients with heart failure, judicious titration of nitroprusside can result in a fall in aortic impedance, increased cardiac output, and reduced ventricular filling pressures without the undesirable effects of a decrease in systemic blood pressure or rise in heart rate. The combined balanced vasodilator effect of nitroprusside can therefore rapidly improve the hemodynamic abnormalities associated with acute heart failure when preload and afterload reduction is desired. Generally, by improving ventricular wall stress and reducing myocardial oxygen consumption, nitroprusside will have a favorable effect on myocardial energetics. Nitroprusside may also improve coronary blood flow and myocardial perfusion by directly reducing coronary vascular resistance and by increasing coronary perfusion pressure. The latter will occur as long as there is a reduction in ventricular diastolic pressure that is greater than aortic coronary diastolic pressure. In patients with occlusive coronary artery disease, care must be taken to avoid excessive reductions in systemic pressure or elevations in heart rate that would reduce coronary perfusion and increase myocardial oxygen demand. Unlike nitroglycerin, nitroprusside may cause "coronary steal" whereby arteriolar dilatation in nonischemic zones diverts coronary flow away from areas of ischemia. The frequency with which this occurs in heart failure is not well documented.

Continuous monitoring of central hemodynamics with an indwelling flow-directed thermodilution pulmonary artery catheter is mandatory to safely and effectively target the optimal dose. In acute heart failure, an arterial catheter for continuous systemic blood pressure recording and monitoring and frequent blood gas determinations is also recommended. It should be recognized, however, that during nitroprusside infusion, the pressure measured in a peripheral artery (usually radial artery) may not reflect a reduction in central aortic pressure because of nitroprusside-induced changes in the amplitude and timing of reflected waves within the central aorta. One must remain cognizant of this when the clinical findings are consistent with systemic hypoperfusion despite a seemingly acceptable peripheral arterial pressure. Nitroprusside can be rapidly titrated to achieve the desired clinical and hemodynamic end points including a reduction in pulmonary capillary wedge pressure to 18–20 mmHg, a decrease in systemic vascular resistance to 1000 to 1200 dynes/s/cm5, reduction in valvular regurgitation, and an improvement in stroke volume, cardiac output, and systemic perfusion while avoiding significant hypotension and tachycardia. Although the target blood pressure is variable depending on the individual patient, a systolic blood pressure of 80 mmHg or greater is usually acceptable. A higher systolic blood pressure may be required in the elderly or in patients with a recent history of hypertension or cerebrovascular disease. The target pulmonary capillary-wedge pressure is usually higher in acute heart failure than in patients with decompensated chronic heart failure. In the latter condition, the stroke volume of the dilated ventricle is not preload-dependent, and therefore relatively normal left ventricular filling pressures can be targeted. In acute heart failure, particularly when myocardial ischemia is present, attention to Starling mechanisms with respect to preload and augmentation of stroke volume remains important. While titrating nitroprusside to achieve hemodynamic goals, doses are rarely greater than 4 µg/kg/min to maintain adequate vasodilation in the acute heart failure setting, and dosing this high should generally be avoided for prolonged periods (more than 72 h) due to the risk of thiocyanate and cyanide toxicity. The most common serious adverse effect of nitroprusside administration in acute heart failure is systemic hypotension. One should be particularly cautious when initiating nitroprusside in a patient with ischemia or infarction and a systolic arterial pressure of less than 100 mmHg. An increase in heart rate during the infusion is an ominous finding and usually presages hypotension. This typically occurs when stroke volume has not increased appropriately, often because of ongoing or worsening ischemia, valvular regurgitation, and inadequate cardiac reserve. A reduction or cessation of the nitroprusside infusion is usually warranted. Alternatively, the addition of a positive inotropic agent such as dobutamine is often advantageous and may allow for the continuation of nitroprusside. Such a combination is commonly used while stabilizing particularly severe, low-output heart failure until more definitive therapy can be instituted. When systemic hypotension and poor peripheral perfusion is present at the outset, nitroprusside should generally be avoided as initial treatment.

As noted above, thiocyanate toxicity is a potentially serious side effect of prolonged nitroprusside infusion and is manifest clinically by nausea, disorientation, psychosis, muscle spasm, and hyperreflexia when plasma thiocyanate concentrations exceed 6 mg/dL. This is uncommon in the management of acute heart failure where nitroprusside therapy is usually a temporary means of support while awaiting definitive therapy. Cyanide toxicity is extremely rare in heart failure management and only occurs during prolonged, high-dose infusions, usually in the setting of significant hepatic dysfunction. The concept of intravenous vasodilator therapy in acute heart failure is based on correction of hemodynamic derangement and stabilization of the patient while a therapeutic plan is devised. The necessity for prolonged treatment (>72 h) often portends a poor prognosis, particularly in the absence of a reversible underlying disorder.

3.1.2. Hydralazine

Hydralazine, like diazoxide, is a direct arteriolar vasodilator with little or no effect on the venous circulation. Thus, the same precautions apply in patients with underlying coronary disease or a dissecting aortic aneurysm, and a beta-blocker should be given concurrently to minimize reflex sympathetic stimulation. The hypotensive response to hydralazine is less predictable than that seen with other parenteral agents and its current use is primarily limited to pregnant women.

Hydralazine is given as an intravenous bolus. The initial dose is 5–10 mg, with the maximum dose being 20 mg. The fall in blood pressure begins within 10–30 min and lasts 2–4 h.

3.2. Potassium-Channel Openers

3.2.1. Minoxidil

In the case of refractory hypertension, powerful additional hypertension agents such as minoxidil may be necessary. Minoxidil represents a third-line antihypertensive drug and should not be used as a first- or second-line drug (due to adverse effects and reflex stimulation of norepinephrine and angiotensin II release). Diuretic therapy is usually needed with diazoxide or minoxidil therapy. Minoxidil may produce pericardial reactions by non-lupus mechanisms.

Bioavailability is 95% and less than 5% from cutaneous application. About 12–20% of the drug is excreted unchanged. Minoxidil sulfate is the active moiety. The glucuronide metabolite appears to have some activity either alone or possibly as a reservoir for endogenous cleavage back to the parent compound. The drug has a half-life of 3–4 h and in case of impaired renal function 9 h. Hemodialysis decreases serum concentration by 24–43%. Minoxidil is also removed by peritoneal dialysis. Accumulation

7. Cardiovascular Drugs

of glucuronide and parent drug occurs, and pharmacologic effect may be enhanced in patients with decreased renal function. Patients with end-stage renal disease should receive halve of the normal doses. In patients being dialyzed, the dose should be administered after dialysis.

In general, lowering the blood pressure with antihypertensive agents, weight loss, or dietary sodium restriction decreases cardiac mass in patients with left ventricular hypertrophy. Regression is largely absent with direct vasodilators (such as hydralazine or minoxidil) despite adequate blood pressure control. The ineffectiveness of direct vasodilators probably reflects the reflex stimulation of norepinephrine and angiotensin II release induced by the these drugs, since these hormones may directly promote the development of left ventricular hypertrophy.

3.2.2. Diazoxide

Diazoxide, in comparison to nitroprusside and nitroglycerin, is an arteriolar vasodilator that has little effect on the venous circulation. Diazoxide is also longer acting and, in the currently recommended doses, requires less monitoring than nitroprusside, since the peak effect is seen within 15 min and lasts for 4–24 h. Diazoxide can be administered as either an intravenous bolus or infusion. A beta-blocker such as propranolol or labetalol is usually given concurrently to block reflex activation of the sympathetic nervous system. This protection, however, is not complete, and it is recommended that diazoxide not be used in patients with angina pectoris, myocardial infarction, pulmonary edema, or a dissecting aortic aneurysm. Diazoxide can also cause marked fluid retention and a diuretic may need to be added if edema or otherwise unexplained weight gain is noted. For these reasons, diazoxide is now rarely used.

Diazoxide has a bioavailability of 85–90% and is excreted unclanged by about 20%. More than 90% are protein bound, which decreases in uremia or hypoalbuminemia. Plasma half-life is 15–30 h and 20–53 h in end-stage renal disease. Decreased binding in uremia or the nephrotic syndrome results in increased free drug in the circulation and increased response. Dose adjustment according to creatinine clearance: (a) >50 mL/min: normal dose; (b) 20–50 mL/min: two-thirds of normal dose; (c) <20 mL/min: one-half to two-thirds normal dose. Hemodialysis requires no additional dose adjustment.

Adverse effects include marked edema (which may require high doses of loop diuretics) and hirsutism.

Medical therapy for insulinoma should be considered in the patient whose insulinoma was missed during pancreatic exploration, who is not a candidate for or refuses surgery, or who has metastatic insulinoma. The therapeutic choices to prevent symptomatic hypoglycemia include diazoxide, verapamil, phenytoin, and the somatostatin analog octreotide. Diazoxide (which must be given in divided doses of up to 1200 mg/d) is the most effective drug for controlling hypoglycemia. However, its use is often limited by marked edema (which may require high doses of loop diuretics) and hirsutism.

3.3. Calcium Channel Blockers

Calcium channel blockers are widely used in the treatment of hypertension, angina pectoris, cardiac arrhythmias, and other disorders and the longer-acting preparations have been prescribed with increasing frequency since 1989.

Calcium channel blockers have become the most popular class of agents used in the treatment of hypertension.

3.3.1. Types of Calcium Channel Blockers

The calcium channel blockers currently available are divided into two major categories based upon their predominant physiologic effects: the dihydropyridines, which preferentially block the L-type calcium channels; and verapamil and diltiazem. The L-type calcium channels are responsible for myocardial contractility and vascular smooth muscle contractility; they also affect conducting and pacemaker cells.

3.3.1.1. DIHYDROPYRIDINES

The dihydropyridines are potent vasodilators that have little or no negative effect upon cardiac contractility or conduction. They can be further divided into three categories based upon half-life and effect on contractility:

1. Short-acting liquid nifedipine.
2. Longer-acting formulations with little cardiac depressant activity: felodipine, isradipine, nicardipine, nifedipine GITS and CC, and nisoldipine.
3. Long-acting agents with no cardiac depressant activity: amlodipine, lacidipine.

3.3.1.2. VERAPAMIL AND DILTIAZEM

Verapamil and, to a lesser extent, diltiazem are less potent vasodilators but have negative effects upon cardiac conduction and contractility.

3.3.2. Side Effects

The side effects that may be seen with the calcium channel blockers vary with the agent that is used. The potent vasodilators can, in 10–20% of patients, lead to one or more of the following: headache, dizziness or lightheadedness, flushing, and peripheral edema. The peripheral edema, which is infrequent with verapamil, is related to redistribution of fluid from the vascular space into the interstitium, possibly induced by vasodilation, which allows more of the systemic pressure to be transmitted to the capillary circulation. In one study of 12 healthy subjects, for example, a single dose of nifedipine increased the foot volume despite also increasing sodium excretion. Thus, treatment of this form of edema with a diuretic will not relieve the edema. On the other hand, edema is much less common when a dihydropyridine is given with an ACE inhibitor. This effect is probably related to venodilation by the ACE inhibitor, which helps remove the fluid sequestered in the capillary bed by the arteriolar dilation from the calcium channel blocker. This form of combination therapy is likely to become much more common since the Food and Drug Administration (FDA) has approved fixed- (low) dose combination preparations of these drugs. The major adverse effect with verapamil is constipation, which can occur in over 25% of patients.

Along with freedom from most of the side effects seen with other classes of antihypertensive agents, calcium antagonists may be unique in not having their antihypertensive efficacy blunted by NSAIDs.

3.3.2.1. EFFECTS ON CARDIAC FUNCTION

Verapamil and, to a lesser degree, diltiazem can diminish cardiac contractility and slow cardiac conduction. As a result, these drugs are relatively contraindicated in

7. Cardiovascular Drugs

patients who are taking beta-blockers or who have severe left ventricular systolic dysfunction, sick sinus syndrome, and second- or third-degree atrioventricular block.

The dihydropyridines have less cardiac depressant activity in vivo for two reasons: (a) the doses employed are limited by the peripheral vasodilation; as a result, plasma levels sufficient to impair contractility and atrioventricular conduction are not achieved; and (b) acute vasodilation leads to a reflex increase in sympathetic activity that can counteract the direct effect of calcium channel blockade.

3.3.3. Specific Drug Interactions (46–48)

3.3.3.1. ISRAPIDINE

Drugs that affect cytochrome CYP (P450) 3A can alter the metabolism of isradipine. Anticonvulsants (such as phenytoin, phenobarbital, and carbamazepine) induce both the intestinal and hepatic form of this isoenzyme. Induction increases the first-pass metabolism of isradipine and decreases its bioavailability. On the other hand, ketoconazole, erythromycin, clarithromycin, cimetidine, grapefruit juice, and other calcium channel blockers can inhibit cytochrome P450 3A. The calcium channel blocker effect is greatest with verapamil, which can slow metabolism of substrates for this isoenzyme by up to 50%. Diltiazem is less potent and other dihydropyridines (such as nicardipine and nisoldipine) appear to have negligible effects. Cytochrome inhibition diminishes first-pass metabolism and increases (as much as twofold) the bioavailability of isradipine. Elimination of absorbed isradipine is also reduced, and the combined effect cause dramatic increases in the plasma level and activity of this drug. Cautious dosing is required in this setting. In addition to being a substrate for CYP3A, isradipine is also capable of inhibiting this isoenzyme. As a result, its coadministration with other drugs that are metabolized by this isoenzyme (such as terfenadine and quinidine) can lead to a clinically important interaction and careful monitoring is important.

3.3.3.2. FELODIPINE (49–51)

Anticonvulsants (phenytoin, phenobarbital, and carbamazepine) can induce intestinal and hepatic cytochrome CYP (P450) 3A. Induction of this enzyme increases the first-pass effect of felodipine and decreases its bioavailability. As a result, higher doses may be required. In comparison, inhibitors of this isoenzyme lead to an increase in plasma drug levels. The effect of grapefruit juice appears to be mediated by selective downregulation of CYP3A in the intestine. The clinical significance of the change in felodipine metabolism with more usual amounts of grapefruit juice ingestion is uncertain. Inhibition of cytochrome CYP3A diminishes the first-pass metabolism of felodipine and increases (as much as twofold) its bioavailability. The elimination of absorbed felodipine is also diminished. The net effect may be a dramatic elevation in the plasma felodipine concentration and in drug activity. Cautious dosing is required in this setting.

3.3.3.3. NICARDIPINE, NIFEDIPINE, NIMODIPINE (52–55)

Drugs that affect cytochrome CYP (P450) 3A can alter the metabolism of nicardipine. Elimination of absorbed nicardipine is also reduced, and the combined effect cause dramatic increases in the plasma level and activity of this drug. Cautious dosing is required.

3.3.3.4. NISOLDIPINE (56,57)

Drugs that affect cytochrome CYP (P450) 3A can alter the metabolism of nisoldipine. Propranolol also slows nisoldipine elimination. It is unlikely that this effect occurs by enzyme inhibition, since these two drugs are metabolized by different cytochrome P450 isoenzymes. Propranolol and presumably other β-blockers may act by decreasing hepatic blood flow.

3.3.3.5. VERAPAMIL (58–60)

Drugs that affect cytochrome CYP (P450) 3A can alter the metabolism of verapamil. It is of interest that verapamil itself has the greatest inhibitory effect of the calcium channel blockers, decreasing the metabolism for substrates of cytochrome CYP3A by up to 50%. As a result, its coadministration with other drugs that are metabolized by this isoenzyme can lead to a clinically important interaction and careful monitoring is important. Examples of this interaction with verapamil include cyclosporine, digoxin, digitoxin, quinidine, terfenadine, and most of the dihydropyridines (such as felodipine, nifedipine, nicardipine, nisoldipine, and isradipine). Moreover, verapamil can displace digitalis from tissue-binding sites and may enhance free digitalis that could cause toxicity.

3.3.3.5.1. Pharmacodynamic Interactions. These include exerting negative inotropic effects and slowing conduction through the atrioventricular node (negative dromotropic action). A number of other cardiovascular drugs may have pharmacodynamic interactions with verapamil (β-blockers have negative inotropic and negative dromotropic effects that may be additive to those of verapamil. Digoxin, which slows AV nodal conduction via its vagotonic activity, can have an additive pharmacologic effect on AV nodal conduction with verapamil, independent of the metabolic interaction described above. Adenosine is a rapidly acting agent that slows conduction through the AV node. Thus, the dose of adenosine necessary to produce AV nodal blockade is lower for patients being treated with verapamil.)

3.4. ACE Inhibitors and AT-1 Antagonists

3.4.1. ACE Inhibitors (Fig. 2)

ACE inhibitors were synthesized as specific inhibitors of the converting enzyme that breaks the peptidyldipeptide bond in angiotensin I, preventing the enzyme from attaching to and splitting the angiotensin I structure. Because angiotensin II cannot be formed and angiotensin I is inactive, the ACE inhibitor paralyzes the renin-angiotensin system, thereby removing the effects of endogenous angiotensin II as both a vasoconstrictor and a stimulant to aldosterone synthesis (61,62).

Interestingly, the plasma angiotensin II levels actually return to previous readings with chronic use of ACE inhibitors whereas the blood pressure remains lowered. This suggests that the antihypertensive effect may involve other mechanisms. Since the same enzyme that converts angiotensin I to angiotensin II is also responsible for inactivation of the vasodepressor hormone bradykinin, by inhibiting the breakdown of bradykinin, ACE inhibitors increase the concentration of a vasodepressor hormone while they decrease the concentration of a vasoconstrictor hormone. The increased plasma kinin

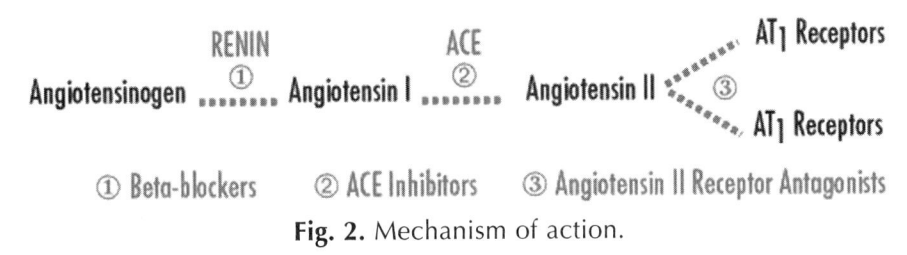

7. Cardiovascular Drugs   245

Angiotensinogen ···RENIN···► Angiotensin I ···ACE···► Angiotensin II ⟨ AT₁ Receptors / AT₁ Receptors

① Beta-blockers   ② ACE Inhibitors   ③ Angiotensin II Receptor Antagonists

Fig. 2. Mechanism of action.

levels may contribute to the improvement in insulin sensitivity observed with ACE inhibitors, but they are also responsible for the most common and bothersome side effect of their use, a dry, hacking cough. ACE inhibitors may also vasodilate by increasing levels of vasodilatory prostaglandins and decreasing levels of vasoconstricting endothelins. Their effects may also involve inhibition of the renin-angiotensin system within the heart and other tissues.

Regardless of the manner in which they work, ACE inhibitors lower blood pressure mainly by reducing peripheral resistance with little, if any, effect on heart rate, cardiac output, or body fluid volumes. After a year of treatment with an ACE inhibitor, the structure and function of subcutaneous resistance vessels were improved whereas no changes were observed with a β-blocker. The lack of a rise in heart rate despite a significant fall in blood pressure has been explained by a blunting of the adrenergic nervous system. ACE inhibitors are widely used in the treatment of hypertension and congestive heart failure *(63,64)*. In addition to efficacy, these agents have the additional advantage of being particularly well tolerated, since they produce few idiosyncratic side effects and do not have the adverse effects on lipid and glucose metabolism seen with diuretics or β-blockers. Although captopril therapy was initially associated with a variety of presumed sulfhydryl group-related complications such as rash, neutropenia, taste abnormalities, and even the nephrotic syndrome, these problems have become uncommon since the maximum dose was reduced to 100 to 150 mg/d. It has also been proposed that ACE inhibitors are associated with an improved quality of life compared to some other antihypertensive drugs, such as propranolol and methyldopa. However, later studies have not confirmed a significant advantage of any antihypertensive drug in terms of quality of life.

In summary, these drugs are widely used for all degrees and forms of hypertension. Their use is likely to increase further because of their particular ability to decrease intrarenal hypertension *(65)*, to unload the hemodynamic burden of congestive heart failure, and to protect against ventricular dysfunction after myocardial infarction.

3.4.1.1. Side Effects (66–71)

Most patients who take an ACE inhibitor experience no side effects nor the biochemical changes often seen with other drugs that may be of even more concern even though they are not so obvious; neither rises in lipids, glucose, or uric acid nor falls in potassium levels are seen, and insulin sensitivity may improve.

ACE inhibitors may cause both specific and nonspecific adverse effects. Among the specific ones are rash, loss of taste, glomerulopathy manifested by proteinuria, and leukopenia. In addition, these drugs may cause a hypersensitivity reaction with angioneurotic edema194. A cough, although often persistent, is infrequently associated with pulmonary dysfunction.

The side effects that do occur are primarily related directly or indirectly to reduced angiotensin II formation. These include hypotension, acute renal failure, hyperkalemia, and problems during pregnancy. There are other complications, cough, angioneurotic edema, and anaphylactoid reactions, that are thought to be related to increased kinins since ACE is also a kininase. This is an important distinction clinically because the side effects related to reduced angiotensin II, but not those related to kinins, are also seen with the angiotensin II receptor antagonists.

3.4.1.1.1. Hypotension. Weakness, dizziness, or syncope may result from an excessive reduction in blood pressure. First-dose hypotension, which can be marked in hypovolemic patients with high baseline renin levels, can be minimized by not beginning therapy if the patient is volume depleted and by discontinuing prior diuretic therapy for 3–5 d. Hypotension can also occur after the initiation of therapy in patients with congestive heart failure. The risk can be minimized by beginning with a very low dose, such as 2.5 mg twice a day (b.i.d.) of enalapril.

3.4.1.1.2. Acute Renal Failure. A decline in renal function, which is usually modest, may be observed in some patients with bilateral renal artery stenosis, hypertensive nephrosclerosis, congestive heart failure, polycystic kidney disease, or chronic renal failure. In each of these disorders, intrarenal perfusion pressure is reduced, a setting in which maintenance of glomerular filtration rate (GFR) is maintained in part by an angiotensin II-induced increase in resistance at the efferent (postglomerular) arteriole. Blocking this response with an ACE inhibitor will sequentially relax the efferent arteriole, lower intraglomerular pressure, and reduce the GFR. The rise in the plasma creatinine concentration generally begins a few days after the institution of therapy, since angiotensin II levels are rapidly reduced. Thus, renal function should be checked at 3–5 d when an ACE inhibitor is begun in a patient who has renal artery stenosis or who is at high risk for this problem (as in an older patient with severe hypertension and atherosclerotic vascular disease). Another rare cause of acute renal failure that is of unproven relation to ACE inhibitors is the development of renal artery thrombosis. This complication appears to occur most often in patients with marked (≥95%) stenotic lesions who have an excessive reduction in blood pressure. It is therefore unclear if there is any specific predisposing effect of the ACE inhibitor.

3.4.1.1.3. Hyperkalemia. Angiotensin II and an elevation in the plasma potassium concentration are the major factors that increase the release of aldosterone, which is the major hormonal stimulus to urinary potassium excretion. In addition to the direct effect of systemic angiotensin II, angiotensin II generated locally within the adrenal zona glomerulosa may mediate the potassium-induced stimulation of aldosterone. Blocking both of these actions with an ACE inhibitor will reduce aldosterone secretion, thereby impairing the efficiency of urinary potassium excretion. The overall incidence of hyperkalemia (defined as a plasma potassium concentration above 5.1 meq/L) is approximately 10%. However, there is a marked variability in risk. ACE inhibitors generally raise the plasma potassium concentration by less than 0.5 meq/L in patients with relatively normal renal function. In contrast, more prominent hyperkalemia may be seen in patients with renal insufficiency, concurrent use of a drug promoting potassium retention such as a potassium-sparing diuretic or an NSAID, or among the elderly.

Among those with renal dysfunction (GFR ≤60 mL/min), limited evidence suggests that increases in serum potassium may be less pronounced with an angiotensin receptor blocker than with an ACE inhibitor (0.12 vs 0.28 meq/L). The use of very low doses of ACE inhibitors may lessen the incidence of hyperkalemia, but still provide some benefit. One well-designed study of 13 patients with proteinuria and mild renal insufficiency evaluated the incidence of hyperkalemia and the antiproteinuric and antihypertensive effects with low- (1.25 mg/d) and high-dose (10 mg/d) ramipril, and placebo. Equivalent antiproteinuric effects were observed with both doses of ramipril (4.4–3.7 gm/d); by comparison, low-dose ramipril did not alter the blood pressure or plasma potassium level, whereas the higher dose resulted in an increase in the plasma potassium (4.5–4.8 meq/L, $p < 0.05$) and a decrease in blood pressure.

3.4.1.1.4. Cough. A dry, hacking cough may develop in 3–20% of patients treated with an ACE inhibitor. The cough has the following clinical features:

1. It usually begins within 1–2 wk of instituting therapy, but can be delayed up to 6 mo.
2. It generally recurs with rechallenge, with either the same or a different ACE inhibitor.
3. It does not occur more frequently in asthmatics than in nonasthmatics but it may be accompanied by bronchospasm.
4. Women are affected more frequently than men.
5. It typically resolves within 1–4 d of discontinuing therapy, but can take up to 4 wk.

The mechanism responsible for the ACE inhibitor-induced cough is not known, but increased local concentrations of kinins, substance P, prostaglandins, or thromboxane may be important.

Both kinins and substance P are metabolized by converting enzyme; thus, their levels are increased by converting enzyme inhibition. Kinins, for example, may induce bronchial irritation and cough via enhanced production of prostaglandins, which may then stimulate afferent C-fibers in the airway. Activation of the arachidonic acid pathway with ACE inhibition may also lead to elevated levels of thromboxane, which can potentiate bronchoconstriction. The possible role of thromboxane in ACE inhibitor-induced cough was evaluated in a double-blind crossover study of nine patients who had developed cough while taking enalapril. The patients were treated with placebo or pico-tamide (600 mg b.i.d.), an agent that inhibits thromboxane synthetase and antagonizes the thromboxane receptor. Active therapy resulting in a significant reduction in thromboxane levels and stopped the cough in eight of the nine patients within 72 h. Inadequate absorption of picotamide occurred in the one nonresponder.

Cough is not a problem with angiotensin II receptor antagonists, such as losartan, which block only the effect of angiotensin II and have no effect on other hormonal mediators. It remains unclear why cough occurs in only some patients treated with ACE inhibitors. It has been suggested that genetic factors may be important. However, common genetic variants for ACE, the B2-bradykinin receptor, or chymase (another enzyme that can convert angiotensin I to angiotensin II) do not explain the variation in susceptibility to cough. Treatment consists of lowering the dose or discontinuing the drug, which will lead to resolution of the cough. Improvement often begins within 4–7 d but may persist for thre 3–4 wk or more in some patients. Patients who have had a good antihypertensive response to the ACE inhibitor can be switched to an angiotensin II receptor antagonist.

3.4.1.1.5. Angioneurotic Edema and Anaphylactoid Reactions. Angioneurotic edema is a rare (0.1–0.2%) but potentially fatal complication of ACE inhibitors. This problem usually appears within hours or at most 1 wk, but can occur as late as 1 yr or more after the onset of therapy. It is typically characterized by swelling of the mouth, tongue, pharynx, and eyelids, and occasionally laryngeal obstruction. Patients should be advised to discontinue the drug and call the physician if they develop facial edema or a sore throat independent of an upper respiratory infection. All ACE inhibitors can induce angioneurotic edema, although it is unclear if they do so with same frequency. The mechanism responsible for the angioneurotic edema is not well understood, but increased kinins may play a role. It is possible, for example, that genetic mild deficiencies in kinin degradation could predispose selected patients to the development of this complication when kinin levels are enhanced following administration of an ACE inhibitor. It is likely, however, that kinins do not provide the entire explanation since some cases of angioneurotic edema have been described with the angiotensin II receptor antagonists that do not raise kinin levels. Another hypothesis is that susceptible patients have a subclinical hereditary or acquired deficiency of complement 1-esterase inactivator, which is another cause of angioneurotic edema. The risk of recurrence of angioedema if ACE inhibitors are continued was addressed in a report of 82 patients who had a first episode of angioedema while on an ACE inhibitor. The overall rate of recurrence during an average follow-up of 2.3 yr was 8.5 per 100 patient-years; however, the risk was much higher in those with continued exposure to ACE inhibitors (18.7 vs 1.8 per 100 patient-years). Review of the medical records revealed that physicians often attributed the angioedema to other causes even after multiple recurrences. Similar factors may contribute to the high incidence of anaphylactoid reactions seen when ACE inhibitors are used in patients treated with high-flux hemodialysis using polyacrylonitrile (PAN) dialyzers.

3.4.1.1.6. Contraindication in Pregnancy. ACE inhibitors are contraindicated in pregnancy, since they are associated with an increased incidence of fetal complications.

3.4.1.1.7. Poisoning. Symptoms of ACE inhibitor overdosing are usually mild. If, however, severe hypotension occurs, intravenous fluids and inotropic support may be required.

3.4.1.2. Drug Interactions

Antacids can decrease the GI absorption of captopril if administered simultaneously. Captopril, and possibly other ACE inhibitors, can enhance the activity of oral antidiabetic agents. Hypoglycemia has occurred when captopril was added to either glyburide or biguanide therapy. Caution should be observed when captopril is added to the regimen of patients receiving these drugs.

Captopril can enhance the effects of antihypertensive agents and diuretics on blood pressure if given concomitantly. This additive effect may be desirable, but dosages must be adjusted accordingly. Patients with hyponatremia or hypovolemia may become hypotensive and/or develop reversible renal insufficiency when given captopril and diuretics concomitantly. Indomethacin has been shown to inhibit the antihypertensive response to captopril. Other NSAIDs, aspirin, and other salicylates may also exert a similar effect on captopril's action, however, other ACE inhibitors may not be affected to the same degree as captopril. It is thought that the antihypertensive action of captopril is highly dependent on its ability to stimulate the synthesis of vasodilatory prostaglandins. NSAIDs inhibit prostaglandin synthesis, thereby attenuating captopril's ability to lower blood pressure. Loss of antihypertensive effect should be considered if an NSAID is added to a regimen that includs captopril. In addition, patients on captopril should be cautioned about routine use of aspirin or over-the-counter NSAIDs.

Many of the ACE inhibitor trials were performed on a background of ASA (acetylsalicyclic acid) suggesting their effects may be additive, although some data also suggest there may be a negative interaction between the two drugs.

Inhibition of ACE results in decreased aldosterone production and potentially decreased potassium excretion, leading to small increases in serum potassium. Hyperkalemia can occur if captopril is given to patients receiving drugs that also increase serum potassium concentration, including potassium-sparing diuretics such as amiloride or spironolactone, potassium salts, or heparin.

Serum digoxin concentrations can rise by 15–30% in patients with congestive heart failure who are given digoxin and captopril concomitantly. However, captopril-induced hyperkalemia can offset the increased digoxin concentrations, and captopril and digoxin have been administered to patients with congestive heart failure with no apparent adverse effects. The clinical significance of this interaction is not clear.

Probenecid decreases the renal tubular secretion of captopril, resulting in higher captopril serum concentrations. If probenecid is given to a patient stabilized on captopril, hypotension may occur. This interaction would appear to be of lesser significance if captopril is added after probenecid therapy is in place.

Captopril can decrease the renal elimination of lithium, which can lead to lithium toxicity. Plasma lithium concentrations should be monitored carefully during concomitant captopril therapy. Clinicians should note that some other antihypertensive agents may also interact with lithium.

3.4.2. Possible Differences Between ACE Inhibitors

It has generally been assumed that the different ACE inhibitors are equally well tolerated. In one large study, for example, enalapril and captopril were equally effective, had the same incidence of usual side effects (such as cough), and the same frequency of drug withdrawal. However, careful quality of life evaluations suggested that patients treated with captopril had a more favorable overall quality-of-life and an increase in general perceived health; these effects were most prominent in those patients who began with a higher quality of life. How this difference might occur is unclear, but differences in penetration into the CNS may be important. The clinical significance of this observation is at present uncertain. Other studies plus the experience of most practitioners do not support the observation that enalapril or other ACE inhibitors lead to an important reduction in the quality of life in many or most patients.

3.4.3. AT-1-Receptor Antagonists

There are a number of approved nonpeptide selective blockers of the binding of angiotensin II to type 1 (AT-1) angiotensin receptors on the cell membrane, thereby inhibiting the action of angiotensin II *(72–74)*. Thus, these drugs, angiotensin II receptor antagonists or blockers (ARBs), represent the third class that antagonizes the renin-angiotensin-aldosterone system: β-blockers reduce the release of renin by inhibiting β-1 receptor stimulation; and the ACE inhibitors block the conversion of inactive angiotensin I to the active hormone angiotensin II. Blockade of the action of angiotensin II leads to elevations in plasma levels of renin, angiotensin I, and angiotensin II. However, this build-up of precursors does not overwhelm the receptor blockade, as evidenced by a persistent fall in both blood pressure and plasma aldosterone levels.

Angiotensin II receptor blockers may offer all of the advantages of ACE inhibitors and fewer side effects *(75–80)*.

3.4.3.1. Side Effects

The angiotensin II receptor antagonists are generally well tolerated. The side-effect profile is similar to that with the ACE inhibitors (e.g., increased incidence of hyperkalemia *(81)* and of acute renal failure in renovascular hypertension), except for those side effects that may be mediated by kinins, particularly cough, which is the most common reason that patients discontinue use of an ACE inhibitor, and much less often angioedema. The incidence of cough with angiotensin II receptor antagonists is similar to that with placebo (3%) and well below that seen with ACE inhibitors (approximately 10%). One large study evaluated patients with a prior history of ACE inhibitor–induced cough; the incidence of recurrent cough was much higher with readministration of an ACE inhibitor (67%) than with either valsartan or hydrochlorothiazide (19%). However, this protection does not appear to be absolute. Thus far, at least 19 cases of angioedema have been described in patients taking losartan; this complication is typically characterized by swelling of the mouth, tongue, pharynx, and eyelids, and occasionally laryngeal obstruction. How this might occur is unclear but nonkinin factors are presumably involved. Another uncommon adverse effect of uncertain origin is dysgeusia.

3.4.3.1.1. Use in Pregnancy. As with ACE inhibitors, angiotensin II receptor antagonists are contraindicated in pregnancy. An additional concern is that AT1 receptor blockade results in the disinhibition of renin release by angiotensin II and increased formation of all angiotensin peptides. These peptides could activate the AT2 receptor, which is known to have high prevalence in the fetus. The availability of the first new class of antihypertensive agents in more than 10 yr has added a great deal of excitement to the treatment of hypertension. It is at present unclear if angiotensin II receptor antagonists will turn out to be a minor addition (an ACE inhibitor without cough, which would still be useful) or a major advance. They may provide a better way to overcome the adverse effects of the renin-angiotensin system. However, outcome data are needed before they are recommended instead of ACE inhibitors.

3.4.3.2. Drug Interactions

Some of the AT-1 blockers are metabolized by the cytochrome P450 (CYP) enzyme system to a significant extent, and as a result, are subject to potential metabolism-related drug interactions. Other drug interaction studies with common medications such as digoxin, warfarin, oral contraceptives, and nifedipine have not revealed any significant drug interactions.

Like nearly all other AT-1 blockers, losartan has relatively poor bioavailability, but its absorption is not significantly affected by food. Following absorption, losartan is converted to an active metabolite, EXP3174, in the liver by the CYP2C9 and possibly CYP3A enzymes. This metabolite is responsible for the majority of the drug's effects. Medications that inhibit the drug-metabolizing enzymes CYP2C9 (Fluvastatin, fluvoxamine, fluoxetine, metronidazole, ritonavir) and possibly CYP3A may inhibit the conversion of losartan to its metabolite, possibly decreasing its effectiveness.

Unlike losartan, valsartan does not require enzymatic conversion to an active form, and valsartan is only minimally metabolized by the body, decreasing the risk of significant drug interactions.

Irbesartan is not a prodrug, but it is metabolized in the liver by the CYP2C9 enzyme. Therefore, drugs that affect this enzyme may interact with irbesartan. Specifically, inducers of CYP2C9 may increase the metabolism and decrease the effectiveness of irbesartan. CYP2C9 inhibitors would be expected to have the opposite effect.

Eprosartan also does not require activation in the body and is not metabolized significantly, lowering the risk of drug interactions.

The effects of candesartan cilexetil are maintained for more than 24 h due to slow dissociation of the drug from the AT1 receptor. Candesartan cilexetil is a prodrug that is converted into the active drug, candesartan, during absorption. Preliminary drug interaction studies have not revealed any significant interactions.

Excretion of lithium reduced (increased plasma-lithium concentration).

4. DIGITALIS

Cardiac glycosides *(82)* are of potential value in most patients with symptoms and signs of systolic heart failure secondary to ischemic, valvular, hypertensive, or congenital heart disease; dilated cardiomyopathies; and cor pulmonale. Improvement of depressed myocardial contractility by glycosides increases cardiac output, promotes diuresis, and reduces the filling pressure of the failing ventricle, with the consequent reduction of pulmonary vascular congestion and central venous pressure. It is widely accepted that cardiac glycosides are of benefit in the treatment of patients with heart failure accompanied by atrial fibrillation or atrial flutter and a rapid ventricular response.

William Withering's monograph in the 18th century contains the first comprehensive description of digitalis glycosides in the treatment of congestive heart failure. The chemical structure of this venerable class of drugs includes a steroid nucleus containing an unsaturated lactone at the C17 position and one or more glycosidic residues at C3. Digoxin is now the most commonly prescribed cardiac glycoside owing to its convenient pharmacokinetics, alternative routes of administration, and the widespread availability of serum drug-level measurements.

4.1. Mechanism of Action

Congestive heart failure: For many years cardiac glycosides have been known to increase the velocity and extent of shortening of cardiac muscle, resulting in a shift upward and to the left of the ventricular function (Frank Starling) curve relating stroke work to filling volume or pressure. This occurs in normal as well as failing myocardium and in atrial as well as ventricular muscle. The positive inotropic effect is due to an increase in the availability of cytosolic Ca^{++} during systole, thus increasing the velocity and extent of sarcomere shortening. This increase in intracellular Ca^{++} is a consequence of cardiac glycoside-induced inhibition of the sarcolemmal Na^+,K^+-ATPase.

Supraventricular Arrhythmias: Direct suppression of the AV node conduction to increase effective refractory period and decrease conduction velocity results in positive inotropic effect, enhanced vagal tone, and decreased ventricular rate to fast atrial arrhythmias. Atrial fibrillation may decrease sensitivity and increase tolerance to higher serum digoxin concentrations.

4.1.1. Pharmacokinetics

The half-life for digoxin elimination of 36–48 h in patients with normal or near-normal renal function permits once-a-day dosing. In the absence of loading doses, near steady-state blood levels are achieved in four to five half-lives, or about 1 wk after initiation of maintenance therapy if normal renal function is present. Digoxin is largely excreted unchanged, with a clearance rate proportional to the GFR, resulting in the excretion of approximately one-third of body stores daily. In patients with heart failure and reduced cardiac reserve, increased cardiac output and renal blood flow in response to treatment with vasodilators or sympathomimetic agents may increase renal digoxin clearance, necessitating dosage adjustment. Digoxin is not removed effectively by peritoneal dialysis or hemodialysis because of its large (4–7 L/kg) volume of distribution. The principal body reservoir is skeletal muscle and not adipose tissue. Accordingly, dosing should be based on estimated lean body mass. Neonates and infants tolerate and may require higher doses of digoxin for an equivalent therapeutic effect than older children or adults. Digoxin crosses the placenta and drug levels in maternal and umbilical vein blood are similar.

Current tablet preparations of digoxin average 70–80% oral bioavailability, with elixir and encapsulated gel preparations approaching 90–100%. Parenteral digoxin is available for intravenous use. Loading or maintenance doses can be given by intravenous injection, which should be carried out over at least 15 min to avoid vasoconstrictor responses to more rapid injection. Intramuscular digoxin is absorbed unpredictably, causes local pain, and is not recommended.

4.2. Drug Interactions (83–91)

4.2.1. Pharmacokinetics

- Cholestyramine, colestipol, kaolin-pectin may reduce digoxin absorption. Separate administration.
- Metoclopramide may reduce the absorption of digoxin tablets.
- Amiodarone reduces renal and nonrenal clearance of digoxin and may have additive effects on heart rate. Reduce digoxin dose by 50% with start of amiodarone.
- Carvedilol may increase digoxin blood levels in addition to potentiating its effects on heart rate.
- Cyclosporine may increase digoxin levels, possibly due to reduced renal clearance.
- Erythromycin, clarithromycin, and tetracyclines may increase digoxin (not capsule form) blood levels in a subset of patients.
- Indomethacin has been associated with isolated reports of increased digoxin blood levels/toxicity.
- Itraconazole may increase digoxin blood levels in some patients; monitor.
- Neomycin can decrease digoxin absorption to a variable degree.
- Propafenone increases digoxin blood levels. Effects are highly variable; monitor closely.

7. Cardiovascular Drugs

- Propylthiouracil (and methimazole) may increase digoxin blood levels by reducing thyroid hormone.
- Quinidine increases digoxin blood levels substantially. Effect is variable (33–50%). Monitor digoxin blood levels/effect closely. Reduce digoxin dose by 50% with start of quinidine. Other related agents (hydroxychloroquine, quinine) should be used with caution.
- Rifampin reduces the intestinal absorption of digoxin, an effect that probably occurs by the induction of intestinal P-glycoprotein. It is likely that anticonvulsants (phenytoin, phenobarbital, and carbamazepine) will cause the same interaction.
- Spironolactone may interfere with some digoxin assays, but may also increase blood levels directly. However, spironolactone may attenuate the inotropic effect of digoxin. Monitor effects of digoxin closely.
- Sulfasalazine can decrease digoxin absorption to a variable degree.
- These medications have been associated with reduced digoxin blood levels, which appear to be of limited clinical significance: aminoglutethimide, aminosalicylic acid, aluminum-containing antacids, sucralfate, sulfasalazine, neomycin, ticlopidine.
- These medications have been associated with increased digoxin blood levels, which appear to be of limited clinical significance: famciclovir, flecainide, ibuprofen, fluoxetine, nefazodone, cimetidine, famotidine, ranitidine, omeprazole, trimethoprim.

4.2.2. Pharmacodynamics

- Amiloride may reduce the inotropic response to digoxin.
- Levothyroxine (and other thyroid supplements) may decrease digoxin blood levels.
- Penicillamine has been associated with reductions in digoxin blood levels.
- Amiodarone reduces renal and nonrenal clearance of digoxin and may have additive effects on heart rate. Reduce digoxin dose by 50% with start of amiodarone.
- Benzodiazepines (alprazolam, diazepam) have been associated with isolated reports of digoxin toxicity.
- Beta-blocking agents (propranolol) may have additive effects on heart rate.
- Calcium preparations: Rare cases of acute digoxin toxicity have been associated with parenteral calcium (bolus) administration.
- Carvedilol may increase digoxin blood levels in addition to potentiating its effects on heart rate.
- Moricizine may increase the toxicity of digoxin (mechanism undefined).
- Succinylcholine administration to patients on digoxin has been associated with an increased risk of arrhythmias.
- Verapamil diltiazem, bepridil, and nitrendipine increased serum digoxin concentrations. Other calcium channel blocking agents do not appear to share this effect. Reduce digoxin's dose with the start of verapamil.
- Drugs that cause hypokalemia (thiazide and loop diuretics, amphotericin B): Hypokalemia may potentiate digoxin toxicity.

4.3. Digitalis Toxicity and Therapeutic Drug Monitoring

Overt digitalis toxicity tends to emerge at two- to threefold higher serum concentrations than the target 1.8 nmol/L, but it must always be remembered that a substantial overlap of serum levels exists among patients exhibiting symptoms and signs of toxicity and those with no clinical evidence of intoxication. If ready access to serum digoxin assays is available, a reasonable approach to the initiation of therapy is to begin at 0.125–0.375 mg/d, depending on lean body mass and estimated creatinine clearance, and to measure a serum digoxin level 1 wk later with careful monitoring of clinical status in the interim. Patients with impaired renal function will not yet have reached steady state and need to be monitored closely until four to five clearance half-lives have elapsed (as long as 3 wk). Oral or intravenous loading with digoxin, although generally safe, is rarely necessary as other safer and more effective drugs exist for short-term inotropic support or for initial treatment of supraventricular arrhythmias.

Blood samples for serum digoxin-level measurement should be taken at least 6–8 h following the last digoxin dose. Serum-level monitoring is justified in patients with substantially altered drug clearance rates or volumes of distribution (e.g., very old, debilitated, or very obese patients). Adequacy of digoxin dosing and risk of toxicity in a given patient should never be based on a single isolated serum digoxin concentration measurement.

Although the incidence and severity of digitalis intoxication are decreasing, vigilance for this important complication of therapy is essential. Disturbances of cardiac impulse formation, conduction, or both are the hallmarks of digitalis toxicity. Among the common electrocardiographic manifestations are ectopic beats of AV junctional or ventricular origin, first-degree atrioventricular block, an excessively slow ventricular rate response to atrial fibrillation, or an accelerated AV junctional pacemaker. These manifestations may require only a dosage adjustment and monitoring as clinically appropriate. Sinus bradycardia, sinoatrial arrest or exit block, and second- or third-degree atrioventricular conduction delay often respond to atropine, but temporary ventricular pacing is sometimes necessary and should be available. Potassium administration is often useful for atrial, AV junctional, or ventricular ectopic rhythms, even when the serum potassium is in the normal range, unless high-grade atrioventricular block is also present. Magnesium may be useful in patients with atrial fibrillation and an accessory pathway in whom digoxin administration has facilitated a rapid accessory pathway-mediated ventricular response. Lidocaine or phenytoin, which in conventional doses have minimal effects on atrioventricular conduction, are useful in the management of worsening ventricular arrhythmias that threaten hemodynamic compromise. Electrical cardioversion can precipitate severe rhythm disturbances in patients with overt digitalis toxicity, and should be used with particular caution.

Potentially life-threatening digoxin or digitoxin toxicity can be reversed by antidigoxin immunotherapy. Purified Fab fragments from digoxin-specific antisera are available at most poison control centers and larger hospitals in North American and Europe. Clinical experience in adults and children has established the effectiveness and safety of antidigoxin Fab in treating life-threatening digoxin toxicity, including cases of massive ingestion with suicidal intent. Doses of Fab are calculated on the basis of a simple formula based on either the estimated dose of drug ingested or the total-body digoxin burden and are administered intravenously in saline over half an hour.

5. NITRATES

Angina pectoris is a symptom complex caused by transient myocardial ischemia. Metabolism in cardiac myocytes is aerobic; as a result, myocardial ischemia occurs when there is an imbalance between oxygen demand and oxygen supply. Myocardial oxygen demand varies with heart rate, contractility, and left ventricular wall stress, which is proportional to left ventricular systolic pressure and left ventricular size. Myocardial oxygen supply is dependent upon coronary blood flow, which is limited in patients with critical coronary artery stenoses or prominent coronary vasoconstriction. In addition, the subendocardium receives most of its blood supply during diastole. Conditions that decrease the duration of diastole, such as tachycardia, make the subendocardium susceptible to ischemia. Thus, the treatment of angina is aimed at decreasing oxygen demand and/or increasing oxygen supply.

Nitrates (as well as β-blocking agents and calcium channel blockers—which are reviewed in the antihypertensives section) are used for pharmacological treatment of angina. As a consequence, the ratio of myocardial oxygen demand to myocardial oxygen supply improves, and myocardial ischemia is alleviated.

Variant angina (also called Prinzmetal's angina) is a form of angina in which angina pectoris spontaneously occurs in association with scapulothoracic (ST) segment elevation on the EKG. Although it was thought to have been first described by Prinzmetal, this form of angina had actually been recognized in the 1930s by other investigators. Prinzmetal proposed that episodic "temporary increased tonus" in a high-grade obstruction of a major coronary artery was responsible for the syndrome of variant angina. It is now accepted that this hypothesis is correct. Coronary vasospasm is a transient, abrupt, marked reduction in the luminal diameter of an epicardial coronary artery that results in myocardial ischemia. This process can usually be reversed by nitroglycerin or a calcium channel blocker. Spasm occurs in the absence of any preceding increase in myocardial oxygen demand and in either normal or diseased vessels. The reduction in diameter is focal and usually at a single site, although spasm in more than one site and diffuse spasm have recently been reported. Spasm typically occurs near an atherosclerotic plaque in a diseased vessel.

The syndrome of unstable angina includes new-onset or crescendo effort angina, rest angina, early post-MI (myocardial infarction) angina, variant angina, and angina occurring soon after percutaneous transluminal coronary angioplasty (PTCA) or coronary artery bypass graft (CABG) surgery.

The primary pathophysiologic event in unstable angina is thought to be a reduction in coronary blood flow due to transient platelet aggregation, coronary thrombosis, or coronary artery spasm. However, small increases in myocardial oxygen demand can also induce this syndrome. Electrocardiography during episodes of unstable angina frequently demonstrates ST segment depressions or T wave changes, although transient ST segment elevations (which express transmural ischemia) can also be observed. Thus, the underlying nature of unstable angina is similar to that of non-Q wave and transmural MI. The principal differences between these disorders are the duration and intermittency of coronary occlusion and the extent of collateral supply to the ischemic area of the myocardium. The major steps involved in the pathogenesis of unstable angina are thought to be plaque rupture followed by thrombus formation.

Alterations of the ST segment include elevation and depression. The most important cause of ST-segment elevation is transmural injury. Outside this setting, ST elevation can be found in combination with other signs of "chronic" or recent infarction and is associated with ventricular asynergy (usually hypokinesia, but also dyskinesia or akinesia). Depression of the ST segment occurs during myocardial ischemia, directly from subendocardial injury or as a mirroring change of ST elevation.

A proximal left anterior descending MI carries a high mortality and is attributed to an occlusion of the left anterior descending before or at the first septal perforator. All of the precordial leads and I and avL show ST segment elevation. The proximal location of occlusion is associated with compromised perfusion to the His-Purkinje conduction tissue owing to loss of septal supply, and often accompanied by a new bundle branch block. Usually left anterior hemiblock or right bundle branch block is present, but bifasicular blocks, left bundle branch block, or Mobitz II atrioventricular block are all possible. Cardiogenic shock is not unexpected in this subgroup, unless there has been effective reperfusion established.

5.1. Nitroglycerin (92–96)

Although the clinical effectiveness of amyl nitrite in angina pectoris was first described in 1867, organic nitrates are still the drugs most commonly used in the treatment of patients with this condition. By their ability to enhance coronary blood flow by coronary vasodilation and to decrease ventricular preload by increasing venous capacitance, sublingual nitrates are indicated for most patients with an acute coronary syndrome. It is now understood that actions by which nitrovasodilators lead to the relaxation of vascular smooth muscle are through mimicking the activity of nitric oxide and its congeners. Nitrogen oxides were originally identified as bioactive factors responsible for endothelium-dependent relaxation of blood vessels. Nitroglycerin is considered a cornerstone of antianginal therapy. The beneficial effect is thought to occur predominantly via reduction in myocardial oxygen demand secondary to venodilation-mediated decrease in preload. In addition, nitrates are clearly capable of arterial, in particular coronary vasodilation, reduction in afterload, improvement in the coronary collateral circulation, redistribution of transmural coronary blood flow from subepicardial to subendocardial regions, relief of coronary spasm, and some antiplatelet activity. Despite extensive clinical use, there is remarkably little objective information documenting the effectiveness of nitroglycerin in unstable angina. Several small trials have evaluated the ability of an open-label infusion of nitroglycerin to reduce the frequency of ischemic chest pain; symptomatic relief was noted in each of the reports. One randomized trial found that, compared to placebo, intravenous nitroglycerin reduced the frequency and duration of ischemic episodes. In addition, a single randomized trial compared the intravenous, oral, and transdermal nitroglycerin preparations. There was no difference in response among the preparations with regard to symptomatic improvement. However, the small size of this study (40 patients) makes it difficult to draw definitive conclusions.

Nitroglycerin administered sublingually remains the drug of choice for the treatment of acute angina episodes and for the prevention of angina. Because sublingual administration avoids first-pass hepatic metabolism, a transient but effective concentration of the drug rapidly appears in the circulation. The half-life of nitroglycerin itself is brief, and it is rapidly converted to two inactive metabolites, both of which are found in the urine after nitroglycerin administration. The liver possesses large amounts of hepatic glutathione organic nitrate reductase, the enzyme that breaks down nitroglycerin, but there is also evidence that blood vessels (veins and arteries) may metabolize nitrates directly. Within 30–60 min, hepatic breakdown has abolished the hemodynamic and clinical effects.

The usual sublingual dose is 0.3–0.6 mg, and most patients respond within 5 min to one or two 0.3-mg tablets. If symptoms are not relieved by a single dose, additional doses of 0.3 mg may be taken at 5-min intervals, but no more than 1.2 mg should be used within a 15-min period. The development of tolerance is rarely a problem with intermittent usage. Sublingual nitroglycerin is especially useful when it is taken prophylactically shortly before physical activities that are likely to cause angina are undertaken. Used for this purpose, it may prevent angina for up to 40 min.

In patients with acute MI, it seems reasonable to conclude that nitroglycerin should usually be given as an intravenous infusion because of the ease of titration, rapidity of action, and uncertainties about dose delivery with the topical or oral preparations. Intravenous nitroglycerin is usually started at a dose of 5–10 µg/min and then rapidly titrated upward as needed. Although some authors recommend that the dose be adjusted to produce a 10–30% reduction in blood pressure, we titrate the dose to relief of symptoms. In general, the dose should not exceed 400 µg/min, with some authors suggesting that the maximal dose should be as low as 40 µg/min.

5.1.1. Nitrate Tolerance (97,98)

The rapid development of tolerance to the venous and arteriolar vasodilating effects of the nitrovasodilators has been known for over a century. Development of nitrate tolerance occurs in most patients within 24 h. Although nitrate tolerance is well documented, the mechanisms responsible are not clearly understood. It can usually be overcome with an increase in dose or the administration of a sulfhydryl donor such as N-acetylcysteine (NAC) to permit the regeneration of reduced sulfhydryl groups. NAC has been shown to potentiate the hemodynamic response to nitroglycerin and to reverse development of nitrate tolerance (positive drug interaction!). The use of NAC was also examined in a study of 200 patients with unstable angina. After a 4-mo follow-up, outcome events (death, MI, or angina requiring revascularization) occurred in 31% receiving nitroglycerin (10 mg), 42% receiving NAC (600 mg), and 39% taking placebo compared to only 13% receiving both drugs. The probability of no failure on medical therapy was significantly higher in the combination-therapy group than in each of the other three groups, primarily because of a reduction in the need for revascularization due to persistent angina. However, the incidence of side effects, particularly headache, was significantly higher in the group taking combination therapy compared to those treated with nitroglycerin alone (31 vs 19%) *(99–101)*.

5.1.2. Side Effects and Contraindications

The primary adverse effects induced by nitrate therapy include hypotension (especially in patients with ventricular ischemia or hypovolemia), headache, flushing, and tachycardia. Hypovolemia or nitrate-induced hypotension respond promptly to volume replacement. Despite presumed correction of preload by the infusion of saline, the antiischemic effect of nitroglycerin persists.

Prolonged infusion of high-dose nitroglycerin may lead to the development both of methemoglobinemia (which can be treated with intravenous methylene blue) and of heparin resistance. In addition, commercial preparations of intravenous nitroglycerin contain alcohol (0.01–0.14 mL/mg of nitroglycerin). Thus, a substantial alcohol load may be delivered to the patient.

Nitrates are contraindicated in patients with hypertrophic cardiomyopathy with outflow tract obstruction (cardiomyopathies are categorized into dilated, restrictive, hypertrophic, and unclassified based on the predominant pathophysiologic characteristics; hypertrophic cardiomyopathy—a genetic background is present in most cases—is a syndrome that results in heart failure due to left ventricular outflow tract obstruction, diastolic cardiac dysfunction, global cardiac ischemia, dysrhythmias, and sudden cardiac death syndrome in a setting of hyperactive autonomic states). Nitrates can induce or increase outflow tract obstruction in this setting and should be used with caution, even in patients not known to have a resting gradient. Nitrates should also be avoided in patients with suspected right ventricular infarction because of the increased risk of inducing hypotension. Further contraindications comprise pericarditis constrictiva, and pericardial effusion with compression of the right ventricle.

Drug interactions have been reported with concomitent use of sildenafil (Viagra®) an inhibitor of phosphodiesterase type 5. Both drugs lead to increased levels of cGMP (cyclic guanosine monophosphate) and to severe vasodilatation with hypotension *(102,103)*.

5.1.3. Action of Nitrates and Other Vasodilatators (Nitroprusside)

Similar to nitroglycerin, nitroprusside causes preload reduction by diminishing heightened venous tone and increasing venous capacitance with a concomitant shift in central blood volume to the periphery. Unique to nitroprusside is its rapid and powerful effect on afterload hemodynamic. In chronic heart failure, both medications (intravenous nitroglycerin and nitroprusside) produce desirable effects on cardiac filling pressures and cardiac output, but the magnitude of the response to nitroprusside appears to be significantly greater, particularly with respect to afterload reduction.

Severe drug-induced hypotension in patients with coronary artery disease may result in reflex tachycardia (e.g., with short-acting drugs like nifedipine), increased cardiac output, and untoward precipitation of angina, and ischemic events (including tachyarrythmias).

In patients with occlusive coronary artery disease, care must be taken to avoid excessive reductions in systemic pressure or elevations in heart rate that would reduce coronary perfusion and increase myocardial oxygen demand. Unlike nitroglycerin, nitroprusside may cause coronary steal whereby arteriolar dilatation in nonischemic zones diverts coronary flow away from areas of ischemia.

6. Diuretics

Diuretics *(104,105)* act by diminishing sodium-chloride reabsorption at different sites in the nephron (Fig. 3), thereby increasing urinary sodium chloride and water losses. The ability to induce negative fluid balance has made diuretics useful in the treatment of a variety of conditions, particularly edematous states and hypertension.

The importance of diuretics in the treatment of the syndrome of congestive heart failure relates to the central role of the kidney as the target organ of many of the neurohumoral and hemodynamic changes that occur in response to a failing myocardium. Diuretics do not influence the natural history of the underlying heart disease responsible for the decline in cardiac output. However, they can improve symptoms of heart

7. *Cardiovascular Drugs*

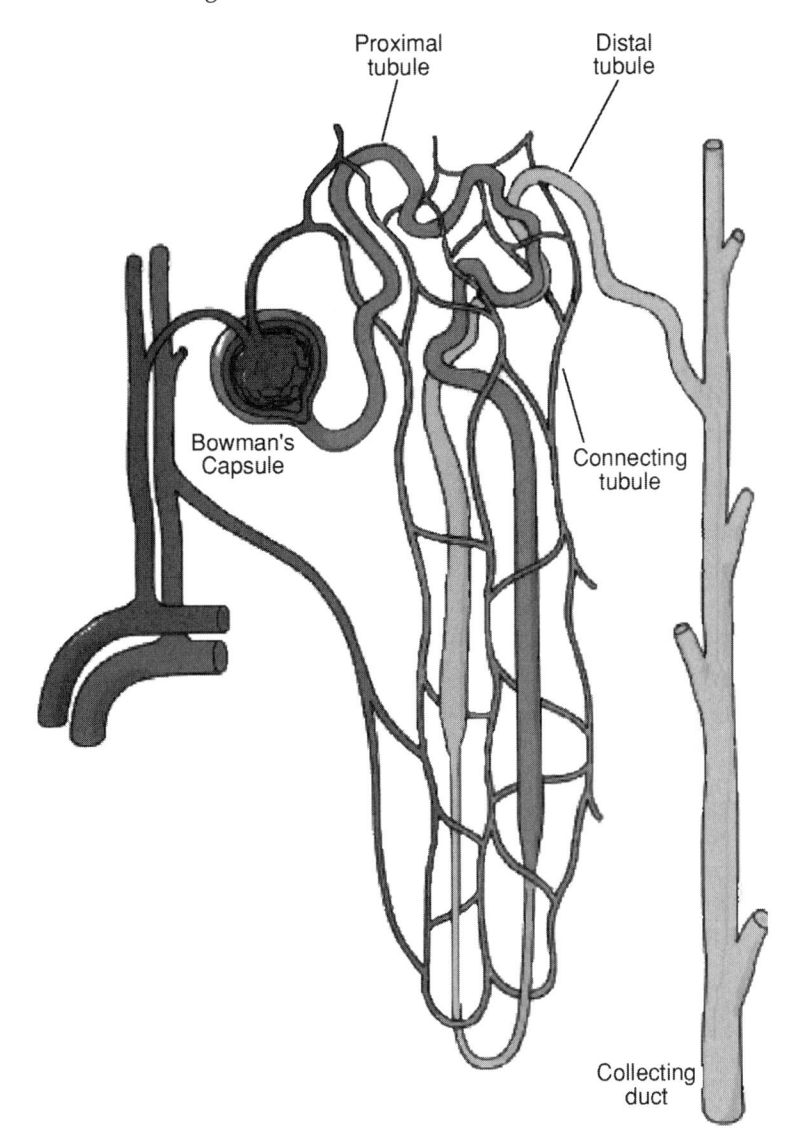

Fig. 3. Parts of a nephron.

failure by acting directly on solute and water reabsorption by the kidney and therefore may slow the progression of cardiac chamber dilation by reducing ventricular filling pressures.

6.1. Mechanisms of Action

The diuretics are generally divided into three major classes, which are distinguished by the site at which they impair sodium reabsorption:

1. Loop diuretics act in the thick ascending limb of the loop of Henle.
2. Thiazide-type diuretics in the distal tubule and connecting segment (and perhaps the early cortical collecting tubule).

3. Potassium-sparing diuretics in the aldosterone-sensitive principal cells in the cortical collecting tubule.
4. Others: acetazolamide *(106)* inhibits the activity of carbonic anhydrase, which plays an important role in proximal bicarbonate, sodium, and chloride reabsorption. As a result, this agent produces both NaCl and NaHCO$_3$ loss. The net diuresis, however, is relatively modest. Mannitol is a nonreabsorbable polysaccharide that acts as an osmotic diuretic, inhibiting sodium and water reabsorption in the proximal tubule and more importantly the loop of Henle. In contrast to other diuretics, mannitol produces a relative water diuresis in which water is lost in excess of sodium and potassium. The major clinical use of mannitol as a diuretic is in the early stages of oliguric, postischemic acute renal failure in an attempt to prevent progression to acute tubular necrosis. It is not generally used in edematous states, since initial retention of the hypertonic mannitol can induce further volume expansion which, in heart failure, can precipitate pulmonary edema.

6.2. Sites of Diuretic Action

1. Proximal tubule high metabolic activity (secretion/resorption)
Recovery of:
   - 65%–80% of sodium and water (Na/Cl cotransport, water follows)
   - 99% of glucose, protein, amino acids recovered
2. Descending limb-Loop of Henle
   - passive diffusion of urea, H$_2$O, Na (thin wall)
   - source of countercurrent multiplier
3. Ascending limb-Loop of Henle
   - strong active transport-Na
   - not permeable to H$_2$O, urea
4. Distal tubule-diluting segment
   - as for ascending limb-loop
5. Distal tubule/Collecting tubule
   - not permeable to urea
   - active sodium resorption
   - sodium/potassium exchange

water permeability under ADH influence

6.3. Thiazide Diuretics

Hydrochlorothiazide (HCTZ) is a thiazide diuretic used in the management of edema and hypertension. In hypertension, thiazide diuretics are often used as initial therapy, either alone or in combination with other agents. Unlike the loop diuretics, their efficacy is diminished in patients with renal insufficiency. HCTZ also has been used to treat diabetes insipidus and hypercalciuria, although these are not FDA-approved indications. HCTZ was approved by the FDA in 1959.

6.3.1. Mechanism of Action

Thiazide diuretics increase the excretion of sodium, chloride, and water by inhibiting sodium ion transport across the renal tubular epithelium. Although thiazides may have more than one action, the major mechanism responsible for diuresis is to inhibit active chloride reabsorption at the distal portion of the ascending limb or, more likely, the early part of the distal tubule (i.e., the cortical diluting segment). Exactly how chloride transport is impaired is unknown. Thiazides also increase the excretion of potassium and bicarbonate, and decrease the elimination of calcium and uric acid. By increasing the sodium load at the distal renal tubule, HCTZ indirectly increases potassium excretion via the sodium/potassium exchange mechanism. Hypochloremia and hypokalemia can cause mild metabolic alkalosis. The diuretic efficacy of HCTZ is not affected by the acid–base balance of the patient. HCTZ is not an aldosterone antagonist, and its main action is independent of carbonic anhydrase inhibition. The antihypertensive mechanism of HCTZ is unknown. It usually does not affect normal blood pressure. Initially, diuretics lower blood pressure by decreasing cardiac output and reducing plasma and extracellular fluid volume. Cardiac output eventually returns to normal, plasma and extracellular fluid values return to slightly less than normal, but peripheral vascular resistance is reduced, resulting in lower blood pressure. These diuretics also decrease the glomerular filtration rate, which contributes to the drug's lower efficacy in patients with renal impairment. The changes in plasma volume induce an elevation in plasma renin activity, and aldosterone secretion is increased, contributing to the potassium loss associated with thiazide diuretic therapy.

6.3.2. Pharmacokinetics

HCTZ absorption from the GI tract varies depending on the formulation and dose. Bioavailability is approximately 50–60%. The drug crosses the placenta but not the blood–brain barrier and is distributed in breast milk. HCTZ is not metabolized and is excreted unchanged in the urine. The half-life of the drug ranges from 5.6 to 14.8 h. The onset of action of the drug is 2 h following oral administration, with peak effects occurring at 4 h. The duration of action ranges from 6 to 12 h.

6.3.3. Contraindications/Precautions

HCTZ-induced fluctuations in serum electrolyte concentration can occur rapidly and precipitate hepatic coma in susceptible patients. Therefore, the drug should be used with caution in patients with hepatic disease. Hyperglycemia, impaired glucose tolerance, and glycosuria can occur during HCTZ therapy, and blood and/or urine glucose levels should be assessed more carefully in patients with diabetes mellitus who are receiving HCTZ.

HCTZ should be used cautiously in patients with renal disease such as severe renal impairment because the drug decreases the GFR and may precipitate azotemia in these patients. Therapy should be interrupted or discontinued if renal impairment worsens, as evidenced by an increase in concentrations of blood urea nitrogen (BUN), serum creatinine, or nonprotein nitrogen. With the exception of metolazone, thiazide diuretics are considered ineffective when the creatinine clearance is less than 30 mL/min.

HCTZ is contraindicated in patients with anuria.

The safety of HCTZ administration during pregnancy has not been established, so the drug should be administered to pregnant women only when absolutely necessary. Thiazides cross the placenta, and jaundice can occur in the fetus or neonate.

HCTZ is classified as pregnancy category D. Thiazide diuretics distribute into breast milk, and it has been recommended by some manufacturers that women should not nurse while receiving thiazide diuretics. The American Academy of Pediatrics recommends breast-feeding be avoided during the first month of lactation in patients receiving thiazide diuretics, because suppression of lactation has been reported. Thiazide diuretics, including HCTZ, should be used with caution in patients with sulfonamide hypersensitivity or carbonic anhydrase inhibitor hypersensitivity because of the risk of cross-sensitivity. Although furosemide and, to a lesser extent, bumetanide are chemically related to the sulfonamides and theoretically should also be used cautiously, in fact, cross-sensitivity with furosemide is an extremely rare occurence. Caution should be used when HCTZ is administered to patients with gout or hyperuricemia since thiazide diuretics have been reported to reduce the clearance of uric acid. HCTZ has been reported to activate or exacerbate systemic lupus erythematosus (SLE).

Patients with severe electrolyte imbalances, such as hyponatremia and hypokalemia, should have their condition corrected before HCTZ is initiated. Initiation of thiazide diuretics under these circumstances can produce life-threatening situations such as cardiac arrhythmias, hypotension, and seizures. HCTZ can cause increase in serum calcium concentrations and should be used with caution in patients with hypercalcemia. Thiazide diuretics have been associated with a slight increase in serum cholesterol and triglyceride concentrations. Data from long-term studies, however, suggest diuretic-induced cholesterol changes are not clinically significant and do not contribute to coronary heart disease risk.

Thiazides should be avoided in neonates with jaundice. Thiazide-induced hyperbilirubinemia is greater in this patient population.

Thiazide diuretics have been reported to cause pancreatitis. They should be used with caution in patients with a history of pancreatitis.

Antihypertensive effects of thiazide diuretics may be enhanced in patients with a sympathectomy.

6.3.4. Drug Interactions

HCTZ can have additive effects when administered with other antihypertensive drugs or diuretics. In some patients, these effects may be desirable, but orthostatic hypotension is possible. Dosages must be adjusted accordingly. In addition, amiloride hydrochloride, spironolactone, and triamterene can reduce the risk of developing hypokalemia because of their potassium-sparing effects; these agents have been used as therapeutic alternatives to potassium supplements.

HCTZ-induced electrolyte disturbances (e.g., hypokalemia, hypomagnesemia, hypercalcemia) can predispose patients to digoxin toxicity, resulting in possibly fatal arrhythmias. Electrolyte balance should be corrected prior to initiating digoxin therapy.

The risk of developing severe hypokalemia can be increased when other hypokalemia-causing agents (e.g., corticosteroids, corticotropin, amphotericin B, other diuretics) are coadministered with HCTZ. Monitoring serum potassium levels and cardiac function is advised, and potassium supplementation may be required.

Concomitant administration of HCTZ to patients receiving nondepolarizing neuromuscular blockers can cause prolonged neuromuscular blockade due to HCTZ-induced hypokalemia. Serum potassium concentrations should be determined and corrected (if necessary) prior to initiation of neuromuscular blockade therapy.

7. Cardiovascular Drugs

Thiazide diuretics reduce lithium renal clearance and can increase lithium serum concentrations. In some cases, thiazide diuretics can be used to counteract lithium-induced polyuria. Lithium dosage should be reevaluated and serum lithium concentrations monitored when a thiazide is added *(107)*.

HCTZ can interfere with the hypoglycemic effects of oral hypoglycemics, which could lead to a loss of diabetic control. Additionally, the concurrent use of diazoxide and thiazide diuretics has resulted in enhanced hyperglycemia.

HCTZ-induced hypovolemia could cause an increased concentration of procoagulant factors in the blood, which could decrease the effects of concomitantly administered anticoagulants and require dosage adjustments of these agents; these effects, however, have not been reported to date.

HCTZ can reduce the renal clearance of amantadine, with subsequent increased serum concentrations and possible toxicity. This interaction has been reported with a combination product of HCTZ and triamterene. Since it is unclear which component was responsible for the interaction, caution should be exercised when administering either drug concurrently with amantadine.

NSAIDs can decrease the diuretic, natriuretic, and antihypertensive actions of diuretics through inhibition of renal prostaglandin synthesis. Concomitant administration of NSAIDs with diuretics also can increase the risk for renal failure secondary to decreased renal blood flow. Patients should be monitored for changes in the effectiveness of their diuretic therapy and for signs and symptoms of renal impairment.

Cholestyramine, an anion-exchange resin, may bind to acidic drugs, such as the thiazide diuretics in the GI tract, and decrease their absorption and therapeutic effectiveness. It is recommended that thiazides be administered at least 4 h before cholestyramine. Although to a lesser extent than cholestyramine, colestipol also has been shown to inhibit the GI absorption and therapeutic response of thiazide diuretics. Administering the diuretic dose at least 2 h before colestipol has been suggested.

6.3.5. Adverse Reactions

Patients receiving HCTZ should be monitored closely for signs of electrolyte imbalance including hyponatremia, hypokalemia, hypomagnesemia, and hypochloremia. Patients should be aware of the symptoms of these disturbances (e.g., lassitude, mental confusion, fatigue, faintness, dizziness, muscle cramps, tachycardia, headache, paresthesia, thirst, anorexia, nausea, or vomiting), and report these signs immediately. Thiazides also can decrease urinary calcium excretion, resulting in hypercalcemia.

Hypokalemia is one of the most common adverse effects associated with thiazide diuretic therapy and can lead to cardiac arrhythmias. This effect is especially important to consider in patients receiving cardiac glycoside therapy because potassium depletion increases the risk of cardiac toxicity. Hyperaldosteronism, secondary to cirrhosis or nephrosis, can predispose patients to hypokalemia when HCTZ is administered. Low dietary-potassium intake, potassium-wasting states, or administration of potassium-wasting drugs also can predispose patients to HCTZ-induced hypokalemia. Patients receiving HCTZ therapy may require supplemental potassium to prevent hypokalemia or metabolic alkalosis.

Hypochloremic alkalosis can occur with hypokalemia during HCTZ therapy, and it is particularly likely to occur in patients with other losses of potassium and/or chloride such as through severe vomiting, diarrhea, excessive sweating, GI drainage, paracentesis, or potassium-losing renal diseases.

Patients receiving HCTZ can develop a dilutional hyponatremia, but it usually is asymptomatic and moderate. Withdrawal of the drug, fluid restriction, and potassium or magnesium supplementation typically will return the serum sodium concentration to normal, but severe hyponatremia can occur. Geriatric patients are especially susceptible to developing hyponatremia, so care should be taken when diuretics are administered to these patients.

HCTZ reportedly has caused azotemia and interstitial nephritis, resulting in reversible renal failure. These effects have occurred mainly in patients with preexisting renal disease.

HCTZ can produce glycosuria and hyperglycemia in diabetic patients, possibly due to potassium depletion. Blood and/or urine glucose levels should be assessed more carefully in diabetic patients receiving HCTZ.

Thiazide diuretics are well known to cause hyperuricemia. The Framingham Study showed that acute gout occurred in only 20% of patients with hyperuricemia. Thiazide diuretics appear to interfere with proximal tubule secretion of uric acid since thiazides are also organic acids and they compete with uric acid for binding at this site. Since thiazides reduce the clearance of uric acid, patients with gout or hyperuricemia may have exacerbations of their disease.

Hypercholesterolemia and/or hypertriglyceridemia have been associated with thiazide diuretic therapy. Although elevations in total cholesterol concentrations of 8% can negate the protection against coronary heart disease provided by a 5-mmHg reduction in blood pressure, data from long-term studies suggest diuretic-induced cholesterol changes are not clinically significant and do not contribute to coronary heart disease risk. After approximately 1 yr of treatment, total serum cholesterol concentrations will subside to baseline or lower, suggesting diuretic-induced cholesterol changes are not a significant coronary heart disease risk factor.

Orthostatic hypotension and hypotension can occur during HCTZ therapy and can be exacerbated by alcohol, narcotics, or antihypertensive drugs.

Thiazide diuretics have been associated with cholestatic jaundice. Caution should be used when thiazides are administered to jaundiced infants due to the risk of hyperbilirubinemia.

Adverse GI effects associated with thiazide therapy include anorexia, gastric irritation, nausea/vomiting, cramps, diarrhea, constipation, sialadenitis, and pancreatitis.

Adverse CNS effects associated with thiazide therapy include dizziness, headache, paresthesias, vertigo, and xanthopsia.

While their incidence is rare, agranulocytosis, aplastic anemia, pancytopenia, hemolysis with anemia, leukopenia, and thrombocytopenia have been reported with thiazide diuretic therapy.

Other adverse effects reported with HCTZ include blurred vision, muscle spasm, impotence, and weakness.

Adverse dermatologic reactions to HCTZ and other thiazide diuretics are uncommon but may occur. These reactions include purpura, photosensitivity, rash, alopecia,

7. Cardiovascular Drugs

urticaria, erythema multiforme including Stevens-Johnson syndrome, exfoliative dermatitis including toxic epidermal necrolysis (TEN), and polyarteritis nodosa.

6.4. Loop Diuretics

6.4.1. Mechanism of Action

Loop diuretics act by inhibition of NaCl reabsorption in the thick ascending limb of the loop of Henle. They inhibit the Na/K/2Cl transport system in the luminal membrane, resulting in:

1. Reduction in sodium chloride reabsorption.
2. Decreases normal lumen-positive potential (secondary to potassium recycling).
3. Positive lumen potential: drives divalent cationic reabsorption (calcium magnesium).
4. Therefore, loop diuretics increase magnesium and calcium excretion.

Hypomagnesemia may occur in some patients. Hypocalcemia does not usually develop because calcium is reabsorbed in the distal convoluted tubule. (In circumstances that result in hypercalcemia, calcium excretion can be enhanced by administration of loop diuretics with saline infusion.)

Since a significant percentage of filtered NaCl is absorbed by the thick ascending limb of loop of Henle, diuretics acting at this site are highly effective.

6.4.2. Properties of Loop Diuretics

These drugs are rapidly absorbed following oral a administration and may be administered by iv. They act rapidly and are eliminated by a renal secretion and glomerular filtration (half-life depends on renal function). Coadministration of drugs that inhibit weak acid secretion (e.g., probenecid or indomethacin) may alter loop diuretic clearance. Other effects include increased renal blood flow, blood flow redistribution within the renal cortex, decreased pulmonary congestion, and the left ventricular filling pressure in congestive heart failure (CHF), which can be observed prior to an increase in urine output.

6.4.3. Clinical Uses

These include acute pulmonary edema, acute hypercalcemia, management of edema, and hyperkalemia (loop diuretics increase potassium excretion; effect increased by concurrent administration of NaCl and water). In acute renal failure, loop diuretics may increase rate of urine flow and increase potassium excretion and may convert oligouric to nonoliguric failure but renal failure duration is usually not affected.

In anion overload (e.g., bromide, chloride, iodide, that are all reabsorbed by the thick ascending loop) administration of loop diuretics may reduce systemic toxicity by decreasing reabsorption; moreover, concurrent administration of sodium chloride and fluid is required to prevent volume depletion.

6.4.4. Adverse Events

Hypokalemia metabolic alkalosis: Increased delivery of NaCl and water to the collecting duct increases potassium and proton secretion. That may cause a hypokalemic metabolic alkalosis. It is managed by potassium replacement and by ensuring adequate fluid intake.

Ototoxicity: Loop diuretics may lead to dose-related hearing loss (is usually reversible). Ototoxicity is more common with decreased renal function and with concurrent administration of other ototoxic drugs such as aminoglycosides.

Hyperuricemia may cause gout. Loop diuretics may cause increased uric acid reabsorption in the proximal tubule, secondary to hypovolemic states.

Hypomagnesemia: Loop diuretics may cause a reduction in sodium chloride reabsorption, decrease normal lumen-positive potential (secondary to potassium recycling), generate positive lumen potential that drives divalent cationic reabsorption (calcium magnesium), and finally, loop diuretics increase magnesium and calcium excretion (hypomagnesemia may occur in some patients that can be reversed by oral magnesium administration)

Allergic reactions with furosemide: skin rash, eosinophilia, interstitial nephritis (less often).

Other adverse events: Dehydration (may be severe); hyponatremia (less common than with thiazides thought may occur in patients who increased water intake in response to a hypovolemic thirst); hypercalcemia may occur in severe dehydration and if a hypercalcemia condition (e.g., oat cell long carcinoma) is also present.

6.4.5. Contraindications/Concerns and Cautions

Obviously it is best not to use this medication in a dehydrated patient if water is being restricted. Weakness or lethargy could be an indicator that blood potassium has dropped too low.

Because of the increased calcium excretion brought on by furosemide (i.e., an increase in urinary calcium levels), there could be a problem using this medication in patients with a history of calcium oxalate bladder stone formation.

It is extremely difficult to overdose with this medication. Toxic doses reported are over 100 times a typical oral dose of medication. It is important to realize that in the treatment of heart failure (this drug's primary use), a crisis can arise at any time.

Taking ginseng may reduce action of loop diuretics resulting in problems with high blood pressure or water retention.

6.4.6. Drug Interactions

One of the most common drug interactions to be aware of is the interaction between furosemide and vasodilating heart medications (especially the ACE inhibitors such as enalapril and captopril). Furosemide may decrease circulating blood volume as it causes a depletion in body water. Thus, water and electrolyte balance must be stable before a vasodilator is added in.

The bronchodilator theophylline may be able to reach higher blood levels when used in conjunction with furosemide. This means that the theophylline dose may need to be reduced.

Loop diuretics can increase the risk of digitalis-induced cardiac toxicity.

Furosemide may lead to displacement of plasma protein binding of warfarin and clofibrate (with elevated plasma levels of these drugs).

Loop diuretics reduce lithium renal clearance and can increase lithium serum concentrations. Furosemide may increase renal toxicity of cephalosporin antibiotics.

Licorice may potentiate the side effects of potassium-depleting diuretics, including loop diuretics.

Furosemide is often used concurrently with digitalis. If furosemide leads to a significant drop in blood potassium levels, this can increase the risk of heart rhythm disturbances and other signs of digitalis toxicity.

Furosemide is often used in combination with prednisone to reduce serum calcium levels. It is possible for this combination of medication to lead to a reduction in potassium level significant enough to require potassium supplementation.

Aminoglycoside antibiotics (amikacin, gentamicin, etc.) have properties that make them toxic to the ear and to the kidney. These properties increase with concomitant use of furosemide.

7. Antihemostatic Drugs

7.1. Anticoagulants

Heparin and warfarin have been the standard anticoagulants used in a variety of clinical settings *(108–110)*.

7.1.1. Mechanisms of Action

The anticoagulant effect of warfarin is mediated by inhibition of the vitamin K–dependent γ-carboxylation of coagulation factors II, VII, IX, and X. This results in the synthesis of immunologically detectable but biologically inactive forms of these coagulation proteins. Warfarin also inhibits the vitamin K–dependent gamma-carboxylation of proteins C and S. Activated protein C in the presence of protein S inhibits activated factor VIII and activated factor V activity. Thus, vitamin K antagonists such as warfarin create a biochemical paradox by producing an anticoagulant effect due to the inhibition of procoagulants (factors II, VII, IX, and X) and a potentially thrombogenic effect by impairing the synthesis of naturally occurring inhibitors of coagulation (proteins C and S) *(111)*. The anticoagulant effect of warfarin is delayed until the normal clotting factors are cleared from the circulation, and the peak effect does not occur until 36–72 h after drug administration. During the first few days of warfarin therapy, prolongation of the PT mainly reflects depression of factor VII, which has a half-life of only 5–7 h; thus, the intrinsic coagulation pathway that does not require factor VII remains intact. Equilibrium levels of factors II, IX, and X are not reached until about 1 wk after the initiation of therapy. For this reason, heparin and warfarin treatment should overlap by 4–5 d when warfarin is initiated in patients with thrombotic disease *(112)*.

7.1.2. Complications and Therapeutic Concerns

The major complication associated with the use of warfarin is bleeding due to excess anticoagulation. In addition, there are major concerns about its use in pregnancy. Finally, there may be a problem with skin necrosis shortly after the institution of warfarin, usually in high doses.

7.1.2.1. Bleeding

The risk of major bleeding episodes in patients treated with warfarin is related to the degree of anticoagulation. Studies in patients with atrial fibrillation indicate that the risk increases substantially at INR values above 4.0. High-risk patients may have bleeding episodes at lower INR values. In order to improve the ability to predict major bleeding, other measurement have been evaluated. For example, one study of 212 outpatients followed for 5 yr reported that the risk of hemorrhage was associated with an increased level of thrombomodulin (>56 µg/L), an endothelium-derived antithrombotic cell-surface glycoprotein that is mainly present on the luminal surface of endothelial cells. The anticoagulant properties of thrombomodulin result from its binding to thrombin and subsequent activation of protein C. However, not all bleeding episodes in anticoagulated patients are due to the anticoagulation. As an example, it should not be assumed that hematuria alone can be explained by chronic stable warfarin therapy. In one report of 243 patients prospectively followed for 2 yr, the incidence of hematuria was similar to that in a control group not receiving warfarin. Furthermore, evaluation of patients who developed hematuria revealed a genitourinary cause in 81% of cases. Infection was most common, but papillary necrosis, renal cysts, and several malignancies of the bladder were also found.

7.1.2.2. USE IN PREGNANCY (113)

Warfarin derivatives are generally felt to be contraindicated during at least the first trimester of pregnancy because of their teratogenic effects. However, the actual risk of embryopathy is unknown. One study, for example, found no congenital abnormalities in 46 women with prosthetic valves who took warfarin during the first trimester. However, other studies have not found such a benign outcome, primarily in patients taking warfarin between the 6th and 12th weeks of pregnancy. In comparison, heparin is a large molecule that does not cross the placenta. Thus, it does not carry the same risk of teratogenicity as warfarin. However, heparin does cause bone loss, which can lead to bone fractures.

7.1.2.3. WARFARIN-INDUCED SKIN NECROSIS (114)

Warfarin-induced skin necrosis typically occurs during the first several days of warfarin therapy, often in association with the administration of large loading doses. The skin lesions occur on the extremities, breasts, trunk, and penis (in males) and marginate over a period of hours from an initial central erythematous macule. Biopsies demonstrate fibrin thrombi within cutaneous vessels with interstitial hemorrhage. Skin necrosis appears to be mediated by the reduction in protein C levels on the first day of therapy, which induces a transient hypercoagulable state. Approximately one-third of patients have underlying protein C deficiency; however, among patients with protein C deficiency, skin necrosis is an infrequent complication of warfarin therapy. Case reports have also described this syndrome in association with an acquired functional deficiency of protein C, heterozygous protein S deficiency, and factor V Leiden.

7.1.3. Warfarin–Drug Interactions

A number of different drugs can interact with warfarin, leading to alterations in its absorption or rate of metabolism *(115–117)*.

7.1.3.1. DECREASED ABSORPTION

The bile acid-binding resins cholestyramine and probably colestipol decrease warfarin absorption. These drugs also enhance warfarin elimination by interrupting its entero-

7. Cardiovascular Drugs

hepatic recirculation. As a result, higher warfarin doses are required as is careful monitoring of the prothrombin time. On the other hand, dosing requirements will fall when resin therapy is discontinued.

7.1.3.2. ALTERED METABOLISM (118,119)

Warfarin is metabolized by the hepatic cytochrome CYP2C9 (P4502C9) isoenzyme, which is inducible by anticonvulsants (including phenobarbital, phenytoin, and carbamazepine), rifampin, glutethimide, and griseofulvin. Coadministration of these drugs enhances warfarin clearance and reversibly increases the dose required for adequate anticoagulation.

Warfarin metabolism can also be inhibited by numerous drugs, potentially requiring a reduction in drug dosage. Examples include amiodarone, disulfiram, acute ethanol ingestion, fluconazole, cimetidine (but not other H-2 blockers), omeprazole, phenylbutazone, oxyphenbutazone, sulfinpyrazone, sulfonamide antibiotics, propafenone, quinolone antibiotics, tamoxifen, disopyramide, miconazole, and clofibrate.

The coadministration of any of these drugs requires close monitoring of the PT to avoid excess anticoagulation. The magnitude of the drug interaction is highly variable. As an example, cimetidine might be expected to have a major effect similar to that seen with other drugs metabolized in the liver (such as lidocaine and propranolol). However, the effect of cimetidine on warfarin clearance is negligible in most patients. Warfarin is administered as a racemic mixture with most of the anticoagulant activity residing in the S-enantiomer. Cimetidine inhibits the relatively inactive R-isomer, resulting in a minimal prolongation of the PT. In contrast, amiodarone, miconazole, phenylbutazone, sulfinpyrazone, and clofibrate preferentially inhibit metabolism of the active stereoisomer via cytochrome CYP2C9 and can therefore have a profound enhancing effect on the degree of anticoagulation.

Quinolone antibiotics have a spectrum of effects on warfarin metabolism. The inhibitory effect is greatest with enoxacin, intermediate with ciprofloxacin and pefloxacin, and negligible with norfloxacin and ofloxacin. The exact warfarin–quinolone drug interaction is unknown. Reduction of intestinal flora responsible for vitamin K production by antibiotics is probable as well as decreased metabolism and clearance of warfarin.

Administration of pulse high-dose intravenous methylprednisolone (500–1000 mg infused IV over 1 h) markedly increased the INR in a prospective study of 10 patients taking chronic oral anticoagulants (fluindione, acenocoumarol). The INR increased from a mean value of 2.8 at baseline to 8.0 (range 5.3–20) after 29 to 156 h. The INR returned to baseline after intravenous vitamin K or discontinuation of the anticoagulant, after 4–12 h and 36–48 h, respectively. Plasma concentrations of fluindione were increased in three of three patients following infusion of methylprednisolone. It was postulated that high-dose methylprednisolone potentiates vitamin K antagonists by inhibiting their cytochrome-P450-dependent catabolism.

7.1.3.3. EFFECT ON ALBUMIN BINDING

Circulating warfarin is tightly bound to albumin. It has been suggested that the coadministration of a nonsteroidal antiinflammatory drug, which is also highly bound, might displace warfarin from its binding sites, leading sequentially to a marked elevation in the unbound and pharmacologically active warfarin concentration and an increased risk of bleeding. Though this mechanism is often cited in the drug interaction literature, it is now known that such effects are of negligible clinical importance. Displacement from protein binding leads to little or no increase in the unbound, pharmacologically active warfarin concentration because of a concurrent rise in warfarin clearance due to increased availability of unbound drug. Thus, a clinically important drug interaction must occur by some other mechanism, such as impaired warfarin metabolism by phenylbutazone and sulfinpyrazone.

Interactions occur during the distribution phase if the drug has a narrow range of safety index and is highly protein bound. For example, Coumadin is an anticoagulant medication that is very highly bound to protein and has a very narrow range-of-safety index. Coumadin interacts with various drugs, vitamins, herbs, and foods via different mechanisms. Some known examples that interact with Coumadin include aspirin, ibuprofen, vitamin K, some types of tea, green leafy vegetables, and so on. These items interact with Coumadin either by enhancing its effectiveness and thus leading to prolonged bleeding, or by decreasing its effectiveness and thus increasing the risk of blood clots in the vessels, both of which may be quite dangerous to the patient. This is why patients who are taking Coumadin need to be exceedingly cautious when taking herbs concurrently. Unfortunately, it is extremely difficult to predict whether an individual herb will interact with Coumadin, because there are very few tests or experiments documenting such interactions. The best precautionary measure is close observation of the patient's condition. If the patient shows abnormal signs of bleeding and bruises, then the dosage of herbs may need to be adjusted and the patient's medical doctor should be contacted immediately.

Herbs with anticoagulant effects include herbs that have blood-activating and blood-stasis-removing functions. Such herbs may interfere with anticoagulant drugs, such as Coumadin, to prolong the bleeding time. Herbs that interfere with Coumadin include Salviae Miltiorrhizae (Dan Shen), Angelica Sinensis (Dang Gui), Ligustici Chuanxiong (Chuan Xiong), Persicae (Tao Ren), Carthamus Tinctorii (Hong Hua), and Hirudo seu Whitmania (Shui Zhi). The synergistic interaction between herbs and Coumadin may be advantageous for the patient as the dosage of both the herbs and the drugs can be reduced without compromising clinical effectiveness.

NSAIDs increase gastric irritation and erosion of the protective lining of the stomach, assisting in the formation of a GI bleed. Additionally, NSAIDs decrease the cohesive properties of platelets necessary in clot formation.

Acetaminophen (paracetamol) use has been associated in epidemiologic studies with an increased risk of developing a prolonged INR. One case control study of 289 patients found that the odds ratio of developing an INR above 6.0 increased with greater acetaminophen intake; a statistically significant odds ratio of 3.5 was observed when weekly consumption exceeded the equivalent of more than seven regular-strength tablets, and rose to 10.0 when weekly consumption exceeded the equivalent of 28 regular-strength tablets. The mechanism by which acetaminophen might potentiate the action of warfarin is not well understood.

7.2. Fibrinolytics

Acute MI usually results from rupture of an atheromatous plaque with subsequent thrombus formation and vessel occlusion.

7. Cardiovascular Drugs

Currently available thrombolytic agents reduce mortality in acute MI. There has been an overall 30% reduction in mortality from 10–15% in the prethrombolytic era to 7–10% today. Accelerated tissue-type plasminogen activator (tPA) appears to produce a greater overall benefit than streptokinase, although it is significantly more expensive. In addition to the agent used, the efficacy of reperfusion therapy is also dependent upon the time at which reperfusion occurs, the degree of flow obtained. The earlier reperfusion occurs, the greater the degree of myocardial salvage that can be achieved. Thus, the benefit is greatest when thrombolytic agents are administered soon after the onset of symptoms, particularly within the first 4 h.

Patients with chest pain suggestive of an acute MI presenting up to 12 h after symptom onset and having electrocardiographic evidence of an acute MI manifested by ST elevation (>1 mm in two contiguous leads in leads I, II, III, aVL, aVF or 2 mm in two contiguous precordial leads) are candidates for thrombolytic therapy. Patients with typical and persistent symptoms in the presence of a new or presumably new left bundle branch block are also considered eligible.

In contrast, thrombolytic therapy is not indicated in patients with unstable angina and no ST elevation because of lack of proven benefit. ST segment depression is also not an indication for thrombolytic therapy unless it represents a true posterior or dorsal MI.

7.2.1. Possible Contraindications for Fibrinolytics (120–122)

- Current use of anticoagulants.
- Known bleeding diathesis (e.g., from significant liver dysfunction).
- Recent stroke.
- Poorly controlled or chronic sustained hypertension (systolic blood pressure >170 mmHg). The presence of hypertension is associated with a higher incidence of stroke due to intracranial hemorrhage.
- Prior central venous or noncompressible puncture, pregnancy, aortic dissection, or neoplasm.
- Streptokinase allergy (tPA can be used in this setting).
- Severe head injury or trauma within 2 wk, including recent surgery (less than 2 wk excluding intracranial or spinal surgery, which may require a longer interval).
- Hemorrhagic retinopathy.

Eligibility for thrombolytic therapy has evolved over the past several years as more information becomes available regarding efficacy and safety. Up to 40% of patients in some series are ineligible for thrombolytic therapy. Active internal bleeding is an absolute contraindication. Patients older than 75 yr may get less overall benefit than younger patients but advanced age is no longer considered a major contraindication for lytic therapy.

7.2.2. Streptokinase

Patients with decreased renal function manifest intrinsic disorders of platelet function. Patients with liver and sometimes those with cardiac disease may have a decreased ability to synthesize vitamin K-dependent clotting factors. Such patients treated with anticoagulants might have a greater tendency to bleed than would normal subjects since there would predictably be a greater overall disruption of hemostasis. The half-life is 0.6 h. The most important adverse effects are bleeding and allergic reaction.

7.2.3. Tissue-Type Plasminogen Activator (Alteplase)

The drug must be given parenterally and in combination with heparin or other antithrobin agents (e.g., hirudin, low molecular weight heparin). The half-life is 0.5–1.2 h. The most important adverse effect is bleeding.

7.3. Antiplatelet Drugs

Platelets play a major role in the thrombotic response to rupture of a coronary artery plaque. Cardiovascular disease, which includes MI, stroke, and peripheral vascular disease, remains far and away the leading the cause of death in the United States and most developed countries, accounting for more than 900,000 deaths annually in the United States alone. The totality of evidence from basic research, observational epidemiologic studies, and randomized clinical trials has provided strong support for the efficacy of antiplatelet drugs in decreasing the risk of cardiovascular disease in a wide range of patient categories *(123–126)*.

7.3.1. Action of Antiplatelet Agents

Antiplatelet agents can interfere with a number of platelet functions including aggregation, release of granule contents, and platelet-mediated vascular constriction. They can be classified according to their mechanism of action.

7.3.1.1. CLASS I

Aspirin *(127,128)* and related compounds (NSAIDs and sulfinpyrazone) block "irreversible" cyclooxygenase (prostaglandin H synthase), the enzyme that mediates the first step in prostaglandin and thromboxane biosynthesis from arachidonic acid.

For drug interactions with aspirin, *see* Chapter 10 on NSAIDs.

7.3.1.1.1. Side Effects. At the recommended dose in these trials, GI side effects (dyspepsia, nausea, vomiting) occur in about 40% of patients (vs 30% in the placebo group) and are dose limiting in 10–20%. GI bleeding is seen in up to 5% per year but frank melena (1% per year) and hematemesis (0.1% per year) are rare. Gout may be aggravated in some patients due to impaired urate excretion. Worsening of bronchospasm and asthma as well as rare anaphylactic reactions have also been observed.

7.3.1.2. CLASS II

Dipyridamole inhibits phosphodiesterase-mediated breakdown of cyclic adenosine monophosphate (AMP), which prevents platelet activation by multiple mechanisms.

7.3.1.2.1. Side Effects. It is possible that dipyridamole may have a deleterious effect because of its potential for inducing coronary steal, which can exacerbate the angina. For these reasons, dipyridamole is not recommended in unstable angina.

Adverse effects at therapeutic doses are usually mild and transient. Vomiting, diarrhea, and symptoms such as dizziness, nausea, headache, and myalgia have been observed. Such effects usually disappear on long-term use of dipyridamole.

As a result of its vasodilating properties, dipyridamole may cause hypotension, hot flushes, and tachycardia. In rare cases, worsening of coronary heart disease has

7. Cardiovascular Drugs

been observed. Hypersensitivity reactions like rash, urticaria, severe bronchospasm, and angioedema have been reported.

In very rare cases, increased bleeding during or after surgery has been observed.

Isolated cases of thrombocytopaenia have been reported in conjunction with treatment with dipyridamole.

Dipyridamole has been shown to be incorporated into gallstones.

7.3.1.2.2. Drug Interactions. Dipyridamole increases plasma levels and cardiovascular effects of adenosine. Adjustment of adenosine dosage should be considered.

When dipyridamole is used in combination with anticoagulants or ASA, the statements on intolerance and risks for these preparations must be observed. Addition of dipyridamole to ASA does not increase the incidence of bleeding events. When dipyridamole was administered concomitantly with warfarin, bleeding was no greater in frequency or severity than that observed when warfarin was administered alone.

Dipyridamole may increase the hypotensive effect of drugs that reduce blood pressure and may counteract the anticholinesterase effect of cholinesterase inhibitors thereby potentially aggravating myasthenia gravis.

7.3.1.3. CLASS III

Ticlopidine and clopidogrel achieve their antiplatelet effect by blocking the binding of ADP to a low-affinity, type 2 purinergic receptor and preventing the activation of the GP IIb/IIIa receptor complex and subsequent platelet aggregation *(129)*.

7.3.1.3.1. Side Effects. Neutropenia *(130)*, which can be quite severe and occurs in approximately 1% of patients, is the most serious side effect of ticlopidine. It usually appears during the first 3 mo of treatment and requires immediate discontinuation of the drug. How this occurs is not well understood but direct suppression of the bone marrow may be involved. Rash (2%), diarrhea (3%), dyspepsia, hepatic dysfunction, and the development of bronchiolitis obliterans organizing pneumonia (BOOP) have also been observed.

Thrombotic thrombocytopenia purpura-hemolytic uremic syndrome (TTP-HUS) *(131)* in a rare complication of ticlopidine therapy. The reported incidence when the drug is used after cardiac stenting is 1 case in 1600 to 1 in 4800. All cases occur within 12 wk. Treatment includes discontinuation of the drug and plasma exchange. Ticlopidine has not yet been approved for use in unstable angina by the FDA but it is recommended by the ACC/AHA Task Force in a dose of 250 mg twice per day in patients notable to take aspirin. Ticlopidine or clopidogrel is also recommended in addition to aspirin when coronary artery stenting is performed. Neutrophil counts should be obtained at baseline, every 2–3 wk during the first 4 mo, and monthly thereafter. Platelet counts should also be obtained at baseline and every week during the first 4 mo of therapy.

Cholesterol Elevation: Ticlopidine therapy causes increased serum cholesterol and triglycerides. Serum total cholesterol levels are increased 8–10% within 1 mo of therapy and persist at that level. The ratios of the lipoprotein subfractions are unchanged.

There were no major adverse events from clopidogrel itself in the CURE trial, although the combination of clopidogrel plus aspirin was associated with a significant increase in major (3.6 vs 2.7%) and minor bleeding (15.3 vs 8.6%). Clopidogrel appears to be associated with fewer complications (e.g., neutropenia, TTP-HUS) than ticlopidine.

One limitation to the use of clopidogrel is its cost, which is about $3 per day in the United States.

7.3.1.3.2. Drug Interactions (Ticlopidine). Therapeutic doses of ticlopidine caused a 30% increase in the plasma half-life of antipyrine and may cause analogous effects on similarly metabolized drugs. Therefore, the dose of drugs metabolized by hepatic microsomal enzymes with low therapeutic ratios or being given to patients with hepatic impairment may require adjustment to maintain optimal therapeutic blood levels when starting or stopping concomitant therapy with ticlopidine. Studies of specific drug interactions yielded the following results:

Aspirin and Other NSAIDs: Ticlopidine potentiates the effect of aspirin or other NSAIDs on platelet aggregation. The safety of concomitant use of ticlopidine and NSAIDs has not been established. The safety of concomitant use of ticlopidine and aspirin beyond 30 d has not been established. Aspirin did not modify the ticlopidine-mediated inhibition of ADP-induced (adenosine 5'-diphosphate) platelet aggregation, but ticlopidine potentiated the effect of aspirin on collagen-induced platelet aggregation. Caution should be exercised in patients who have lesions with a propensity to bleed, such as ulcers. Long-term concomitant use of aspirin and ticlopidine is not recommended.

Antacids: Administration of ticlopidine after antacids resulted in an 18% decrease in plasma levels of ticlopidine.

Cimetidine: Chronic administration of cimetidine reduced the clearance of a single dose of ticlopidine by 50%.

Digoxin: Coadministration of ticlopidine with digoxin resulted in a slight decrease (approximately 15%) in digoxin plasma levels. Little or no change in therapeutic efficacy of digoxin would be expected.

Theophylline: In normal volunteers, concomitant administration of ticlopidine resulted in a significant increase in the theophylline elimination half-life from 8.6 to 12.2 h and a comparable reduction in total plasma clearance of theophylline.

Phenobarbital: In six normal volunteers, the inhibitory effects of ticlopidine on platelet aggregation were not altered by chronic administration of phenobarbital.

Phenytoin: In vitro studies demonstrated that ticlopidine does not alter the plasma protein binding of phenytoin. However, the protein-binding interactions of ticlopidine and its metabolites have not been studied in vivo. Several cases of elevated phenytoin plasma levels with associated somnolence and lethargy have been reported following coadministration with ticlopidine. Caution should be exercised in coadministering this drug with ticlopidine, and it may be useful to remeasure phenytoin blood concentrations.

Propranolol: In vitro studies demonstrated that ticlopidine does not alter the plasma protein-binding of propranolol. However, the protein-binding interactions of ticlopidine and its metabolites have not been studied in vivo. Caution should be exercised in coadministering this drug with ticlopidine.

Other Concomitant Therapy: Although specific interaction studies were not performed, in clinical studies ticlopidine was used concomitantly with β-blockers, calcium channel blockers, and diuretics without evidence of clinically significant adverse interactions.

7.3.1.3.3. Contraindications. The use of ticlopidine is contraindicated in the following conditions:

7. Cardiovascular Drugs

- Hypersensitivity to ticlopidin.
- Presence of hematopoietic disorders such as neutropenia and thrombocytopenia or a past history of either TTP (thrombotic thrombocytopenia purpura) or aplastic anemia.
- Presence of a hemostatic disorder or active pathological bleeding (such as bleeding peptic ulcer or intracranial bleeding).
- Patients with severe liver impairment.

7.3.1.3.4. Drug Interaction (Clopidogrel). The safety of chronic concomitant administration of aspirin and clopidogrel has not been established. The concomitant use of heparin and clopidogrel should be undertaken with caution, as the safety has not been established.

During drug-interaction studies, no clinically significant drug–drug interactions were observed with clopidogrel and aspirin (administered as 500 mg twice a day for 1 d), heparin, atenolol, nifedipine, estrogen, digoxin, or theophylline. The pharmacodynamic activity of clopidogrel was not significantly influenced by coadministration of phenobarbital or cimetidine. Coadministration of clopidogrel with naproxen resulted in increased occult GI blood loss. There are no known drug or laboratory test interactions with clopidogrel.

Cytochrome P450 System: At high concentrations in vitro, clopidogrel inhibited the activity of CYP450 2C9, which could result in higher plasma levels of drugs metabolized by this isozyme, such as phenytoin, tamoxifen, tolbutamide, warfarin, torsemide, fluvastatin, and many NSAIDs, but there are no data with which to predict the magnitude of such interactions.

Experience from the CAPRIE study indicated that clopidogrel can be safely administered long term (e.g., up to 3 yr) with many other commonly prescribed medications without evidence of clinically significant interactions. These medications include diuretics, β-blocking agents, ACE inhibitors, calcium antagonists, cholesterol-lowering agents, coronary vasodilators, antidiabetic agents, antiepileptic agents, and hormone replacement therapy.

7.3.1.4. CLASS IV

Anti-IIb/IIIa antibodies (abciximab) and receptor antagonists (tirofiban, eptifibatide) inhibit the final common pathway of platelet aggregation and may also prevent initial adhesion to the vessel wall.

7.3.1.4.1. Side Effects. One complication of abciximab therapy is thrombocytopenia, occurring within 24 h of initiating therapy. The reported incidence is 0.8–1.6% (vs 0.7% for placebo). Although the mechanism is unknown, platelet transfusions are effective. Another concern is excessive bleeding if emergency bypass surgery is required after the administration of abciximab. A paucity of data exists, but one report suggested that routine platelet transfusions prevented major bleeding and reduced excessive blood transfusions.

8. LIPID-LOWERING DRUGS

Lipid-altering agents encompass several classes of drugs that include HMG-CoA reductase (hydroxymethylglutaryl CoA reductase) inhibitors or statins, fibric acid derivatives, bile acid sequestrants, nicotinic acid, and probucol. These drugs differ with respect to mechanism of action and to the degree and type of lipid lowering. Thus, the indications for a particular drug are influenced by the underlying lipid abnormality. The mechanisms of benefit seen with lipid lowering are incompletely understood. Regression of atherosclerosis occurs in only a minority of patients; furthermore, the benefit of lipid lowering is seen in as little as 6 mo, before significant regression could occur. Thus, other factors must contribute; these include plaque stabilization, reversal of endothelial dysfunction, and decreased thrombogenicity *(132)*.

8.1. Statins

The HMG-CoA reductase inhibitors *(133,134)* represent a major therapeutic advance in lipid-regulating pharmacological therapy because of their increased efficacy, tolerability, and ease of administration. Currently available statins include lovastatin, pravastatin, simvastatin, fluvastatin, and atorvastatin. These agents are competitive inhibitors of HMG-CoA reductase, the rate-limiting step in cholesterol biosynthesis. Fluvastatin dosed at 20–40 mg/d, lovastatin dosed at 10–80 mg/d, pravastatin dosed at 10–40 mg/d, or simvastatin dosed at 5–40 mg/d may be expected to decrease low-density lipoprotein (LDL) cholesterol 20–40% *(135–140)*.

The resultant reduction in intracellular cholesterol in the liver stimulates the up-regulation of the B/E receptor and increases clearance of lipoproteins containing apo B or apo E from the plasma compartment. Although the predominant effect is to decrease circulating LDL cholesterol, VLDL and IDL particles are also removed. Inhibition of the synthesis of apo B–containing lipoproteins has also been postulated as a potential mechanism for these agents, but this hypothesis remains controversial. Potential beneficial nonlipid effects include a reduction in plasminogen activator inhibitor 1 (PAI-1) in patients with hypercholesterolemia, reported with lovastatin and pravastatin, which provides a hemostatic mechanism for clinical improvement with HMG-CoA reductase inhibitor therapy *(141)*.

8.1.1. Side Effects

Adverse reactions occur less frequently with the statins than with the other classes of lipid-lowering agents. The side effects of the HMG-CoA reductase inhibitors are minimal. The major clinical problems that have been reported are hepatotoxicity and myopathy *(142,143)*.

Serum liver enzyme levels were greater than three times the upper limit of normal in less than 2% of subjects who received maximum-dosage lovastatin in the 1-yr Expanded Clinical Evaluation of Lovastatin (EXCEL) study, and at the usual dosage, the incidence was less than 1%. Most cases of transaminase elevation appear to occur within the first 3 mo of therapy. Rhabdomyolysis has been documented in approximately 0.1% of subjects receiving lovastatin monotherapy and appears to occur at about the same frequency for all the HMG-CoA reductase inhibitors. However, the exact incidence of myopathy, as defined by creatine kinase elevation, that is attributable to HMG-CoA reductase inhibitor use is difficult to establish: In subjects who continued in the EXCEL study a second year, creatine kinase elevations above the upper limit of normal were reported in 50–67% of the groups receiving various dosages of lovastatin and 54% of the placebo group.

7. Cardiovascular Drugs

Despite initial concern based on inhibitors of enzymes of cholesterol synthesis other than HMG-CoA, no evidence of increased lens opacity has been reported with the use of HMG-CoA reductase inhibitors. Although it has been postulated that the lipophilic agents, lovastatin and simvastatin, may have a greater potential for sleep disturbances than the hydrophilic fluvastatin and pravastatin, because the former cross the blood–brain barrier, the incidence of sleep disturbances is uncommon with either lipophilic or hydrophilic agents.

Atorvastatin is more lipophilic than other agents, leading to concern that it may be associated with a higher incidence of adverse reactions relative to other agents with long-term safety data and proven efficacy in randomized trials (such as pravastatin and simvastatin). This concern was mitigated by a review of pooled data involving more than 4000 patients treated with atorvastatin and a trial of 2856 patients randomized to atorvastatin or simvastatin. The overall adverse-event profile was similar to that observed for other statins. There is, however, one case report of a patient previously treated safely with simvastatin who developed acute hepatitis when atorvastatin was administered.

8.1.2. Drug Interactions

Risk for myopathy may be increased when an HMG-CoA reductase inhibitor is combined with a fibric-acid derivative, nicotinic acid, cyclosporine, or erythromycin *(144)*.

Cerivastatin has recently been withdrawn from market worldwide because of increased risk for myopathy in particular in combination with fibric-acid derivatives.

8.1.2.1. FIBRIC-ACID DERIVATIVES *(145)*
(GEMFIBROZIL, FENOFIBRATE, BEZAFIBRATE) AND NIACIN (NICOTINIC ACID)

Although there is no experience with the use of atorvastatin given concurrently with fibric-acid derivatives and niacin, the benefits and risks of such combined therapy should be carefully considered. The risk of myopathy during treatment with other drugs in this class is increased with concurrent administration.

In a crossover study in 20 healthy male volunteers given concomitant single doses of pravastatin and gemfibrozil, there was a significant decrease in urinary excretion and protein binding of pravastatin. In addition, there was a significant increase in AUC, C_{max}, and T_{max} for the pravastatin metabolite SQ 31,906. Combination therapy with pravastatin and gemfibrozil is generally not recommended.

Pravastatin and fluvastatin are not extensively metabolized by the cytochrome CYP3A4 system; as a result, they have few interactions with other drugs unlike other statins. Several studies have noted no increase in the risk of myositis when pravastatin was used in conjunction with sustained release niacin or cyclosporine; similar considerations appear to apply to fluvastatin. In contrast, lovastatin in high dose (40–80 mg/d) is associated with an appreciable risk of myositis in patients also receiving cyclosporine. However, this combination is usually well tolerated if only low doses of lovastatin are used (10 mg or 20 mg/d): muscle toxicity occurs in only 0–2% of cases. Similar results have been reported with low-dose simvastatin.

Concomitant therapy with other lipid metabolism regulators: Combined drug therapy should be approached with caution as information from controlled studies is limited.

8.1.2.2. BILE ACID SEQUESTRANTS

Patients with mild to moderate hypercholesterolemia: LDL-C reduction was greater when atorvastatin 10 mg and colestipol 20 g were coadministered (−45%) than when either drug was administered alone (−35% for atorvastatin and −22% for colestipol).

8.1.2.3. PATIENTS WITH SEVERE HYPERCHOLESTEROLEMIA

LDL-C reduction was similar (−53%) when atorvastatin 40 mg and colestipol 20 g were coadministered when compared with that of atorvastatin 80 mg alone. Plasma concentration of atorvastatin was lower (approximately 26%) when atorvastatin 40 mg plus colestipol 20 g were coadministered compared with atorvastatin 40 mg alone.

Concomitant administration resulted in an approximately 40–50% decrease in the mean AUC of pravastatin. However, when pravastatin was administered 1 h before or 4 h after cholestyramine or 1 h before colestipol and a standard meal, there was no clinically significant decrease in bioavailability or therapeutic effect.

However, the combination drug therapy was less effective in lowering the triglycerides than atorvastatin monotherapy in both types of hypercholesterolemic patients. When atorvastatin is used concurrently with colestipol or any other resin, an interval of at least 2 h should be maintained between the two drugs, since the absorption of atorvastatin may be impaired by the resin.

8.1.2.4. COUMARIN ANTICOAGULANTS

Atorvastatin had no clinically significant effect on PT when administered to patients receiving chronic warfarin therapy. In a study involving 10 healthy male subjects given pravastatin and warfarin concomitantly for 6 d, bioavailability parameters at steady state for pravastatin (parent compound) were not altered. Pravastatin did not alter the plasma protein-binding of warfarin. Concomitant dosing did increase the AUC and C_{max} of warfarin but did not produce any changes in its anticoagulant action (i.e., no increase was seen in mean PT after 6 d of concomitant therapy). However, bleeding and extreme prolongation of PT has been reported with another drug in this class. Patients receiving warfarin-type anticoagulants should have their PTs closely monitored when pravastatin is initiated or the dosage of pravastatin is changed.

8.1.2.5. DIGOXIN

Coadministration of multiple doses of atorvastatin and digoxin increased steady-state plasma digoxin concentrations by approximately 20%. Patients taking digoxin should be monitored closely and appropriately. In a crossover trial involving 18 healthy male subjects given pravastatin and digoxin concurrently for 9 d, the bioavailability parameters of digoxin were not affected. The AUC of pravastatin tended to increase, but the overall bioavailability of pravastatin plus its metabolites SQ 31,906 and SQ 31,945 was not altered.

8.1.2.6. ORAL CONTRACEPTIVES

Coadministration of atorvastatin with an oral contraceptive, containing 1 mg norethindrone and 35 µg ethinyl estradiol, increased plasma concentrations (AUC levels) of norethindrone and ethinyl estradiol by approximately 30 and 20%, respectively. These increases should be considered when selecting an oral contraceptive.

7. Cardiovascular Drugs

8.1.2.7. ANTACIDS

Administration of aluminum- and magnesium-based antacids suspension, with atorvastatin decreased plasma concentrations of atorvastatin by approximately 35%. LDL-C reduction was not altered but the triglyceride-lowering effect of atorvastatin may be affected.

8.1.2.8. CIMETIDINE

Administration of cimetidine with atorvastatin did not alter plasma concentrations or LDL-C-lowering efficacy of atorvastatin, however, the triglyceride-lowering effect of atorvastatin was reduced from 34 to 26%. The AUC_{0-12h} for pravastatin when given with cimetidine was not significantly different from the AUC for pravastatin when given alone. A significant difference was observed between the AUCs for pravastatin when given with cimetidine compared to when administered with antacid.

In a study with healthy subjects, coadministration of maximum doses of both atorvastatin (80 mg) and terfenadine (120 mg), a CYP 3A4 substrate, was shown to produce modest increases in AUC values. The QTc interval remained unchanged. However, since an interaction between these two drugs cannot be excluded in patients with predisposing factors for arrhythmia (e.g., preexisting prolonged QT interval, severe coronary artery disease, hypokalemia), caution should be exercised when these agents are coadministered.

8.1.2.9. ANTIPYRINE

Antipyrine was used as a nonspecific model for drugs metabolized by the microsomal hepatic enzyme system (cytochrome P450 system). Atorvastatin had no effect on the pharmacokinetics of antipyrine, thus interactions with other drugs metabolized via the same cytochrome isozymes are not expected. Since concomitant administration of pravastatin had no effect on the clearance of antipyrine, interactions with other drugs metabolized via the same hepatic cytochrome isozymes are not expected.

8.1.2.10. ERYTHROMYCIN

In healthy individuals, plasma concentrations of atorvastatin increased approximately 40% with coadministration of atorvastatin and erythromycin, a known inhibitor of cytochrome P450 3A4.

8.1.2.11. OTHER CONCOMITANT THERAPY

Caution should be exercised with concomitant use of immunosuppressive agents and azole antifungals. Some investigators have measured cyclosporine levels in patients on pravastatin, and to date, these results indicate no clinically meaningful elevations in cyclosporine levels. In one single-dose study, pravastatin levels were found to be increased in cardiac transplant patients receiving cyclosporine.

8.2. Fibrates

Three fibrates *(146,147)* are currently available in the United States: gemfibrozil, clofibrate, and fenofibrate. The mechanism of action of the fibric-acid derivatives is complex and has not been completely elucidated. The major effect is a decrease in VLDL (very-low-density lipoprotein) secondary to increased lipoprotein lipase activity; lipoprotein lipase hydrolyzes triglyceride from VLDL to form IDL (intermediate-density lipoprotein), which is either removed by the B/E receptor through apo E-mediated recognition and binding or collect more cholesterol esters from HDL to become LDL. The fibrates may also exert a peripheral effect by decreasing plasma levels of free fatty acids.

In addition to their effects on lipoprotein levels, fibric-acid derivatives may alter the composition of lipoproteins. As noted above, gemfibrozil and bezafibrate have been shown to decrease the concentration of small, dense LDL. The fibrates may thus protect against coronary atherosclerosis not only by reducing LDL cholesterol level but also by shifting LDL particles to a less atherogenic phenotype.

Additionally, the fibric-acid derivatives provide nonlipid benefits, such as improvements in coagulation and fibrinolysis. A reduction in platelet aggregability and reactivity in response to epinephrine has been documented with gemfibrozil. Gemfibrozil has also been shown to decrease the activity of PAI-1, thereby potentially improving fibrinolytic efficacy. Bezafibrate has been reported to decrease circulating levels of fibrinogen; fibrinogen has been directly associated with risk for coronary artery disease in epidemiological studies.

Clofibrate should not be used since it has been associated with cholangiocarcinoma and other GI cancers. Other fibrates that are available worldwide include bezafibrate and ciprofibrate.

8.2.1. Side Effects

The side effects of the fibric-acid derivatives are generally mild and are encountered in approximately 5–10% of patients treated with these agents. The majority of complaints are of nonspecific GI symptoms such as nausea, flatulence, bloating, and dyspepsia. Increased lithogenicity of bile has been reported with clofibrate therapy but has not been clearly demonstrated with the other fibrates. Fibrate monotherapy rarely results in muscle toxicity, although mild elevations of creatine kinase may occasionally occur. However, the risk for myopathy is increased when a fibrate is used in combination with an HMG-CoA reductase inhibitor, as described above. Although recent studies have demonstrated that this combination may be used without severe muscle toxicity, great caution is required, and careful patient education and surveillance are prerequisites.

8.2.2. Drug Interactions

An important drug interaction is that fenofibrate increases the clearance of cyclosporine. In one series of 43 heart transplant recipients, for example, fenofibrate therapy led to a 30% reduction in cyclosporine levels. Five of these patients had an episode of acute rejection that was associated with decrease in cyclosporine levels on the visit before the episode. A small elevation in the plasma creatinine concentration of 0.34 mg/dL (30 µmol/L), which did not become apparent for at least 6 mo, was also noted. Fibrates are primarily excreted by the kidneys; therefore, the dosage and dosing interval should be reduced in patients with renal insufficiency to avoid myositis. The dosing of bezafibrate, for example, should be reduced with renal insufficiency. Bezafibrate, like other fibrates, interacts with warfarin. As a result, the warfarin dose should be reduced by 30% in patients treated with this drug.

8.3. Probucol

Probucol is a complex agent that cannot be readily classified with the other lipid-regulating drugs in terms of structure or mechanism of action. It is a bisphenol derivative that is similar in structure to butylated hydroxytoluene, a compound with powerful antioxidant activity that has also been demonstrated to decrease the early microcirculatory changes induced by hypercholesterolemia in rabbits *(119)*.

The mechanism of action by which probucol lowers lipid levels has not been completely elucidated. Probucol does not appear to decrease the production of lipoproteins nor does it alter plasma clearance through the B/E receptor pathway.

Probucol dosed at 1 gm/d decreases LDL cholesterol 5–15% and decreases HDL cholesterol 20–30%. Triglyceride is usually not affected. The effect on HDL cholesterol appears to be greater in patients with higher pretreatment levels of HDL cholesterol and is of concern because of the inverse relation between HDL cholesterol level and incidence of coronary artery disease established in epidemiological studies.

The side effects of probucol appear to be minimal. Probucol is highly lipophilic, so its absorption is enhanced after a fatty meal; therefore, administration should be separated from meals to prevent drug toxicity. Mild gastrointestinal symptoms are occasionally reported. The main clinical concern with probucol use is the possible potentiation of rhythm disorders associated with prolongation of repolarization. In experimental animals, increased incidence of sudden cardiac death with probucol administration was thought to be caused by induced ventricular arrhythmias. Although no clear correlation between probucol use and sudden cardiac death has been established in humans, the QT interval should be monitored, especially in patients with baseline prolongation or receiving concomitant sotalol, quinidine, procainamide, tricyclic antidepressants, phenothiazines, or other agents known to increase the QT interval.

8.4. Bile Acid Sequestrants

Cholestyramine is a polymeric resin, administered orally to bind bile acids. Originally, cholestyramine was used to treat pruritis secondary to cholestasis, but its main use today is to treat hypercholesterolemia with concomitant hypertriglyceridemia. Cholestyramine also has been used to treat clostridium difficile enterocolitis, although traditional antibiotics are more effective. Colestipol hydrochloride is an oral antilipemic agent. It is a nonabsorbable bile acid sequestrant similar in action to cholestyramine. Colestipol and cholestyramine appear to be equal in their cholesterol-lowering effects. Since the development and release of HMG-CoA reductase inhibitors, colestipol use has declined. Colestipol, however, is not absorbed and has a safer toxicity profile than do other antilipemics, thus making it a desirable agent in children and pregnant women. Colestipol was approved by the FDA in 1977.

By releasing chloride, colestipol combines with bile acids in the intestine to form insoluble, nonabsorbable complexes that are excreted in the feces along with unchanged resin. Since cholesterol is the major precursor of bile acids, the removal of bile acids from the enterohepatic circulation increases the catabolism of cholesterol to form bile acids. The loss of bile acids stimulates a compensatory increase in the hepatic production of cholesterol. It is postulated that the increased hepatic production of cholesterol falls short of the amount lost, leading to a net decrease in circulating cholesterol. This effect, however, has not been clearly shown. It is likely that colestipol's cholesterol-lowering effect is related to increased catabolism of LDL. Clinically, colestipol lowers LDL and total cholesterol, but has little effect on HDL cholesterol. Triglycerides increase with colestipol therapy. Thus, colestipol is appropriate for type II hyperlipoproteinemia in patients without hypertriglyceridemia.

Colestipol can bind to substances other than bile acids, especially if they undergo enterohepatic recirculation as does digitoxin. Whereas colestipol has been used clinically to accelerate the clearance of digitoxin in cases of toxicity, charcoal and Fab fragments are probably preferred agents for this use. Other agents that bind readily with colestipol include chenodiol, chlorothiazide, digoxin, fat-soluble vitamins, penicillin G, and tetracycline.

8.4.1. Pharmacokinetics

Since colestipol is not absorbed orally, serum concentrations and half-life parameters do not apply. Colestipol is not affected by digestive enzymes. It is eliminated in the stool. Reduction of the plasma cholesterol concentration usually is seen within 24–48 h of starting therapy, and maximum effects are achieved within 1 mo.

8.4.2. Contraindications/Precautions

Colestipol is contraindicated in patients with cholelithiasis or complete biliary obstruction. In these conditions, secretion of bile acids into the GI tract is impaired. Colestipol is also contraindicated in patients with primary biliary cirrhosis since it can further raise serum cholesterol.

Colestipol is relatively contraindicated in constipated patients because of the danger of fecal impaction. Colestipol is relatively contraindicated in patients with coronary artery disease or hemorrhoids because constipation can aggravate these conditions.

Because colestipol can bind with vitamin K, colestipol is relatively contraindicated in patients with any preexisting bleeding disorder or coagulopathy (*see* Interactions).

Because colestipol can bind with exogenous thyroid hormones if administered simultaneously (*see* Interactions), colestipol is relatively contraindicated in patients with hypothyroidism.

Colestipol is relatively contraindicated in patients with renal disease because colestipol releases chloride, which can increase the risk of developing hyperchloremic metabolic acidosis.

It is unknown whether or not cholestipol causes fetal harm if taken during pregnancy. Adequate studies have not been done. Cholestipol should only be used during pregnancy if the potential benefits justify the potential added risk to the fetus.

8.4.3. Drug Interactions

Colestipol can bind with and possibly decrease the oral absorption of carbamazepine, thiazide diuretics, oral furosemide, oral penicillin G, propranolol, oral tetracyclines, orally administered vancomycin, and fat-soluble vitamins including vitamin A, vitamin D, and vitamin K or orally administered phytonadione. Colestipol can bind with and delay or prevent absorption of thyroid hormones including dextrothyroxine. Colestipol also can bind with ursodiol. Staggering the doses of these agents by several hours should prevent binding with colestipol.

7. Cardiovascular Drugs

Cholestyramine can decrease the serum concentrations of imipramine. Though it is logical to conclude that staggering the times of administration may avoid this interaction, doing so did not prevent a similar interaction between cholestyramine and doxepin even when the doses were separated by 6 h. Until more data are available, clinicians should avoid using cholestyramine in patients stabilized on doxepin or imipramine.

Colestipol may affect the hypoprothrombinemic actions of warfarin. Colestipol can bind with vitamin K in the diet, impairing vitamin K absorption, which, in turn, may increase warfarin's hypoprothrombinemic effect. Conversely, colestipol can bind with warfarin directly and impair warfarin bioavailability, although the effects of colestipol on warfarin absorption are less pronounced than the ability of cholestyramine to bind with warfarin. To avoid altering warfarin pharmacokinetics, doses of warfarin and colestipol should be staggered by at least 4–6 h. Colestipol should be prescribed cautiously to any patient receiving warfarin, although colestipol may be an acceptable alternative to cholestyramine in a patient receiving warfarin who also requires therapy with a bile acid sequesterant.

Colestipol can bind with digitoxin and enhance digitoxin clearance. Because digitoxin undergoes enterohepatic recirculation, staggering the administration times of each agent may not prevent this drug interaction. Colestipol should be used cautiously in patients receiving digitoxin. Patients should be observed for loss of digitalis effect if colestipol is added or for digitalis toxicity if colestipol is discontinued in a patient stabilized on cardiac glycosides. Digoxin also may be similarly affected, albeit to a lesser degree since it undergoes less enterohepatic recirculation than digitoxin.

Cholestyramine has been shown to reduce the bioavailability of glipizide but appears to have no effect on tolbutamide absorption. The effect of cholestyramine on the bioavailability of other oral sulfonylureas is unknown.

Cholestyramine enhances the clearance of methotrexate from the systemic circulation. This interaction has actually been used therapeutically in patients with methotrexate toxicity, although activated charcoal is more effective.

8.4.4. Adverse Reactions

The most common adverse reactions to colestipol therapy are GI related. Constipation occurs in 10% of patients. It is usually mild and transient but can produce fecal impaction, requiring medical attention. Every effort should be made to avert possible constipation; the patient should be instructed to drink plenty of water and include additional fiber in the diet. Colestipol can worsen preexisting constipation or aggravate hemorrhoids. Bleeding hemorrhoids or blood in the stool occur infrequently and may result from severe constipation. Other adverse GI reactions include abdominal pain, eructation, flatulence, nausea/vomiting, diarrhea, or steatorrhea.

There have been rare reports of cholelithiasis, cholecystits, GI bleeding, or peptic ulcer. A causal effect has not been established.

Because colestipol can bind with and impair the absorption of dietary vitamin K, hypoprothrombinemia can occur.

Other adverse reactions have been reported with colestipol. Cardiovascular effects are rare such as angina and tachycardia. There have been infrequent reports of a hypersensitivity rash, with urticaria and dermatitis. Reports include musculoskeletal aches and pains in the extremities, joint pain and arthritis, and backache. Neurologic effects include headache and occasional reports of dizziness or lightheadedness, and insomnia. Other infrequent effects include anorexia, shortness of breath, and swelling of the hands or feet.

8.5. Niacin

Niacin, also known as vitamin B_3 has initially been used as a natural cholesterol-lowering agent that often rivals prescription drugs in mild to moderate cases. Three forms of niacin supplements, each with a specific therapeutic role, are commercially available: nicotinic acid (also called nicotinate), niacinamide, and inositol hexaniacinate, a compound of niacin and inositol (another B-family vitamin).

Normally, enough niacin from foods is absorbed to carry out basic functions, working on the cellular level to keep the digestive system, skin, and nerves healthy. This vitamin is also critical to releasing energy from carbohydrates and helping to control blood-sugar levels. Interestingly, niacin is also synthesized from tryptophan, an amino acid found in eggs, milk, and poultry.

In a recent study of people with high cholesterol, niacin not only reduced LDL and triglycerides by 17 and 18%, respectively, but it also increased HDL by 16%. Although both nicotinic acid and inositol hexaniacinate have cholesterol-benefiting actions, inositol hexaniacinate is the preferred form, because it does not cause skin flushing and poses much less risk of liver damage with long-term use.

Niacin improves circulation by relaxing arteries and veins, and disorders characterized by circulation difficulties may benefit as a result. In those suffering from Raynaud's disease, for example, niacin's ability to improve blood flow to the extremities may counter the numbness and pain in the hands and feet that occurs when blood vessels overreact to cold temperatures. The calf cramping and other painful symptoms of intermittent claudication, another circulation disorder, may lessen under the vessel-relaxing influence of niacin as well. The inositol hexaniacinate form of niacin works best for circulation-related discomforts.

Niacinamide can help treat osteoarthritis and rheumatoid arthritis, insulin-dependent diabetes, insomnia, and migraine headaches.

8.5.1. Precautions

High doses (75 mg or more) of niacin can cause side effects. The most common side effect is called "niacin flush." It is harmless unless with concurrent asthma; so people with asthma should not take niacin supplements at high dosages. At very high doses like those used to lower cholesterol, liver damage and gastroduodenal ulcers can occur. Patients with liver disease or gastric ulcera should not take niacin supplements.

8.5.2. Drug Interactions

Taking aspirin before taking niacin may reduce the flushing associated with niacin. However, large doses of aspirin may prolong the length of time of action.

Niacin binds bile acid sequestrants (cholesterol-lowering medications such as colestipol and cholestyramine) and may decrease their effectiveness; therefore, niacin and these medications should be taken at different times of the day.

7. Cardiovascular Drugs

When niacin is taken at the same time as another class of cholesterol-lowering medications, the HMG-CoA reductase inhibitors or statins, the likelihood for serious side effects, such as muscle inflammation or liver toxicity, is increased. In severe cases, kidney failure may occur.

Doses of niacin that are high enough to reduce cholesterol levels may raise blood sugar and lead to a loss of blood sugar control. However, one study suggests that niacin may actually benefit patients with recent onset of Type 1 diabetes. People taking insulin, metformin, glyburide, glipizide, or other similar medications used to treat high blood sugar levels should monitor their blood sugar levels closely.

Niacin should not be taken at the same time as tetracycline, an antibiotic, because it interferes with the absorption and effectiveness of this medication. Niacin either alone or in combination with other B vitamins should be taken at different times from tetracycline.

When niacin is taken with certain blood pressure medications (such as prazosin, doxazosin, and guanabenz), the likelihood of side effects from these medications is increased.

The use of nicotine patches with niacin may increase the chances of or worsen the flushing reactions associated with this supplements.

REFERENCES

1. Vaughan-Williams EM. A classification of antiarrhythmic action reassessed after a decade of new drugs. J Clin Pharmacol 24:129–147 (1984).
2. Members of the Sicilian Gambit. Antiarrhythmic therapy: a pathophysiological approach. Armonk, NY: Futura Publishing, 1994:41.
3. Velebit V, Podrid PJ, Lown B, Cohen BH, and Graboys TB. Aggravation and provocation of ventricular arrhythmias by antiarrhythmic drugs. Circulation 65:886–894 (1982).
4. The Cardiac Arrhythmia Suppression Trial Investigators (CAST). Preliminary report: effect of encainide and flecainide on mortality in a randomized trial arrhythmia suppression after myocardial infarction. N Engl J Med 10:406–412 (1989).
5. The Cardiac Arrhythmia Suppression Trial II Investigators. Effect of the antiarrhythmic agent moricizine on survival after myocardial infarction. N Engl J Med 327:227–233 (1992).
6. Julian DG, Camm AJ, Frangin G, Janse MJ, Munoz A, Schwartz PJ, and Simon P. Randomised trial of effect of amiodarone on mortality in patients with left-ventricular dysfunction after recent myocardial infarction: EMIAT. Lancet 349:667–674 (1997).
7. Boutitie F, Boissel J-P, Connolly SJ, Camm AJ, Cairns JA, Julian DG, et al., and the EMIAT and CAMIAT Investigators. Amiodarone Interaction with β-blockers: analysis of the merged EMIAT (European Myocardial Infarct Amiodarone Trial) and CAMIAT (Canadian Amiodarone Myocardial Infarction Trial) databases. Circulation 99:2268–2275 (1999).
8. Pratt CM, Camm AJ, Cooper W, Friedman PL, MacNeil DJ, Moulton KM, et al., for the SWORD Investigators. Mortality in the Survival with Oral d-Sotalol (SWORD) trial: why did patients die? Am J Cardiol 81:869–876 (1998).
9. MacMillan LB, Hein L, Smith MS, Piascik MT, and Limbird, LE. Central hypotensive effects of the alpha-2a-adrenergic receptor subtype. Science 273:801–803 (1996).
10. Link RE, Desai K, Hein L, Stevens ME, Chrusinski A, Bernstein D, et al. Cardiovascular regulation in mice lacking alpha-2 adrenergic receptor subtypes b and c. Science 273:803–805 (1996).

11. Kasiske BL, Ma JZ, Kalil RS, and Louis TA. Effects of antihypertensive therapy on serum lipids. Ann Intern Med 122:133–141 (1995).
12. Carruthers G, Dessain P, Fodor G, Newman C, Palmer W, and Sim D. Comparative trial of doxazosin and atenolol on cardiovascular risk reduction in systemic hypertension. Am J Cardiol 71:575–581 (1993).
13. Levy D, Walmsley P, and Levenstein M, for the Hypertension and Lipid Trial Study Group. Principal results of the Hypertension and Lipid Trial (HALT): a multicenter study of doxazosin in patients with hypertension. Am Heart J 131:966–973 (1996).
14. ALLHAT Collaborative Research Group. Major cardiovascular events in hypertensive patients randomized to doxazosin vs chlorthalidone: the antihypertensive and lipid-lowering treatment to prevent heart attack trial (ALLHAT). JAMA 283:1967–1975 (2000).
15. Lasagna L. Diuretics versus alpha-blockers for treatment of hypertension (editorial). JAMA 283:2013–2014 (2000).
16. Khouri AF and Kaplan NM. Alpha-blocker therapy of hypertension. JAMA 266:394–398 (1991).
17. Editorial. Alpha-blockade for hypertension: indifferent past, uncertain future. Lancet 1:1055–1056 (1989).
18. Materson BJ, Reda DJ, Cushman WC, Massie BM, Freis ED, Kochar MS, et al. Single-drug therapy for hypertension in men. A comparison of six antihypertensive agents with placebo. N Engl J Med 328:914–921 (1993).
19. Dollery CT, Frishman WH, and Cruickshank JM. Current cardiovascular drugs, 1st ed. London: Current Science, 1993:83.
20. Frishman W. Acebutolol. Cardiovasc Rev Rep 6:979–983 (1985).
21. Leibowitz D. Sotalol: a novel beta blocker with class III antiarrhythmic activity. J Clin Pharmacol 33:508–512 (1993).
22. Laßnig E, Auer J, Berent R, Mayr H, and Eber B. Beta-blockers and heart failure. J Clin Basic Cardiol 4:11–14 (2001).
23. Woosley RL, Kornhauser D, Smith R, Reele S, Higgins SB, Nies AS, et al. Suppression of chronic ventricular arrhythmias with propranolol. Circulation 60:819–827 (1979).
24. Koch-Weser J. Drug therapy: metoprolol. N Engl J Med 301:698–703 (1979).
25. Koch-Weser J and Frishman WH. beta-Adrenoceptor antagonists: new drugs and new indications. N Engl J Med 305:500–506 (1981).
26. Opie LH. Drugs and the heart. Part 1. Beta blocking agents. Lancet 1:693–698 (1980).
27. Dobbs JH, Skoutakis VA, Acchardio SR, and Dobbs BR. Effects of aluminum hydroxide on the absorption of propranolol. Curr Ther Res 21:877–882 (1977).
28. Hibbard DM, Peters JR, and Hunninghake DB. Effects of cholestyramine and colestipol on the plasma concentrations of propranolol. Br J Clin Pharmacol 18:337–342 (1984).
29. Somogyi A and Muirhead M. Pharmacokinetic interactions of cimetidine. Clin Pharmacokinet 12:321–366 (1987).
30. Feely J, Wilkinson GR, and Wood AJ. Reduction of liver blood flow and propranolol metabolism by cimetidine. N Engl J Med 304:692–695 (1981).
31. Zhou HH, Anthony LB, Roden DM, and Wood AJ. Quinidine reduces clearance of (+)-propranolol more than (−)-propranolol through marked reduction in 4-hydroxylation. Clin Pharmacol Ther 47:686–693 (1990).
32. Hii JT, Duff HJ, and Burgess ED. Clinical pharmacokinetics of propafenone. Clin Pharmacokinet 21:1–10 (1991).
33. Vestal RE, Kornhauser DM, Hollifield JW, and Shand DG. Inhibition of propranolol metabolism by chlorpromazine. Clin Pharmacol Ther 25:19–24 (1979).
34. Vestal RE, Kornhauser DM, Hollifield JW, and Shand DG. Inhibition of propranolol metabolism by chlorpromazine. Clin Pharmacol Ther 25:19–24 (1979).

35. Holtzman JL, Kvam DC, Berry DA, Mottonen L, Borrell G, Harrison LI, et al. The pharmacodynamic and pharmacokinetic interaction of flecainide acetate with propranolol: effects on cardiac function and drug clearance. Eur J Clin Pharmacol 33:97–99 (1987).
36. Branch RA, Shand DG, Wilkinson GR, and Nies AS. The reduction of lidocaine clearance by dl-propranolol: an example of hemodynamic drug interaction. J Pharmacol Exp Ther 184:515–519 (1973).
37. Branch RA, Shand DG, Wilkinson GR, and Nies AS. The reduction of lidocaine clearance by dl-propranolol: an example of hemodynamic drug interaction. J Pharmacol Exp Ther 184:515–519 (1973).
38. Ochs HR, Carstens G, and Greenblatt DJ. Reduction in lidocaine clearance during continuous infusion and by coadministration of propranolol. N Engl J Med 303:373–377 (1980).
39. van Harten J, van Brummelen P, Lodewijks MTM, Danhof M, Breimer DD. Pharmacokinetics and hemodynamic effects of nisoldipine and its interaction with cimetidine. Clin Pharmacol Ther 43:332–341 (1988).
40. Kirch W, Kleinbloesem CH, and Belz GG. Drug interactions with calcium antagonists. Pharmacol Ther 45:109–136 (1990).
41. Cohn JN, Franciosa JA, and Francis GS. Nitroprusside infusion in acute myocardial infarction. Acta Med Scand 652(Suppl):125–127 (1981).
42. Merillon JP, Fontenier G, Lerallut JF, Jaffrin MY, Chastre J, Assayag P, et al. Aortic input impedance in heart failure: comparison with normal subjects and its changes during vasodilator therapy. Eur Heart J 5:447–455 (1984).
43. Yin FC, Guzman PA, Brin KP, Maughan WL, Brinker JA, Traill TA, et al. Effect of nitroprusside on hydraulic vascular loads on the right and left ventricle of patients with heart failure. Circulation 67:1330–1339 (1983).
44. Pepine CJ, Nichols WW, Curry RC Jr, and Conti CR. Aortic input impedance during nitroprusside infusion. J Clin Invest 64:643–654 (1979).
45. duCailar J, Mathier-Daude JC, Kienlen J, and Chardon P. Blood and urinary cyanide concentrations during long-term sodium nitroprusside infusions. Anesthesiology 51:363–364 (1979).
46. Somogyi A and Muirhead M. Pharmacokinetic interactions of cimetidine. Clin Pharmacokinet 12:321–366 (1987).
47. Bailey DG, Arnold MO, Munoz C, and Spence JD. Grapefruit juice-felodipine interaction: mechanism, predicability, and effect of naringin. Clin Pharmacol Ther 53:637–642 (1993).
48. Kirch W, Kleinbloesem CH, and Belz GG. Drug interactions with calcium antagonists. Pharmacol Ther 45:109–136 (1990).
49. Capewell S, Freestone S, Critchley JAJH, and Pottage A. Reduced felodipine bioavailability in patients taking anticonvulsants. Lancet 2:480–482 (1988).
50. Dunselman PH and Edgar B. Felodipine clinical pharmacokinetics. Clin Pharmacokinet 21:418–430 (1991).
51. Lown KS, Bailey DG, Fontana RJ, Janardan SK, Adair CH, Fortlage LA, et al. Grapefruit juice increases felodipine oral availability in humans by decreasing intestinal CYP3A protein expression. J Clin Invest 99:2545–2553 (1997).
52. Schwartz JB, Upton RA, Lin ET, Williams RL, and Benet LZ. Effect of cimetidine or ranitidine administration on nifedipine pharmacokinetics and pharmacodynamics. Clin Pharmacol Ther 43:673–680 (1988).
53. Howden CW. Clinical pharmacology of omeprazole. Clin Pharmacokinet 20:38–49 (1991).
54. Soons PA, van den Berg G, Danhof M, van Brummelen P, Jansen JB, Lamers CB, et al. Influence of single- and multiple-dose omeprazole treatment on nifedipine pharmacokinetics and effects in healthy subjects. Eur J Clin Pharmacol 42:319–324 (1992).

55. Muck W, Wingender W, Seiberling M, Woelke E, Ramsch KD, and Kuhlmann J. Influence of the H2-receptor antagonists cimetidine and ranitidine on the pharmacokinetics or nimodipine in healthy volunteers. Eur J Clin Pharmacol 42:325 (1992).
56. Friedel HA and Sorkin EM. Nisoldipine. A preliminary review of its pharmacodynamic and pharmacokinetic properties, and therapeutic efficacy in the treatment of angina pectoris, hypertension and related cardiovascular disorders. Drugs 36:682–731 (1988).
57. van Harten J, van Brummelen P, Lodewijks MT, Danhof M, Breimer DD. Pharmacokinetics and hemodynamic effects of nisoldipine and its interaction with cimetidine. Clin Pharmacol Ther 43:332–341 (1988).
58. Rutledge DR, Pieper JA, and Mirvis DM. Effects of chronic phenobarbital on verapamil disposition in humans. J Pharmacol Exp Ther 246:7–13 (1988).
59. Venkatesan K. Pharmacokinetic drug interactions with rifampicin. Clin Pharmacokinet 22:47–65 (1992).
60. Lai WT, Lee CS, Wu JC, Shen SH, and Wu SN. Effects of verapamil, propranolol, and procainamide on adenosine-induced negative dromotropism in human beings. Am Heart J 132:768–775 (1996).
61. Croog SH, Levine S, Testa MA, Brown B, Bulpitt CJ, Jenkins CD, et al. The effects of antihypertensive therapy on the quality of life. N Engl J Med 314:1657–1664 (1986).
62. Boissel JP, Collet JP, Lion L, Ducruet T, Moleur P, Luciani J, et al. A randomized comparison of the effect of four antihypertensive monotherapies on the subjective quality of life in previously untreated asymptomatic patients: field trial in general practice. J Hypertens 13:1059–1067 (1995).
63. Kostis JB, Shelton B, Gosselin G, Goulet C, Hood WB Jr, Kohn RM, et al. Adverse effects of enalapril in the studies of left ventricular dysfunction (SOLVD). Am Heart J 131:350–355 (1996).
64. Auer J, Berent R, and Eber B. Long term ACE inhibitor therapy in patients with heart failure or left ventricular dysfunction. J Evidence-Based Healthcare 5:22–23 (2001).
65. Toto RD, Mitchell HC, Lee H-C, Milam C, and Pettinger W. Reversible renal insufficiency due to angiotensin converting enzyme inhibitors in hypertensive nephrosclerosis. Ann Intern Med 115:513–519 (1991).
66. Rose BD. Clinical physiology of acid-base and electrolyte disorders, 4th ed. New York: McGraw-Hill, 1994.
67. Reardon LS. Hyperkalemia in outpatients using angiotensin-converting enzyme inhibitors. Arch Intern Med 158:26–32 (1998).
68. Textor SC, Bravo EL, Fouad FM, and Tarazi RC. Hyperkalemia in azotemic patients during angiotensin-converting enzyme inhibition and aldosterone reduction with captopril. Am J Med 73:719–725 (1982).
69. Israili ZH and Hall WD. Cough and angioneurotic edema associated with angiotensin-converting enzyme inhibitor therapy. A review of the literature and pathophysiology. Ann Intern Med 117:234–242 (1992).
70. Brown NJ, Snowden RN, and Griffin MR. Recurrent angiotensin-converting enzyme inhibitor associated angioedema. JAMA 278:232–233 (1997).
71. Lip GYH and Ferner RE. Poisoning with anti-hypertensive drugs: angiotensin converting enzyme inhibitors. J Hum Hypertens 9:711–715 (1995).
72. Burnier M and Brunner HR. Angiotensin II receptor antagonists. Lancet 35:637–645 (2000).
73. Grossman E, Peleg E, Carroll J, Shamiss A, and Rosenthal T. Hemodynamic and humoral effects of the angiotensin II Antagonist losartan in essential hypertension. Am J Hypertens 7:1041–1044 (1994).
74. Kassler-Taub K, Littlejohn T, Elliott W, Ruddy T, and Adler E, for the Irbesartan/Losartan Study Investigators. Comparative efficacy of two angiotensin II receptor antagonists,

irbesartan and losartan, in mild-to-moderate hypertension. Am J Hypertens 11:445–453 (1998).

75. Andersson OK and Neldam S. The antihypertensive effect and tolerability of candesartan cilexetil, a new generation angiotensin II antagonist, in comparison with losartan [see comments]. Blood Press 7:53–59 (1998).

76. Pitt B, Poole-Wilson PA, Segal R, Martinez FA, Dickstein K, Camm AJ, et al. Effect of losartan compared with captopril on mortality in patients with symptomatic heart failure: randomised trial the Losartan Heart Failure Survival Study ELITE II. Lancet 355:1582–1587 (2000).

77. Goldberg AI, Dunlay MC, and Sweet CS. Safety and tolerability of losartan potassium, an angiotensin II receptor antagonist, compared with hydrochlorothiazide, atenolol, felodipine ER, and angiotensin-converting enzyme inhibitors for the treatment of systemic hypertension. Am J Cardiol 75:793–795 (1995).

78. Faison EP, Snavely DB, Thiyagarajan B, and Nelson EB. The incidence of cough with the angiotensin II receptor antagonist, losartan, is significantly less than with angiotensin converting enzyme inhibitors and is similar to that of placebo (abstract). Am J Hypertens 7: 34A (1994).

79. van Rijnsoever EW, Kwee-Zuiderwijk WJ, and Feenstra J. Angioneurotic edema attributed to the use of losartan. Arch Intern Med 158:2063–2065 (1998).

80. Heeringa M and Van Puijenbroek EP. Reversible dysgeusia attributed to losartan (letter). Ann Intern Med 129:72 (1998).

81. Bakris GL, Siomos M, Richardson D, Janssen I, Bolton WK, Hebert L, et al. ACE inhibition or angiotensin receptor blockade: impact on potassium in renal failure. Kidney Int 58:2084–2092 (2000).

82. The Digitalis Investigation Group. The effect of digoxin on mortality and morbidity in patients with heart failure. N Engl J Med 336(8):525–533 (1997).

83. Lindenbaum J, Maulitz RM, and Butler VP. Inhibition of digoxin absorption by neomycin. Gastroenterology 71:399–404 (1976).

84. Lindenbaum J, Rund DH, Butler VP Jr, Tse-Eng D, and Saha, JR. Inactivation of digoxin by the gut flora: reversal by antibiotic therapy. N Engl J Med 305:789–794 (1981).

85. Nademanee K and Kannan R. Amiodarone-digoxin interaction: clinical significance, time course of development, potential pharmacokinetic mechanisms and therapeutic implications. J Am Coll Cardiol 4:111–116 (1984).

86. Doering W. Quinidine-digoxin interaction. Pharmacokinetics, underlying mechanism, and clinical implications. N Engl J Med 301:400–404 (1979).

87. Hager WD, Fenster P, Mayersohn M, Perrier D, Graves P, Marcus FI, et al. Digoxin-quinidine interaction. N Engl J Med 300:1238–1241 (1979).

88. Fromm MF, Kim RB, Stein CM, Wilkinson GR, and Roden DM. Inhibition of P-glycoprotein-mediated drug transport. A unifying mechanism to explain the interaction between digoxin and quinidine. Circulation 99:552–557 (1999).

89. Waldorff S, Hansen PB, Egeblad H, Berning J, Buch J, Kjaergard H, et al. Interactions between digoxin and potassium-sparing diuretics. Clin Pharmacol Ther 33:418–423 (1983).

90. Dorian P, Strauss M, Cardella C, David T, East S, and Ogilvie R. Digoxin-cyclosporine interaction: severe digitalis toxicity after cyclosporine treatment. Clin Invest Med 11:108–112 (1988).

91. Leibovitz A, Bilchinsky T, Gil I, and Habot B. Elevated serum digoxin level associated with coadministered fluoxetine. Arch Intern Med 158:1152–1153 (1998).

92. DePace NL, Herling IH, Kotler ML, Hakki AH, Spielman SR, and Segal BL. Intravenous nitroglycerin for rest angina. Potential pathophysiologic mechanisms of action. Arch Intern Med 142:1806–1809 (1982).

93. Kaplan K, Divison R, Parker M, Przybylek J, Teagarden JR, and Lesch M. Intravenous nitroglycerin for treatment of unstable angina unresponsive to standard nitrate therapy. Am J Cardiol 51:694 (1983).
94. Karlberg KE, Saldeen T, Wallin R, Henriksson P, Nyquist O, and Sylven C. Intravenous nitroglycerin reduces ischaemia in unstable angina pectoris: a double-blind placebo-controlled study. J Intern Med 243:25–31 (1998).
95. Curfman GD, Heinsimes JA, Lozner EC, and Fung HL. Intravenous nitroglycerin in the treatment of spontaneous angina pectoris: a prospective randomized trial. Circulation 67: 276–282 (1983).
96. Horowitz JD. Role of nitrates in unstable angina pectoris. Am J Cardiol 70:64B (1992).
97. Packer M, Lee WH, Kessler PD, Gottlieb SS, Medina N, and Yushak M. Prevention and reversal of nitrate tolerance in patients with congestive heart failure. N Engl J Med 317: 799–804 (1987).
98. May DC, Popma JJ, Black WH, Schaefer S, Lee HR, Levine BD, et al. In vivo induction and reversal of nitroglycerin tolerance in human coronary arteries. N Engl J Med 317: 805–809 (1987).
99. Winniford MD, Kennedy PL, Wells PJ, and Hillis LD. Potentiation of nitroglycerin-induced coronary dilation by N-acetylcysteine. Circulation 73:138–142 (1986).
100. Horowitz JD, Henry CA, Syrjanen ML, Louis WJ, Fish RD, Smith TW, et al. Combined use of nitroglycerin and N-acetylcysteine in the management of unstable angina pectoris. Circulation 77:787–794 (1988).
101. Ardissino D, Merlini PA, Savonitto S, Demicheli G, Zanini P, Bertocchi F, et al. Effect of transdermal nitroglycerin or N-acetylcysteine, or both, in the long-term treatment of unstable angina pectoris. J Am Coll Cardiol 29:941–947 (1997).
102. Jackson G. Erectile dysfunction and cardiovascular disease. Int J Clin Pract 53:363–368 (1999).
103. DeBusk R, Drory Y, Goldstein I, Jackson G, Kaul S, Kimmel SE, et al. Management of sexual dysfunction in patients with cardiovascular disease: recommendations of The Princeton Consensus Panel. Am J Cardiol 86:175–181 (2000).
104. Rose BD. Diuretics. Kidney Int 39:336–352 (1991).
105. Bronner F. Renal calcium transport: mechanisms and regulation. An overview. Am J Physiol 257:F707–F711 (1989).
106. Leaf A, Schwartz WB, and Relman AS. Oral administration of a potent carbonic anhydrase inhibitor ("Diamox"). I. Changes in electrolyte and acid-base balance. N Engl J Med 250: 759–764 (1954).
107. Batlle DC, von Riotte AB, Gaviria M, and Grupp M. Amelioration of polyuria by amiloride in patients receiving long-term lithium therapy. N Engl J Med 312:408–414 (1985).
108. Freedman MD. Oral anticoagulants: pharmacodynamics, clinical indications and adverse effects. J Clin Pharmacol 32:196–209 (1992).
109. Hirsh J, Dalen JE, Anderson DR, Poller L, Bussey H, Ansell J, et al. Oral anticoagulants: mechanism of action, clinical effectiveness, and optimal therapeutic range. Chest 114:445S–469S (1998).
110. Altman R, Rouvier J, and Gurfinkel E. Oral anticoagulant treatment with and without aspirin. Thromb Haemost 74:506–510 (1995).
111. Clouse LH and Comp PC. The regulation of hemostasis: the protein C system. N Engl J Med 314:1298–1304 (1986).
112. Gage BF, Fihn SD, and White RH. Management and dosing of warfarin therapy. Am J Med 109:481–488 (2000).
113. Sbarouni E and Oakley CM. Outcomes of pregnancy in women with valve prosthesis. Br Heart J 71:196–201 (1994).

114. Bauer KA. Coumarin-induced skin necrosis. Arch Dermatol 129:766–768 (1993).
115. Weser JK and Sellers E. Drug interactions with coumarin anticoagulants. N Engl J Med 285:547–558 (1971).
116. MacLeod SM and Sellers EM. Pharmacodynamic and pharmacokinetic drug interactions with coumarin anticoagulants. Drugs 11:461 (1976).
117. Serlin MJ and Breckenridge AM. Drug interactions with warfarin. Drugs 25:610–620 (1983).
118. Aithal GP, Day CP, Kesteven PJ, and Daly AK. Association of polymorphisms in the cytochrome P450 CYP2C9 with warfarin dose requirement and risk of bleeding complications. Lancet 353:717–719 (1999).
119. Taube J, Halsall D, and Baglin T. Influence of cytochrome P-450 CYP2C9 polymorphisms on warfarin sensitivity and risk of over-anticoagulation in patients on long-term treatment. Blood 96:1816–1819 (2000).
120. Hennekens CH, O'Donnell CJ, Ridker PM, and Marder VJ. Current issues concerning thrombolytic therapy for acute myocardial infarction. J Am Coll Cardiol 25(Suppl):18S (1995).
121. The GUSTO Investigators. An international randomized trial comparing four thrombolytic strategies for acute myocardial infarction. N Engl J Med 329:673–682 (1993).
122. Holmes DR Jr, Califf RM, and Topol EJ. Lessons we have learned from the GUSTO trial. J Am Coll Cardiol 25(Suppl):10S (1995).
123. Balsano F, Rizzon P, Violi F, Scrutinio D, Cimminiello C, Aguglia F, et al. Antiplatelet treatment with ticlopidine in unstable angina. Circulation 82:17–26 (1990).
124. Cairns JA, Theroux P, Lewis HD, Ezekowitz M, and Meade TW. Antithrombotic agents in coronary artery disease. Chest 119:228S–252S (2001).
125. Mehta J, Mehta P, Pepine CJ, and Conti CR. Platelet function studies in coronary artery disease. X. Effect of dipyridamole. Am J Cardiol 47:1111–1114 (1981).
126. Antiplatelet Trialists' Collaboration. Collaborative overview of randomised trials of antiplatelet therapy-I: prevention of death, myocardial infarction, and stroke by prolonged antiplatelet therapy in various categories of patients. BMJ 308:81–106 (1994).
127. Patrono C. Aspirin as an antiplatelet drug. N Engl J Med 330:1287–1294 (1994).
128. Wallentin LC, and the RISC Group. Aspirin (75 mg/day) after an episode of unstable coronary artery disease: long-term effects on the risk for myocardial infarction, occurrence of severe angina and the need for revascularization. J Am Coll Cardiol 18:1587–1593 (1991).
129. Sharis PJ, Cannon CP, and Loscalzo J. The antiplatelet effects of ticlopidine and clopidogrel. Ann Intern Med 129:394–405 (1998).
130. Ono K, Kurohara K, Yoshihara M, Shimamoto Y, Yamaguchi M, et al. Agranulocytosis caused by ticlopidine and its mechanism. Am J Hematol 37:239–242 (1991).
131. Steinhubl SR, Tan WA, Foody JM, and Topol EJ, for the EPISTENT investigators. Incidence and clinical course of thrombotic thrombocytopenic purpura due to ticlopidine following coronary stenting. JAMA 281:806–810 (1999).
132. Larsen ML and Illingworth DR. Drug treatment of dyslipoproteinemia. Med Clin North Am 78:225–245 (1994).
133. Brown AS, Bakker-Arkema RG, Yellen L, Henley RW Jr, Guthrie R, Campbell CF, et al. Treating patients with documented atherosclerosis to National Cholesterol Education Program-recommended low-density-lipoprotein cholesterol goals with atorvastatin, fluvastatin, lovastatin and simvastatin. J Am Coll Cardiol 32:665–672 (1998).
134. Auer J and Eber B. Current aspects of statins. J Clin Basic Cardiol 2:203–208 (1999).
135. Brown G, Albers JJ, Fisher LD, Schaefer SM, Lin JT, Kaplan C, et al. Regression of coronary artery disease as a result of intensive lipid-lowering therapy in men with high levels of apolipoprotein B. N Engl J Med 323:1289–1298 (1990).
136. Auer J, Berent R, and Eber B. Lessons learned from trials with statins. Clin Card 24:277–280 (2001).

137. Bakker-Arkema RG, Davidson MH, Goldstein RJ, Davignon J, Isaacsohn JL, Weiss SR, et al. Efficacy and safety of a new HMG CoA reductase inhibitor, atorvastatin, in patients with hypertriglyceridemia. JAMA 276:128–133 (1996).
138. Dart A, Jerums G, Nicholson G, d'Emden M, Hamilton-Craig I, Tallis G, et al. A multicenter, double-blind, one-year study comparing safety and efficacy of atorvastatin versus simvastatin in patients with hypercholesterolemia. Am J Cardiol 80:39 (1997).
139. Grundy SM. HMG-CoA reductase inhibitors for treatment of hypercholesterolemia. N Engl J Med 319:24–33 (1988).
140. Auer J, Berent R, and Eber B. Focus on statins: lipid lowering mechanisms and beyond. Preventive Cardiol 4:89–92 (2001).
141. Auer J, Berent R, Weber T, and Eber B. Clinical significance of pleiotropic effects of statins: lipid reduction and beyond. Curr Med Chem 9:1831–1850 (2002).
142. Schmassmann-Suhijar D, Bullingham R, Gasser R, et al. Rhabdomyolysis due to interaction of simvastatin with mibefradil. Lancet 351:1929–1930 (1998).
143. Pierce LR, Wysowski DK, and Gross TP. Myopathy and rhabdomyolysis with lovastatin-gemfibrozil combination therapy. JAMA 264:71–75 (1990).
144. Athyros VG, Papageorgiou AA, Hatzikonstandinou HA, Didangelos TP, Carina MV, Kranitsas DF, et al. Safety and efficacy of long-term statin-fibrate combination in patients with refractory familial combined hyperlipidemia. Am J Cardiol 80:608–613 (1997).
145. Rosenson RS and Frauenheim WA. Safety of combined pravastatin-gemfibrozil therapy. Am J Cardiol 74:499–500 (1994).
146. Boissonnat P, Salen P, Guidollet J, Ferrera R, Dureau G, Ninet J, et al. The long-term effects of the lipid-lowering agent fenofibrate in hyperlipidemic heart transplant recipients. Transplantation 58:245–247 (1994).
147. Monk JP and Todd JP. Bezafibrate: a review of its pharmacodynamic and pharmacokinetic properties, and therapeutic use in hyperlipidaemia. Drugs 33:539–576 (1987).

PART III
Antibiotics

Chapter 8

Antimicrobial Drugs

Amanda J. Jenkins, PhD and Jimmie L. Valentine, PhD

1. INTRODUCTION

Infectious disease may be defined as a disease that is transmissible or likely to spread *(1)*. In industrial Europe, diseases such as tuberculosis were scourges and doctors and scientists of the day concentrated their efforts to treat and understand these illnesses. In modern times, the types of infectious disease affecting the human population may have changed due to the eradication of diseases such as smallpox, but these diseases still result in significant morbidity and mortality worldwide *(2)*. In the present chapter, we describe most infectious diseases affecting the Western world, with current treatment and antimicrobial options. Thereafter, we discuss the classification, pharmacokinetics, metabolism, drug and herbal interactions, assays, and forensic implications of the antimicrobials.

1.1. Bacterial and Viral Meningitis

Meningitis is an infection of the arachnoid matter in the brain and cerebrospinal fluid (CSF) present in the subarachnoid space *(3)*. Once the infection has broken through the protective meninges membranes it may be rapidly spread throughout the brain by the CSF. If the infection spreads into the brain it may result in a condition known as meningoencephalitis. Meningitis is generally classified into bacterial or viral, although a third category, chronic meningitis, may also be used. Bacteria such as *Escherichia coli, Haemophilus influenzae, Neisseria meningitides*, and pneumococcus usually cause bacterial meningitis or acute pyogenic meningitis. *E. coli* is usually the cause of the infection in the neonate, with *H. influenzae* the culprit in infants and young children. *N. meningitidis* is often the cause of disease in teenagers and young adults and is most often responsible for the spread of the disease since it may be transmitted through the air. Clinically, patients present with fever, headache, sensitivity to light, stiff neck,

From: *Handbook of Drug Interactions: A Clinical and Forensic Guide*
A. Mozayani and L. P. Raymon, eds. © Humana Press Inc., Totowa, NJ

and irritability. Approximately 10–15% of cases are fatal *(4)*. A spinal tap yields cloudy CSF. Treatment is with antibiotics such as aminoglycosides, cephalosporins, chloramphenicol, penicillins, and tetracyclines. Appropriate antibiotic therapy reduces the risk of dying to less than 15%. However, even with treatment, a possible complication of recovery may be hydrocephalus. This development is most common with pneumococcal meningitis. In the immunosuppressed patient, diagnosis may be more difficult as other bacteria may cause the disease and the patient may present with atypical CSF findings.

The causative agent in viral or lymphatic meningitis may not be identified but approximately 90% of cases are caused by enteroviruses such as coxsackieviruses. Common viruses include herpes simplex type II, mumps, and Epstein-Barr virus. Clinical presentation is similar to bacterial meningitis but the course is generally less severe.

1.1.1. Chronic Meningitis

This form of meningitis takes longer to become apparent and is usually caused by *Mycobacterium tuberculosis*. In these cases, the meninges are filled with a gelatin- or fibrous-like substance. Clinically, an individual may present with symptoms of lethargy, headache, vomiting, and mental confusion. One complication of this form of meningitis is that the long-term inflammatory reaction in the subarachnoid space may produce endarteritis, which may result in an infarction.

1.2. Escherichia coli

E. coli is a bacterium with many strains. The majority of strains pose little danger to humans but one strain, *E. coli* serotype O157:H7 is a major cause of food-borne illness *(5)*. It is a gram-negative rod-shaped bacterium producing Shiga toxin. Diagnosis is by detection of the bacterium in the feces. There are approx 73,000 cases annually in the United States. The major source of the bacterium in industrialized countries is ground beef but other sources include unpasteurized milk and juice. The bacterium is water-borne, with transmission occurring by drinking contaminated water or contact with contaminated lakes, ponds, and swimming pools. Clinically, *E. coli* produces bloody diarrhea and abdominal cramps with little fever. Occasionally no symptoms result from the infection. Resolution may take 5–10 d. In some individuals, infection with this strain may cause a hemolytic uremic syndrome resulting in destruction of red blood cells and kidney failure. This complication occurs at a frequency of 2–7%.

Most people do not require treatment and there is no evidence that antibiotic treatment improves the course of the illness. If antibiotic treatment is provided, common antibiotics include aminoglycosides, fluoroquinolones, penicillins, sulfonamides, and trimethoprim-sulfamethoxazole.

Hemolytic uremic syndrome is life threatening and requires intensive medical care. Long-term consequences of *E. coli* infection are related to the severe uremic complication. Approximately 30% of individuals who develop this syndrome will have kidney disease in later years.

Other strains of *E. coli* also produce disease and are referred to as diarrheagenic or non-Shiga toxin-producing *E. coli*. These serotypes are classified into four groups, namely enterotoxigenic (ETEC), enteropathogenic, enteroinvasive, and enteroaggregative *(6)*. The incidence of these strains causing disease is unknown since most laboratories do not have the ability to identify the organisms. Clinical symptoms include watery or bloody diarrhea, abdominal cramps with or without fever, chills, loss of appetite, and muscle aches. ETEC is the main cause of traveler's diarrhea. It is also transmitted by contaminated food or water. As with Shiga toxin *E. coli*, treatment is usually supportive. ETEC may be resistant to antibiotics such as trimethoprim-sulfamethoxazole and ampicillin. Fluoroquinolones may be effective treatment.

1.3. Streptococcal Disease (Groups A and B)

Group A *streptoccoccus* is a bacterium found in the throat and skin. Infections are known as "strep throat." Although a relatively mild disease, these microorganisms may cause more severe illness to spread through direct contact with mucus of an infected person. Treatment with antibiotics such as macrolides, penicillins, quinolones, quinupristin/dalfopristin, teicoplanin, and tetracyclines is effective. Symptoms range from no illness to severe with necrotizing faciitis and toxic shock syndrome (TSS). These latter conditions are known as invasive Group A streptococcal disease. There were approximately 9400 cases of invasive disease in the United States in 1999 *(7)*. Invasive disease results when bacteria enter areas of the body where they are usually absent. Necrotizing faciitis describes the destruction of muscle and skin tissue. Early symptoms include fever, pain, and redness. Treatment may involve surgery to remove necrosed tissue. Streptococcal TSS results in a rapid decrease in blood pressure and organ failure. Signs include shock, fever, dizziness, and confusion. Approximately 20% of individuals with necrotizing faciitis and more than 50% of TSS patients die *(8)*.

If an individual becomes sensitized to streptococcal antigens, rheumatic fever may result. This is a systemic, nonsuppurative inflammatory disease *(3)*. This disease affects the joints, lungs, blood vessels, and the heart. Although an individual may acquire this disease at any age, more than 90% of cases occur between the ages of 5–15 yr *(3)*. Treatment with antibiotics has reduced the death rate significantly over the last 50 yr. Deaths caused by this disease are due to heart damage with involvement of the heart valves.

Group B *streptococcus* is a bacterium that may cause illness especially in the young and elderly. It is the cause of the most common life-threatening infections in newborn babies such as sepsis, meningitis, and pneumonia. In pregnant women, the most common infections include sepsis, amnionitis, and urinary tract infections *(9)*. In other adults, blood, skin, or soft-tissue infections and pneumonia result from exposure to this bacterium. The bacteria may be transmitted from the gastrointestinal and genital tracts intrapartum. The mode of transmission in nonpregnant adults is not known.

Approximately 17,000 cases occur annually in the United States *(10)*. About 16% of adults and 5% of infants with the infection die. Long-term effects may include children with learning problems and hearing and sight loss due to meningitis. Treatment is with antibiotics such as penicillin or ampicillin, which may be administered intravenously.

1.4. **Haemophilus influenzae**

Haemophilus influenzae is a gram-negative coccobacillus. The bacterium enters the human body through the nasopharynx. The bacteria may colonize and remain for months without causing any symptoms. In some individuals, however, the organism causes an invasive infection. The mode of transmission to the blood is unknown but may result in meningitis, epiglottitis, pneumonia, arthritis, and cellulitis *(11)*. Between 2 and 5% of people die with invasive *H. influenzae* disease. Diagnosis should include serotyping a culture since type b is the only form preventable by vaccine. Antimicrobial therapy usually involves 10- to 14-d treatment with chloramphenicol or a cephalosporin such as cefotaxime *(12)*. Other drugs that have been utilized in therapy include bacitracin, penicillins, chloramphenicol, macrolides, quinolones, rifampin, sulfonamides, tetracyclines, and trimethoprin-sulfamethoxazole. Strains of *H. influ*enzae resistant to ampicillin are common throughout the United States and therefore this medication should be avoided.

1.5. Hepatitis

Several hepatitis causing viruses are known, including A, B, C, D, and E. Clinically, patients present with symptoms such as fever, lethargy, nausea, loss of appetite, abdominal pain, and jaundice. The course of disease caused by viral infection of the liver is categorized into several clinical syndromes, namely, the carrier state, acute hepatitis, chronic hepatitis, and fulminant hepatitis *(3)*. The latter results in massive necrosis of the liver and is primarily associated with hepatitis B virus (HBV).

Hepatitis A virus (HAV) is an RNA picornavirus, which may result in infection in humans after an incubation period of 15–50 d *(13)*. The probability of symptoms is age dependent with >70% of infections in young children being asymptomatic. Jaundice is a frequent symptom in adults. Illness may last for about 2 mo although some individuals have prolonged or relapsing illness up to 6 mo. The virus replicates in the liver and is excreted in the feces of an infected individual. A person is most likely to transmit the disease in the 2-wk period before the onset of jaundice. The disease is transmitted by the fecal–oral route and more rarely by transfusion with blood collected from an infected person. Hepatitis A is diagnosed by identification of IgM-anti-Hepatitis A antibody as it cannot be clinically differentiated from other types of viral hepatitis. Approximately 100 people die per year in the United States as a result of liver failure from hepatitis A. A vaccine is available for prophylaxis and may also be administered within 2 wk after contact with an HAV-infected person.

HBV, the most well known hepatitis-causing virus, has a core of double-stranded DNA. It is estimated that more than 1 million people in the United States who have chronic HBV infection are potentially infectious *(14)*. Immunization is the most effective prevention. Transmission is typically by the percutaneous route, blood and blood products, hypodermic needles, and dental and surgical instruments *(3)*. The virus is present in semen, menstrual blood, urine, and feces *(3)*. Like HAV, diagnosis is made by identification of specific serum markers. The incubation period of HBV ranges from 1 to 6 mo and the individual antigen and antibody titers vary throughout the course of the disease. For example, when the patient is asymptomatic markers such as HbsAg are detected but as symptoms appear anti-Hbe and anti-HBs are measured.

Hepatitis C virus (HCV) is an RNA virus that has infected an estimated 4 million Americans *(15)*. HCV is diagnosed by identification of anti-HCV, typically by immunoassay followed by specific confirmation by immunoblot assay. Alternatively, RNA gene amplification techniques may be utilized. Many people with acute HCV are asymptomatic. Less than 30% develop jaundice. Progression to chronic liver disease may take many years after exposure. Cirrhosis may occur in 10–20% of individuals with chronic HCV. Antiviral therapy such as α-interferon is recommended for patients with chronic HCV who are at high risk for developing cirrhosis (e.g., alcoholics). Alternative therapy using a combination of interferon and ribavirin has FDA (Food and Drug Administration) approval for use in patients who have relapsed after interferon treatment.

Hepatitis D virus (HDV) is a single-strand RNA virus that requires the presence of HBV to replicate. Infection may be acquired with HBV or as a superinfection in individuals with chronic HBV infection *(16)*. The former category of individuals generally develops more severe acute disease and is at greater risk of developing fulminant hepatitis than the latter. Transmission of HDV is similar to the other viruses although sexual transmission appears to be less efficient than for HBV. The type of antibodies detected in serum of infected individuals is dependent on whether the virus has been acquired as a coinfection with HBV. In people who are coinfected both IgM anti-HDV, and IgG anti-HDV are detected. Hepatitis Delta Antigen can be detected in serum in only about 25% of patients with HDV-HBV infection. There is currently no treatment available to prevent HDV infection in an individual with chronic HBV.

Hepatitis E virus (HEV) is a spherical single stranded RNA virus that is the major cause of non-A, non-B hepatitis. The incubation period is 15–60 d after HEV exposure. Although symptoms of HEV exposure are similar to other types of viral hepatitis, less common symptoms include diarrhea and a urticarial rash. There is no evidence of chronic infection with HEV. IgM and IgG anti-HEV are produced after HEV infection. Currently there are no commercially available tests to identify HEV in the United States although serologic tests using enzyme immunoassays and Western Blot techniques are utilized in research laboratories. Transmission of this virus is mainly by the fecal–oral route. Person-to-person transmission is relatively rare with this hepatitis virus *(17)*.

Additional drug therapy for hepatitis includes the immunoglobulins, entecavir (HBV), and lamivudine.

1.6. Herpes

Herpes simplex virus (HSV) type I causes an oral infection, known as "fever blisters" *(18)*. Herpes simplex type II is commonly associated with herpes genitalis. The latter is caused by HSV II in approximately 80% of cases. Herpes genitalis is a sexually transmitted disease. Two forms are recognized clinically (primary and recurrent) but both forms result in vesicular and ulcerative lesions. The initial infection is associated with more numerous painful lesions, fever, and headache due to lack of immunity. Recurrent lesions tend to be less severe and less far-reaching with little systemic illness *(19)*. Transmission to neonates is possible in infected pregnant women. If a woman is infected near the time of delivery, there is a 1:2 likelihood of the newborn developing neonatal herpes *(3)*. This disease is potentially fatal due to the resulting generalized severe encephalitis. Other diseases caused by the HSV include HSV I encephalitis resulting in hemorrhagic necrosis, and herpetic viral meningitis (HSV II).

There is no cure for genital herpes but antimicrobial treatments such as acyclovir, dicofovir, docosanol, famiciclovir, fomivirsen, foscarnet, ganciclovir, idoxuridine, penciclovir, trifuridine, valacyclovir, valganciclovir, and vidarabine can prevent and shorten recurrent episodes.

1.7. Legionnaires' Disease

Legionellosis is a disease caused by the bacterium *Legionella pneumophilia*, which is found in water systems. The infection may present as Legionnaires' disease (LD) or Pontiac fever (PF). The former is the more severe form that is characterized by pneumonia, fever, chills, and a cough, whereas PF presents as an acute flu-like illness with fever and muscle aches. Other Legionella species may also cause these conditions but in the United States more than 90% of cases are caused by *L. pneumophilia (20)*. Fewer than 20,000 cases of LD and PF occur each year in the United States but 5–15% of LD cases are fatal. Person-to-person transmission does not occur and infection is caused by inhalation of contaminated aerosols. PF generally does not require treatment as individuals usually recover in a few days. LD may be effectively treated with erythromycin. Rifampin may be coadministered in severe cases. Other drugs include the macrolides, quinolones, quinupristin/dalfopristin, and tetracyclines.

1.8. Salmonellosis

The estimated incidence of salmonellosis is about 1.4 million cases per year in the United States, with about 500 fatalities *(21)*. Salmonellosis is an infection caused by the gram-negative bacterium *Salmonella*. This bacterium includes three species, *Salmonella typhi*, *Salmonella cholerae-suis*, and *Salmonella enteriditis*. The bacteria are transmitted to humans by eating food contaminated with the organism, usually from animal feces. There are several distinct clinical syndromes caused by this bacterium. The most severe is typhoid fever, which is caused exclusively by *S. typhi*. Other conditions include gastroenteritis; bacteremia; enteric fevers; localized infections in bones, joints, etc.; and asymptomatic carriers. Gastroenteritis is the most common form of infection and involves fever, diarrhea, and abdominal cramps. The illness resolves in 4–7 d and most individuals recover without treatment providing dehydration is prevented. Antibiotics are not usually necessary unless the infection extends beyond the intestinal tract. Ampicillin, gentamicin, trimethoprim-sulfamethoxazole, or ciprofloxacin may be administered. Other medications include aminopenicillins, chloramphenicol, fluoroquinolones, polymixin B, and the tetracyclines. Clinical signs of typhoid fever include lethargy, fever with bacteremic chills, and abdominal pain. By the second week the spleen enlarges and a rash may appear. The fever is now persistent. If untreated, the fever is accompanied by confusion and delirium by the third week of the disease. Complications include infective endocarditis and intestinal hemorrhage and perforation *(3)*.

1.9. Toxic Shock Syndrome

TSS is caused by a bacterium, *Staphylococcus aureus*. In the United States, the incidence of this illness is 1–2 per 100,000 women 15–44 yr of age *(22)*. This organism flourishes in skin and mucous membranes. It has been associated with the use of tampons and barrier contraceptive devices. It may also occur as a complication of surgery or abscesses. Symptoms include rash, fever, diarrhea, and muscle pains. More serious symptoms include hypotension and multisystem failure. Approximately 5% of TSS cases result in death. Treatment includes an antibiotic regimen using drugs such as the macrolides, penicillin G, quinolones, quinupristin/dalfopristin, teicoplanin, or the tetracyclines.

1.10. Tuberculosis

In 2000, there were at least 16,000 reported tuberculosis (TB) cases in the United States *(23)*. TB is a chronic granulomatous disease caused by the bacterium *Mycobacterium tuberculosis (3)*. The bacteria may infect any part of the body but typically involves the lungs. Most infections are acquired by direct transmission of airborne droplets of organisms from an individual with active TB by inhalation to another. After exposure, most people are able to resist disease and the bacteria become inactive, but viable organisms may remain dormant in the lungs for many years. This is called latent TB infection *(3)*. These individuals have no symptoms, do not have active disease, and therefore cannot transmit the organisms to other people. However, they may develop disease if untreated. TB disease occurs when the immune system is unable to prevent the bacteria from multiplying. People with weak immune systems are susceptible to development of the disease. These include individuals with diabetes mellitus, silicosis, substance abuse, severe kidney disease, or leukemia. Symptoms depend on the area of the body where the bacteria are growing. In the lungs, the individual may develop a cough (and may cough up blood) and pain in the chest. Other symptoms include weight loss, weakness or fatigue, chills, fever, and night sweats. TB may be treated with several drugs including amikacin, aminosalicylic acid, capreomycin, cycloserine, ethambutol, ethionamide, isoniazid, kanamycin, pyrazinamide, rifampin, and streptomycin. The most common drugs used to treat this communicable disease are isoniazid (INH), rifampin, ethambutol, pyrazinamide, and streptomycin. Treatment usually involves taking multiple medications.

2. CLASSIFICATION OF ANTIMICROBIALS

There have been a number of attempts to classify antibiotics or antivirals based upon both chemical structure *(24)* and mechanism of action *(25,26)*. The former method fails with regard to many of the newer antibiotics and antivirals whereas the latter type of classification system based on mechanism of action is sometimes deficient because the mechanism of action of all antibiotics is not clearly elucidated. The antivirals are different but like the antibiotics their purpose is to disrupt the normal physiological status of the parasitic organism (a virus, in the case of antivirals). Thus, the best method for classifying antimicrobials (a term used here to include both antibiotics and antivirals) combines elements of both types of classification. This can be illustrated in Fig. 1, which shows antibiotics that inhibit bacterial cell wall synthesis (the mechanism of action) may have both similar and dissimilar chemical structures. For example, the penicillins and cephalosporins, with their common β-lactam ring, have similar chemical structures whereas vancomycin is dissimilar, yet all have a mode of action that involves inhibition of bacterial cell wall synthesis. Table 1 lists the major classifications of antimicrobials with regard to chemical structure and/or mechanism of action.

3. PHARMACOKINETICS OF ANTIMICROBIALS

Classical pharmacokinetics of therapeutic drugs describes the rate of absorption, distribution, and elimination following drug administration. Antimicrobials, however,

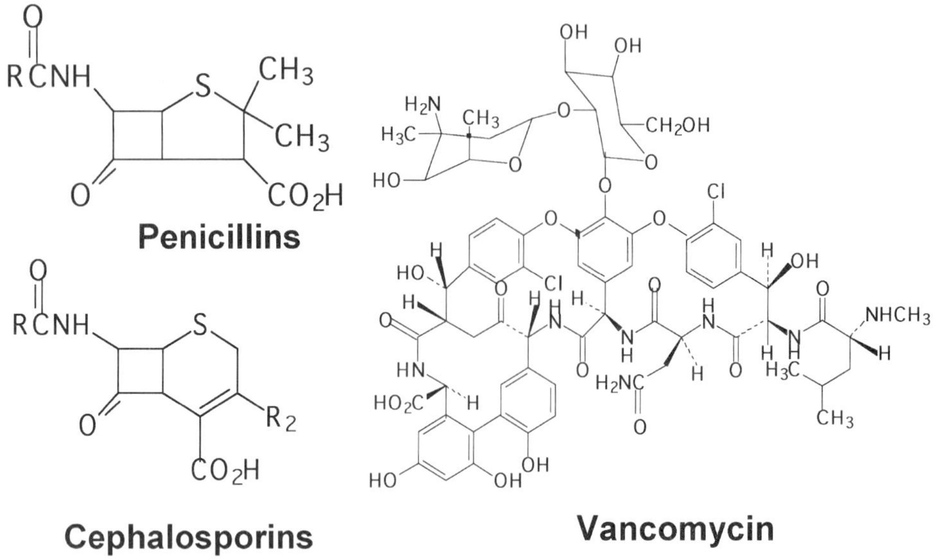

Fig. 1. Chemical structure of antibiotics.

must be considered differently than most therapeutic drugs since although the host is administered the drug, the microbe must also absorb, distribute, and eliminate the drug, at a rate that is usually independent of the host. For many therapeutic drugs where absorption is comparable, the observed pharmacological effects can be correlated with the rate drug is removed from the central compartment (systemic circulation) through processes of metabolism, redistribution, or elimination. This is the basis for performing therapeutic monitoring and adjusting a patient's dose based upon a determination of the drug or a metabolite in a physiological fluid that can describe what is happening in the central compartment. An example is digoxin, whose blood level can be measured and a therapeutic range established that should produce the desired effect, i.e., increase the strength of contractility in the failing heart, without producing the toxic effect of arrhythmia. In contrast, the observed pharmacological effect with an antimicrobial depends upon the parasite (microbe) suffering a toxic effect such as inhibition of growth or cellular disruption without concurrent toxic effects to the host, not just disappearance from the central compartment of the host. Thus, it often becomes difficult to equate the experimentally determined pharmacokinetics of an antibiotic with a therapeutic response. Rather, therapeutic monitoring of antimicrobials is more often done to prevent a toxic response in the host. For example, monitoring the peak and trough levels of aminoglycosides to prevent oto- or nephrotoxicity in the host. A typical clinical protocol utilizes two serum concentrations to define the therapeutic range to prevent the known toxicities. A so-called "peak" level is obtained 30 min following dosing and a "trough" level determined 30 min prior to the next dose. For gentamicin, these levels should be in the range of 6–10 µg/mL for the peak level and 0.5–2 µg/mL for the trough level. For such levels to be meaningful, they should be drawn when the drug is near a steady-state concentration, usually after three or more doses.

8. Antimicrobial Drugs

Table 1
Classification of Antimicrobial Agents

Classification: Mechanism of Action	Classification: Chemical Structure	Examples
Inhibit bacterial cell wall synthesis	β-Lactams; azoles	Penicillins, cephalosporins, vancomycin, cycloserine, bacitracin, azole antifungals (clotrimazole, fluconazole, itraconazole, ketoconazole)
Affect permeability of bacterial cell membrane and lead to leakage of intracellular compounds	Detergents, polyenes	Polymyxin, polyene antifungals (nystatin, amphotericin B)
Affect function of 30S and 50S ribosomal subunits causing a reversible inhibition of protein synthesis	Macrolides, tetracyclines	Chloramphenicol, tetracyclines, macrolides (erythromycin, clarithromycin, azithromycin) clindamycin, pristinamycins (quinupristin/dalfopristin)
Binding to 30S ribosomal subunit altering protein synthesis leading to bacterial cell death	Aminoglycosides	Aminoglycosides (gentamicin, tobramycin, kanamycin, streptomycin), spectinomycin
Inhibit bacterial nucleic acid metabolism via inhibition of polymerase (rifamycins) or topoisomerases (quinolones)	Rifamycins, Quinolones	Rifamycins (rifampin, rifabutin, rifapentine), quinolones
Antimetabolites—blocking essential enzymes of bacterial folate metabolism	Sulfonamides	Trimethoprim/sulfamethoxazole, sulfonamides
Antivirals: Type 1: Nucleic acid analogs that inhibit viral DNA a. polymerase or b. reverse transcriptase	Pyridine nucleosides	Acyclovir, ganciclovir Zidovudine, lamivudine
Type 2: Nonnucleoside reverse transcriptase inhibitors		Nevirapine, efavirenz, delavirdine
Type 3: Inhibitors of essential viral enzymes, e.g., a. HIV protease or b. influenza neuraminidase		Sauuinavir, indinavir, ritonavir, nelfinavir, amprenavir, lopinavir Amantadine, rimantadine, zanamivir

3.1. Host–Parasite Considerations

Coupled with the host–parasite pharmacokinetic descriptions, the phagocytic complex produced by the immune response of the patient (host) toward the parasite must also be considered. That is, once the host in response to a parasitic invasion mobilizes an immune response, will the phagocytic complex absorb the antimicrobial agent and will its typical mechanism of action be operative within the complex? In short, the answer to this question is that antimicrobial agents work in concert with the immune system as evidenced by the fact that a person that is immune compromised will often not respond in the desired manner to antimicrobial therapy. This is indirect evidence that antimicrobials penetrate phagocytes and augment destruction of the microorganism. Some direct evidence also exists that antibiotics are absorbed into phagocytes. Tulkens *(27)* discussed evidence that beta-lactams diffuse into but do not accumulate in phagocytes because of their acidic character and aminoglycosides being too polar to readily cross membranes are taken up slowly by endocytosis resulting exclusively in lysosomal localization. This investigator also discussed licosaminides, macrolides, and fluoroquinolones that accumulate in phagocytes, with the two former antibiotics exhibiting accumulation in both cytosolic and lysosomal localization, whereas the fluoroquinolones appear to be entirely soluble in bacterial cells. Using a *S. aureus*-infected line of macrophages, the author was able to demonstrate that the macrolides and to a greater extent the fluoroquinolones reduced the original inoculum.

Another factor that must be considered is the presentation of the antimicrobial agent to the loci of infection. Such sites of infection might occur in soft tissues, joints, or bones that have limited blood perfusion. Similarly, the central nervous system (CNS) has limited availability to most antimicrobials due to the blood–brain barrier. Some of the antimicrobials exist as anions at physiological pH and are actively transported out of the CNS following passive diffusion into the CNS. Thus the net concentration gradient favors passage of the antibiotic out of the CNS. With an inflamed meninges passive diffusion of many antimicrobials into the CNS occurs at an increased rate shifting the net concentration gradient in favor of agent into the CNS. But as the CNS infection is arrested, the gradient in the opposite direction is restored. With such inaccessible sites, successful therapy will depend upon achieving what is referred to as the minimum inhibitory concentration, the so-called MIC. The concept of MIC relates to the lowest concentration of antibiotic that will prevent visible growth of bacteria in serially diluted concentrations of the bacteria in either agar or broth. Passive diffusion of the antibiotic to the site of infection at or above the MIC would be expected to produce inhibition of bacterial growth. Recently, evidence has been reported that a sub-MIC level might enhance phagocytosis by macrophages. Nosanchuk et al. *(28)* demonstrated that the major antifungal drugs used in the treatment of cryptococcosis, amphotericin B and fluconazole, would enhance phagocytosis of macrophages at subinhibitory concentration. The results suggest that the normal mechanism of action, altering cell wall permeability or inhibiting cell wall synthesis, respectively (Table 1) can cooperate with humoral and cellular immune defense systems in controlling fungal infection even at sub-MIC concentrations. Thus, as emphasized above, a functional immune system is important to the therapeutic effectiveness of the antimicrobial agent.

3.2. Antimicrobial Absorption

In general, enteral, parenteral, and topical administration can be used with most classes of antimicrobials, although there are exceptions based upon physicochemical properties of the specific agent. All routes of administration, with the exception of intravenous, will have a distinct absorption phase, that is, a lag time until the antimicrobial

8. Antimicrobial Drugs

reaches its maximum concentration in blood plasma, often referred to as C_{pmax}, following administration.

The enteral route of administration offers the most complex set of physiological barriers to absorption. One of the most formidable barriers is pH found in various segments of the gastrointestinal tract. The effect of pH is basically twofold. First, the antimicrobial drug may be labile to acid or base hydrolysis. Typically, pH in the stomach is acidic (approximately 2.0) and that of the intestine is basic (approximately 8.0). For example, penicillin G is rapidly hydrolyzed by stomach acid and less than one-third of it would be absorbed. Converting penicillin G to the potassium salt forms penicillin VK, which is acid resistant and permits adequate oral bioavailability. The second factor related to pH is the relationship that exists between it and the acid dissociation constant (pK_a) of the antimicrobial drug. Depending upon the pK_a of an antimicrobial, the possibility exists that the antimicrobial will become ionized. Since the unionized form generally is required for passive diffusion across the lipid membranes that constitute the gastrointestinal tract, bioavailability of the dosage form can be limited. Sulfonamides illustrate this principle since most members of the class have a pK_a value in the range of 4.9–7.7 *(24)*. Applying the principles of the Henderson-Hasselbach equation,

$$pK_a - pH = \log (\text{ionized drug/unionized drug})$$

It is apparent that at the intestinal pH of approximately 8.0, it would be anticipated that the sulfonamides would exist mainly as the unionized form and be absorbed via passive diffusion. This is in fact the case for all the sulfonamides, which are absorbed well when given orally, the exception being sulfasalazine, which is a prodrug designed to be metabolized in the distal portion of the small intestine and colon for a local action. Once the sulfonamide is absorbed into the systemic circulation where the pH is 7.4, it exists mainly in the unionized form and can cross other membrane barriers in the body as well as penetrate the microbial organism via passive diffusion as described in the subsequent section.

pK_a of the antimicrobial agent may also determine whether it can form complexes with other coadministered drugs. For example, fluoroquinolones such as ofloxacin, lomefloxacin, norfloxacin, and ciprofloxacin have ionizable groups with pK_a values close to neutrality *(25)*. The optimum pH for complexation with iron (III) was found to be 3.8 *(26)*. Thus, it would be expected that concurrent administration of iron with a fluoroquinone would reduce the bioavailability of both drugs due to complexation in the acid environment of the stomach.

Oral absorption of tetracyclines can be inhibited by virtue of the fact that because of their chemical structure, sites for chelation are present. Thus concurrent administration of over-the-counter antacids containing calcium, aluminum, zinc, silicate, or bismuth subsalicylate *(27)* or formulations of iron or vitamins containing iron *(28)* will form chelated complexes that are not absorbed across gastric mucosa. In a similar manner, calcium contained in dairy products will form chelation complexes that will inhibit absorption of the tetracyclines *(29)*.

Another barrier to antimicrobial absorption is metabolism of the administered drug by isozymes found in the wall and clefts of the gastrointestinal tract. Such metabolism would convert the nonpolar, lipid-soluble antimicrobial into a polar, more water-soluble metabolite. Because of the change in physicochemical properties, the metabolite would not be available for passive diffusion across the lipoid membranes of the gastrointestinal tract. Specific examples of this barrier to absorption are given in the subsequent section on Antimicrobial Metabolism.

3.3. Antimicrobial Distribution

Following the absorptive process, the antimicrobial agent is transported throughout the body via systemic circulation. The blood pH 7.4 and the inherent pK_a of the antimicrobial drug will determine the unionized to ionized ratio. That portion of the antimicrobial drug that is ionized can be bound to blood proteins, the most notable being albumin, through electrostatic interactions. That portion that is unionized or often termed the "free drug" is available to diffuse across cellular membranes. This "free drug" is also referred to as the "pharmacologically active" portion of the absorbed drug since in order to interact with a receptor to produce an effect, the drug has to transverse the protective cellular membrane. As noted above, with antimicrobial drugs it is advantageous for no host pharmacological action to occur; rather it is hoped that the microbe will be the recipient of the toxic effects of the antimicrobial agent. In *E. coli* it has been shown that the intracellular pH and the pK_a of the sulfonamide determine the passive diffusion rate across the bacteria membrane *(30)*.

Antimicrobial agents must reach deep-seated parts of the body that harbinger microbes if they are to be effective. Some examples will illustrate this principle. First, antimicrobial agents must penetrate into the mucus and crypts of the gastrointestinal tract to eradicate *Campylobacter pylori*. Such penetration by the antimicrobial agent has been determined by physicochemical properties of the antimicrobial, such as pK_a, stability and activity over a wide range of pH, and lipid solubility *(31)*. A second example is penetration of antimicrobials into infections involving cysts in patients with autosomal-dominant polycystic kidney disease *(32)*. In 10 patients with this disease, blood, urine, and cyst fluid was analyzed at either surgery or autopsy for antibiotic concentrations. Drugs active against anaerobes, such as metronidazole and clindamycin, were present in therapeutic concentrations in the cysts. Ampicillin, trimetoprim-sulfamethoxazole, erythromycin, vancomycin, and cefotaxime were likewise found in the cysts but not aminoglycosides. These authors suggested that this was due to the favorable physicochemical properties of the penetrating drugs, viz, pK_a and lipid solubility. A third example will illustrate how a concomitantly administered drug can enhance the bioavailability of an antimicrobial agent into a deep-seated area of the body. Patients undergoing cataract surgery were given an intravenous infusion of ceftazidime, cefotaxime, aztreonam, or ceftriaxone along or without oral acetazolamide *(33)*. Difference in aqueous humor concentration with concurrent administration of acetazolamide was statistically significant demonstrating that transmembrane penetration of antimicrobials into a deep-seated compartment like the eye can be accomplished. A fourth example illustrates that antimicrobial agents can penetrate into bone that has limited vascular circulation *(34)*. Two groups of patients each containing four persons received either 1 g oxacillin or 1 g cefazolin preoperatively then had cervical discs removed and concentration of antibiotic measured. Two other groups of four persons each received 2 g of drug instead of the 1 g given the other groups. Antibiotic levels were detected in all discs but were only quantifiable in the 2-g-dosed groups. This study demonstrated that larger doses of an antimicrobial agent would be required to treat a bone infection.

8. Antimicrobial Drugs

Table 2
Cytochrome Isoforms Metabolizing Antimicrobials

Antimicrobial Chemical Structure	Cytochrome (CYP) Isoform Responsible for Metabolism
Azoles	2C9, 2C19 (fluconazole)
Macrolides	3A4
Rifamycins	2C9, 2C19, 3A4 (rifampicin an inducer)
Quinolones	1A2
Sulfonamides	2C9
Pyridine nucleotides	1A2, 3A4 (zidovudine)
	3A4 (nevirapine, saquinavir, indinavir, ritonavir, nelfinavir)
	3A4 (efavirenz an inducer)

3.4. Host Metabolism of Antimicrobials

Metabolism of antimicrobial agents in the host (human patient) occurs by either Phase I (oxidative) and/or Phase II (conjugation) mechanisms. Metabolism of the β-lactam antimicrobials occurs mainly as a result of parasite enzymes as discussed in a subsequent section. Most Phase I metabolism of antimicrobials in humans occurs through a superfamily of mixed-function monooxygenase enzymes termed the cytochromes P450 or abbreviated CPY *(35)*. The different cytochromes are divided into families based upon their protein and DNA homology *(36)*. Six of these enzyme families mediate the oxidative metabolism of most drugs, viz, CYP1A2, CYP2C9, CYP2C19, CYP2D6, CYP2E1, and CYP3A4 *(37)*. These families of isoenzymes are well known for many clinically relevant drug–drug interactions *(38–42)* and most have rather specific drug substrates. Many antimicrobials discussed in the present context are metabolized by either CYP1A2, CYP2C9, CYP2C19, and/or CYP3A4. Table 2 is a current listing of those antimicrobials known to be metabolized by these isoforms. Phase II metabolism of some antimicrobials is accomplished by glucuronide conjugation with the uridine 5'-diphospho-glucuronosyltransferase (UGT) family of enzymes. Various isoforms exist for the UGT family, with each isoform exhibiting substrate specificity for different drugs *(43,44)*. The multigene superfamily of human UGT includes more than 24 genes and cDNAs, of which 16 are functional and encode full-length proteins *(45,46)*, 8 are encoded by the UGT1A locus (1A1, 1A3, 1A4, 1A6, 1A7, 1A8, 1A9, 1A10) *(47, 48)*, and 8 are encoded by UGT2 genes (2A1, 2B4, 2B7, 2B10, 2B11, 2B15, 2B17, and 2B28) *(49)*. At the present time, those antimicrobials that are known to form glucuronides have not been characterized for the specific UGT isoform responsible for the transformation. For, example, zidovudine (AZT) is metabolized to its inactive glucuronide by UGT and this conversion can be inhibited by fluconazole *(50)*, presumably by competitive inhibition. Two other types of Phase II metabolism have been reported but not fully examined to date, viz, glutathione conjugation with activated sulfonamides *(51,52)* and N-acetylation of amantadine *(53,54)*.

From a number of studies, information is available on which CYP family a particular therapeutic drug is a substrate. For example, tolbutamide, an oral hypoglycemic drug which is structurally similar to the sulfonamides, is known to be a substrate for CYP2C9 producing hydroxytolbutamide as the metabolite *(55)*. Thus, it would be reasonable to expect that coadministration of a sulfonamide and tolbutamide might alter the metabolic degradation of the latter due to competitive inhibition of CYP2C9. This has been demonstrated both in vivo *(56)* and in vitro *(57)*. In the former study, the area under the curve (AUC) for tolbutamide was increased fivefold when coadministered with sulfaphenazole, a sulfonamide used in tuberculosis. In the latter study, sulfaphenazole was shown to possess the greatest inhibition of tolbutamide in human liver CYP2C9 followed by sulfadiazine, sulfamethizole, sulfisoxazole, and sulfamethoxazole.

CYP2C9 is involved mostly in metabolism of polar acidic drugs *(58)* and is competitively inhibited by the sulfonamides listed above, tolbutamide, nonsteroidal antiinflammatory drugs *(59,60)*, COX-2 inhibitors *(61,62)*, phenytoin, selective serotonin reuptake inhibitors (SSRIs), *(63)*, and warfarin *(64)*. The other major cytochrome family responsible for antimicrobial metabolism, CYP3A4, is responsible for metabolism of about 50% of all therapeutic agents *(65)*. Both CYP2C9 and CYP3A4 are found in human liver and intestine *(66)*, but evidence to date indicates that CYP3A4 is the predominant form present in intestine and is inducible with rifampin *(67)*. Because each cytochrome family has many different therapeutic drugs as substrates, there exists the potential for administration of an antimicrobial to affect the metabolism of a concurrently administered therapeutic agent by competitive inhibition that may result in one of the following:

1. Increasing therapeutic drug concentration.
2. Decreasing therapeutic drug concentration.
3. Increasing antimicrobial concentration.
4. Decreasing antimicrobial concentration.

In instances 1 and 2, the severity of the observed effect will depend upon the therapeutic index of the drug. For example, if the therapeutic drug has a very small therapeutic to toxic ratio, the coadministration of an antimicrobial drug may have a deleterious effect if both are metabolized by the same cytochrome isoenzyme system. This narrow range of toxic to therapeutic ratio was brought to light with the prokinetic agent, cisapride, used for the treatment of gastrointestinal disorders, particularly gastroesophageal reflux in adults and children. Cisapride is metabolized by CYP3A4 *(68)*. Coadministration with the macrolide antibiotics produced potentially fatal arrhythmias *(69–71)*. This was shown to be due to an increase of unmetabolized cisapride due to competition between the macrolide antibiotic and cisapride for the CYP3A4 isozyme.

A similar situation was discovered when the antifungal drug, ketoconazole, was ingested concurrently with the nonsedating antihistamine, terfenadine. Fatal cardiac arrhythmias occurred *(72)* and were found to be due to a competition for CYP3A4 metabolism wherein terfenadine's metabolism was blocked *(73)*. This increase in terfenadine concentration unmasked its ability to block fast potassium channels in the heart resulting in cardiac conduction delays *(74)*.

Though many examples could be cited concerning alterations of a therapeutic drug's effect when coadministered with an antimicrobial agent, examination of cyclosporine will be instructive and illustrate the clinical problem *(75)*. Cyclosporine, a common immunosuppressive drug, is administered after human organ transplants. Rifampicin decreases cyclosporine blood concentrations below the limit of detection of many assays, whereas erythromycin and ketoconazole increase its concentration. Similarly, sulfadimidine and trimethoprim have been reported to increase cyclosporine levels.

8. Antimicrobial Drugs

Other macrolide antibiotics and azole antifungal agents as well as fluoroquinolones increase cyclosporine levels. Obviously, concomitant use of these antimicrobial agents with cyclosporine would require adjustment of the cyclosporine dose to achieve optimal immunosuppression.

In some cases, two different classes of antimicrobial agents might be concurrently administered. For example, in the treatment of TB sometimes two different rifamycins may be coadministered with a macrolide. This can be illustrated by rifampicin and rifabutin, both of which are inducers of CYP3A4, decreasing the blood level of clarithromycin (a macrolide antibiotic), which is also metabolized by CPY3A4 *(76)*.

Erythromycin has been suggested as a probe to determine the extent of CYP3A4 activity in an individual. The underlying concept is that a person's CYP3A4 activity could be determined and used as a predictor of potential drug interactions, since CYP3A4 has such a prominent role in the metabolism of drugs. In the so-called erythromycin breath test *(77)*, a subject is administered ^{14}C-N-methyl-erythromycin (3μCi) intravenously. The radiolabeled CO_2 from N-demethylation mediated by CYP3A4 is determined in subsequent breath samples. Although this test has been widely explored, it has been found that oral probes will augment the information obtained by intravenous labeled erythromycin since CYP3A4 is also found in intestinal epithelium. The benzodiazepine, midazolam, is often used for this test *(78,79)*. An interesting use of the erythromycin breath test has been to investigate variations in CYP3A4 metabolism in HIV patients *(80)*. This study suggested that HIV patients had greater variability in hepatic activity of CYP3A4 and this may explain the variations often seen in the plasma concentrations of protease inhibitors like indinavir.

3.5. Elimination of Antimicrobials

Antimicrobials are eliminated from the body by a variety of pathways including excretion into the urine, bile, sweat, milk, and feces depending upon their physicochemical properties. Renal elimination occurs for many of the antimicrobials by several mechanisms, viz, glomerular or tubular, but there also exists a possibility of passive reabsorption occurring in the proximal tubule. If the antimicrobial is not bound to blood proteins, it can be effectively removed by glomerular filtration that is facilitated using passive diffusion of the unionized drug with a molecular size less than that of proteins. In general, the rate of clearance of the glomerulus is about 120 mL/min; therefore, if the observed clearance of the antimicrobial is greater than 120 mL/min, a combination of glomeruli and tubular excretion must be occurring. If the antimicrobial is ionized at physiological pH, it could be excreted by an active transport system in either the proximal or distal tubule. Examples of antimicrobials excreted by both passive glomerular and active proximal tubular secretion are the penicillins and cephalosporins. For example, penicillin G has a renal clearance rate of >200 mL/min and approximates that of plasma flow since both passive and active renal transport is occurring. Probenecid will effectively compete with penicillin G for active transport in the tubule and results in an increased blood level of penicillin G and a prolonged half-life. In a similar way, many of the pyridine nucleotides antimicrobials, such as acyclovir, ganciclovir, and zidovudine, are actively transported in the renal tubule *(81)*. As an example, valaciclovir, a prodrug form of acyclovir, has its renal excretion altered by coadministration of either cimetidine or probenecid, the former most likely due to inhibition of liver CYP3A4 and the latter due to competition for active tubular excretion *(82)*.

4. ANTIMICROBIAL METABOLISM IN THE MICROBE

Metabolism of antimicrobials, as noted above, may occur in both host (patient) and microorganism. The microbial metabolism may be beneficial to the microorganism by rendering the toxic drug harmless to the microorganism or detrimental by incorporating the drug into the respiratory, metabolic, or structural pathways of the microorganism, so bringing about its ultimate demise. An example of the former is the production of beta-lactamase by bacteria that opens the β-lactam ring of penicillins and cephalosporins and produces an inactive antibiotic. The latter type of microbial metabolism is summarized in Table 1 where antimicrobial agents cause inhibition of growth or antimicrobial cell death by a variety of incorporation mechanisms.

To prevent the microorganism from metabolizing the β-lactam antimicrobial, a β-lactamase inhibitor, such as clavulanic acid, sulbactam, or tazobactam can be coadministered. In general, the observed antimicrobial action is greater than if the β-lactam antimicrobial was given as a single agent. Some examples are ampicillin-sulbactam, ticarcillin-clavulanate, amoxicillin-clavulanate, and piperacillin-tazobactam *(83)*.

5. DRUG INTERACTIONS

Psychotropic drugs are known to have many varied interactions with antimicrobial agents *(84,85)*. Several examples with the antifungal agent, itraconazole, a known inhibitor of CYP3A4, will be utilized as an example. Haloperidol plasma concentrations were increased in schizophrenic patients concurrently treated with itraconazole *(86)*. The resultant increase in plasma concentrations produced significant neurological side effects. The increase in plasma concentration of alprazolam during concurrent administration of itraconazole produced significantly depressed psychomotor function in test subjects *(87)*.

Psychotropic drugs are often used in the pharmacological treatment of emotional disorders of HIV-infected patients. Such patients may also be receiving antidepressant, antifungal, antiviral, and protease inhibitor drugs. For example, in vitro CYP3A4 metabolism of the antidepressant trazodone suggested that biotransformation to its major metabolite, meta-chlorophenylpiperazine, was inhibited by the antifungal, ketoconazole, as well as the protease inhibitors ritonavir and indinavir *(88)*.

Multidrug antiviral regimens are typically used to treat HIV-infected patients in addition to the antibiotics and therapeutic drugs discussed above. For example, a patient is often treated with one or more nucleoside reverse transcriptase inhibitors (zidovudine, didanosine, zalcitabine, lamivudine, or abacavir) and a protease inhibitor (saquinavir, ritonavir, indinavir, nelfinavir, or amprenavir) or alternately with two nucleoside reverse transcriptase inhibitors and a nonnucleoside reverse transcriptase inhibitor (nevirapine, delavirdine, or efavirenz) *(89)*. The protease inhibitors are metabolized by CYP3A4 and several of the reverse transcriptase inhibitors are inducers of various cytochromes, including CYP3A4. Therefore combinations of antiviral drugs have the potential for drug interactions. Inhibition of CYP3A4 may sometimes be an advantage. For example, higher plasma levels of the HIV protease inhibitor, saquinavir, which is metabo-

8. Antimicrobial Drugs

lized by CYP3A4, can be achieved by combining the drug with CYP3A4 inhibitors like ritonavir or ketoconazole *(90)*. But conversely, it cannot be coadministered with therapeutic agents that are likewise metabolized by CYP3A4, such as terfenadine or cisapride.

The widespread use of drugs for gastrointestinal disorders, such as antacids and H_2 histamine receptor-blocking agents such as ranitidine, have been reported to alter the bioavailability of many antimicrobials *(91,92)*. The prokinetic agent cisapride is an example of a therapeutic drug used to treat gastrointestinal disorders. Due to competition for CYP3A4 with other concomitantly administered drugs, toxic effects could be unmasked. Such interactions are potentially harmful to the patient. In one study, interaction between erthyromycin and cisapride produced prolongation of the QT interval and clinically cardiac arrhythmias were observed. Other antimicrobials such as fluconazole or miconazole did not produce QT elongation when administered with cisapride *(93)*. Because the azole antifungal agents are inhibitors of CYP3A4, their concurrent use with cisapride is not recommended *(74)*.

The HCG-CoA reductase inhibitors commonly used to block cholesterol biosynthesis are metabolized by CYP3A4. Therefore, their concurrent use with the antimicrobials that are also metabolized by CYP3A4 should be avoided *(94)*.

Information is now being published that the drug sildenafil (Viagra) is predominately metabolized by CYP3A4 *(95)*. Therefore, any other drug that is metabolized by CYP3A4, including the antimicrobials discussed above, has the potential to impair sildenafil biotransformation.

6. HERBAL AND NATURAL PRODUCT INTERACTIONS

Many patients using antimicrobials may also use over-the-counter herbal preparations to augment their health needs. Even though use of herbal products has become widespread in recent years, there is little scientific information available on how these substances affect prescribed and over-the-counter drugs. Early reports indicate that the herbal products may either induce CYP3A4 or be metabolized by this isoenzyme and hence have the potential to inhibit the metabolism of drugs. For example, the naphtodiantrons found in St. John's wort appear to induce CYP3A4 and would therefore have the potential to decrease the blood concentrations of any antimicrobial also metabolized by CYP3A4. However, this flavonoid constitutes only about 0.1–0.5% of the St. John's wort *(96)*. Thus the contribution to clinical inhibition would be questionable but not unexpected depending upon the method of manufacturing the herbal preparation. Using midazolam as the probe for CYP3A4, one group has suggested that this herb when ingested in the dose recommended for depression is unlikely to inhibit CYP3A4 activity *(97)*. However, another study has demonstrated that using only one probe for CYP3A4 activity may not give a true picture of metabolism in a patient *(98)*.

Recently, it has been found that garlic supplements interact with some antiretroviral medications. In one study *(99)*, the area under the serum concentration curve for saquinavir was decreased approximately 51% when concurrently used with a garlic supplement. Such a drop in serum levels was sufficient to cause treatment failures.

A common natural product interference is between endogenous constituents of grapefruit juice and antimicrobials. A number of flavones have been demonstrated to be present in grapefruit juice. For example, kaempferol, naringenin, and quercetin are three such flavones and all are metabolized by CYP3A4 *(100,101)*. The bioavailability of erythromycin has been shown to increase as a result of the inhibitor effect of grapefruit juice on intestinal CYP3A4 *(43)*. Similar results have been demonstrated with saquinavir and amprenavir *(44)*. Several investigators have shown that the inhibitor effect of grapefruit juice occurs only with the oral dose and not an intravenous dose of the therapeutic drug *(46,47,70)*. Such information suggests that inhibition of CYP3A4 occurs in the gastrointestinal tract as opposed to the liver. Thus the increase in the observed bioavailability of the studied antimicrobials apparently is due to reduced metabolism of the parent drugs in the gastrointestinal tract. Similar results would be anticipated with any orally administered microbial that is metabolized by CYP3A4 and to a lesser extent by those metabolized by CYP2C9. This is because the flavanoids found in grapefruit juice seem to be more selective to inhibiting CYP3A4 than CYP2C9 *(73)*. There may also be some selectivity of inhibition based upon the particular flavones studied. For example, Obach *(71)* has examined some individual flavones found in grapefruit juice, viz, hyperforin, I3,II8-biapigenin, hypericin, and quercetin for their inhibition of CYP2C9, CYP3A4, and several other cytochromes. The biflavone, I3,II-8-biapigenin, demonstrated the greatest potency toward CYP2C9 and CYP3A4.

7. Assays for Antimicrobials

A variety of assays are available both for determining the sensitivity of a strain of bacteria to antibiotic susceptibility as well as for determining the level of the antimicrobial in a physiological fluid. The earliest antibiotic assays evolved from attempts to qualitatively demonstrate antimicrobial activity in biological fluids *(102)*. For clinical purposes there are two distinct requirements. First, there is a need to know if a bacterium is sensitive or resistant to the proposed antibiotic treatment. This type of assay has been a mainstay of clinical laboratories for a number of years. The patient's blood or urine is cultured on agar plates along with various antibiotic standards and controls. Replication of the bacteria would be an indication of resistance to the proposed antibiotic treatment whereas inhibition of growth would indicate sensitivity *(103)*. For those antimicrobials with a narrow therapeutic index, blood level monitoring is advisable.

Commercially available immunoassays exist for some antimicrobials, such as the aminoglycosides. The aminoglycosides have also been analyzed by chromatographic methods *(104–108)*. The macrolide antibiotics, because of their large molecular size, lend themselves to analysis with high-performance liquid chromatography (HPLC) with either electrochemical or ultraviolet detection. Erythromycin propionyl ester and its free base *(109–112)*, clarithromycin *(113)*, and its biological active hydroxy metabolite may all be determined in biological fluids using HPLC. Chromatographic methods have been utilized for analysis of many of the antivirals *(114–119)*.

8. Implications for Toxicological and Forensic Investigations

Antimicrobials are inherently nontoxic agents. However, as the foregoing discussion indicates, when combined with a variety of therapeutic drugs, some potentially toxic and even fatal effects are possible. This is largely due to the fact that most antimicrobials are metabolized by CYP3A4 isoenzymes that also metabolize over 50% of all therapeutic drugs. When competition for the saturable CYP3A4 occurs, toxic effects of the therapeutic drug, effects not usually seen when given alone, are unmasked. Most toxicology and forensic laboratories do not normally analyze for the antimicrobial drugs in general toxicology screens. The main reason is that separate and distinct assays are required for most members of this group. Many antimicrobials have their origin from natural sources and hence are large complex molecules not readily lending themselves to most toxicological and forensic analytical methods. However, when investigative or medical records indicate that a toxic or presumed toxic event followed a combination of a therapeutic and antimicrobial drug, there must be careful consideration of the toxic effect of the therapeutic agent due to competition by the antimicrobial for CYP3A4. Some suspicion may already be raised with an elevation of the concentration of the therapeutic drug in the biological fluid. However, the interpretation of the reason for the elevated level might be incorrect if it is assumed *a priori* that the patient or decedent has taken an overdose of the therapeutic drug.

REFERENCES

1. The Little Oxford Dictionary, 4th edition, compiled by George Ostler, G. Oxford, England: Oxford University Press, 1970.
2. Casarett and Doull's Toxicology the basic science of poisons, fourth edition, Amdur MO, Doull J, and Klaassen CD, eds. Elmsford, NY: Pergamon, 1991.
3. Robbins SL and Kumar V. Basic pathology, 4th ed. Philadelphia: Saunders Company, 1987.
4. www.cdc.gov/ncidod/dbmd/diseaseinfo/meningococcal_t.htm. 11/30/01
5. Mead PS and Griffin PM. *Escherichia coli* O157:H7. Lancet 352:1207–1212 (1998).
6. www.cdc.gov/ncidod/dbmd/diseaseinfo/diarrecoli_t.htm. 11/30/01
7. www.cdc.gov/ncidod/dbmd/diseaseinfo/groupastreptococcal_t.htm. 11/30/01
8. www.cdc.gov/ncidod/dbmd/diseaseinfo/groupastreptococcal_g.htm. 11/30/01
9. Schuchat A. Group B streptococcus. Lancet 353:51–56 (1999).
10. www.cdc.gov/ncidod/dbmd/diseaseinfo/groupbstrep_t.htm. 11/30/01
11. Shapiro ED and Ward JI. The epidemiology and prevention of disease caused by *Haemophilus influenzae* type b. Epidemiol Rev 13:113–142 (1991).
12. Peltola HH. *H. influenzae* in the post-vaccination era. Lancet 341:864–865. (1993).
13. www.cdc.gov/mmwr/preview/mmwrhtml/rr4812a1.htm 11/30/01
14. Hepatitis B virus: a comprehensive strategy for eliminating transmission in the United States through universal childhood vaccination: recommendations of the immunization practices advisory committee. MMWR November 22, 1991 40(RR-13):1–19.
15. Recommendations for prevention and control of Hepatitis C virus (HCV) infection and HCV-related chronic disease. MMWR October 16, 1998 47(RR19):1–39.
16. www.cdc.gov/ncidod/diseases/hepatitis/slideset/hep_d/slide_1.htm. 11/30/01
17. Labrique AB, Thomas DL, Stoszek SK, and Nelson KE. Hepatitis E: an emerging infectious disease. Epidemiol Rev 21:162–179 (1999).
18. www.cdc.gov/nchst/dstd/Fact_Sheets/facts_Genital_Herpes.htm 11/30/01
19. Mertz G and Corey L. Genital herpes simplex virus infections in adults. Urol Clin North Am 11:103 (1984).
20. www.cdc.gov/ncidod/dbmd/diseaseinfo/legionellosis_g.htm 11/30/01
21. CDC. Multidrug-resistant *Salmonella* serotype enteritidis infection associated with consumption of raw shell eggs—United States, 1994–1995. MMWR 45:737–742 (1996).
22. Hajjeh RA, Reingold A, Weil A, Shutt K, Schuchat A, and Perkins BA. Toxic shock syndrome in the United States: surveillance update, 1979–1996. Emerg Infect Dis J 5:807–810 (1999).

23. www.cdc.gov/nchstp/tb/faqs/qa.htm 11/30/01
24. Berdy J. Recent developments of antibiotic research and classification of antibiotics according to chemical structure. Adv Appl Microbiol 18:309–406 (1974).
25. Cuddy PG. Antibiotic classification: implications for drug selection. Crit Care Nur Quart 20:89–102 (1997).
26. Fish DN, Piscitelli SC, and Danziger LH. Development of resistance during antimicrobial therapy: a review of antibiotic classes and patient characteristics in 173 studies. Pharmacother 15:279–291 (1995).
27. Tulkens PM. Intracellular distribution and activity of antibiotics. Eur J Clinic Microbiol Infect Dis 10:100–106 (1991).
28. Nosanchuk JD, Cleare W, Franzot SP, and Casadevall A. Amphotericin B and fluconazole affect cellular charge, macrophage phagocytosis, and cellular morphology of *Cryptococcus neoformans* at subinhibitory concentrations. Antimicro Agents Chemother 43:233–239 (1999).
29. Mengeles Mengelers MJ, Hougee PE, Jannsen LH, and Van Miert AS. Structure–activity relationships between antibacterial activities and physicochemical properties of sulfonamides. J Vet Pharmacol Ther 20:276–283 (1997).
30. Ouedraogo G, Morliere P, Santus R, and Miranda-Castell JV. Damage to mitochrondria of cultured human skin fibroblasts photosensitized by fluoroquinolones. J Photochem Photobiol B- Biology 58:20–25 (2000).
31. Lee DS, Han HJ, Kim K, Park WB, Cho JK, and Kim JH. J Pharm Biomed Anal 12:157–164 (1994).
32. Neuvonen PJ. Interactions with absorption of tetracyclines. Drugs 11:45–54 (1976).
33. Venho VMK, Salonen RO, and Mattila MJ. Modification of the pharmacokinetics of doxycycline in man by ferrous sulfate or tissues. Chemother 21:8–18 (1975).
34. Jung H, Peregrina AA, Rodriguez JM, and Moreno-Esparza R. The influence of coffee with milk and tea with milk on the bioavailability of tetracycline. Biopharm Drug Dis 18:459–463 (1997).
35. Buttner D and Buttner H. pH dependency in uptake of sulfonamides by bacteria. Chemother 26:153–163 (1980).
36. McNulty CA, Dent JC, Ford GA, and Wilkinson SP. Inhibitory antimicrobial concentrations against *Campylobacter pylori* in gastric mucosa. J Antimicro Chemother 22:729–738 (1988).
37. Bennett WM, Elzinga L, Pulliam JP, Rashad AL, and Barry JM. Cyst fluid antibiotic concentrations in autosomal-dominant polycystic kidney disease. Am J Kidney Dis 6:400–404 (1985).
38. Voutsinas P, Kavouklis E, Voutsinas D, Kontoghiorgi K, and Giamarellou H. The effect of acetazolamide on the kinetics of four newer beta-lactams in the aqueous humor. Clin Microbiol Infect 7:70–74 (2001).
39. Rhoten RL, Murphy MA, Kalfas IH, Hahn JF, and Washington JA. Antibiotic penetration into cervical discs. Neurosurg 37:418–421 (1995).
40. Gonzalez FJ. Human cytochrome P450: problems and prospects. Trends Pharmacol Sci 13:346–352 (1992).
41. Nelson DR, Koymans L, Kamataki T, Stegeman JJ, Fyereisen R, Waxman PJ, et al. P450 super-family: update on new sequences, gene mapping, accession numbers and nomenclature. Pharmacogenet 6:1–42 (1996).
42. Caraco Y. Genetic determinants of drug responsiveness and drug interactions. Ther Drug Monitor 20:517–524 (1998).
43. Wienkers LC. Problems associated with in vitro assessment of drug inhibition of CYP3A4 and other P-450 enzymes and its impact on drug discovery. J Pharmacol Toxicol Meth 45:79–84 (2001).

8. Antimicrobial Drugs

44. Guengerich FP. Uncommon P450-catalyzed reactions. Curr Drug Metab 2:93–115 (2001).
45. Dresser GK, Spence JD, and Bailey DG. Pharmacokinetic-pharmacodynamic consequences and clinical relevance of cytochrome P450 3A4 inhibition. Clin Pharmacokinet 38:41–57 (2000).
46. Wood MJ. Interactions of antibiotics with other drugs. J Antimicro Chemother 20:628–630 (1987).
47. O'Reilly RA. Warfarin metabolism and drug–drug interactions. Adv Exp Med Biol 214: 205–212 (1987).
48. Burchell B, Brierley CH, and Rance D. Specificity of human UDP-glucuronosyltransfereases and xenobiotic glucuronidation. Life Sci 57:1819–1831 (1995).
49. Clarke DJ and Burchell B. The uridine diphosphate glucuronosyltransferase multigene famil: function and regulation. In: Kauffman FC, ed. Handbook of experimental pharmacology. Conjugation-deconjugation reactions in drug metabolism and toxicity. Berlin: Springer-Verlag, 1994:3–43.
50. Gagné J-F, Montminy V, Belanger P, Journaut K, Gaucher G, and Guillemette C. Common human UGT1A polymorphisms and the altered metabolism of irinotecan active metabolite 7-ethyl-10-hydroxycamptothecin (SN-38). Mol Pharmacol 62:608–617 (2002).
51. Tukey RH and Strassburg CP. Human UDP-glucuronosyltransferases: metabolism, expression and disease. Annu Rev Pharmacol Toxicol 40:581–616 (2000).
52. Ritter JK, Chen F, Sheen YY, Tran HM, Kimura S, Yeatman MT, et al. A novel complex locus UGT1 encodes human bilirubin, phenol and other UDP-glucuronosyltransferase isozymes with identical carboxyl termini. J Biol Chem 267:3257–3261 (1992).
53. Gong QH, Cho JW, Hang T, Potter C, Gholami N, Basu NK, et al. Thirteen UDPglucuronosyltransferase genes are encoded at the human UGT1 gene complex locus. Pharmacogenetics 11:357–682 (2001).
54. Tukey RH, Strassburg CP, and Mackenzie PI. Pharmacogenomics of human UDP-glucuronosyltransferases and irinotecan toxicity. Mol Pharmacol 62:446–450 (2002).
55. Trapnell CB, Kelecker RW, Jamis-Dow C, and Collins JM. Antimicro Agents Chemother 42:1592–1596 (1998).
56. Zhao Z, Koeplinger KA, Peterson T, Conradi RA, Burton PS, Suarato A, et al. Mechanis, structure-activity studies, and potential applications of burch glutathione S-transferase-catalyzed cleavage of sulfonamides. Drug Met Disp 27:992–998 (1999).
57. Koeplinger KA, Zhao Z, Peterson T, Leone JW, Schwende FS, Heinrikson RL, et al. Activated sulfonamides are cleaved by glutathione-S-transferases. Drug Met Disp 27:986–991 (1999).
58. Bras AP, Hoff HR, Aoki FY, and Sitar DS. Amantadine acetylation may be effected by acetyltransferases other than NAT1 or NAT2. Can J Physiol Pharmacol 76:701–706 (1998).
59. Bras APM, Jänne J, Porter CW, and Sitar DS. Spermidine/spermine N^1-acetyltransferase catalyzes amantadine acetylation. Drug Met Dis 29:676–680 (2001).
60. Thomas RC and Ikeda GJ. The metabolic fate of tolbutamide in man and in the rat. J Med Chem 9:507–510 (1966).
61. Veronese ME, Miners JO, Randles D, Gregov D, and Birkett DJ. Validation of the tolbutamide metabolic ratio for population screening with use of sulfaphenazole to produce model phenotypic poor metabolizers. Clin Pharmacol Ther 47:403–411 (1990).
62. Komatsu K, Ito K, Nakajima Y, Kanamitsu S-I, Imaoka S, Funae Y, et al. Prediction of in vivo drug–drug interactions between tolbutamide and various sulfonamides in humans based on in vitro experiments. Drug Metab Disp 28:475–481 (2000).
63. Miners JO and Birkett DJ. Cytochrome P4502C9: an enzyme of major importance in human drug metabolism. Brit J Clin Pharmacol 45:525–538 (1998).

64. Leeman T, Transon C, and Dayer P. Cytochrome P450TB (CYP2C): a major monooxygenase catalyzing diclofenac 4'-hydroxylation in human liver. Life Sci 52:29–34 (1992).
65. Newlands AJ, Smith DA, Jones BC, and Hawksworth GM. Metabolism of non-steroidal anti-inflammatory drugs by cytochrome P450 2C. Brit J Clin Pharmacol 34:152P (1992).
66. Tang C, Shou M, Rushmore TH, Mei Q, Sandhu P, Woolf EJ, et al. In-vitro metabolism of celecoxib, a cyclooxygenase-2 inhibitor, by allelic variant forms of human liver microsomal cytochrome P450 2C9: correlation with CYP2C9 genotype and in-vivo pharmacokinetics. Pharmacogenet 11:223–235 (2001).
67. Tang C, Shou M, Mei Q, Rushmore TH, and Rodrigues AD. Major role of human liver microsomal cytochrome P450 2C9 (CYP2C9) in the oxidative metabolism of celecoxib, a novel cyclooxygenase-II inhibitor. J Pharmacol Ther 293:453–459 (2000).
68. Schmider J, Greenblatt DJ, von Moltke LL, Karsov D, and Shader RI. Inhibition of CYP2C9 by selective serotonin reuptake inhibitors in vitro: studies of phenytoin p-hydroxylation. Br J Clin Pharmacol 44:495–498 (1997).
69. Steward DJ, Haining RL, Henne KR, Davis G, Rushmore TH, Trager WF, et al. Genetic association between sensitivity to warfarin and expression of CYP2C9*3. Pharmcogenetics 7:361–367 (1997).
70. Tang W and Stearns RA. Heterotropic cooperativity of cytochrome P450 3A4 and potential drug-drug interactions. Current Drug Metab 2:185–198 (2001).
71. Obach RS, Zhang Q-Y, Dunbar D, and Kaminsky LS. Metabolic characterization of the major human small intestinal cytochrome P450s. Drug Met Disp 29:347–352 (2001).
72. Kolars JC, Schmiedlin-Ren P, Schuetz JD, Fang C, and Watkins PB. Indentification of rafampin-inducible P450IIIA4 (CYP 3A4) in human small bowel enterocytes. J Clin Invest 90:1871–1878 (1992).
73. Desta Z, Soukhova N, Mahal SK, and Flockhart DA. Interaction of cisapride with the human cytochrome P450 system: metabolism and inhibition studies. Drug Metabol Disp 28:789–800 (2000).
74. Michalets EL and Williams CR. Drug interactions with cisapride: clinical implications. Clin Pharmacokinet 39:49–75 (2000).
75. Piquette RK. Torsade de pointes induced by cisapride/clarithromycin interaction. Ann Pharmacother 33:22–26 (1999).
76. Wysowski DK and Bacsanyi J. Cisapride and fatal arrhythmia. N Engl J Med 335:290–291 (1996).
77. Monahan BP, Ferguson CL, Killeavy ES, Lloyd BK, Troy J, and Cantilena LR Jr. Torsades de pointes occurring in association with terfenadine use. J Am Med Assoc 264:2788–2790 (1990).
78. Woolsey RL, Chen Y, Freiman JP, and Gillis RA. Mechanism of the cardiotoxic actions of terfenadine. J Am Med Assoc 269:1532–1536 (1993).
79. Honig PK, Wortham DC, Zamani K, Conner DP, Mullin JC, and Cantilena LR. Terfenadine-ketoconazole interaction: pharmacokinetic and electrocardiographic consequences. J Am Med Assoc 269:1513–1518 (1993).
80. Yee GC and McGuire TR. Pharmacokinetic drug interactions with cyclosporine (Part I). Clin Pharmacokinet 19:319–332 (1990).
81. Rodvold KA. Clinical pharmacokinetics of clarithromycin. Clin Pharmackinet 37:385–398 (1999).
82. Rivory LP, Slaviero KA, Hoskins JM, and Clarke SJ. The erythromycin breath test for the predicition of drug clearance. Clin Pharmacokinet 40:151–158 (2001).
83. McCrea J, Prueksaritanont T, Gertz BJ, Carides A, Gillen L, Antonello S, et al. Concurrent administration of the erythromycin breath test (EBT) and oral midazolam as in vivo probes for CYP3A4 activity. J Clin Pharmacol 39:1212–1220 (1999).

8. Antimicrobial Drugs

84. Ananth J and Johnson K. Psychotropic and medical drug interactions. Psychother Psychosomat 58:178–196 (1992).
85. Shader RI, von Moltke LL, Schmider J, Harmatz JS, and Greenblatt DJ. The clinician and drug interactions—an update. J Clin Psychopharmacol 16:197–201 (1996).
86. Yasui N, Kondo T, Otani K, Furukori H, Mihara K, Suzuki A, et al. Effects of itraconazole on the steady-state plasma concentrations of haloperidol and its reduced metabolite in schizophrenic patients: in vivo evidence of the involvement of CYP3A4 for haloperidol metabolism. J Clin Psychopharmacol 19:149–154 (1999).
87. Yasui N, Kondo T, Otani K, Furukori H, Kaneko S, Ohkubo T, et al. Effect of itraconazole on the single oral dose pharmacokinetics and pharmacodynamics of alprazolam. Psychopharmacol 139:269–273 (1998).
88. Zalma A, vonMoltke LL, Granda BW, Harmatz JS, Shader RI, and Greenblatt DJ. In vitro metabolism of trazodone by CYP3A4: inhibition by ketoconazole and human immunodeficiency viral protease inhibitors. Biol Psychiatr 47:655–661 (2000).
89. Barry M, Mulcahy F, Merry C, Gibbons S, and Back D. Pharmacokinetics and potential interactions amongst antiretroviral agents used to treat patients with HIV infection. Clin Pharmacokinet 36:289–304 (1999).
90. Vella S and Florida M. Saquinavir. Clinical pharmacology and efficacy. Clin Pharmacokinet 34:189–201 (1998).
91. Deppermann KM, Lode H, Hoffken G, Tschink G, Kalz C, and Koeppe P. Influence of ranitidine, pirenzepine, and aluminum magnesium hydroxide on the bioavailability of various antibiotics, including amoxicillin, cephalexin, doxycycline, and amoxicillin-calvulanic acid. Antimicro Agents Chemother 33:1901–1907 (1989).
92. Lode H. Drug interactions with quinolones. Rev Infect Dis 10:S132–S136 (1988).
93. Laine K, Forsstrom J, Gronroos P, Irjala K, Kailajarvi M, and Scheinin M. Frequency and clinical outcome of potentially harmful drug metabolic interactions in patients hospitalized on internal and pulmonary medicine wards: focus on warfarin and cisapride. Ther Drug Monitor 22:503–509 (2000).
94. Ucar M, Mjorndal T, and Dahlqvist R. HNG-CoA reductase inhibitiors and myotoxicity. Drug Safety 22:441–457 (2000).
95. Warrington JS, Shader RI, von Moltke LL, and Greenblatt DJ. In vitro biotransfromation of sildenafil (Viagra): identification of human cytochromes and potential drug interactions. Drug Metab Disp 28:392–397 (2000).
96. Kinirons MT, O'Shea D, Kim RB, Groopman JD, Thummel KE, Wood AJ, et al. Failure of erythromycin breath test to correlate with midazolam clearance as a probe of cytochrome P4503A. Clin Pharmacol Ther 66:224–231 (1999).
97. Slain D, Pakyz A, Israel DS, Monroe S, and Polk RE. Variability in activity of hepatic CYP3A4 in patients infected with HIV. Pharmacother 20:898–907 (2000).
98. Takeda M, Khamdang S, Naridawa S, Kimura H, Kobayashi Y, Yamamoto T, et al. Human organic anion transporters and human organic cation transporters mediate renal antiviral transport. J Pharmacol Exp Ther 300:918–924 (2002).
99. Piscitelli SC. The effect of garlic supplements on the pharmacokinetics of saquinavir. Clin Infect Dis 34:234–238 (2002).
100. De Bony F, Tod M, Bidault R, On NT, Posner J, and Rolan P. Multiple interactions of cimetidine and probenecid with valaciclovir and its metabolite acyclovir. Antimicro Agents Chemother 46:458–463 (2000).
101. Lister PD, Prevan AM, and Sanders CC. Importance of β-lactamase inhibitor pharmacokinetics in the pharmacodynamics of inhibitor-drug combinations: studies with piperacillin-tazobactam and piperacillin-sulbactam. Antimicro Agents Chemother 41:721–727 (1997).

102. Sabath LD. The assay of antimicrobial compounds. Human Pathol 7:287–295 (1976).
103. Edberg SC and Chu A. Determining antibiotic levels in the blood. Am J Med Technol 41: 99–105 (1975).
104. Isoherranen N and Soback S. Chromatographic methods for analysis of aminoglycoside antibiotics. J AOAC Internatl 82:1017–1045 (1999).
105. Soltes L. Aminoglycoside antibiotics—two decades of their HPLC bioanalysis. Biomed Chromatog 13:3–10 (1999).
106. Adams E, Van Vaerenbergh G, Roets E, and Hoogmartens J. Analysis of amikacin by liquid chromatography with pulsed electrochemical detection. J Chromatog 819:93–97 (1998).
107. Preu M, Guyot D, and Petz M. Development of a gas chromatography-mass spectrometry method for the analysis of aminoglycoside antibiotics using experimental design for the optimisation of the derivatisation reactions. J Chromatog 818:95–108 (1998).
108. Tawa R, Matsunaga H, and Fujimoto T. High-performance liquid chromatographic analysis of aminoglycoside antibiotics. J Chromatog 812:141–150 (1998).
109. Stubbs C and Kanfer I. High-performace liquid chromatography of erythromycin propionyl ester and erythromycin base in biological fluids. J Chromatog 427:93–101 (1988).
110. Croteau D, Vallee F, Bergeron MG, and LeBel M. High-performance liquid chromatographic assay of erythromycin and its esters using electrochemical detection. J Chromatog 419:205–212 (1987).
111. Stubbs C, Haigh JM, and Kanfer I. Determination of erythromycin in serum and urine by high-performance liquid chromatography with ultra-violet detection. J Pharm Sci 74: 1126–1128 (1985).
112. Chen ML and Chiou WL. Analysis of erythromycin in biological fluids by high-performance liquid chromatography with electrochemical detection. J Chromatog 278:91–100 (1983).
113. Chu SY, Sennello LT, and Sonders RC. Simultaneous determination of clarithromycin and 14®-hydroxyclarithromycin in plasma and urine using high-performance liquid chromatography with electrochemical detection. J Chromatog 571:199–208 (1991).
114. Zhang S, Yuan Z, Liu H, Zou H, Xiong H, and Wu Y. Electophoresis 21:2995–2998 (2000).
115. Merodio M, Campanero MA, Mirshahi T, Mirshahi M, and Irache JM. Development of a sensitive method for the determination of ganciclovir by reversed-phase high-performance liquid chromatography. J Chromatog 870:159–167 (2000).
116. Pham-Huy C, Stathoulopoulou F, Sandouk P, Scherrmann JM, Palombo S, and Girre C. Rapid determination of valaciclovir and acyclovir in human biological fluids by high-performance liquid chromatography using isocratic elution. J Chromatog B Biomed Sci Appl 732:47–53 (1999).
117. Eisenberg EJ and Cundy KC. High-performance liquid chromatographic determination of cytosine-containing compounds by precolumn fluorescence derivatization with phenacyl bromide: application to antiviral nucleosides and nucleotides. J Chromatog B Biomed Appl 679:119–127 (1996).
118. Frijus-Plessen N, Michaelis HC, Foth H, and Kahl GF. Determination of 3'-azido-3'-deoxythymidine, 2',3'-dideoxycytidine, 3'fluoro-3'-deoxythymidine and 2',3'-dideoxyinosine in biological samples by high-performance liquid chromatography. J Chromatog 534: 101–107 (1990).
119. Unadkat JD, Crosby SS, Wang JP, and Hertel CC. Simple and rapid high-performance liquid chromatographic assay for zidovudine (azidothymidine) in plasma and urine. J Chromatog 430:420–423 (1988).

Chapter 9

Drug Interactions with Medications Used for HIV/AIDS

Michael Frank, MD

1. INTRODUCTION AND OVERVIEW OF AIDS TREATMENT

The last decade has seen a combination of astounding successes and continuing challenges in the field of HIV treatment. The death rate as a result of AIDS in the United States has decreased significantly and consistently since 1996, because of current therapies (1). Unfortunately, the successes witnessed in the developed world have not been matched in the developing world where new treatments have generally not been available, such as in sub-Saharan Africa where over 20 million persons are believed to be infected with HIV. The decline in AIDS mortality in the United States has been seen in all racial/ethnic groups and both genders (1). Declining mortality has not been accompanied by decreases in incidence of HIV infection, however, so that the overall prevalence of HIV infection continues to rise. This is especially true for African Americans and for women, who have faster rising rates of HIV infection. Even with the dramatically increasing numbers of HIV-infected women, the incidence of HIV infection in newborns continues to fall as a result of effective antiretroviral treatment of pregnant HIV-infected women to prevent transmission to their babies.

Successful treatment of HIV infection, however, is now increasingly appreciated to have unanticipated adverse effects as well. These include some long-term toxicities of the medications, and interactions both between the medications and between the HIV medications and other medications that a person may be taking. As persons living with HIV continue to live longer, they run a higher risk of needing treatment for other common medical conditions whose prevalence increases with age, and consequently the likelihood of drug interactions will also increase.

From: *Handbook of Drug Interactions: A Clinical and Forensic Guide*
A. Mozayani and L. P. Raymon, eds. © Humana Press Inc., Totowa, NJ

Treatment for HIV infection and AIDS involves two broad areas *(2)*. The first is the use of medications to prevent or treat the opportunistic infections that may occur as a result of the immune system being compromised by HIV infection. Consensus guidelines for primary and secondary prophylaxis of opportunistic infections are available on the Internet *(3)*. The most commonly used medications for opportunistic infection prophylaxis include trimethoprim-sulfamethoxazole, dapsone, and azithromycin. Many others also may be used for treatment or prophylaxis of infections. The most important for our purposes here include clarithromycin, the antimycobacterials rifampin and rifabutin, the antifungals fluconazole, itraconazole, and ketoconazole, the antiparasitic atovaquone, and the antiviral ganciclovir. Drug interactions can be especially problematic when treating tuberculosis coincident with HIV *(4)*.

The major thrust of medical management of HIV infection now is actual treatment of the HIV infection itself with antiretroviral medications. A detailed description of antiretroviral therapy can be found in recent guidelines *(5)*. Whereas diagnostic testing for HIV infection depends on the demonstration of HIV antibody by enzyme-linked immunosorbent assay and confirmatory Western blot testing, monitoring of HIV treatment depends on following levels of HIV virus by quantitative polymerase chain reaction for viral RNA. With use of an appropriate combination of antiretrovirals, and strict adherence to the regimen, the majority of patients can achieve reductions in plasma HIV viral load to levels below the level of detection of current assays (<50 copies/mL). Successful treatment for HIV always involves a regimen of multiple different medications, because of the ease with which HIV can develop resistance to regimens of only a single or even two active drugs. Thus persons being treated for HIV are always on a multiple medication regimen, and the potential for drug interactions is always present *(6,7)*.

Antiretroviral drugs presently available can be divided into three general classes: nucleoside analog reverse transcriptase inhibitors, nonnucleoside reverse transcriptase inhibitors, and protease inhibitors. Currently available nucleoside analogs (and their brand names) include zidovudine (Retrovir), didanosine (Videx), zalcitabine (Hivid), stavudine (Zerit), lamivudine (Epivir), abacavir (Ziagen), and tenofovir (Viread). Strictly speaking, tenofovir is a nucleotide analog, since it has already undergone the first of three phosphorylations required for activation of the nucleosides. Also available are combinations of zidovudine and lamivudine together (Combivir) and zidovudine, lamivudine, and abacavir together (Trizivir). Available nonnucleoside reverse transcriptase inhibitors are nevirapine (Viramune), delaviridine (Rescriptor), and efavirenz (Sustiva). Protease inhibitors include saquinavir (Invirase, Fortovase), ritonavir (Norvir), indinavir (Crixivan), nelfinavir (Viracept), amprenavir (Agenerase), and ritonavir/lopinavir (Kaletra).

For a patient starting out with a totally susceptible virus, many different drug combination regimens have been shown to be similarly effective. Choosing the combination of specific drugs for treatment of a specific patient is an individualized decision that depends on many factors, including the patient's baseline viral load and immune status, results of resistance testing of the patient's viral isolate, other medical conditions or medications, the number of doses/day and the number of pills/dose the patient is able and willing to comply with, anticipated adverse effects, and known or expected antiviral synergistic or antagonistic effects. The most commonly used regimens for treating HIV involve a combination of two nucleoside analogs with either a nonnucleoside reverse transcriptase inhibitor or a protease inhibitor (*see* Table 1). For example, com-

Table 1
Recommended Regimens for Initial Therapy of HIV Infection (5)

	Column A	Column B
Strongly recommended choices	Zidovudine + Lamivudine Stavudine + Lamivudine Zidovudine + Didanosine Stavudine + Didanosine	Efavirenz Nelfinavir Indinavir Ritonavir + Lopinavir Ritonavir + Indinavir Ritonavir + Saquinavir
Recommended as alternatives only	Zidovudine + Zalcitabine	Abacavir Nevirapine Delaviridine Ritonavir Saquinavir Nelfinavir + Saquinavir

Recommended regimens include one choice from Column A combined with one choice from Column B.

monly used initial treatment regimens typically combine either zidovudine/lamivudine (Combivir) or stavudine and lamivudine, with either efavirenz, or nelfinavir, or ritonavir/lopinavir (Kaletra). The last is a medication that combines the protease inhibitors ritonavir and lopinavir inside the same capsule, actually taking advantage of the interaction of the two drugs to simplify dosing. Indeed the use of ritonavir as a "booster" to enhance levels of other drugs is now common in the management of HIV infection (8).

2. Mechanisms of Pharmacokinetic Interactions

Interactions among drugs used in the treatment of HIV and AIDS are due to a variety of mechanisms (6,8). Moreover, for some drugs, interactions may be effected through more than one pathway. Also, some drugs have active metabolites, so that changes in metabolism of the parent drug may not be associated with the same magnitude of change in drug activity. Finally, because of the sometimes multiple and often not yet clearly elucidated ways that drugs can interact, predicting the outcome of a drug interaction in humans based on in vitro or animal model data can be problematic. This is especially true if trying to predict the effect of interactions between three or more drugs, based on data from two-way interactions, as is often the case in management of patients with AIDS.

The vast majority of drug interactions in HIV/AIDS are due to effects on the hepatic cytochrome P450 system, and especially the CYP3A4 isoenzyme (9). All of the currently available protease inhibitors and nonnucleoside reverse transcriptase inhibitors are metabolized through this system, as are many of the drugs used for prophylaxis or treatment of HIV-associated opportunistic infections. In addition to being substrates for these enzymes, most of these drugs also result in inhibition or induction (or even both) of one or more of the P450 isoenzymes (6,9). Some drugs such as rifampin, rifabutin, nevirapine, and efavirenz are primarily inducers of the P450 system and tend to thus increase the metabolism of other drugs, thereby lowering their levels. Other drugs, such as delaviridine, indinavir, saquinavir, itraconazole, and clarithromycin, are primarily inhibitors of this pathway and so usually increase levels of other drugs metabolized by the same enzyme. Finally, some drugs, such as ritonavir, nelfinavir, and amprenavir, have more complicated effects, being inhibitors of certain isoenzymes and inducers of others. These drugs thus raise levels of some coadministered drugs and decrease levels of others. In fact, the same drug may actually be both an inducer and an inhibitor of the same isoenzyme, making its effects on the metabolism of another drug dependent on the time frame of its administration and whether steady state has been achieved. Obviously the effects of such an interaction can be very difficult to predict.

Ritonavir is one of the most potent inhibitors of the P450 system yet found, and is a good example of the complexity of these interactions. It is both a substrate for and a very potent inhibitor of the CYP3A4 isoenzyme, much more so than delaviridine, indinavir, nelfinavir, or amprenavir, which are all more potent than saquinavir *(10,11)*. However, like nevirapine, efavirenz, and the rifamycins, it also induces CYP3A4, thereby inducing its own metabolism as well as that of other drugs. In addition, it both inhibits and induces other isoenzymes such as CYP2C19 and 2D6, and so may interact with a wide variety of drugs metabolized through any of these pathways *(12)*.

Two other points need to be made regarding the cytochrome P450 system and drug interactions. The first is that the same enzymes are present in the intestines as well as the liver, so that the site of cytochrome P450 interaction may be the intestine as the drugs are being absorbed, and not just the liver *(13)*. Second, these enzymes also metabolize, and can be induced or inhibited by, a wide variety of other substances besides those traditionally thought of as drugs. For example, many "natural" supplements or herbal medications such as St. John's wort, garlic supplements, and even grapefruit juice have significant effects on intestinal or hepatic cytochrome P450 system enzymes, and consequently on the pharmacokinetics of some antiretrovirals *(14–16)*.

But although the P450 system is the primary means of drug interactions in HIV/AIDS, there are several other possible pathways. The P-glycoprotein multidrug transporter is a membrane protein, which acts as an efflux transporter for a number of drugs and other molecules and is present in intestinal mucosa as well as several other sites in the body. It is increasingly being recognized as playing an important role in drug kinetics and distribution, and as a common pathway for potential drug interactions. For example, changes in activity of intestinal P-glycoprotein can result in changes of blood levels of orally administered drugs. Protease inhibitors and other drugs such as rifampin that have effects on the P450 system may also be substrates for, or inhibitors or inducers of, the P-glycoprotein pathway *(17,18)*.

Glucuronidation is another pathway for metabolism of some drugs including digoxin, zidovudine, and the estrogens in oral contraceptives. The enzyme responsible, glucuronyl-transferase, can be increased by rifampin and by certain protease inhibitors such as ritonavir and nelfinavir, which could lead to reduced levels of other drugs metabolized through this pathway *(19,20)*. Changes in absorption of a drug can also result from changes in gastric pH (and thereby solubility) caused by another drug, or from actual chelation inside the gastrointestinal tract by the other drug *(21,22)*. The nucleoside analog antiretrovirals require activation by phosphorylation before they can inhibit HIV reverse transcriptase. Depending on their base, they may compete for the same phosphorylation enzyme and thus may competitively inhibit the activation of each other. For example, the combination of zidovudine and stavudine is actually antagonistic for this reason (23). Finally, though it is uncommon for the drugs that are the subject of this chapter, one drug may reduce the renal clearance of another, thereby increasing its blood levels (24).

3. Specific Pharmacokinetic Interactions

Specific interactions for drugs used in the management of HIV infection and AIDS are listed in Table 2. Included are the currently available antiretrovirals that have drug interactions, and the most significant drugs used for prevention or treatment of opportunistic infections. Listed for each drug are affected drugs according to the direction of the effect, with reference numbers.

4. Pharmacodynamic Interactions

In addition to the aforementioned interactions, where one drug affects the concentration of another, drugs may interact by modifying the effect of another without at all changing its concentration (6,7). A prime example of this relevant to HIV treatment is also one of the most basic principles of successful antiretroviral therapy, namely the use of combination therapy. By appropriately combining different antiretroviral drugs, we achieve additive, or in some cases synergistic, anti-HIV activity (2,5). It is important to note, however, that this is not an automatic result of combining just any two drugs. Some combinations of drugs do not provide additive activity, and some may in fact even be antagonistic. For example, both the combination of zidovudine and stavudine, and the combination of indinavir and saquinavir, have been shown to be antagonistic (23,86).

Hydroxyurea has no direct antiviral activity on its own. It does, however, inhibit cellular ribonucleotide reductase activity, thereby decreasing intracellular levels of the deoxynucleoside triphosphates that are required for reverse transcription of the viral genome, and theoretically enhancing the activity of nucleoside analog reverse transcriptase inhibitors, especially didanosine. Hydroxyurea used to be given along with didanosine to potentiate its antiviral activity (87). This practice is no longer recommended because it also resulted in increased toxicity, including increased risks of cytopenias, hepatitis, and episodes of fatal pancreatitis (5,88,89).

Pharmacodynamic interactions often result in additive toxicity of medications when drugs that have overlapping adverse effects are used together. This is especially seen with toxicities that are related to total dose or duration of the offending agents, such as bone marrow toxicity or chronic peripheral neuropathy. For example, rates of anemia and neutropenia are increased when zidovudine is used concurrently with ganciclovir or sulfonamides, and an unacceptably high rate of peripheral neuropathy precludes the combination of zalcitabine with either stavudine or didanosine (2,7,90–92). Nucleoside analogs, especially stavudine, have been associated with mitochondrial dysfunction and a rare syndrome of lactic acidosis and hepatic steatosis, which can be life threatening (93–95). This syndrome appears to be more common when multiple nucleoside analogs are used together, and the combination of stavudine and didanosine may be particularly problematic, especially in pregnant women (96,97). Other examples of additive toxicities involving drugs used in the management of HIV/AIDS are listed in Table 3.

Table 2
Specific Pharmacokinetic Drug Interactions
with Drugs Used in the Management of HIV/AIDS

Drug Generic (Trade) Names	Increases Levels of	Decreases Levels of
Amprenavir (Agenerase)	Astemizole (5)	Delaviridine (25)
	Atorvastatin (5)	Indinavir (26)
	Bepridil (5)	Methadone (27)
	Cisapride (5)	
	Ergotamines (5)	
	Ketoconazole (5)	
	Lovastatin (5)	
	Midazolam (5)	
	Rifabutin (5)	
	Sildenafil (5)	
	Simvastatin (5)	
	Terfenadine (5)	
	Triazolam (5)	
Atovaquone (Mepron)	Zidovudine (28)	
Clarithromycin (Biaxin)	Astemizole (7)	
	Cisapride (7)	
	Delaviridine (2)	
	Saquinavir (5)	
	Terfenadine (7)	
Delaviridine (Rescriptor)	Alprazolam (2)	
	Amphetamines (2)	
	Astemizole (5)	
	Cisapride (5)	
	Clarithromycin (5)	
	Dapsone (5)	
	Ergotamines (5)	
	Indinavir (29)	
	Lovastatin (5)	
	Midazolam (5)	
	Nelfinavir (5)	
	Nifedipine (2)	
	Quinidine (5)	
	Rifabutin (30)	
	Ritonavir (5)	
	Saquinavir (31)	
	Sildenafil (5)	
	Simvastatin (5)	
	Terfenadine (5)	
	Triazolam (5)	
	Warfarin (5)	
Didanosine (Videx)		Ciprofloxacin (21)
		Dapsone (32)
		Delaviridine (33)
		Ethambutol (4)
		Indinavir (6)
		Itraconazole (34)
		Ketoconazole (35)
		Tetracycline (2)

9. HIV/AIDS Drugs

Table 2 (*continued*)

Drug Generic (Trade) Names	Increases Levels of	Decreases Levels of
Efavirenz (Sustiva)	Astemizole *(5)* Buproprion *(36)* Cisapride *(5)* Ergotamines *(5)* Midazolam *(5)* Nelfinavir *(37)* Ritonavir *(38)* Terfenadine *(5)* Triazolam *(5)*	Amprenavir *(39,40)* Clarithromycin *(3,5)* Indinavir *(41)* Lopinavir *(6)* Methadone *(27)* Oral contraceptives *(5)* Rifabutin *(42)* Saquinavir *(6,43)* Warfarin *(5)*
Fluconazole (Diflucan)	Astemizole *(7)* Cisapride *(7)* Methadone *(27)* Rifabutin *(44)* Terfendadine *(7)* Triazolam *(45)* Warfarin *(46)* Zidovudine *(47)*	
Ganciclovir (Cytovene)	Didanosine *(7)*	
Indinavir (Crixivan)	Amprenavir *(5)* Astemizole *(5)* Atorvastatin *(5)* Cisapride *(5)* Clarithromycin *(5)* Ergotamines *(5,48)* Estrogens *(5)* Ketoconazole *(5)* Lovastatin *(5)* Midazolam *(5)* Nelfinavir *(5)* Rifabutin *(49)* Saquinavir *(5)* Sildenafil *(5,50)* Simvastatin *(5)* Terfenadine *(5)* Triazolam *(5)*	
Itraconazole (Sporanox)	Amprenavir *(6)* Astemizole *(7)* Cisapride *(7)* Cyclosporine *(51)* Digoxin *(51)* Indinavir *(6)* Midazolam *(7)* Nelfinavir *(6)* Rifabutin *(7)* Saquinavir *(6)* Terfendadine *(7)* Tolbutamide *(51)* Triazolam *(7)* Warfarin *(51)*	

(*continued*)

Table 2 (*continued*)

Drug Generic (Trade) Names	Increases Levels of	Decreases Levels of
Ketoconazole	Amprenavir *(5)* Astemizole *(7)* Cisapride *(7)* Indinavir *(5)* Midazolam *(7)* Nelfinavir *(6)* Nevirapine *(5)* Saquinavir *(5)* Terfenadine *(7)* Triazolam *(7)*	
Lopinavir/ritonavir (Kaletra)	Saquinavir *(26)* *See* ritonavir	Amprenavir *(26)* Ritonavir *(26)* *See* ritonavir
Nelfinavir (Viracept)	Amprenavir *(26)* Astemizole *(5)* Atorvastatin *(5)* Buproprion *(36)* Cisapride *(5)* Ergotamines *(5)* Indinavir *(26)* Ketoconazole *(5)* Lovastatin *(5)* Midazolam *(5)* Rifabutin *(52)* Saquinavir *(5)* Sildenafil *(5)* Simvastatin *(5)* Terfenadine *(5)* Triazolam *(2)*	Delaviridine *(53)* Methadone *(27)* Oral contraceptives *(20)* Phenytoin *(54)*
Nevirapine (Viramune)		Clarithromycin *(5)* Efavirenz *(26)* Indinavir *(55)* Ketoconazole *(5)* Lopinavir *(5,26)* Methadone *(27,56)* Nelfinavir *(2)* Oral contraceptives *(5)* Rifabutin *(2)* Rifampin *(2)* Saquinavir *(57)*
Rifabutin (Mycobutin)		Amprenavir *(58,59)* Clarithromycin *(7)* Delaviridine *(30)* Efavirenz *(3)* Indinavir *(49,60)* Nelfinavir *(52)* Nevirapine *(4)* Saquinavir *(61–63)*

9. HIV/AIDS Drugs

Table 2 (*continued*)

Drug Generic (Trade) Names	Increases Levels of	Decreases Levels of
Rifampin		Amprenavir *(5,64)*
		Atovaquone *(3)*
		Clarithromycin *(7)*
		Delaviridine *(5,63)*
		Efavirenz *(5,65)*
		Indinavir *(5,64)*
		Lopinavir *(5)*
		Methadone *(27)*
		Midazolam *(7)*
		Nelfinavir *(5,64)*
		Nevirapine *(5,66)*
		Ritonavir *(5,63,64)*
		Saquinavir *(5,62,64,67)*
		Triazolam *(7)*
		Warfarin *(7)*
		Zidovudine *(68)*
Ritonavir (Norvir, also in Kaletra)	Alprazolam *(6,69)*	Alprazolam *(6,69)*
	Amiodarone *(5)*	Atovaquone *(5)*
	Amitriptyline *(2)*	Divaproex *(5)*
	Amprenavir *(5,70)*	Lamotrigine *(5)*
	Astemizole *(5)*	Methadone *(5,27)*
	Atorvastatin *(5,6)*	Morphine *(2)*
	Bepridil *(5)*	Naproxen *(2)*
	Buproprion *(36)*	Oral contraceptives *(19)*
	Cisapride *(5)*	Phenytoin *(5,6,78)*
	Clarithromycin *(3,7)*	Theophylline *(5,83)*
	Clozapine *(5)*	Warfarin *(5,84)*
	Desipramine *(5)*	
	Efavirenz *(5)*	
	Ergotamines *(5,71)*	
	Fentanyl *(7)*	
	Flecainide *(5)*	
	Fluoxetine *(72)*	
	Indinavir *(5,73,74)*	
	Ketoconazole *(5)*	
	Lopinavir *(5)*	
	Lovastatin *(5)*	
	MDMA *(75)*	
	Meperidine *(7)*	
	Midazolam *(5)*	
	Nelfinavir *(5,76,77)*	
	Phenytoin *(6,78)*	
	Pimozide *(2)*	
	Pravastatin *(6)*	
	Propafenone *(5)*	
	Propoxyphene *(7)*	
	Quinidine *(5)*	
	Rifabutin *(3,63,64,79)*	

(*continued*)

Table 2 (*continued*)

Drug Generic (Trade) Names	Increases Levels of	Decreases Levels of
Ritonavir (Norvir, also in Kaletra) *(continued)*	Saquinavir *(5,43,80,81)* Sildenafil *(5,82)* Simvastatin *(5,6)* Terfenadine *(5)* Triazolam *(5)*	
Saquinavir (Fortovase, Invirase)	Astemizole *(5)* Cisapride *(5)* Clarithromycin *(5)* Ergotamines *(5)* Ketoconazole *(5)* Lovastatin *(5)* Midazolam *(5)* Rifabutin *(5,26)* Sildenafil *(5,82)* Simvastatin *(5)* Terfenadine *(5)*	Amprenavir *(26)*
Stavudine (Zerit)		Zidovudine *(23)*
Tenofovir (Viread)	Didanosine *(85)*	
Trimethoprim-sulfamethoxazole	Lamivudine *(24)*	
Zidovudine (Retrovir, also in Combivir, Trizivir)		Stavudine *(23)*

Table 3
Drugs with Overlapping/Additive Toxicities,
Grouped According to Organ System Affected *(2,5–7)*[a]

Bone Marrow	Peripheral Neuropathy	Hepatic
Zidovudine Sulfonamides Dapsone Ganciclovir Pyrimethamine 5-FU Hydroxyurea cytotoxic chemotherapy	Stavudine Didanosine Zalcitabine Isoniazid Metronidazole Alcohol Vincristine cis-Platinum Phenytoin	Any antiretroviral, but especially nevirapine, ritonavir, NRTIs Rifamycins Isoniazid Pyrazinamide Sulfonamides Azole antifungals Hydroxyurea
Pancreatitis	**Renal**	**Gastrointestinal**
Didanosine Zalcitabine Stavudine Pentamidine Alcohol Hydroxyurea Valproic acid	Indinavir Amphotericin Pentamidine Foscarnet Aminoglycosides	All antiretrovirals, especially PIs Macrolides Rifamycins

[a] NRTIs denotes nucleoside analog reverse transcriptase inhibitors; PIs denotes protease inhibitors.

Internet Resources

The field of management of HIV/AIDS is a rapidly changing one, with new drugs continually being developed. Keeping up with all of the new information in the field, including new data on potential drug interactions, is a challenge. In addition to the references at the end of this chapter, the following Internet sites are recommended:

http://www.aidsinfo.nih.gov
http://www.medscape.com/Home/Topics/AIDS/AIDS.html
http://www.retroconference.org
http://www.hopkins-aids.edu
http://hivinsite.ucsf.edu/InSite
http://www.iapac.org/index.html

References

1. CDC. HIV and AIDS—United States, 1981–2000. MMWR 50:430–434 (2001).
2. Mullin SM, Jamjian CM, and Spruance SL. Antiretroviral adverse effects and interactions: clinical recognition and management. In: Sande MA and Volberding PA, eds. The medical management of AIDS. Philadelphia: Saunders, 1999:79–96.
3. 2001 USPHS/IDSA Guidelines for the prevention of opportunistic infections in persons infected with human immunodeficiency virus. From the website, http://www.aidsinfo.nih.gov/guidelines.
4. Burman WJ, Gallicano K, and Peloquin C. Therapeutic implications of drug interactions in the treatment of human immunodeficiency virus-related tuberculosis. Clin Infect Dis 28: 419–430 (1999).
5. Guidelines for the use of antiretroviral agents in hiv-infected adults and adolescents, February 4, 2002. From the website, http://www.aidsinfo.nih.gov/guidelines.
6. Piscitelli SC and Gallicano KD. Interactions among drugs for HIV and opportunistic infections. N Engl J Med 344:984–996 (2001).
7. Piscitelli SC, Flexner C, Minor JR, Polis MA, and Masur H. Drug interactions in patients infected with human immunodeficiency virus. Clin Infect Dis 23:685–693 (1996).
8. Gerber JG. Using pharmacokinetics to optimize antiretroviral drug–drug interactions in the treatment of human immunodeficiency virus infection. Clin Infect Dis 30(Suppl 2):S123–S129 (2000).
9. Michalets EL. Update: clinically significant cytochrome P-450 drug interactions. Pharmacotherapy 18:84–112 (1998).
10. Eagling VA, Back DJ, and Barry MG. Differential inhibition of cytochrome P450 isoforms by the protease inhibitors ritonavir, saquinavir, and indinavir. Br J Clin Pharmacol 44: 190–194 (1997).
11. Cheng C-L, Smith DE, Carver PL, et al. Steady-state parmacokinetics of delaviridine in HIV-positive patients: effect on erythromycin breath test. Clin Pharmacol Ther 61:531–543 (1997).
12. Kumar GN, Rodrigues AD, Buko AM, and Denissen JF. Cytochrome P450-mediated metabolism of the HIV-1 protease inhibitor ritonavir (ABT-538) in human liver microsomes. J Pharmacol Exp Ther 277:423–431 (1996).
13. Kupferschmidt HH, Fattinger KE, Ha HR, Follath F, and Krahenbuhl S. Grapefruit juice enhances the bioavailability of the HIV protease inhibitor saquinavir in man. Br J Clin Pharmacol 45:355–359 (1998).

14. Roby CA, Anderson GD, Kantor E, Dryer DA, and Burstein AH. St. John's wort: effect on CYP3A4 activity. Clin Pharmacol Ther 67:451–457 (2000).
15. Foster BC, Gallicano K, Cameron W, and Choudhri SH. Constituents of garlic inhibit cytochrome P450 3A4-mediated drug metabolism. Can J Infect Dis 9(Suppl A):472P (1998).
16. Bailey DG, Malcolm J, Arnold MJ, and Spence JD. Grapefruit juice–drug interactions. Br J Clin Pharmacol 46:101–110 (1998).
17. Greiner B, Eichelbaum M, Fritz P, et al. The role of intestinal P-glycoprotein in the interaction of digoxin and rifampin. J Clin Invest 104:147–153 (1999).
18. Lee CG, Gottesman MM, Cardarelli CO, et al. HIV-1 protease inhibitors are substrates for the MDR1 multidrug transporter. Biochemistry 37:3594–3601 (1998).
19. Ouellet D, Hsu A, Qian J, et al. Effect of ritonavir on the pharmacokinetics of ethinyl oestradiol in healthy female volunteers. Br J Clin Pharmacol 46:111–116 (1998).
20. Pai VB and Nahata MC. Nelfinavir mesylate: a protease inhibitor. Ann Pharmacother 33:325–329 (1999).
21. Sahai J, Gallicano K, Oliveras L, et al. Cations in the didanosine tablet reduce ciprofloxacin bioavailability. Clin Pharmacol Ther 53:292–297 (1993).
22. Piscitelli SC, Goss TF, Wilton JH, et al. Effects of ranitidine and sucralfate on ketoconazole bioavailability. Antimicrob Agents Chemother 35:1765–1771 (1991).
23. Hoggard PG, Kewn S, Barry MG, Khoo SH, and Back KJ. Effects of drugs on 2,3-dideoxy-2,3-didehydrothymidine phosphorylation in vitro. Antimicrob Agents Chemother 41:1231–1236 (1997).
24. Moore KHP, Yuen GJ, Raasch RH, et al. Pharmacokinetics of lamivudine administered alone and with trimethoprim-sulfamethoxazole. Clin Pharmacol Ther 59:550–558 (1996).
25. Tran JQ, Petersen C, Garrett M, et al. Pharmacokinetic interactions between delaviridine and reduced-dose amprenavir in HIV-negative adults following multiple dosing. In: Abstracts of the 39th Annual Meeting of the Infectious Diseases Society of America. San Francisco, October 25–28, 2001, Abstract 481 (2001).
26. Schutz M and Wendrow A. Quick reference guide to antiretrovirals. From the website http://www.medscape.com/Medscape/HIV/TreatmentUpdate/1998/tu01/public/toc-eng.tu01.html (2001).
27. Gourevitch MN. Interactions between HIV-related medications and methadone. Mount Sinai J Med 68:227–228 (2001).
28. Lee BL, Tauber MG, Sadler B, et al. Atovaquone inhibits the glucuronidation and increases the plasma concentrations of zidovudine. Clin Pharmacol Ther 59:14 (1996).
29. Ferry JJ, Herman BD, Carel BJ, Carlson GF, and Batts DH. Pharmacokinetic drug-drug interaction study of delaviridine and indinavir in healthy volunteers. J Acquir Immune Defic Syndr Hum Retrovirol 18:252–259 (1998).
30. Borin MT, Chambers JH, Carel BJ, et al. Pharmacokinetic study of the interactions between rifabutin and delaviridine mesylate in HIV-1 infected patients. Antiviral Res 35:53–63 (1997).
31. Cox SR, Ferry JJ, Batts DH, et al. Delaviridine and marketed protease inhibitors: pharmacokinetic interaction studies in healthy volunteers: In: Programs and abstracts of the 4th Conference on Retroviruses and Opportunistic Infections. Washington, DC, January 22–26, 1997, Abstract 133 (1997).
32. Metroka CE, McMechan MF, Andrada R, et al. Failure of prophylaxis with dapsone in patients taking dideoxyinosine. N Engl J Med 325:737 (1991).
33. Morse GD, Fischl MA, Shelton MJ, et al. Single dose pharmacokinetics of delaviridine mesylate and didanosine in patients with human immunodeficiency virus infection. Antimicrob Agents Chemother 41:169 (1997).
34. May DB, Drew RH, Yedinak KC, et al. Effect of simultaneous didanosine administration on itraconazole absorption in healthy volunteers. Pharmacotherapy 14:509 (1994).

35. Knupp CA, Brater DC, Relue J, et al. Pharmacokinetics of didanosine and ketoconazole after administration to patients seropositive for the human immunodeficiency virus. J Clin Pharmacol 33:912 (1993).
36. Hesse LM, von Moltke LL, Shader RI, and Greenblatt DJ. Ritonavir, efavirenz, and nelfinavir inhibit CYP2B6 activity in vitro: potential drug interactions with buproprion. Drug Metab Disp 29:100–102 (2001).
37. Fiske WD, Benedek IH, White SJ, et al. Pharmacokinetic interaction between efavirenz and nelfinavir mesylate in healthy volunteers. In: Programs and abstracts of the 5th Conference on Retroviruses and Opportunistic Infections. Chicago, IL, February 1–5, 1998, Abstract 144 (1998).
38. Fiske W, Benedek IH, Joseph JL, et al. Pharmacokinetics of efavirenz and ritonavir after multiple oral doses in healthy volunteers, in Conference Record of the 12th World AIDS Conference. Geneva, June 28–July 3, 1998, Abstract 827 (1998).
39. Falloon J, Piscitelli S, Vogel S, Sadler H, Mitsuya M, Kavlick MF, et al. Combination therapy with amprenavir, abacavir, and efavirenz in human immunodeficiency virus-infected patients failing a protease inhibitor regimen: pharmacokinetic drug interactions and antiviral activity. Clin Infect Dis 30:313–318 (2000).
40. Duval X, Le Moing V, Longuet P, Leport C, Vilde JL, Lamotte C, et al. Efavirenz-induced decrease in plasma amprenavir levels in human immunodeficiency virus-infected patients and correction by ritonavir. Antimicrob Agents Chemother 44:2593 (2000).
41. Fiske WD, Mayers D, Wagner K, et al. Pharmacokinetics of DMP 266 and indinavir multiple oral doses in HIV-1 infected individuals. In: Programs and abstracts of the 4th Conference on Retroviruses and Opportunistic Infections. Washington, DC, January 22–26, 1997, Abstract 169 (1997).
42. Benedek IH, Fiske WD, White SJ, et al. Pharmacokinetic interaction between multiple doses of efavirenz and rifabutin in healthy volunteers. Clin Infect Dis 27:1008 (1998).
43. Piketty C, Race E, Castiel P, Belec L, Peytavin G, Si-Mohammed A, et al. Efficacy of a five-drug combination including ritonavir, saquinavir, and efavirenz in patients who failed on a conventional triple-drug regimen: phenotypic resistance to protease inhibitors predicts outcome of therapy. AIDS 13:F71–F77 (1999).
44. Trapnell CB, Narang PK, Li R, and Lavelle JP. Increased plasma rifabutin levels with concomitant fluconazole therapy in HIV-infected patients. Ann Intern Med 124:573–576 (1996).
45. Varhe A, Olkkola KT, and Nevmonen PJ. Effect of fluconazole dose on the extent of fluconazole-triazolam interaction. Br J Clin Pharmacol 42:465–470 (1996).
46. Crussell-Porter LL, Rindone JP, Ford MA, and Jaskar DW. Low-dose fluconazole therapy potentiates the hypoprothrombinemic response of warfarin sodium. Arch Intern Med 153: 102–104 (1993).
47. Sahai J, Gallicano K, Pakuts A, and Cameron DW. Effect of fluconazole on zidovudine pharmacokinetics in patients infected with human immunodeficiency virus. J Infect Dis 169: 1103–1107 (1994).
48. Rosenthal E, Sala F, and Chichmanian R-M. Ergotism related to concurrent administration of ergotamine tartrate and indinavir. JAMA 281:987 (1999).
49. Indinavir pharmacokinetics study group. Indinavir (MK 639) drug interactions studies. In: Program and abstracts of the XI International AIDS Conference. Vancouver, B.C., July 7–12, 1996, Abstract MoB174 (1996).
50. Merry C, Barry MG, Ryan M, et al. Interaction of sildenafil and indinavir when coadministered to HIV positive patients. AIDS 13:F101–F107 (1999).
51. Karyotakis NC and Anaissie EJ. The new antifungal azoles: fluconazole and itraconazole. Curr Opin Infect Dis 7:658–666 (1994).

52. Kerr B, Lee C, Yuen G, et al. Overview of in vitro and in vivo drug interactions studies of nelfinavir mesylate, a new HIV-1 protease inhibitor. In: Programs and abstracts of the 4th Conference on Retroviruses and Opportunistic Infections. Washington, DC, January 22–26, 1997, Abstract 373 (1997).

53. Cox SR, Schneck DW, Herman BD, et al. Delaviridine and nelfinavir: a pharmacokinetic drug-drug interaction study in healthy adult volunteers. In: Programs and abstracts of the 5th Conference on Retroviruses and Opportunistic Infections. Chicago, February 1–5, 1998, Abstract 345 (1998).

54. Honda M, Yasuoka A, Aoki M, and Oka S. A generalized seizure following initiation of nelfinavir in a patient with human immunodeficiency virus type 1 infection, suspected due to interaction between nelfinavir and phenytoin. Intern Med 38:302–303 (1999).

55. Murphy RL, Sommadossi JP, Lamson M, et al. Antiviral effect and pharmacokinetic interaction between nevirapine and indinavir in persons infected with human immunodeficiency virus type 1. J Infect Dis 179:1116–1123 (1999).

56. Clarke SM, Mulcahy FM, Tjia J, et al. Pharmacokinetic interactions of nevirapine and methadone and guidelines for use of nevirapine to treat injection drug users. Clin Infect Dis 33:1595–1597 (2001).

57. Sahai J, Cameron W, Salgo M, et al. Drug interaction study between saquinavir and nevirapine. In: Programs and abstracts of the 4th Conference on Retroviruses and Opportunistic Infections. Washington, DC, January 22–26, 1997, Abstract 178 (1997).

58. Polk RE, Israel DS, Patron R, et al. Pharmacokinetic interaction between 141W94 and rifabutin and rifampin after multiple dose administration. In: Programs and abstracts of the 5th Conference on Retroviruses and Opportunistic Infections. Chicago, February 1–5, 1998, Abstract 340 (1998).

59. Sadler B, Gillotin C, Chittick GE, and Symonds WT. Pharmacokinetic drug interactions with amprenavir. In: Conference record of the 12th World AIDS Conference. Geneva, June 28–July 3, 1998, Abstract 12389 (1998).

60. Hamzeh F, Benson C, Gerber J, et al. Steady-state pharmacokinetic interaction of modified-dose indinavir and rifabutin. In: Programs and abstracts of the 8th Conference on Retro-viruses and Opportunistic Infections. Chicago, IL, February 4–8, 2001, Abstract 742 (2001).

61. Sahai J, Stewart F, Swick L, et al. Rifabutin reduces saquinavir plasma levels in HIV-infected patients. In: Programs and abstracts of the 36th Interscience Conference on Antimicrobial Agents and Chemotherapy. Washington, DC, Abstract A27 (1996).

62. Jorga K and Buss NE. Pharmacokinetic drug interactions with saquinavir soft gel capsule. In: Programs and abstracts of the 39th Interscience Conference on Antimicrobial Agents and Chemotherapy. San Francisco, September 26–29, 1999, Abstract 20 (1999).

63. Centers for Disease Control. Notice to readers: updated guidelines for the use of rifabutin or rifampin for the treatment and prevention of tuberculosis among HIV-infected patients taking protease inhibitors or nonnucleoside reverse transcriptase inhibitors. MMWR 49:185–189 (2000).

64. Centers for Disease Control. Prevention and treatment of tuberculosis among patients infected with human immunodeficiency virus: principles of therapy and revised recommendations. MMWR 47(RR-20):1–58 (1998).

65. Benedek IH, Joshi A, Fiske WD, et al. Pharmacokinetic interaction between efavirenz and rifampin in healthy volunteers. In: Conference record of the 12th World AIDS Conference. Geneva, June 28–July 3, 1998 (1998).

66. Ribera E, Pou L, Lopez RM, et al. Pharmacokinetic interaction between nevirapine and rifampicin in HIV-infected patients with tuberculosis. J Acquir Immune Defic Syndr 28:450–453 (2001).

9. HIV/AIDS Drugs

67. Veldkamp AI, Hoetelmans MW, Beijnen JH, et al. Ritonavir enables combined therapy with rifampin and saquinavir. Clin Infect Dis 29:1586 (1999).
68. Gallicano KD, Sahai J, Shukla VK, et al. Induction of zidovudine glucuronidation and amination pathways by rifampicin in HIV-infected patients. Br J Clin Pharmacol 48:168–179 (1999).
69. Greenblatt DJ, von Moltke LL, Harmatz JS, et al. Alprazolam-ritonavir interaction: implications for product labeling. Clin Pharmacol Ther 67:335–341 (2000).
70. Degen O, Kurowski M, Van Lunzen J, Schewe CK, and Stelbrink H-J. Amprenavir and ritonavir: intraindividual comparison of different doses and influence of concomitant NNRTI on steady-state pharmacokinetics in HIV-infected patients. In: Programs and abstracts of the 8th Conference on Retroviruses and Opportunistic Infections. Chicago, February 4–8, 2001, Abstract 739 (2001).
71. Montero A, Giovannoni AG, and Tvrde PL. Leg ischemia in a patient receiving ritonavir and ergotamine. Ann Intern Med 130:329–330 (1999).
72. DeSilva KE, Le Flore DB, Marston BJ, and Rimland D. Serotonin syndrome in HIV-infected individuals receiving antiretroviral therapy and fluoxetine. AIDS 15:1281–1285 (2001).
73. Hsu A, Granneman GR, Cao G, et al. Pharmacokinetic interaction between ritonavir and indinavir in healthy volunteers. Antimicrob Agents Chemother 42:2784–2791 (1998).
74. van Heeswijk RPG, Veldkamp AI, Hoetelmans RMW, et al. The steady state plasma pharmacokinetics of indinavir alone and in combination with a low dose of ritonavir in twice daily dosing regimens in HIV-1 infected individuals. AIDS 13:F95–F99 (1999).
75. Henry JA and Hill IR. Fatal interaction between ritonavir and MDMA. Lancet 352:1751–1752 (1998).
76. Kurowski M, Kaeser B, Mroziekiewicz A, et al. The influence of low doses of ritonavir on the pharmacokinetics of nelfinavir 1250 mg bid. In: Programs and abstracts of the 40th Interscience Conference on Antimicrobial Agents and Chemotherapy. Toronto, September 17–20, 2000, Abstract 333 (2000).
77. Flexner C, Hsu A, Kerr B, et al. Steady-state pharmacokinetic interactions between ritonavir, nelfinavir, and the nelfinavir active metabolite M8 (AG1402). In: Conference record of the 12th World AIDS Conference. Geneva, June 28–July 3, 1998, Abstract 42265 (1998).
78. Hsu A, Granneman GR, and Bertz RJ. Ritonavir: clinical pharmacokinetics and interactions with other anti-HIV agents. Clin Pharmacokinet 35:275–291 (1998). [Erratum, Clin Pharmacokinet 35:473.]
79. Cato A, Cavanaugh J, Shi H, et al. The effect of multiple doses of ritonavir on the pharmacokinetics of rifabutin. Clin Pharmacol Ther 63:414–421 (1998).
80. Hsu A, Granneman GR, Cao G, et al. Pharmacokinetic interactions between two human immunodeficiency virus protease inhibitors, ritonavir and saquinavir. Clin Pharmacol Ther 63:453–464 (1998).
81. Merry C, Barry MG, Mulcahy FM, et al. Saquinavir pharmacokinetics alone and in combination with ritonavir in HIV-1 infected patients. AIDS 11:F29–F33 (1997).
82. Muirhead GJ, Wulff MB, Fielding A, Kleinermans D, and Buss N. Pharmacokinetic interactions between sildenafil and saquinavir/ritonavir. Br J Clin Pharmacol 50:99–107 (2000).
83. Hsu A, Granneman GR, Witt G, Cavanaugh JH, and Leonard J. Assessment of multiple doses of ritonavir on the pharmacokinetics of theophylline. In: Program and abstracts of the XI International AIDS Conference. Vancouver, B.C., July 7–12, 1996, 89 (1996).
84. Knoell KR, Young TM, and Cousins ES. Potential interaction involving warfarin and ritonavir. Ann Pharmacother 32:1299–1302 (1998).
85. Flaherty JF, Kearney B, Wolf J, et al. Coadministration of tenofovir DF and didanosine: a pharmacokinetic and safety evaluation. In: Programs and abstracts of the 41st Interscience

Conference on Antimicrobial Agents and Chemotherapy. Chicago, IL, December 16–19, 2001, Abstract 1729 (2001).
86. Merrill DP, Manion KJ, Chou TC, and Hirsch MS. Antagonism between human immunodeficiency virus type 1 protease inhibitors indinavir and saquinavir in vitro. J Infect Dis 176:265–268 (1997).
87. Rutschmann OT, Opravil M, Iten A, et al. A placebo-controlled trial of didanosine plus stavudine, with and without hydroxyurea, for HIV infection. The Swiss HIV Cohort Study. AIDS 12:F71–F77 (1998).
88. Goodrich J and Khardori N. Hydroxyurea toxicity in human immunodeficiency virus-positive patients. Clin Infect Dis 29:692–693 (1999).
89. Weissman SB, Sinclair GI, Green CL, and Fissell WH. Hydroxurea-induced hepatitis in human immunodeficiency virus-positive patients. Clin Infect Dis 29:223–224 (1999).
90. Hochster H, Dieterich D, Bozzette S, et al. Toxicity of combined ganciclovir and zidovudine for cytomegalovirus disease associated with AIDS: an AIDS clinical trials group study. Ann Intern Med 113:111–117 (1990).
91. Causey D. Concomitant ganciclovir and zidovudine treatment for cytomegalovirus retinitis in patients with HIV infection: an approach to treatment. J Acquir Immune Defic Syndr 4(Suppl 1):S16–S21 (1991).
92. Burger DM, Meenhorst PL, Koks CHW, and Beijnen JH. Drug interactions with zidovudine. AIDS 7:445–460 (1993).
93. Fortgang IS, Belitsos PC, Chaisson RE, and Moore RD. Hepatomegaly and steatosis in HIV-infected patients receiving nucleoside analog antiretroviral therapy. Am J Gastroenterol 90:1433–1436 (1995).
94. Boxwell DE and Styrt BA. Lactic acidosis in patients receiving nucleoside reverse transcriptase inhibitors. In: Programs and abstracts of the 39th Interscience Conference on Antimicrobial Agents and Chemotherapy. San Francisco, CA, September 26–29, 1999, Abstract 1284 (1999).
95. Lonergan JT, Behling C, Pfander H, et al. Hyperlactatemia and hepatic abnormalities in 10 human immunodeficiency virus-infected patients receiving nucleoside analogue combination regimens. Clin Infect Dis 31:162–166 (2000).
96. Lonergan JT, Havlir D, and Barber E, and Mathews WC. Incidence of symptomatic hyperlactatemia in HIV-infected adults on NRTIs. In: Programs and Abstracts of the 9th Conference on Retroviruses and Opportunistic Infections. Seattle, WA, February 24–28, 2002, Abstract 35 (2002).
97. Bristol-Myers Squibb Company. Healthcare provider important drug warning letter. January 5, 2001.

PART IV
Nonsteroidal Antiinflammatory Drugs

Chapter 10

Nonsteroidal Antiinflammatory Drugs

Cyclooxygenase Inhibitors, Disease-Modifying Antirheumatic Agents, and Drugs Used in Gout

Imad K. Abukhalaf, PhD,
Daniel A. von Deutsch, DDS, PhD, MSCR,
Mohamed A. Bayorh, PhD, and Robin R. Socci, PhD

Nonsteroidal antiinflammatory drugs (NSAIDs) can be divided into two major groups: cyclooxygenase (COX) inhibitors and noncyclooxygenase inhibitors. COX inhibitors represent a wide range of therapeutic agents. Non-COX inhibitors represent the disease-modifying antirheumatic drugs (DMARDs), and the agents used in gout.

Pharmacologically, the term NSAIDs should include both COX inhibitors and non-COX inhibitors. However, the generic term NSAIDs has come to refer to COX inhibitors only. Thus, to prevent any confusion, and in accordance with the most commonly utilized terminology, in this chapter, the terms NSAIDs and COX inhibitors will be used interchangeably.

This chapter discusses various aspects of the pharmacology of NSAIDs, DMARDs, and the agents used in gout.

1. COX INHIBITORS/NONSTEROIDAL ANTIINFLAMMATORY DRUGS

COX inhibitors are among the most widely used over-the-counter (OTC) therapeutic agents in the world. Other common designations for COX inhibitors are antipyretic

From: *Handbook of Drug Interactions: A Clinical and Forensic Guide*
A. Mozayani and L. P. Raymon, eds. © Humana Press Inc., Totowa, NJ

analgesics, antiinflammatory agents, antiinflammatory analgesics, and to a lesser extent nonnarcotic analgesics. Although there are several NSAID preparations available on the market, none of these agents is ideal for controlling or modifying the signs and symptoms of inflammation. These agents provide only symptomatic relief but do not slow the progression of the underlying disease. Although these agents are commonly referred to as NSAIDs, most of them exert not only antiinflammatory effect, but antipyretic and analgesic effects as well. These agents are used to treat mild to moderate pain and elevated body temperature, arthritis and other inflammatory disorders, as well as gout and hyperuricemia. A significant number of NSAIDs are available as OTC medications and are commonly taken for minor aches and pains.

Although not all NSAIDs are Food and Drug Administration (FDA) approved for the treatment of rheumatic diseases, most of them are effective in rheumatoid arthritis, osteoarthritis, and localized musculoskeletal syndromes such as sprains, strains, and lower back pain.

1.1. Functional Classification of NSAIDs

COX enzyme occurs in two isoenzymes, COX-1 and COX-2 *(1)*. COX-1 is a constitutive enzyme expressed in most tissues and in blood platelets. COX-2 is an inducible enzyme (inducible by cytokines, growth factors, and tumor promoters) and present mainly in inflammatory cells and is responsible for the production of prostaglandins, which function as chemical mediators in the inflammatory process. The antiinflammatory effect of NSAIDs is usually the result of their inhibition of COX-2 whereas their unwanted effects are primarily the result of their inhibition of COX-1. Investigations conducted recently by Deininger and colleagues *(2)* and others have shown that COX-2 positive cells accumulate in tumor cells, single macrophages, and microglial cells in the immediate surrounding necrotic area (the investigators concluded that further research was needed to determine whether COX-2 is part of the tumor's response to necrosis, or if it is involved in the development of necrosis).

Newer NSAIDs, like celecoxib and rofecoxib, are selective inhibitors of COX-2. They are approved by the FDA for the treatment of osteoarthritis and/or rheumatoid arthritis. Generally, NSAIDs are classified according to their selectivity to inhibit COX *(3,4)*. Those that inhibit both COX-1 and COX-2 are referred to as nonselective COX inhibitors, whereas the new-generation NSAIDs that selectively inhibit COX-2 are referred to as COX-2 selective inhibitors (Table 1).

1.2. Chemistry

With the exception of nabumetone, which is a ketone prodrug, all nonselective COX inhibitors that are available in the United States are weak organic acids. As shown in Table 1, they are categorized into several classes of compounds. These are: salicylic acids, acetic acid derivatives, propionic acid derivatives, fenamic acid derivatives, oxicams, *para*-phenolic acid derivatives, and pyrozalones. This dissimilarity in the chemical structure of NSAIDs results in a protean spectrum of pharmacokinetic properties.

1.3. Pharmacokinetics

The fact that NSAIDs have wide range of pharmacokinetic properties does not mean that they do not share common characteristics. For instance, most of these drugs

Table 1
Cyclooxygenase Inhibitors

Nonselective Inhibitors									Selective COX-2 Inhibitors
Salicylates									
Acetylated Salicylates	Nonacetylated Salicylates	Acetic Acid Derivatives	Propionic Acid Derivatives	Fenamic Acid Derivatives	Pyrazalones	Enolic Acids (Oxicams)	Aminophenols		
Aspirin	Sodium salicylate	Indomethacin	Ibuprofen	Mefenamic	Azapropazone[b]	Piroxicam	Phenacetin[b]		Celecoxib
Diflunisal	Calcium salicylate	Sulindac	Naproxen	Meclofenamic	Phenylbutazone[b]	Meloxicam	Acetaminophen		Rofecoxib
	Choline salicylate	Tolmetin	Fenoprofen	Flufenamic[b]	Oxyphenbutazone[b]	Tenoxicam[b]			
	Choline magnesium salicylate	Diclofenac	Ketoprofen						
	Magnesium salicylate	Etodolac	Flurbiprofen						
	Salicyl salicylate	Nabumetone[a]	Oxaprozin						
		Ketorolac	Tiaprofen[b]						
			Carprofen[b]						

[a] Prodrug.
[b] Not available or no longer available in the United States.

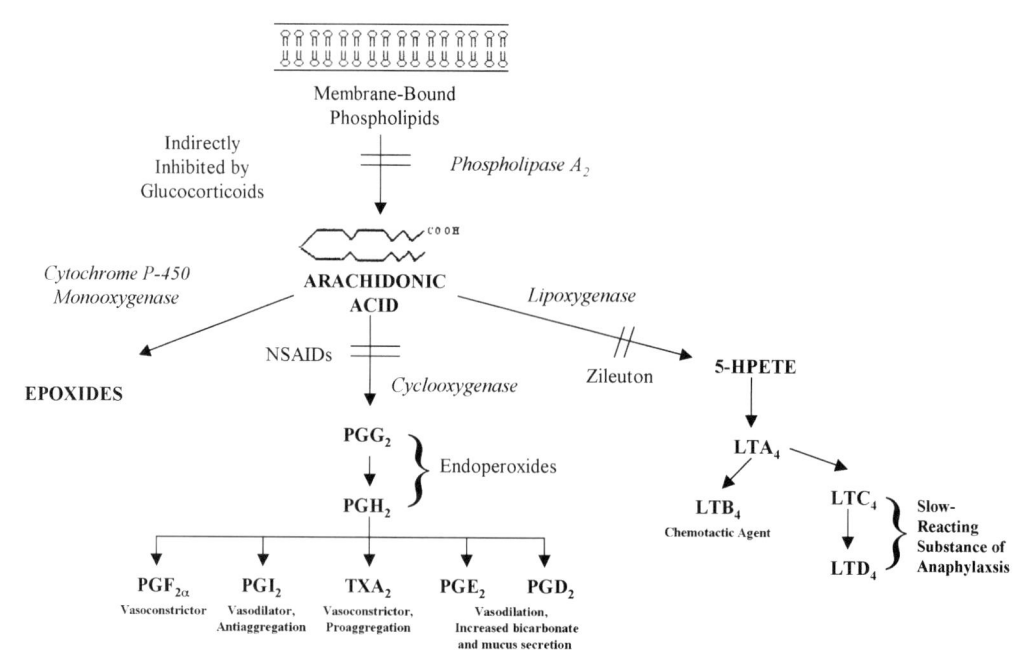

Fig. 1. Biosynthetic pathways for eicosanoid synthesis. Some prostaglandins are tissue-specific. NSAIDs = nonsteroidal anti-inflammatory agents; PGs, prostaglandins; TXA_2, thromboxane A_2; HPETE, hydroperoxyeicosatetraenoic acid; LT, leukotriene.

are well absorbed, and food does not substantially change their bioavailability. Additionally, most of these agents are highly protein-bound usually to albumin. Most NSAIDs are extensively metabolized, some by both phase I and phase II biotransformation reactions, whereas others by phase II conjugation reactions only. CYP3A or CYP2C are the main cytochrome P450 enzyme families responsible for most of phase I biotransformation reactions involving NSAIDs. Although some NSAIDS (and their metabolites) undergo enterohepatic circulation, generally, elimination of NSAIDs occurs primarily by renal excretion.

1.4. Pharmacodynamics and Their Antiinflammatory Effect

As mentioned above, ecosanoids, particularly prostaglandins, are important chemical mediators that play a major role in the inflammatory process. Inhibiting the biosynthesis of these eicosanoids results in the disruption of the biochemical events that lead to inflammation. The main antiinflammatory effect of NSAIDs is mediated primarily by the inhibition of prostaglandin synthesis. Specifically, NSAIDs inhibit COX, the enzyme that catalyzes the formation of prostaglandin endoperoxides PGG_2 and PGH_2 from arachidonic acid. As a result, the synthesis of all prostaglandins derived from these endoperoxides is inhibited (Fig. 1). This does not mean, however, that COX inhibition is NSAIDs' only antiinflammatory mechanism of action; other mechanisms of action do contribute to the overall antiinflammatory activity of some NSAIDs (5). The leukotrienes are major products of the lipoxygenase pathway. Leukotrienes (LT) C_4 and D_4 are potent bronchoconstrictors and are the primary components of the slow-reacting substance of anaphylaxis that is secreted in asthma and anaphylaxis. Leukotriene B_4 is a potent chemotactic agent for polymorphonuclear leukocytes (PMNs) and macrophages. Lipoxygenase inhibitors, such as zileuton, and the leukotriene receptor antagonist zafirlukast are used to alleviate the symptoms of asthma and anaphylaxis. Such mechanisms will be discussed with individual agents discussed in this chapter.

1.4.1. Antipyretic Effects of NSAIDs

Control of the body's temperature occurs in the thermoregulatory center in the hypothalamus. This center regulates the balance between the loss of body heat and heat production. Fever occurs when this balance is altered in favor of heat production. The inflammatory process and/or bacterial endotoxins cause(s) the release of interleukin-1 (IL-1) from macrophage which, in turn, induces the biosynthesis of E-type prostaglandins (PGE_n) in the hypothalamus, causing an increase in the body's temperature (fever) by raising the "thermostatic set-point." NSAIDs can reset the body's "thermostatic set-point" through the inhibition of COX, hence PGE_n biosynthesis. This action results in dilating superficial blood vessels and increased sweating, followed by a drop in temperature. NSAIDs have no effect on normal body temperature.

1.4.2. Analgesic Effects of NSAIDs

Tissue damage and inflammation result in the production of prostaglandins. Some of these prostaglandins, e.g., PGE_2, sensitize nociceptors to the actions of bradykinin, histamine, and 5-hydroxytryptamine, and other chemical mediators (6). Thus, the severity of pain associated with inflammatory diseases such as arthritis, bursitis, and with some forms of cancer (metastatic cancer of bone) can effectively be alleviated with NSAIDs. Additionally, by inhibiting COX, NSAIDs are very effective in alleviating headaches resulting from the vasodilatory effects of PGE_2. NSAIDs can also be used in combination with opioids resulting in a reduction of the required effective dose of opiates by 30%.

In addition to the effects that NSAIDs have locally in alleviating pain, there is growing evidence that NSAIDs are acting, in part, through a centrally mediated component (7). The exact mechanism(s) by which NSAIDs act centrally remain(s) unclear. In addition to NSAIDs' ability to inhibit COX, they may act through monoaminergic control system. Prostaglandins such as PGE_2 have been shown to augment the action of excitatory neural mediators such as calcitonin gene-related peptides through mediating their release. By inhibiting the action of COX centrally, NSAIDs block PGE_2-mediated interference with the down regulation of nociception, thereby reducing the magnitude and duration of pain. In the spinal cord, results from current research suggest that COX-2, and not COX-1, inhibitors attenuate pain by reducing prostaglandin-induced spinal excitability.

1.5. Common Adverse Effects of NSAIDs

Adverse effects of NSAIDs are common especially in individuals taking high doses over long periods of time (8). Common adverse effects are often encountered in the gastrointestinal (GI) tract, skin, kidney, and to a lesser extent in liver, spleen, blood, and bone marrow. The severity and frequency of occurrence of these effects vary greatly among NSAIDs.

1.5.1. On the Gastrointestinal Tract

The most common adverse effects (approximately threefold that of non-NSAIDs users) associated with the use of NSAIDs are GI tract disturbances that include dyspepsia, diarrhea or constipation, nausea, and vomiting *(9)*. The extent of gastric damage in chronic users may go unnoticed, potentially leading to erosive gastritis, peptic ulceration, and serious hemorrhage. The risk of such damage in chronic users has been determined to be approximately one out of five. The risk of gastric bleeding from commonly prescribed NSAIDs varies greatly. Due to the seriousness and frequency of the GI irritation associated with NSAIDs, warnings regarding the risks of serious GI injury are now included with the NSAID package inserts as required by the FDA.

The mechanism by which NSAIDs cause GI tract damage is a result of its inhibition of COX-1 resulting in inhibiting the production of PGE_2, which is responsible for regulating gastric acid secretion and mucosal protection. The effect of NSAIDs on gastric damage can be reduced by oral administration of prostaglandin analogs such as misoprostol.

1.5.2. On the Skin

The second most common adverse effect associated with the use of NSAIDs is skin reactions, which can range from mild rashes, photosensitivity, and urticaria to more serious conditions. Fortunately, potentially fatal skin-related adverse reactions are rare. Sulindac and mefenamic acid have particularly high incidences of skin reactions, with frequencies of occurrence of 5–10% and 10–15%, respectively.

1.5.3. On the Renal System

Generally, normal use of NSAIDs has little impact on kidney function. However, some individuals suffer acute reversible renal insufficiency, which usually ends when drug administration is stopped. The basis behind these renal effects is that PGE_2 and PGI_2 influence renal vasodilation and inhibit the actions of antidiuretic hormone (ADH). This results in decreased water reabsorption, and thus enhanced water excretion. Inhibiting prostaglandin biosynthesis by NSAIDs results in renal vasoconstriction, increased water reabsorption, hence increased water retention. Unlike normal usage, chronic treatment with NSAIDs can result in more serious adverse effects such as chronic nephritis and renal papillary necrosis. The combination of these two conditions results in "analgesic nephropathy."

1.6. Common Drug Interactions

NSAIDs interact with several therapeutic agents and with themselves *(10)*. For example, aspirin has been known to dissociate other NSAIDs from the plasma protein-binding sites. The most important drug interactions involving NSAIDs are those with heparin and oral anticoagulants. The concomitant administration of NSAIDs with heparin or oral anticoagulants such as warfarin has been known to increase the risk of bleeding. This is because of the NSAIDs ability to inhibit platelet aggregation and displace these agents (anticoagulants) from their plasma protein-binding sites, thus potentiating their effect(s). Other drug interactions include sulfonamides, which can be also displaced from their plasma protein-binding sites by salicylates. This leads to increased blood concentrations of free sulfonamides and therefore increased toxicity associated

10. Nonsteroidal Antiinflammatory Drugs

with these agents. Likewise, the combination of NSAIDs with lithium or methotrexate can lead to increased toxicity associated with these agents as their rate of excretion is reduced, thus increasing their plasma levels. Additionally, the coadministration of any of the NSAIDs and probenecid results in potentiation of the NSAID effect. Patients who combine NSAIDs with these agents should be monitored closely for titration of dosage.

Other drug interactions involving NSAIDs are those with loop diuretics and antihypertensive drugs. The concomitant administration of NSAID and a diuretic or an antihypertensive agent leads to decreased efficacies of these agents. In such cases, patients should be monitored closely for drug effectiveness.

1.7. Nonselective COX Inhibitors

1.7.1. Salicylates

Available salicylate preparations include acetyl salicylic acid, sodium salicylate, salicylic acid, magnesium salicylate, methylsalicylate, salicylamide, 5-aminosalicylate, and diflunisal. The most frequently used members of this class of drugs are acetyl salicylic acid (aspirin) and sodium salicylate *(11,12)*. Until the advent of ibuprofen, aspirin was the standard against which all NSAIDs were measured.

Like most other NSAIDs, the analgesic, antipyretic, and antiinflammatory actions of salicylates are primarily attributed to their ability to inhibit COX. The action of salicylates is exerted both in the periphery and at the thermoregulatory center in the brain.

1.7.1.1. ACETYLATED SALICYLATES

1.7.1.1.1. Aspirin (Acetyl Salicylic Acid)

1. **Absorption, Distribution, and Metabolism:** As with all acidic drugs, aspirin (and other salicylates) absorption is influenced by pH. Aspirin is rapidly absorbed in the stomach and upper small intestine in the nonionized form. Alkalinization of the gastric juice and the use of enteric-coated or buffered aspirin preparations result in reduced gastric irritation and decreased rate (not extent) of absorption without reducing its clinical effectiveness. Aspirin, like most NSAIDs, is transported bound to albumin (90%). It is distributed across membranes by passive diffusion. It crosses the placenta and can be detected in milk, other bodily fluids, and tissues.

   Once absorbed, aspirin undergoes rapid hydrolysis of its components, salicylate and acetic acid, by the actions of tissue and plasma esterases to its components salicylate and acetic acid. This accounts for its short (15-min) plasma half-life. Half-lives of salicylates and other NSAIDs are shown in Table 2. Most of aspirin's therapeutic effects are attributed to its salicylate metabolite. Approximately 13% of a given salicylate therapeutic dose is eliminated in the urine, and the rest undergoes several routes of biotransformation reactions before elimination, of which 50% is conjugated to glycine, 20% is glucuronated at the hydroxyl-group site, 12% is glucuronated at the carboxyl-group site, and the rest (less than 5%) is oxidized into gentisic acid.

   When plasma concentration of salicylate exceeds 300 µg/mL (total body load of 600 mg), the metabolic enzyme system responsible for salicylate metabolism becomes saturated resulting in a longer half-life for the drug. At this point, elimination of salicylate conjugates by the kidney changes from first-order to zero-order kinetics. This means that any additional amount of salicylate beyond this point will result in a disproportionate increase in salicylate concentration. Consequently, salicylate half-life increases from 3–5 h at the lower analgesic doses to 12–15 h at the higher antiinflammatory doses.

Table 2
Half-Lives of Nonsteroidal Antiinflammatory Drugs

Drug	Half-Life (Hours)
A. Nonselective COX Inhibitors	
Aspirin	0.25
Salicylate[a]	2–19
Diclofenac	1.1
Diflunisal	13
Etodolac	6.5
Fenoprofen	2.5
Flurbiprofen	3.8
Ibuprofen	2
Indomethacin	4–5
Ketoprofen	1.8
Ketorolac	4–10
Meclofenamate	3
Meloxicam	20
Nabumetone[b]	26
Naproxen	14
Oxaprozin	58
Piroxicam	57
Sulindac	8
Tolmetin	1
B. Selective COX Inhibitors	
Celecoxib	11
Rofecoxib	17

[a]Major antiinflammatory metabolite of aspirin.
[b]Nabumetone is a prodrug; the half-life is for its active metabolite.

2. **Pharmacologic Actions and Therapeutic Indications:** Aspirin possesses antiinflammatory, analgesic, and antipyretic properties. Among all NSAIDs, aspirin is the only agent that irreversibly inhibits COX by acetylating the serine residue(s) at or near the active site of the enzyme (13). In addition, it interferes with the functions of inflammatory chemical mediators resulting in inhibiting granulocyte adherence to damaged vasculature, stabilizing lysosomal membranes, and inhibiting the migration of PMNs to the inflammation site (14). Inhibition of such events results in the cessation of the inflammatory process.

As an analgesic, aspirin is indicated for reducing pain of mild to moderate intensity. It is ineffective in cases of severe visceral pain. By inhibiting prostaglandin synthesis, PGE_2 will not be available to sensitize the nerve endings to the actions of bradykinin, histamine, and other chemical mediators of inflammation, and thus sensation of pain is inhibited.

As an antipyretic, aspirin is indicated for reducing elevated body temperature. It has virtually no effect on normal body temperature. This effect is mediated by COX inhibition in the thermoregulatory center in the hypothalamus. This results in the inhibition of PGE_2, which is normally secreted by white blood cells in response to inflammation or infection. Additionally, aspirin inhibits IL-1 (a cytokine released from macrophages during inflammation). Such actions culminate in vasodilation of superficial blood vessels and therefore, increased heat dissipation.

In significantly lower doses, aspirin is a very effective antithrombotic agent indicated in the prophylaxis of myocardial infarction, stroke, and other thromboembolic disorders *(15)*. It is well documented that the protaglandin thromboxane A_2 enhances platelet aggregation, a primary event in thrombus formation. At low doses, aspirin inhibits the production of thromboxane A_2 in platelets (by irreversibly inhibiting COX) resulting in reduced platelet aggregation *(16)*.

3. **Preparations and Dosage:** Aspirin is commercially available in many forms such as tablets, chewable tablets, chewing gum, controlled-release tablets, enteric-coated tablets, and solutions. Generally, the dosage of aspirin needed to inhibit platelet aggregation is significantly less than that needed for analgesic or antipyretic effect, which in turn, is less than the dose needed to relieve inflammation caused by arthritic and other inflammatory disorders. For the relief of mild pain or fever, the optimal dose for adults and adolescents ranges from 325 to 650 mg every 4 h, or 500 mg every 3 h, or 1000 mg every 6 h. For children ages 2–14, the optimal dose ranges from 10 to 15 mg/kg/dose every 4 h, up to 80 mg/kg/d.

   For the relief of mild to moderate pain associated with inflammation, as in osteoarthritis or rheumatoid arthritis, the maximum dosage for adults should not exceed 6 g/d. For children, the dose ranges from 10 to 80 mg/kg/d, in divided doses every 4–6 h. On the other hand, if indicated for the treatment of juvenile rheumatoid arthritis, the dose ranges from 60 to 110 mg/kg/d in divided doses every 6–8 h. For the treatment of acute rheumatic fever, however, the dose for adult ranges from 5 to 8 g/d in divided doses. As for children, the initial dose should not exceed 100 mg/kg/d in divided doses for the first 2 wk, then a maintenance dose of 75 mg/kg/d in divided doses for the next 4–6 wk.

   To reduce the severity of or prevent acute myocardial infarction, aspirin is indicated in a dose of 160 mg/d. To reduce the risk of myocardial infarction for patients with unstable angina or previous myocardial infarction, aspirin should be administered in a dose of 325 mg/d.

   As discussed previously, when aspirin is taken in antiinflammatory doses, the half-life of its primary active metabolite, salicylic acid, changes to 12 h or more. In this case, frequent dosing may not be necessary. It is clinically acceptable for patients who are on high-dose regimen to divide their total daily dosage of aspirin into only three portions taken after meals.

4. **Contraindications:** Aspirin is contraindicated in patients who are allergic to aspirin or its derivatives and components, to tartrazine dye, and in people with asthma, or bleeding disorders such as hemophilia and peptic ulcers. Aspirin is also contraindicated in children with flu symptoms or chickenpox, because aspirin may increase the risk of Reye's syndrome. There has been no evidence that aspirin exerts any harmful effects on the unborn fetus.

5. **Adverse Effects:** Adverse effects associated with aspirin are dose-dependent. At therapeutic doses, aspirin can cause gastrointestinal distress and ulceration. High antiinflammatory doses can cause tinnitus. Regular use of large doses can cause decreased blood iron levels (from bleeding), leukopenia, thrombocytopenia, ecchymosis, rash, urticaria, angioedema, and salicylism, which is characterized by dizziness, tinnitus, vomiting, diarrhea, confusion, central nervous system (CNS) depression, diaphoresis, headache, hyperventilation, and lassitude. As mentioned above, treatment with aspirin should be avoided with children to eliminate the risk of Reye's syndrome. Table 3 illustrates the toxic effects associated with various doses of aspirin.

Table 3
Toxic Effects of Salicylates

Dose (g)	Plasma Concentration (mg/dL)	Pharmacologic Effect	Toxic Effect
0.080–0.160	0–5	Antiplatelet	Impaired Hemostasis, Hypersensitivity Reactions,
0.650–0.975	5–10	Analgesic Antipyretic	Gastric Intolerance, Bleeding
3–6	10–50	Antiinflammatory	Tinnitus
6–10	50–80	Salicylism	Hyperventilation, Respiratory Alkalosis
10–20	80–110	Salicylism	Fever, Dehydration, Metabolic Acidosis
20–30	>110	Salicylism	Shock, Coma, Respiratory & Renal Failure, Death

6. **Treatment of Aspirin Toxicity and Salicylism:** Treatment should start with measuring plasma salicylate levels and urine pH. As shown in Table 3, serious toxicity becomes imminent if the amount ingested exceeds 150 mg/kg. If ingestion is recent, gastric lavage is recommended. In serious cases, intravenous administration of fluid to maintain high urine volume is necessary. Infusion of sodium bicarbonate to alkalinize the urine, ventilatory assistance, correction of acid-base and electrolyte imbalance is of utmost importance.

   At the cellular level as the dose of aspirin is increased, there is an uncoupling of the ability of the electron transport chain to convert the energy of the normally established proton gradient across the inner mitochondrial membrane into adenosine 5"triphosphate (ATP). This occurs by allowing protons to cross the otherwise impermeable mitochrondrial membrane thus collapsing of the proton gradient. Since electron transport continues, but phosphorylation of adenosine 5'-triphosphate (ADP) to ATP is prevented, there is an increase in metabolism to reestablish the proton gradient as well as increased oxygen consumption. The result is increased acidosis, and in response, hyperventilation and respiratory alkalosis. The eventual result is respiratory and metabolic acidoses.

7. **Drug Interactions:** Administering aspirin concomitantly with other drugs/drug classes may produce undesirable adverse effects *(17)*. These drugs/drug classes include:
   a. Heparin or other anticoagulants: It is well documented that the combination of aspirin and heparin, coumarin, or any other anticoagulant results in increased risk of bleeding and prolongation of bleeding time.
   b. Antacids and activated charcoal: They have been shown to reduce the rate of aspirin absorption.
   c. Urine acidifiers such as ascorbic acid, sodium phosphate, and ammonium chloride: They decrease the rate of excretion of salicylic acid by increasing the rate of its reabsorption.
   d. Urine alkalinizers (i.e., methotrexate): They increase the rate of aspirin excretion.
   e. Alcohol: Concomitant administration of alcohol and aspirin results in increased risk of bleeding.

f. Penicillin: Aspirin increases the half-life of penicillin because it competes with penicillin on the active secretory transporters in the renal tubules.
   g. Vancomycin: Coadministration of aspirin and vancomycin results in increased risk of ototoxicity.
   h. ACE (angiotensin-converting enzyme) inhibitors (i.e., enalapril): Concomitant administration of aspirin and ACE inhibitors results in decreased antihypertensive effect.
   i. Corticosteroids: They increase the rate of excretion of aspirin resulting in reduced plasma levels.
   j. Carbonic anhydrase inhibitors (i.e., acetazolamide): Although they increase excretion of aspirin, they also potentiate its toxicity by inducing metabolic acidosis and enhancing its penetration into the tissues.
   k. Nizatidine: Results in increased plasma levels of aspirin.
   l. Methotrexate: Aspirin has been shown to decrease the rate of excretion of methotrexate resulting in higher plasma levels and increased methotrexate toxicity.
   m. Sulfonylureas (i.e., tolbutamide): Large doses of aspirin may enhance the effects of sulfonylureas.

1.7.1.1.2. Diflunisal. Diflunisal is a difluorophenyl derivative of salicylic acid that is not metabolized into salicylic acid. It is more potent than aspirin as an antiinflammatory and analgesic agent. On the other hand, unlike aspirin, it does not exert antipyretic effect. Diflunisal undergoes enterohepatic circulation and is also found in the milk of lactating women. Additionally, its side effects are those common to NSAIDs but to a lesser extent. Diflunisal metabolism is subject to saturation kinetics. Because its clearance is dependent on renal function, it is contraindicated in patients with compromised renal function. Additionally, it is contraindicated in patients with asthma attacks, rhinitis, NSAID-precipitated urticaria, and in patients sensitive to diflunisal.

1. **Preparations and Dosage:** Diflunisal is available in 250- and 500-mg tablets. For the relief of mild to moderate pain, diflunisal is started with a 1-g dose followed by 0.5 g every 8–12 h. Maximum dosage should not exceed 1.5 g/d. As an antiinflammatory agent for patients with osteoarthritis or reuhmatoid arthritis, diflunisal is initiated as 0.5 or 1 g/d in divided doses twice a day provided that the daily dosage does not exceed 1.5 g.
2. **Drug Interactions:** Diflunisal interacts with several drug/drug classes, which include:
   a. Antacids: Concomitant administration of diflunisal and antacids results in decreased plasma levels of diflunisal.
   b. NSAIDs: Diflunisal should not be taken with other NSAIDs for this may result in increased risk of gastrointestinal irritation and bleeding.
   c. Acetaminophen: Long-term use of both diflunisal and acetaminophen may increase the risk of adverse renal effects.
   d. Beta-blockers: Diflunisal has been shown to impair the antihypertensive effects of beta-blockers and other antihypertensive agents.
   e. Concomitant use of diflunisal with either cefamandole, cefoperazone, cefotetan, valproic acid, or plicamycin may result in increased risk of hypoprothrombinemia.
   f. The use of diflunisal with colchicines, glucocorticoids, potassium supplements, alcohol, or the long-term use of corticotropin have been shown to increase the risk of gastrointestinal irritation and bleeding.
   g. Cyclosporin and gold compounds: Coadministration of either compound with diflunisal increases the risk of nephrotoxicity.

h. Digoxin, methotrexate, phenytoin, insulin, oral antidiabetic agents, or loop diuretics: The administration of any of these agents with diflunisal results in increased plasma concentration of these drugs, which may lead to increased toxicity associated with these agents.
i. Heparin, oral anticoagulants, thrombolytic agents: Diflunisal administration with any of these drugs/drug classes may result in prolonged prothrombin time, and increased risk of bleeding.
j. Probenecid: It increases plasma concentrations of diflunisal.

1.7.1.2. NONACETYLATED SALICYLATES

Nonacetylated salicylates agents include salicylsalicylate (salsalate), magnesium salicylate, sodium salicylate, calcium salicylate, choline salicylate, and combined choline magnesium salicylate. These agents possess significant antiinflammatory activity. As analgesics, however, they are less effective than aspirin. Because they are less effective inhibitors of COX, their side effects regarding GI irritation and peptic ulceration are attenuated rendering them suitable for patients with asthma and with individuals who are prone to bleeding and/or GI disorders.

1.7.2. Acetic Acid Derivatives

1.7.2.1. INDOMETHACIN

Indomethacin is an indole acetic acid derivative. It is 20–30 times more potent than aspirin in its antiinflammatory, analgesic, and antipyretic effects. This is attributable not only to COX inhibition, but also to its ability to reduce polymorphonuclear cell migration and decrease T- and B-cell proliferation, which are key events in the inflammatory process. It is also believed to inhibit the production of arachidonic acid (primary precursor of eicosanoids) by inhibiting phospholipases A and C *(18)*. It also influences the intracellular cyclic-AMP (adenosine monophosphate) concentrations by inhibiting phosphodiesterase.

Like most other NSAIDs, indomethacin is well absorbed. It is metabolized in the liver and undergoes extensive enterohepatic circulation. It appears in the breast milk of lactating women. Indomethacin and its inactive metabolites are excreted unchanged in bile and urine. It is indicated for the symptomatic relief of osteoarthritis, rheumatoid arthritis, and ankylosing spondylitis. It is also very effective in the management of acute gouty arthritis. It is the drug of choice for the treatment of patent ductus arteriosus, which is maintained by continual synthesis of prostacyclin and PGE_2 *(19)*. It is also used in the management of Bartter's syndrome, which involves a deficiency in renal chloride reabsorption and overproduction of prostaglandins, and Sweet's syndrome, which is acute febrile neurophilic dermatosis.

1. **Preparations and Dosage:** Indomethacin is available in 25- and 50-mg capsules, 75-mg sustained-release capsules, and 25-mg/5 mL suspension also for oral use. Additionally, 50-mg suppositories and 1-mg indomethacin per vial for intravenous use (after suspension) are also available.

    For the symptomatic relief of osteoarthritis, rheumatoid arthritis, or ankylosing spondylitis in adults, indomethacin is administered in 25- to 50-mg tablets (or oral suspension) twice to four times a day. The dosage can be increased by 25 or 50 mg/d every week as long as the total dose does not exceed 200 mg/d. After clinically acceptable response is achieved, the dose should be reduced to the minimum required to maintain the same response. Suppositories can be given in 50-mg doses up to four times a day.

For the symptomatic relief of juvenile arthritis, indomethacin is administered 1.5 to 2.5 mg/kg/d in divided doses (three to four times per day) not to exceed 4 mg/kg/d or 150 to 200 mg/d. When a clinically acceptable response is achieved, the dose is reduced to the minimum dose needed to maintain that response.

For the symptomatic relief of acute gouty arthritis in adults, the usual loading dose is 100 mg followed by 50 mg three times a day. Maximum dosage should not exceed 200 mg/d. When a clinically acceptable response is achieved, dosage should be tapered until the drug is discontinued. If suppositories are used, 50 mg four times a day is the recommended regimen. Suppository use should be avoided when possible to avoid rectal irritation and bleeding.

For the treatment of patent ductus arteriosus in premature infants weighing 500–1750 g, initial loading dose of 0.2 mg/kg over 5–10 s, followed by 0.25 mg/kg given at 12- to 24-h intervals, if needed. For neonates who are less than 7 d old, the follow-up dosage is reduced to 0.2 mg/kg. For neonates under 2 d old, the follow-up dosage is reduced to 0.1 mg/kg, if needed.

2. **Contraindications and Adverse Effects:** Indomethacin is strictly contraindicated in pregnancy, especially during the third trimester to prevent indomethacin-induced premature closure of the ductus arteriosus. It is also contraindicated in patients allergic to indomethacin, iodides, other NSAIDs, or their components. Adverse effects associated with indomethacin include abdominal pain, diarrhea, vomiting, pancreatitis, and GI bleeding. Headaches (in some cases associated with dizziness and confusion) have been reported in 15–25% of patients. Hematinic adverse effects were reported including agranulocytosis, aplastic anemia, bone marrow depression, hemolytic anemia, and iron-deficiency anemia. Hyperkalemia and hypoglycemia were also reported. Because it can be excreted in the breast milk of lactating mothers, it may cause seizures in infants.
3. **Drug Interactions:** The agents that interact with diflunisal (listed earlier), also interact with indomethacin. Other drugs/drug classes that interact with indomethacin include:
    a. Aminoglycosides: increased risk of aminoglycoside toxicity as a result of its increased concentration in the plasma.
    b. Bone marrow depressants: may result in increased leukopenic and thrombocytopenic effects of these agents.
    c. Probenecid: significantly prolongs indomethacin's half-life resulting in increased indomethacin toxicity.
    d. Zidovudine: the coadministration of zidovudine and indomethacin results in increased toxicity of both drugs.
    e. Lithium: increased plasma lithium concentration and thus increased lithium toxicity.
    f. Platelet aggregation inhibitors: may result in increased risk of GI irritation and hemorrhage.
    g. Diflunisal: increases plasma indomethacin concentration resulting in increased toxicity.

1.7.2.2. Diclofenac

Diclofenac is a phenylacetic acid derivative that possesses antiinflammatory, analgesic, and antipyretic properties with potency equal to that of indomethacin. This is attributable not only to its effectiveness in inhibiting COX but its ability to decrease the bioavailability of arachidonic acid by enhancing its conversion to triglycerides. Like most other NSAIDs, diclofenac is rapidly absorbed following oral administration, and undergoes extensive first-pass metabolism resulting in a systemic bioavailability of approximately 50%. It is one of the few NSAIDs that accumulates in the synovial fluid with half-life in this compartment double that of the plasma. It is metabolized in the liver principally by CYP3A4 and its inactive metabolites are excreted primarily in urine and to a lesser extent in the bile. Its side effects are those common to NSAIDs, which include GI distress, hemorrhage, and to a lesser extent peptic ulceration. This drug is more commonly associated with increased plasma aminotransferase levels than any other NSAID. Other adverse effects such as dizziness, drowsiness, headache, bradycardia, glaucoma, tinnitus, and leukocytosis have been reported although to a lesser extent.

1. **Preparations, Therapeutic Indications, and Contraindications:** Diclofenac sodium is available in 25-, 50-, and 75-mg enteric-coated tablets. Extended-release tablets and rectal suppositories are available for adults. Diclofenac is indicated primarily as an anti-inflammatory agent in the treatment of rheumatoid arthritis, osteoarthritis, and ankylosing spondylitis *(20)*. Additionally, it is used as an analgesic in the management of patients with dysminorrhea and/or chronic lower back pain.

    Diclofenac is contraindicated in patients with active bleeding or ulcers, asthma attacks, rhinitis, NSAID-induced urticaria, or allergy to diclofenac or other NSAIDs.

2. **Dosages:** For the relief of pain and inflammation in rheumatoid arthritis, 75 or 100 mg of diclofenac sodium, as extended-release tablets, is administered daily (or 75 mg twice a day). If regular tablets are used, the loading dose should be 150–200 mg/d in divided doses. The maintenance dose is 75–100 mg/d in divided doses. The maximum dose should not exceed 225 mg/d. Sometimes rectal suppositories are used to replace tablets in the last oral dose. In such case, 50–100 mg of diclofenac is given.

    For the relief of pain and inflammation of osteoarthritis, diclofenac tablets are given in the amount of 100–150 mg/d in divided doses. The maximum dose should not exceed 150 mg/d.

    To relieve pain in ankylosing spondylitis, diclofenac tablets are given in the amount of 100–125 mg/d in four or five divided doses.

    For the relief of pain associated with dysmenorrhea, diclofenac tablets (50-mg) are given twice a day; if necessary, 100 mg can be given as a loading dose only. If the patients are elderly or have serious renal dysfunction, dosage may be reduced.

3. **Drug Interactions:** Plasma levels of diclofenac are increased by the coadministration of cimetidine. Cimetidine, a histamine receptor antagonist, also binds to cytochrome P450 and diminishes the activity of hepatic microsomal mixed-function oxidases. Diclofenac also interacts with the drug/drug classes that interact with indomethacin (detailed previously).

1.7.2.3. SULINDAC

Sulindac is a pyrroleacetic acid derivative. It is a prodrug that is metabolized into an active sulfide metabolite that possesses significant antiinflammatory activity. It is very well absorbed when administered orally. Because the metabolite undergoes extensive enterohepatic circulation, it has a relatively long half-life (Table 2). It occurs in two enantiomers with the S (–) enantiomer being more active as COX inhibitor than the R (+) enantiomer.

As with other NSAIDs the use of sulindac is associated with GI distress although to a lesser extent than indomethacin or aspirin. However, like diclofenac, it is associated with increased plasma levels of aminotransferases. Additionally, among all NSAIDs, it is the most commonly associated with cholestatic liver damage. Other less common adverse effects observed with sulindac include thrombocytopenia, agranulocytosis, and nephrotic syndrome.

1. **Preparations, Therapeutic Indications, and Contraindications:** Sulindac is available in 100- and 200-mg tablets. Sulindac is indicated for the treatment of rheumatoid arthritis, osteoarthritis, ankylosing spondylitis, acute gout, tendinitis, and brusitis. It has also been shown to suppress familial intestinal polyposis.

    Sulindac is contraindicated in patients with angioadema, asthma, bronchospasm, nasal polyps, rhinitis, or NSAID-induced urticaria.

2. **Dosage:** To decrease pain and inflammation in ankylosing spondylitis, bursitis, osteoarthritis, and rheumatoid arthritis, sulindac is administered in a dose of 150–200 mg twice a day. This dosage is to be adjusted based on the patient's response up to a maximum of 200 mg twice a day.

    For the relief of symptoms of acute gouty arthritis, and tendinitis, sulindac is given as 200 mg twice a day for 7–14 d. This dosage should be decreased to the lowest effective dosage after obtaining a clinically satisfactory response. In elderly patients, if necessary, the dosage should be reduced to half of the usual adult dosage.

3. **Drug Interactions:** Like diclofenac and other NSAIDs, sulindac interacts with several therapeutic agents. In addition to the interactions shown with diflunisal, diclofenac, and other NSAIDs, sulindac interacts with the following drugs/drug classes:

    a. Ranitidine and cimetidine: Coadministration of sulindac with either of these agents leads to increased bioavailability of these agents.

    b. Dimethyl sulfoxide (DMSO): Coadministration of DMSO and sulindac leads to decreased effectiveness of the latter.

1.7.2.4. TOLMETIN

Tolmetin is a pyrroleacetic acid derivative. It is more potent antiinflammatory agent than aspirin but less than endomethacin *(21)*. Due to its short half-life (Table 2) and thus the need for frequent dosing, it fell into disfavor. Adverse effects associated with tolmetin are similar to those with other NSAIDs. These include GI distress, nausea, abdominal pain, diarrhea, headache, drawsiness, hypertension, dysuria, hematuria, and less frequently hepatitis.

Unlike most other NSAIDs, it does not displace anticoagulants such as warfarin from plasma protein-binding sites. However, it does prolong bleeding time presumably by prolonging prothrombin time and inhibiting the production of thromboxane A_2 in the platelets (like aspirin).

1. **Preparations, Therapeutic Indications, and Contraindications:** Tolmetin is available in 200- and 600-mg capsules. As with most other NSAIDs, tolmetin is indicated in patients with rheumatoid arhritis, osteoarthritis, and ankylosing spondylitis. It is ineffective in the treatment of acute gout. It is contraindicated in patients with angioadema, asthma, bronchospasm, nasal polyps, rhinitis, or NSAID-induced urtichaira.

2. **Dosage:** For the relief of pain associated with rheumatoid arthritis and osteoarthritis, tolmetin is administered in a dosage of 400 mg three times a day. The total daily maintenance dosage ranges from 600 to 1800 mg administered in divided doses either three or four times a day. The maximum dosage for rheumatoid arthritis is 2000 mg/d, whereas that of osteoarthritis is 1600 mg/d.

For the relief of juvenile rheumatoid arthritis in children over 2 yr of age, tolmetin is initially given in the amount of 20 mg/kg/d in divided doses three or four times a day. The maintenance dose is 15–30 mg/kg/d in divided doses. The maximum dose is 30 mg/kg/d.

3. **Drug Interactions:** Drug interactions involving tolmetin are similar to those of other NSAIDs detailed above. Tolmetin also interacts with the drug/drug classes shown below:
   a. ACE inhibitors: Concomitant administration of ACE inhibitors and tolmetin may result in decreased efficacy of the former and possibly reduced renal function.
   b. Alendronate: It may increase the GI distress associated with tolmetin.
   c. Antineoplastics, antithymocyte globulin, and strontium-89 chloride: Coadministration of any of these agents with tolmetin may increase the risk of bleeding.
   d. Cidofovir: It may contribute to increasing risk of nephrotoxicity.

1.7.2.5. ETODOLAC AND ITS PREPARATIONS, THERAPEUTIC INDICATIONS, AND CONTRAINDICATIONS

Etodolac is a pyranoindoleacetic acid derivative. It possesses antiinflammatory, analgesic, and antipyretic properties. It is significantly more selective COX-2 inhibitor than COX-1. It is well and rapidly absorbed. Its adverse effects, contraindications, and drug interactions associated with etodolac are similar to other NSAIDs.

Etodolac is available in 200- and 300-mg capsules. It is indicated mainly for analgesia and for the treatment of osteoarthritis. Generally, it is less effective than other NSAIDs in the treatment of rheumatoid arthritis. It is contraindicated in patients who are allergic to etodolac or its components or in patients with angioedema, bronchospasm, rhinitis, nasal polyps, and/or NSAID-induced urticaria.

For the treatment of osteoarthritis, 800–1200 mg etodolac is administered per day in divided doses. Maintenance dose ranges from 600 to 1200 mg/d in divided doses. The maximum daily dose is 1200 mg. For patients weighing less than 132 pounds (60 kg), the maximum dose is 20 mg/kg/d. If extended-release tablets are given, the adult dose normally ranges from 400 to 1000 mg/d.

As an analgesic, a loading dose of 400 mg is used, then 200–400 mg every 6–8 h. For patients weighing 132 pounds (60 kg) or more, the maximum dose is 1200 mg/d. For patients weighing less than 132 pounds, the maximum dose is 20 mg/kg/d.

1.7.2.6. NABUMETONE

Nabumetone, a naphthylalkanone derivative, is the only nonacid COX inhibitor available in the United States *(22)*. It is a ketone prodrug that is metabolized to the active acetic acid form. It has a relatively long half-life (Table 2) permitting a once- or twice-a-day dosing regimen. Unlike many other NSAIDs, it does not undergo enterohepatic circulation.

Its adverse effects and contraindications are similar to other NSAIDs. Additionally, it has been reported to cause muscle spasms, myalgia, alopecia, jaundice, photosensitivity, pruritus, and rash. Blood urea nitrogen (BUN), serum creatinine, and electrolyte levels must be monitored in patients taking nabumetone for early signs of impaired renal functions, especially in elderly patients or those who have compromised hepatic or renal functions.

1. **Preparations, Therapeutic Indications, and Contraindications:** Nabumetone is available in 500- and 750-mg tablets. It is primarily indicated in the treatment of rheumatoid arthritis.

10. Nonsteroidal Antiinflammatory Drugs

2. **Dosage:** For the relief of symptoms of acute and chronic osteoarthritis and rheumatoid arthritis, nabumetone is initially given in a 1-g dose per day or in divided doses twice daily. This is increased to 1.5–2 g/d in divided doses preferably twice daily. The maintenance dose is adjusted according to the clinical response. The maximum dose should not exceed 2 g/d.

*1.7.2.7. K*ETOROLAC

Ketorolac is a pyrrolopyrrole compound. It possesses antiinflammatory, analgesic, and antipyretic properties. It is used, however, for systemic analgesia mainly in the management of short-term acute postoperative pain. The adverse effects associated with ketorolac, its drug interactions profile, and contraindications are similar to those of other NSAIDs. It has been reported, however, that the use of ketorolac for more than 5 d is associated with a significant increase in renal impairment and peptic ulcerations. For this reason, it is no longer available in the Canada and some European markets.

1. **Preparations, Therapeutic Indications, and Contraindications:** Ketorolac is available as 10-mg tablets. It is also available in injectable form in 15-mg/mL, 30-mg/mL, and 60-mg/2mL preparations. It can be administered orally, intravenously, or more commonly, intramuscularly. It is indicated for the management of acute postoperative pain for a period not exceeding 5 d.

    It is not recommended in obstetrics or for preoperative analgesia or for long-term treatment.
2. **Dosages:** For the acute management of pain, ketorolac is given orally four to six times per day for no longer than 5 d. If given intramuscularly, a loading dose of 30–60 mg of ketorolac followed by a maintenance dose of 15–30 mg every 6 h is recommended. The maximum daily dose is 150 mg the first day and 120 mg thereafter.

1.7.3. Propionic Acids

*1.7.3.1. I*BUPROFEN

Ibuprofen is a phenylpropionic acid derivative. It possesses antiinflammatory, analgesic, and antipyretic properties. It is extensively metabolized in the liver into inactive metabolites. Ibuprofen has had an excellent safety record and is available under several trade names for analgesia as OTC medications. It replaced aspirin as the gold standard against which other NSAIDs are compared. It has a relatively short half-life (Table 2) and, like diclofenac, it accumulates in the synovial fluid for prolonged periods of time.

Its GI adverse effects are similar to aspirin, but they occur less frequently. Other adverse effects are rash, pruritus, headache, tinnitus, and fluid retention nephritis. Acute renal failure has also been reported.

1. **Preparations, Therapeutic Indications, and Contraindications:** Ibuprofen is available as 400-, 600-, and 800-mg tablets. It is indicated for the treatment of osteoarthritis, rheumatoid arthritis, and dysmenorrhea. OTC preparations are used for the treatment of headaches, dysmenorrhea, and musculoskeletal pain. It is contraindicated in patients with angioedema, bronchospasm, nasal polyps, asthma attacks, rhinitis, NSAID-induced urticaria, or in patients allergic to ibuprofen or other NSAIDs.
2. **Dosage:** For the relief of pain associated with rheumatoid arthritis and osteoarthritis, ibuprofen is given as 300, 400, 600, or 800 mg three to four times daily. The maximum range per day is 1.2–3.2 g. To relieve pain associated with primary dysmenorrhea,

the normal dose is 400 mg every 4 h as needed. To relieve minor aches and pains, and to reduce fever, a dose of 200–400 mg every 4–6 h is the standard, up to a maximum dose of 1.2 g/d. For the relief of pain associated with juvenile arthritis, children are given 30–70 mg/kg/d in divided doses either three or four times daily. A dose of 20 mg/kg/d is given for a mild form of the disease. To reduce fever in children between 6 mo and 12 yr old, they are given 5–10 mg/kg every 4–6 h, up to a maximum dose of 40 mg/kg/d.

3. **Drug Interactions:** Ibuprofen interacts with other therapeutic agents such as:
   a. Acetaminophen: Long-term use of both ibuprofen and acetaminophen may lead to increased risk of nephrotoxicity.
   b. Antihypertensives: The coadministration of antihypertensive agent with ibuprofen may lead to decreased efficacy of the former.
   c. Alcohol and other NSAIDs: The administration of ibuprofen with any other NSAID has been shown to increase the risk of bleeding and GI adverse effects.
   d. Bone marrow depressants: The concomitant administration of ibuprofen and bone marrow depressants may cause increased leukopenic and thrombocytopenic effects of the latter.
   e. Cefamandole, cefoperazone, and cefotetan, plicamycin, and valproic acid: Administration of any of these agents with ibuprofen may increase the risk of hypoprothrombinemia, ulceration, and bleeding.
   f. Colchicine, platelet aggregation inhibitors, corticosteroids, potassium supplements: The coadministration of any of these agents with ibuprofen may increase the risk of GI adverse effects and in some cases GI bleeding.
   g. Cyclosporin: The concomitant administration of ibuprofen and cyclosporin may increase the risk of nephrotoxicity. This may also result in increased plasma levels of cyclosporin.
   h. Digoxin: The administration of ibuprofen and digoxin may lead to increased blood levels of digoxin and thus increased risk of digitalis toxicity.
   i. Diuretics (including loop-potassium-sparing, and thiazide): The administration of any of these agents with ibuprofen may result in decreased efficacies of these agents.
   j. Gold compounds and nephrotoxic drugs: May result in increased risk of adverse renal effects.
   k. Heparin, oral anticoagulants, and thrombolytics: Increased anticoagulant effects and thus increased risk of hemorrhage.
   l. Insulin, and oral antidiabetic drugs: The combination of ibuprofen and any of these agents may result in increased hypoglycemic effects of these agents.
   m. Lithium: The combination of ibuprofen and lithium may lead to increased blood levels of lithium.
   n. Methotrexate: Ibuprofen and other NSAIDs are contraindicated in patients taking methotraxate because such a combination may result in decreased methotrexate clearance, and thus increased risk of methotrexate toxicity.
   o. Probenecid: The coadministration of probenecid and ibuprofen may result in increased blood levels and toxicity of the latter.

1.7.3.2. NAPROXEN

Naproxen is phenylpropionic acid derivative that possesses antiinflammatory, analgesic, and antipyretic properties. It has a relatively long half-life rendering it suitable for once- or twice-a-day dosing regimen. Naproxen undergoes phase I and phase II biotransformation reactions and is excreted in the form of inactive conjugates or free acid. Upper GI adverse effects associated with naproxen are significantly less than those with aspirin but double those of ibuprofen *(23)*. The adverse effects associated with NSAIDs have been observed with naproxen. However, naproxen has had a very good safety record and has been available as an OTC medication for several years.

1. **Preparations, Therapeutic Indications, and Contraindications:** Naproxen is available as a free acid in 250-, 375-, and 500-mg tablets, 375- and 500-mg delayed-release tablets, 375- and 500-mg controlled-release tablets, or as an oral suspension (125 mg/5 mL). In the form of naproxen sodium, it is available as 250- and 500-mg tablets by prescription or OTC in 200-mg tablets. Naproxen is indicated for the treatment of osteoarthritis, rheumatoid arthritis, ankylosing spondylitis, juvenile arthritis, acute tendinitis, and bursitis. It is also indicated as an analgesic for musculoskeletal back pain and dysmenorrhea. Because naproxen has the ability to inhibit the migration of polymorphonuclear leukocytes, it is also indicated for the treatment of acute gouty arthritis. Its contraindications are similar to other NSAIDs detailed earlier in the chapter.
2. **Dosage:** For the relief of mild to moderate musculoskeletal inflammation, including ankylosing spondylitis, osteoarthritis, and rheumatoid arthritis, naproxen in the form of tablets, delayed-release tablets, or oral suspension is given in the amount of 250–500 mg twice a day, up to a maximum of 1500 mg/d. Naproxen sodium, in the form of extended-release tablets, is given in a dose of 750 to 1000 mg/d, up to a maximum of 1500 mg/d. If regular naproxen tablets are used, the normal dose is 275–550 mg twice daily, up to a maximum of 1650 mg/d. The combination of naproxen tablets and suppositories is possible, however, the combined dose (oral plus suppository) should not exceed 1500 mg/d.

    To relieve symptoms of juvenile rheumatoid arthritis and other inflammatory conditions in children, they are given naproxen at 10 mg/kg/d in divided doses twice daily as either oral suspension or tablets.

    To relieve symptoms of acute gouty arthritis, adults receiving delayed-release tablets, oral suspension, or regular tablets of naproxen are given an initial dose of 750 mg followed by 250 mg every 8 h until symptoms subside. Adults receiving extended-release tablets of naproxen sodium are given an initial dose of 1000–1500 on the first day, then 1000 mg daily until symptoms subside. The dose should not exceed more than 1500 mg/d. Adults given naproxen sodium tablets receive an initial dose of 825 mg followed by 275 mg every 8 h until symptoms subside.

    For the relief of mild to moderate pain, including acute tendinitis and bursitis, and dysmenorrhea, adults receiving delayed-release tablets of naproxen are normally given an initial dose of 1000 mg every day, to be increased as prescribed, up to a maximum of 1500 mg/d. Adults receiving extended-release tablets of naproxen sodium are given an initial dose of 1100 mg every day, to be increased as prescribed, up to a maximum of 1500 mg/d. Adults receiving oral suspension or regular tablets of naproxen are given an initial dose of 500 mg followed by 250 mg every 6–8 h, up to a maximum of 1250 mg/d. Adults receiving tablets of naproxen sodium are given an initial dose of 550 mg followed by 275 mg every 6–8 h, up to a maximum of 1375 mg/d.

    To relieve fever, mild to moderate musculoskeletal inflammation, and mild to moderate pain, adults receiving OTC tablets of naproxen sodium are usually given 220 mg every 8–12 h or 440 mg followed by 220 mg 12 h later. The maximum dose is 660 mg/d for 10 d unless directed otherwise by a physician. The dose for patients over the age of 65 is reduced to 220 mg every 12 h, up to a maximum of 440 mg for 10 d.
3. **Drug Interactions:** Drug interactions involving naproxen are similar to other NSAIDs.

1.7.3.3. FENOPROFEN

Fenoprofen is a propionic acid derivative. It has analgesic and antiinflammatory properties. It has a relatively short half-life (Table 2). The adverse effects associated with fenoprofen are similar to those with other NSAIDs but to a lesser extent. Among all NSAIDs, fenoprofen is most closely associated with toxic effects of interstitial nephritis.

1. **Preparations, Therapeutic Indications, Contraindications, and Drug Interactions:** Fenoprofen, as fenoprofen calcium, is available in 200- and 300-mg capsules and 600-mg tablets. It is indicated for the relief of pain, stiffness, and inflammation from rheumatoid arthritis, and osteoarthritis. It is also used as an analgesic in dysmenorrhea and musculoskeletal pain. Contraindications and drug interactions are the same of those described for other NSAIDs.
2. **Dosage:** To manage mild to moderate pain, adults receiving capsules or tablets of fenoprofen calcium are given 200 mg every 4–6 h as needed.

    To relieve pain, stiffness, and inflammation from rheumatoid arthritis or osteoarthritis, adults receiving capsules or tablets of fenoprofen calcium are given 300 to 600 mg three or four times daily, up to a maximum dose of 3200 mg/d.

1.7.3.4. FLURBIPROFEN

Flurbiprofen is a propionic acid derivative. It is one of the newest nonselective COX inhibitors to be approved in the United States. It undergoes enterohepatic circulation and its R (+) and S (–) enantiomers are extensively metabolized by phase I and phase II biotransformation reactions. Its adverse effects are typical of other NSAIDs.

1. **Preparations, Therapeutic Indications, Contraindications, and Drug Interactions:** Flurbiprofen is available in 50- and 100-mg tablets. It is indicated for the treatment of acute or chronic osteoarthritis, and rheumatoid arthritis. As with most other NSAIDs, it is contraindicated in patients with angioedema, bronchospasm, nasal polyps, asthma attacks, rhinitis, NSAID-induced urticaria, or in patients allergic to flurbiprofen or other NSAIDs.
2. **Dosage:** To treat acute or chronic rheumatoid arthritis and osteoarthritis, adults receiving extended-release capsules are given 200 mg daily in the evening. If, on the other hand, tablets are to be used, patients are given an initial dose of 200 to 300 mg/d in divided doses twice to four times a day, up to a maximum dose of 300 mg/d.

1.7.3.5. KETOPROFEN

Ketoprofen is a propionic acid derivative. Its antiinflammatory and analgesic activities are attributed to its ability to inhibit COX as well as 5-lipoxygenase. Additionally, it has been shown to stabilize lysosomal membranes. As with most other NSAIDs, it is rapidly absorbed. It is metabolized in the liver and undergoes enterohepatic circulation. Its GI and CNS adverse effects are typical of other NSAIDs.

1. **Preparations, Therapeutic Indications, Contraindications, and Drug Interactions:** Ketoprofen is available in 25-, 50-, and 75-mg capsules. It is indicated for the management of osteoarthritis and rheumatoid arthritis. It is also used in gout and for primary dysmenorrhea. Its contraindications and drug interactions are typical of other propionic acid derivatives such as ibuprofen and flurbiprofen.

10. Nonsteroidal Antiinflammatory Drugs 357

2. **Dosage:** For the management of osteoarthritis and rheumatoid arthritis, the usual dose is 75 mg three times a day or 50 mg four times a day. If extended-release caplets are use, the dose is 200 mg once a day. For primary dysmenorrhea, the usual dose is 25–50 mg every 6–8 h as necessary.

1.7.3.6. OXAPROZIN

Oxaprozin is a propionic acid derivative. It possesses antiinflammatory as well as uricosuric properties rendering it more useful in the treatment of gout than any other NSAID. It has a very long half-life (Table 2), which makes it suitable for once-daily dosing regimen.

1. **Preparations, Therapeutic Indications, Contraindications, and Drug Interactions:** Oxaprozin is available in 600-mg caplets and 600-mg tablets. It is indicated for the treatment of rheumatoid arthritis and osteoarthritis. Its contraindications and drug interactions are typical of other propionic acid derivatives.
2. **Dosage:** To treat rheumatoid arthritis, patients are given 1200 mg every day with the dosage adjusted based on the patient's response, up to a maximum of either 1800 mg/d in divided doses twice or thrice a day.

To treat osteoarthritis, patients are given 600–1200 mg every day, up to a maximum of either 1800 mg/d in divided doses twice or three times a day. An initial loading dose of 1200–1800 mg can be given to speed up the onset of action. In patients with renal impairment, the initial dose should be limited to 600 mg every day.

1.7.4. Fenamic Acids

1.7.4.1. MECLOFENAMATE AND MEFENAMIC ACID

These agents are derivatives of fenamic acid. The antiinflammatory effect of meclofenamate and mefenamic acid is attributed to their ability to inhibit COX and phospholipase A_2. These agents undergo phase I and phase II biotransformation reactions. Conjugated metabolites are excreted in urine and unconjugated metabolites are excreted in the feces. They are not superior to other NSAIDs in their antiinflammatory effects. The adverse effects associated with these agents are similar to other NSAIDs. The use of mefenamic acid, in particular, is associated with high incidence of skin reactions. Their GI adverse effects (particularly diarrhea) associated with these agents are more severe and frequent than with other NSAIDs. For this reason they have not received widespread clinical use for the treatment of inflammatory disorders.

1. **Preparations, Therapeutic Indications, Contraindications, and Drug Interactions:** Meclofenamate is available in 50- and 100-mg capsules. Mefenamic acid is available as 250-mg capsules. Although both agents can be used for the treatment of rheumatoid arthritis and osteoarthritis, because of the high incidence of toxicity associated with these drugs they fell into disfavor. Most commonly, they are indicated as analgesics to relieve the pain associated with dysmenorrhea. They are contraindicated in pregnancy and should not be used for more than a week.
2. **Dosage:** The loading dose of mefenamic acid is 500 mg for the first day, then 250 mg every 6 h thereafter for no more than a week. To relieve pain and inflammation of rheumatoid arthritis and osteoarthritis, meclofenamate is given as 50–100 mg every 6–8 h

as needed, up to a maximum of 400 mg/d. To treat primary dysmenorrhea, meclofenamate is given as 100 mg three times a day for up to 6 d.

1.7.5. Enolic Acids (Oxicams)

1.7.5.1. MELOXICAM

Meloxicam is an enolcarboxamide, an oxicam derivative. Although meloxicam inhibits both COX-1 and 2, it is slightly COX-2 selective *(24)*. Unlike most other NSAIDs, meloxicam is slowly absorbed. It has a relatively long half-life (Table 2). Although it has been used in Europe and the Middle East for some time, it has been recently been approved for use in the United States.

1. **Preparations, Therapeutic Indications, Adverse Effects, Contraindications, and Drug Interactions:** It is available in 3.5-, 7.5-, and 15-mg tablets. It is indicated for the treatment of osteoarthritis. Its adverse effects and contraindications are similar to those described for other NSAIDs. Recently, it has been shown to decrease the diuretic effect of furosemide. Other drug interactions are similar to those associated with other NSAIDs.
2. **Dosage:** To relieve pain due to osteoarthritis, the dose is 7.5 mg a day, up to a maximum of 15 mg a day.

1.7.5.2. PIROXICAM AND ITS PREPARATIONS, THERAPEUTIC INDICATIONS, CONTRAINDICATIONS, AND DRUG INTERACTIONS

Piroxicam is an oxicam. Like most of the NSAIDs discussed thus far, piroxicam's antiinflammatory, analgesic, and antipyretic activities are attributed to its ability to nonselectively inhibit COX-1 and -2. At high concentrations, it has been shown to inhibit the migration of polymorphonuclear leukocytes. Unlike meloxicam, piroxicam is rapidly absorbed. Due to its enterohepatic circulation, it has a very long half-life (ranges from 30 to 85 h) (Table 2), which permits a once-a-day dosing regimen. It is extensively metabolized in the liver and metabolites are excreted in urine and feces. The adverse effects associated with piroxicam are typical of other NSAIDs.

Piroxicam is available in 10- and 20-mg capsules. It is indicated for the treatment of rheumatoid arthritis and osteoarthritis. Drug interactions and contraindications are similar to other NSAIDs.

1.7.6. Aminophenols

1.7.6.1. ACETAMINOPHEN

Acetaminophen is a *para*-aminophenol derivative. It possesses analgesic and antipyretic properties. Although it is a weak COX inhibitor, it is not an NSAID *per se*. It has virtually no antiinflammatory effects and lacks platelet inhibitory effects.

Acetaminophen is available as OTC medication under several trade names. The mechanism behind its analgesic and antipyretic effects is not well understood, but believed to be the result of its inhibitory effects on COX in the CNS rather than the periphery. Orally administered acetaminophen is rapidly and completely absorbed. Its half-life is relatively short (2 h). Acetaminophen is extensively metabolized by hepatic microsomal conjugation enzymes and is converted to glucuronide and sulfate conjugates. These metabolites are pharmacologically inactive and are readily excreted in urine.

In therapeutic doses, acetaminophen is virtually void of any significant adverse effects. It is significantly safer than aspirin. With larger doses, however, abdominal pain, dizziness, nausea, vomiting, and disorientation have been reported. With massive doses (overdose), hepatic toxicity and liver failure may occur *(25,26)*.

1. **Mechanism Behind Acetaminophen Toxicity:** Less than 5% of ingested acetaminophen undergoes phase I biotransformation reactions. These reactions, catalyzed by the microsomal CYP450 enzyme system, yield *N*-acetyl-*para*-benzoquinone (NABQ). NABQ is a very reactive electrophile that is neutralized by intracellular glutathione. As long as intracellular glutathione is available, virtually no hepatic damage occurs. However, if acetaminophen is taken in massive doses (10–15 g or higher), conjugation pathways become saturated, which leads to the accumulation of NABQ *(27)*. When the intracellular glutathione pool is depleted, this very reactive compound will bind to nucleophilic groups on the cellular proteins and causes lipid peroxidation, resulting in hepatotoxicity and sometimes death. Agents such as *N*-acetylcysteine and cysteamine can be used within hours of acetaminophen overdose to protect victims from hepatotoxicity.

2. **Preparations, Therapeutic Indications, and Contraindications:** Acetaminophen is available in 160-, 325-, 500-, and 650-mg capsules or tablets. It is also available as extended-release tablets, elixirs, solutions, suspensions, suppositories, chewable tablets, and sprinkles. Additionally, acetaminophen is available in combination with other agents such as caffeine, phenyltoloxamine, antihistamines, and codeine. Generally, it is indicated for the relief of minor to moderate pain associated with headache, musculoskeletal ache, toothache, menstrual cramps, minor arthritis, and common cold. Because it possesses antipyretic properties, acetaminophen is also indicated to reduce fever.

    Acetaminophen is considered the analgesic and antipyretic of choice for children with viral infections because acetaminophen, unlike aspirin, does not increase the risk of Reye's syndrome. It is contraindicated in patients allergic to acetaminophen or its components and in patients with hepatic disease.

3. **Dosage:** For the relief of mild to moderate pain associated with headache, muscle ache, backache, minor arthritis, common cold, toothache, menstrual cramps, or to reduce fever, the usual dose ranges from 325 to 650 mg every 4–6 h. Also, it can be given in a dose of 1000 mg three or four times a day, or two extended-release caplets every 8 h, up to a maximum of 4000 mg/d. Dosages for children of various ages are shown in Table 4.

4. **Drug Interactions:** Acetaminophen interacts with a number of drugs/drug classes. These include:
    a. Oral contraceptives: Oral contraceptives have been known to decrease the efficacy of acetamenophen.
    b. Propranolol: The concomitant administration of propranolol and acetaminophen results in increased effectiveness of the latter.
    c. Anticholinergics: Anticholinergics interfere with (slow down) the absorption of acetaminophen and thus retard its onset of action.
    d. Barbiturates, hydantoins, rifampin, sulfinpyrazone, isoniazid, and carbamazepine: The coadministration of any of these agents with acetaminophen may result in decreased therapeutic effects and increased hepatotoxic effects of acetaminophen.
    e. Probenecid: Concomitant administration of acetaminophen and probenecid may result in increased therapeutic efficacy of the former.
    f. Loop diuretics and lamotrigine: acetaminophen may decrease the therapeutic effects of these agents.

Table 4
Acetominophen Dosages for Children of Various Ages

Age (years)	Dosage Every 4 h (mg)	Maximum No. of Doses per 24 h
0–3 mo	40	5
4–11 mo	80	5
1	120	5
2–3	160	5
4–5	240	5
6–8	320	5
9–10	400	5
11	480	5
12–14	640	5
>14	650	5

g. Zidovudine: The coadministration of acetaminophen and zidovudine may result in decreased effects of the latter.

h. Alcohol: Chronic alcohol consumption depletes liver mitochondrial GSH (reduced glutathione) and induces cytochrome P450. Both actions increase the hepatotoxic effects of NABQ.

1.7.7. Other Nonselective COX Inhibitors

Other nonselective COX inhibitors include azapropazone, carprofen, flufenamic acid, phenacetin, phenylbutazone, tenoxicam, and tiaprofen. These agents are not available in the United States and will not be discussed further in this chapter.

1.8. COX-2 Selective Inhibitors

1.8.1. Celecoxib

Celecoxib is a pyrazole derivative. It is a highly selective COX-2 inhibitor. Its potency as an inhibitor of COX-2 is at least 300 times more than that of COX-1 *(28)*. It is well absorbed and highly protein-bound. Its half-life is 11 h (Table 2). There is no evidence that celecoxib has any effect on platelet aggregation. Because it has virtually no effect on COX-1, GI adverse effects (such as peptic ulceration) associated with this agent are minimal compared to nonselective COX inhibitors *(29)*. Other (non-GI) adverse effects associated with this drug are comparable to other NSAIDs. It is primarily metabolized by CYP2C9 in the liver.

1. **Preparations, Therapeutic Indications, and Contraindications:** Celecoxib is available in 100-, and 200-mg capsules. It is indicated for the relief of pain associated with osteoarthritis and rheumatoid arthritis *(30)*. As an adjunct medication, it is used to reduce adenomatous colorectal polyps in patients with familial adenomatous polyposis. It is contraindicated in patients allergic to aspirin, celecoxib or its components, or other NSAIDs. It is also contraindicated in patients who are sensitive to sulfonamide derivatives or those who have a history of NSAID-induced nasal polyps with bronchospasms.

10. *Nonsteroidal Antiinflammatory Drugs*   361

2. **Dosage:** To relieve pain associated with osteoarthritis, the dose is 200 mg every day or 100 mg twice a day. To relieve pain from rhematoid arthritis, the dose is 100–200 mg twice a day up to 400 mg/d.

   As an adjunct medication to reduce adenomatous colorectal polyps in patients with familial adenomatous polyposis, adults are given 400 mg twice a day. For patients with hepatic impairment, the daily dosage should be reduced. For patients weighing less than 50 kg, the therapy should be started with the lowest recommended dose.

3. **Drug Interactions:** Celecoxib interacts with the following drugs/drug classes:
   a. ACE inhibitors: Celecoxib has been shown to decrease the antihypertensive effects of ACE inhibitors, which may result in increased risk of renal failure.
   b. Aspirin: Concomitant administration of celecoxib and aspirin results in increased risk of GI complications and bleeding.
   c. Lithium: Celecoxib may cause increased plasma lithium levels.
   d. Oral anticoagulants: Celecoxib potentiates warfarin effect by increasing prothrombin time and thus the risk of bleeding.
   e. Fluconazole: The coadministration of fluconazole and celecoxib results in increased plasma levels of the latter.
   f. Furosemide and thiazide diuretics: Celecoxib has been shown to decrease the diuretic effects of these drugs, which may result in increased risk of renal failure.
   g. Fluconazole: Concomitant administration of celecoxib and fluconazole results in increased plasma levels of celecoxib.

1.8.2. Rofecoxib

Rofecoxib is a furanone derivative. It is highly selective COX-2 inhibitor *(31,32)*. It possesses antiinflammatory properties and appears to have analgesic and antipyretic effects as well. It is well-absorbed. It is less protein-bound than celecoxib. Its relatively long half-life (17 h) allows for a once-a-day dosing regimen. Like celecoxib, because it is selective COX-2 inhibitor, the GI adverse effects associated with this agent are minimal. Its other adverse effects are typical of other NSAIDs. Rofecoxib is metabolized primarily by cytosolic hepatic enzymes. At the time of writing this chapter, it was reported that the FDA is investigating reports that rofecoxib may be linked to rare cases of aseptic (nonbacterial) meningitis in humans.

1. **Preparations, Therapeutic Indications, and Contraindications:** Rofecoxib is available in 12.5- and 25-mg tablets and oral suspensions of 12.5 mg/5 mL and 25 mg/5 mL. It is indicated for the treatment of osteoarthritis and for the management of acute pain and primary dysmenorrhea *(33,34)*. As with celecoxib, rofecoxib is contraindicated in patients allergic to aspirin, rofecoxib or its components, or other NSAIDs. It is also contraindicated in patients who have a history of NSAID- or iodide-induced nasal polyps, angioedema, asthma, bronchospasm, rhinitis, or urticaria.
2. **Dosage:** To treat osteoarthritis, adults receiving oral suspension or tablets are given an initial dose of 12.5 mg every day, which may be increased, if needed, to 25 mg every day, up to a maximum of 50 mg/d. To manage acute pain and primary dysmenorrhea, adults are given 50 mg of rofecoxib in an oral suspension or tablet form every day for up to 5 d.
3. **Drug Interactions:** In addition to the drugs/drug classes listed under celecoxib, rofecoxib interacts with the following agents:
   a. Methotrexate: As with most COX inhibitors, the coadministration of rofecoxib and methotrexate increases the plasma levels of methotrexate.

b. Rifampin: It has been shown to decrease the plasma levels, and probably effectiveness, of rofecoxib.

c. Cimetidine: The coadministration of cimetidine and rofecoxib results in increased plasma levels of the rofecoxib.

1.8.3. Other COX-2 Selective Inhibitors

There are a number of COX-2 selective inhibitors that are still under investigation. Of these, valdecoxib appears to be the most promising *(35)*. Recombinant enzyme assays suggest that valdecoxib is a significantly more potent and selective COX-2 inhibitor than celecoxib or rofecoxib.

1.9. Selecting the Right NSAID

Prescription and OTC NSAIDs are available from many different sources and in many strengths. Patients should take the minimum dosage to which they achieve a satisfactory clinical response. As with other medications, there is substantial individual variation in clinical response to NSAIDs. For this reason, patients should be aware that what works for others may not work for them and vice versa. Additionally, patients who are on other medications such as warfarin should consider NSAIDs (ibuprofen or tolmetin) that do not interact with oral anticoagulants. Also, if compliance is a problem, NSAIDs that do not require frequent dosing may increase compliance. Furthermore, there is no relationship between the price of the NSAID and its clinical effectiveness *(36)*. Likewise, there is no relationship between the price of the NSAID and the incidence of adverse effects. Although newer NSAIDs may not be associated with significant GI adverse effects, they may exert toxic effects in other ways.

2. DISEASE-MODIFYING ANTIRHEUMATIC DRUGS (DMARDs)

Unlike COX inhibitors, which only provide symptomatic relief and do not influence the progression of the disease, most DMARDs have been shown to slow the progression of bone and cartilage damage in osteoarthritis and rheumatoid arthritis *(37,38)*. These agents may induce remission but cannot repair existing damage. The effects of some of these medications may take up to 6 mo before they become evident *(39,40)*. This is why these medications are sometimes referred to as "slow-acting drugs." The various DMARD subclasses are shown in Table 5. These therapeutic agents are used for the treatment of patients with severe rheumatic disorders that have not responded adequately to COX inhibitors *(41)*.

2.1. Immunosuppressive Drugs

2.1.1. Methotrexate

Methotrexate is an antineoplastic and immunomodulating agent that has several mechanisms of action *(42)*. As a folic acid analog, it inhibits dihydrofolate reductase, thereby limiting the availability of tetrahydrofolate for DNA synthesis. Thus, the replication of T lymphocytes and other rapidly dividing cells that play a role in the inflammatory process is inhibited. Additionally, it interferes with the migration of PMNs to the site of inflammation. Methotrexate also reduces the production of free radicals and inhibits the production of some cytokines *(43)*.

Table 5
Disease Modifying Antirheumatic Drugs

Immunosuppressants	Antimalarial	Alkylating Agents	Gold	Anti-TNF-α	Interleukin Receptor Antagonists	Other
Methotrexate Cyclosporin Azathioprine Leflunomide	Chloroquine Hydroxychloroquine	Chlorambucil Cyclophosphamide	Aurothiomalate Aurothioglucose Auranofin	Infliximab Etanercept	Anakinra	Penicillamine Sulfasalazine[a]

[a]Prodrug.

Methotrexate is approximately 70% absorbed when taken orally. Compared to other DMARDs, it is well tolerated. Its adverse effects include GI toxicity including ulcerative colitis and diarrhea, nausea, mucosal ulcers, cytopenias, liver cirrhosis, acute pneumonia-like syndrome, and dose-related hepatotoxicity.

2.1.1.1. Preparations, Therapeutic Indications, Dosage, and Contraindications

Methotrexate is available in 2.5-mg tablets. It is indicated for the treatment of rheumatoid arthritis. The dose ranges between 7.5 and 20 mg once per week. The most common dosage, though, is 15 mg per week. It is contraindicated in pregnancy, breast-feeding mothers, and patients hypersensitive to methotrexate or its component.

2.1.1.2. Drug Interactions

Methotrexate interacts with a number of drugs/drug classes including:

1. Bone marrow depressants: The combination of bone marrow depressants and methotrexate may result in the potentiation of the effects of these agents.
2. Folic acid: The administration of folic acid and methotrexate may decrease the effect of the latter.
3. Hepatotoxic agents: Concomitant administration of hepatotoxic agents and methotrexate increases the risk of hepatotoxicity.
4. Neomycin: It has been shown to decrease the absorption of many drugs including methotrexate.
5. Conventional NSAIDs: The combination of methotrexate and any of the COX inhibitors may increase the risk of methotrexate toxicity.
6. Sulfonamides: The concomitant administration of sulfonamides and methotrexate increases the risk of hepatotoxicity.
7. Vaccines: The combination of killed-virus or live-virus vaccine with methotrexate may increase the risk of infection.

2.1.2. Cyclosporin

Cyclosporin is an immunosuppressant *(44)*. It exerts its effect by inhibiting the proliferation of T lymphocytes, inhibiting the release of interleukin-2 and tumor necrosis factor-α (TNF-α). The cyclosporin-binding protein, cyclophilin, may play a role in cyclosporin's actions. It is indicated for the treatment of rheumatoid arthritis. It is also indicated for the prevention of graft rejection. The main adverse effects associated with cyclosporin are nephrotoxicity, liver dysfunction, and in some cases lymphoma.

2.1.2.1. Preparations, Therapeutic Indications, and Dosage

Cyclosporin is available in 25-mg and 100-mg capsules and 100-mg/mL oral solution. It is indicated for the treatment of severe and active rheumatoid arthritis. Adults receive 25 mg/kg/d in divided doses every 12 h. After 8 wk, this dose should be increased by 0.5–0.75 mg/kg/d, and again after 12 wk. The maximum dosage is 4 mg/kg/d.

Cyclosporin is contraindicated in patients with compromised renal function, neoplastic diseases, and uncontrolled hypertension. It is also indicated in patients who are hypersensitive to cyclosporin or any of its components.

2.1.2.2. Drug Interactions

Cyclosporin interacts with a wide array of therapeutic agents including aminoglycosides, amphotericin B, calcium channel blockers, erythromycin and other antibiotics, oral contraceptives, colchicines, sulfonamides, digoxin, foscarnet, HMG-CoA reductase inhibitors (statins), various NSAIDs, probucol, terbinafine, and metoclopramide. Most of the drug interactions involving cyclosporin result in increased toxicity especially nephrotoxicity.

2.1.3. Azathioprine

Azathioprine is an immunosuppressive agent. It is a purine analog whose primary metabolite, 6-thioinosinic acid, inhibits the synthesis of inosinic acid and suppresses T- and B-cell functions. It is primarily indicated to prevent graft rejection. It is also indicated for the treatment of severe cases of rheumatoid arthritis and other inflammatory diseases such as systemic lupus erythematosus. Like other DMARDs, it has a slow onset of action. As with other immunosuppressant agents, the main adverse effects associated with azothioprine are bone marrow suppression, increased risk of infections, and less frequently malignancies.

2.1.3.1. PREPARATIONS, THERAPEUTIC INDICATIONS, AND DOSAGE

Azathrioprine is available as azathioprine sodium in 50-mg tablets. It is indicated for the treatment of rheumatoid arthritis. Adults are given an initial dose of 1 mg/kg/d (50–100 mg/kg/d) as either a single dose or divided into two doses per day, for 6–8 wk. If there are no therapeutic effects and/or adverse effects from the initial dose, the dosage should be increased 0.5 mg/kg every 4–6 wk up to 2.5 mg/kg. The optimal dose is 2–2.5 mg/kg/d. If the patient also takes allopurinol, the dosage must be reduced to 25–33% of the usual dosage.

Azathioprine is contraindicated in patients who are hypersensitive to the drug.

2.1.3.2. DRUG INTERACTIONS

Azathioprine interacts with several therapeutic agents, including ACE inhibitors, and agents that affect bone marrow development. It also interacts with allopurinol, anticoagulants, methotrexate, cyclosporin, and nondepolarizing neuromuscular blockers.

2.1.4. Leflunomide

Leflunomide is a new orally administered immunosuppressive agent that has proven effective in the treatment of rheumatoid arthritis. Its efficacy is comparable to that of methotrexate. Its active metabolite (A77-1726) inhibits the *de novo* synthesis of ribonucleotides resulting in arresting the cell cycle at the G_1 phase. This prevents the proliferation of activated T lymphocytes and interferes with the functions of B cells. The main adverse effects associated with leflunomide are diarrhea and elevation plasma levels of liver enzymes. It can be taken concomitantly with methtrexate in patients who did not respond to the latter agent alone.

2.1.4.1. PREPARATIONS, INDICATIONS, AND DOSAGE, AND CONTRAINDICATIONS

Leflunomide is available in 10-, 20-, and 100-mg tablets. It is indicated for the treatment of rheumatoid arthritis. The loading dose is 100 mg/d followed by a maintenance dose of 20 mg/d. The 10-mg tablet is used for dose adjustment, if necessary.

Leflunomide is contraindicated in pregnancy and in patients hypersensitive to leflunomides or its components.

2.1.4.2. Drug Interactions

Leflunomide interacts with a number of drug/drug classes including azathiprine, charcoal, cholestyramine, cyclosporin, ethanol, fosphenytoin, isoniazid, ketoconazole, methotrexate, NSAIDs, phenytoin, rifampin, sulfasalazine, tacrine, tolbutamide, troglitazone, live-virus vaccines, and warfarin.

2.2. Gold

Like methotrexate, gold preparations have been shown to reduce pain and slow the progression of bone and articular destruction *(45)*. Its mechanism of action is not fully understood. However, it is believed to inhibit the lysosomal enzymes, reduce histamine release from mast cells, and suppress the phagocytic activity of polymorphonuclear leukocytes. Typical of most DMARDs, it has a slow onset of action with a latency period of 3–4 mo. Due to its toxic effects, it has a high rate of discontinuance. However, if clinical response is achieved without serious toxicity, it can be continued indefinitely. Its total-body half-life is approximately 1 yr. It accumulates in the synovial membranes, liver, kidney, adrenal glands, spleen, bone marrow, and lymph nodes. It persists in the renal tubules for many years. There is no correlation between gold salt concentration and therapeutic or toxic effects.

The main adverse effects associated with gold therapy include pruritic dermatitis, eosinophelia, thrombocytopenia, leukopenia, diarrhea, metallic taste in the mouth, skin pigmentation, blood dyscrasias, and rarely proteinuria.

2.2.1. Preparations and Contraindications

Aurothiomalate is available in 25- and 50-mg ampules. Aurothioglucose is available as a 500-mg/10 mL multidose vial. Both aurothiomalate and aurothioglucose are parenteral gold preparations usually given by deep muscular injection. Auranofin is an oral preparation that is available in 3-mg capsules. Gold therapy is indicated for patients with active rheumatoid arthritis and in patients who have not responded to conventional NSAIDs. Adults are given auranofin at an initial dose of 6 mg every day or 3 mg twice daily. If necessary, the maintenance dose can be raised to 9 mg/d after 3 mo of treatment. In children age 6 and older, the initial dose is 0.1 mg/kg/d and the maintenance dose is 0.15 mg/kg/d, up to a maximum of 0.2 mg/kg/d. Drug must be discontinued if clinical response is not achieved after 3 mo at 9 mg/d.

Parenteral gold is given intramuscularly in doses of 50 mg/wk for 20 wk. If clinical response is achieved without serious adverse effects, the drug can be continued indefinitely by lengthening the dosing intervals from weekly to biweekly, and then to a monthly dosing regimen.

Gold therapy is contraindicated in pregnancy, and in patients with colitis, bone marrow aplasia, serious liver and kidney disease, and blood dyscrasias.

2.2.2. Drug Interactions

The concomitant administration of gold salts and phenytoin may result in increased plasma phenytoin levels.

2.3. Alkylating Agents

Chlorambucil and cyclophosphamide are the most frequently used alkylating agents in patients with rheumatoid arthritis. Cyclophosphamide and the primary metabolite of chlorambucil interfere with cell replication by crosslinking to their DNA. They are indicated for the management of rheumatoid arthritis, and in patients with systemic lupus erythomatosus and/or vasculitis. Their main adverse effects include leukemia, and dose-dependent infertility and bone marrow suppression.

2.3.1. Preparations and Dosage

Chlorambucil is available in 2-mg tablets. The usual oral dosage is 0.1–0.2 mg/kg/d for 3–6 wk. This usually amounts to 4–10 mg/d for the average patient. The entire daily dose may be given at one time. The dosage must be carefully adjusted according to the response of the patient and must be reduced as soon as there is an abrupt fall in white blood cell count.

Cyclophosphamide is available in 25- or 50-mg tablets. For rheumatoid arthritis, cyclophosphamide is given as 50–150 mg daily in a single dose. It should be taken with breakfast, and lots of fluid should be taken throughout the day.

2.3.2. Drug Interactions

Chlorambucil interacts with a number of therapeutic agents including anticoagulants, barbiturates, digoxin, filgrastim (G-CSF), immunosuppressive agents, NSAIDs, platelet inhibitors, salicylates, sargramostim (GM-CSF), strontium-89 chloride, thrombolytic agents, and live-virus vaccines.

Cyclophosphamide interacts with anthracyclines, anticoagulants, antithymocyte globulin, barbiturates, bupropion, carbamazepine, cocaine, desmopressin, digoxin, etanercept, filgrastim (G-CSF), fosphenytoin, immunosuppressive agents, infliximab, mibefradil, mitotane, mivacurim, NSAIDs, phenytoin, platelet inhibitors, rifabutin, rifampin, rifapentine, salicylates, sargramostim (GM-CSF), St. John's wort, strontium-89 chloride, succinylcholine, tamoxifen, thrombolytic agents, trastuzumab, and live-virus vaccines.

2.4. Antimalarial Agents

Chloroquine and its major metabolite hydroxychloroquine are the main antimalarial drugs used in rheumatoid arthritis. They have been shown to cause remission of rheumatoid arthritis but are incapable of retarding the progression of the bone and articular damage. In addition to rheumatoid arthritis, they are also indicated in systemic lupus erythematosus. The mechanisms of their antiinflammatory actions are not well understood. However, they are believed to decrease leukocyte migration and interfere with the action of acid hydrolases and the functions of T lymphocytes. Also they are believed to inhibit DNA synthesis. Hydroxychloroquine is preferred over chloroquine in the treatment of rheumatoid arthritis and systemic lupus erythematosus because it causes less ocular toxicity than chloroquine.

2.4.1. Preparations and Dosage

Chloroquine phosphate is available in 250- and 500-mg tablets. Hydroxychloroquine sulfate is available in 200-mg tablets. For treatment of rheumatoid arthritis, adults receive a daily dose of 400–600 mg either as one dose or divided into two. If side effects occur, a temporary reduction in the initial dose can be made and a few days later the dose can gradually be increased. If a good response is obtained after 4–12 wk, then the dosage is reduced by 50% and continued at a maintenance dose of 200–400 mg/d. Doses must be taken with food or glass of milk or water.

2.4.2. Drug Interactions

Chloroquine and hydroxychloroquine interact with botulinum toxin Types A and B, digoxin, kaolin (pectin), and penicillamine. Chloroquine also interacts with cimetidine, mefloquine, praziquantel, prilocaine, and rabies vaccine. Hydroxychloroquine also interacts metropolol.

2.5. Sulfasalazine

Sulfasalazine is a sulfonamide. It is a prodrug that is metabolized into 5-aminosalisylic acid and sulfapyridine. Its mechanism of action is not well understood. It is believed, however, that sulfapyridine and/or the parent compound are responsible for the drug's antirheumatic effect. Adverse effects associated with sulfasalazine include rashes, nausea, vomiting, chills, depression, fatigue, headaches, and less frequently agranulocytosis aplastic anemia and leukopenia.

2.5.1. Preparations, Therapeutic Indications, Dosage, and Contraindications

Sulfasalazine is available as 500-mg enteric-coated tablets. It is indicated for rheumatoid arthritis, ankylosing spondylitis, inflammatory bowel diseases, and juvenile arthritis. For rheumatoid arthritis, adults initially are given 500–1000 mg every day for 1 wk. Then, the dose can be increased by 500 mg/d every week, up to a maximum of 2000 mg/d in divided doses. If clinical response is not achieved after 12 wk of therapy, the dose can be increased to 3000 mg/d. The maintenance dose is 1000 mg every 12 h, up to a maximum of 3000 mg/d.

2.5.2. Drug Interactions

1. Bone marrow depressants: Concomitant administration of sulfasalazine and any bone marrow depressant may result in increased leukopenic and thrombocytopenic effects of both agents.
2. Hepatotoxic drugs: Coadministration of sulfasalazine and any hepatotoxic agent may result in increased hepatotoxicity.
3. Methotraxate: Coadministration of methotrexate with sulfasalazine results in the potentiation of the effects of the former.
4. Folic acid: Sulfasalazine has been known to increase folic acid absorption.
5. Digoxin: Sulfasalzine may inhibit digoxin absorption and thus limit its bioavailability.
6. Hydantoin, oral anticoagulants, and oral antidiabetic drugs: Sulfasalazine is known to potentiate the therapeutic and toxic effects of these agents.

2.6. D-Penicillamine

D-Penicillamine is a metabolite of the antibiotic agent penicillin and an analog of the sulfhydryl-containing amino acid cysteine. Its mechanism of action is not well understood. It is believed, however, to interfere with the synthesis of collagen, DNA, and mucopolysaccharides. As with other DMARDs, it is slow acting with a latency period of 3–4 mo. Because it interferes with the absorption of many therapeutic agents, it fell into disfavor. It is indicated in patients with active and severe rheumatoid arthritis who have not had adequate response to conventional NSAIDs or gold therapies. Its adverse effects include dermatitis, anorexia, vomiting, proteinuria, leukopenia, thrombocytopenia, aplastic anemia, autoimmune disease, and metallic taste.

10. Nonsteroidal Antiinflammatory Drugs

Patients on penicillamine should be closely monitored. Blood and platelet count should be performed every fortnight. It is contraindicated in pregnancy and in patients with renal insufficiency. Because penicillamine is a metal-chelating agent, it should not be given in combination with gold. Also, it should not be combined with phenylbutazone or other cytotoxic agent.

2.6.1. Drug Interactions

Penicillamine interacts with aluminum hydroxide, antimalarial agents, antineoplastic agents, gold compounds, immunosuppressive agents, iron salts, polysaccharide-iron complex, and pyridoxine (vitamin B_6).

2.7. Anti-TNF-α Agents

2.7.1. Infliximab

It is a chimeric mouse–human monoclonal antibody that is specific to human TNF-α. It binds TNF-α, thus blocking it from binding to its receptor. This prevents the induction of the release of proinflammatory cytokines. As a result, a significant reduction in the migration of proinflammatory cells to the inflammation site is achieved. It is indicated in combination to methotrexate for the treatment of rheumatoid arthritis *(46–48)*. It has been shown that such combination is significantly more effective in retarding the progression of the articular damage than methotrexate alone. The main adverse effects associated with infliximab are upper respiratory tract infection, headaches, nausea, cough, sinusitis, and rash.

2.7.1.1. Preparations, Therapeutic Indications, and Contraindications

Infliximab is available in 100-mg vials that must be diluted with 10 mL sterile water. This preparation should be further diluted in a total volume of 250 mL normal saline. It is indicated for the treatment of rheumatoid arthritis and Crohn's disease. The dose is 5 mg/kg given as a single intravenous infusion followed by additional 5 mg/kg at 2 and 6 wk after the first infusion. Maintenance dose is every 8 wk. It is contraindicated in patients who are allergic to infliximab, its components, and/or murine proteins. Infliximab should not be infused with any other medication or through plasticized polyvinyl chloride infusion devices.

2.7.1.2. Drug Interactions

Infliximab interacts with anakinra, immunosuppressive agents, toxoids, and live-virus vaccines.

2.7.2. Etanercept

Etanercept is a chimeric recombinant fusion protein combining the p75 region of tumor necrosis factor receptor and the Fc region of IgG_1. It binds specifically to TNF-α and blocks it from binding to its receptor. As with infliximab, this results in a significant reduction in the release of proinflammatory cytokines and decreased number of migrating proinflammatory cells to the inflammation site. Etanercept is as effective as methotrexate. However, it has the advantage of an earlier onset of action. It is indicated to patients with rheumatoid arthritis who have not had adequate response to other DMARDs *(49–51)*. It is typically administered subcutaneously, 25 mg twice a week. Its adverse effects are similar to those of infliximab.

2.7.2.1. Preparations, Therapeutic Indications, and Contraindication

Etanercept is available in 25-mg single-use vials usually given subcutaneously twice weekly for the treatment of active rheumatoid arthritis alone or in combination with methotrexate. Also, it can be used for the treatment of juvenile arthritis. It is contraindicated in patients who are sensitive to etanercept, its components, and/or hamster proteins.

2.7.2.2. Drug Interactions

Etanercept interacts with anakinra, azathioprine, cyclophosphamide, leflunomide, methotrexate, toxoids, and live-virus vaccines.

2.8. Interleukin-1 Receptor Antagonists
2.8.1. Anakinra

Anakinra represents the first of a new class of DMARDs. This recombinant IL-1 receptor antagonist received FDA approval for the treatment of rheumatoid arthritis in November of 2001. Anakinra acts by competitively inhibiting the binding of IL-1 (one of the primary proinflammatory cytokines/chemical mediators associated with rheumatoid arthritis) to the IL-1 receptor. This results in a significant reduction of macrophages and lymphocytes in the synovial tissue. Multicenter clinical trials have shown that anakinra is effective in reducing joint pain and swelling either as a monotherapy or in combination with methotrexate.

2.8.1.1. Therapeutic Indications and Contraindications

Anakinra is indicated for the reduction of signs and symptoms of rheumatoid arthritis in patients who have not responded to other DMARDs. The dosing regimen for adults is 100 mg/d given subcutaneously. It is contraindicated in patients who are hypersensitive to *E. coli* proteins and/or latex. Also, anakinra should not be given intramuscularly or intravenously or to patients with renal impairment.

Generally, adverse reactions are rare. However, some patients may experience headache, GI disturbances, sinusitis, infection, itching due to reaction at the injection site, diarrhea, and erythema.

2.8.1.2. Drug Interactions

Anakinra has been shown to interact with infliximab and etanercept. As a result, the coadministration of either of these agents with anakinra is not recommended. Additionally, because anakinra interferes with the immune response mechanisms, live-virus vaccines should not be given to patients receiving anakinra.

3. Drugs Used in Gout

Gout is a metabolic disorder characterized by elevated levels of uric acid in the plasma (hyperuricemia). Because uric acid (a product of purine metabolism) is poorly soluble in the blood, monosodium urate crystals accumulate in tissues particularly in the joints and kidneys. This deposition of urate crystals triggers an inflammatory process characterized by the phogocytosis of these urate crystals by synoviocytes, the release of chemotactic mediators, and the migration of PMNs into the affected joint. Acute gouty attacks can involve any joint especially the first metatarso-phalangeal joint.

10. Nonsteroidal Antiinflammatory Drugs

Table 6
Drugs Used in Gout

Treatment of Acute Gouty Attack	Treatment of Chronic Gout	
Indomethacin[a] Colchicine	Uricosuric Agents Probencid Sulfinpyrazone Oxaprozin[b]	Inhibitors of UA Synthesis Allopurinol

[a]Other NSAIDs are effective; salicylates are not recommended.
[b]An NSAID.

3.1. Treatment of Acute Gouty Attacks

The main strategy behind the treatment of acute gouty attacks is to reduce the inflammation as fast as possible. This is usually accomplished by the utilization of COX inhibitors or colchicine (Table 6).

3.1.1. Indomethacin

Although most NSAIDs are effective in treating acute gouty episodes, indomethacin is the drug of choice for treatment of acute gout. In this context, indomethacin not only inhibits the production of prostaglandins, but also inhibits the phagocytosis of the monosodium urate crystals by the mononuclear phagocytes. The dosing schedule is 50 mg every 6 h until an adequate response is achieved, then the dose is reduced to 25 mg three times a day for 5 d. The pharmacology of indomethacin is discussed in detail elsewhere in this chapter.

3.1.2. Colchicine

Colchicine has proven effective in alleviating pain and inflammation associated with acute gouty attacks. The mechanism of action behind its antiinflammatory effect is its ability to bind tubulin protein of cells in the immune system (such as PMNs), thus interfering with their migration, phagocytosis, and the release of proinflammatory mediators such as leukotriene B_4. Adverse reactions associated with colchicine include diarrhea, nausea, hair loss, and rarely dose-dependent bone marrow suppression.

3.1.2.1. Preparations and Dosage

Colchicine is available in 0.5-, 0.6-, and 6-mg tablets and in injectable form (1 mg per vial). For the prevention of acute gouty attacks, oral colchicine is given as 0.5–0.6 mg every day. The same dose can be given two or three times a day. It can also be given as 0.5–1 mg on the first day, followed by 0.5 mg every 2 h until pain is alleviated. Parenteral colchicine can be given in an intravenous infusion as 0.5–1 mg every day or twice a day. The maximum amount should not exceed 4 mg/d.

3.1.2.2. Drug Interactions

Colchicine interacts with a number of therapeutic agents including anticoagulants, antineoplastics, cyclosporin, NSAIDs, and vitamin B_{12}.

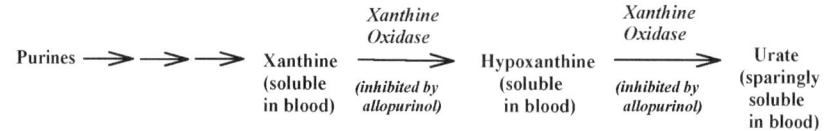

Purines →→→ Xanthine (soluble in blood) —Xanthine Oxidase (inhibited by allopurinol)→ Hypoxanthine (soluble in blood) —Xanthine Oxidase (inhibited by allopurinol)→ Urate (sparingly soluble in blood)

Fig. 2. Inhibition of purine metabolism by allopurinol.

3.2. Management of Chronic Gouty Arthritis

The strategy behind the treatment of chronic gouty arthritis is to keep uric acid levels in the blood below saturation (6 mg/dL or less) to prevent its accumulation in tissues *(52,53)*. This can be accomplished by either reducing the rate of production of uric acid with allopurinol or increasing the rate of uric acid excretion by uricosuric agents (Table 6).

3.2.1. Allopurinol

Allopurinol is a purine analog. As a hypoxanthine isomer, it reduces uric acid synthesis by competitively inhibiting zanthine oxidase. This results in decreased plasma uric acid levels and increased xanthine and hypoxanthine levels that are more soluble in plasma and are readily excreted (Fig. 2). The main adverse effects associated with allopurinol are GI intolerance, diarrhea, vomiting, and nausea *(54)*.

3.2.1.1. Preparations, Therapeutic Indications, Dosage, and Contraindications

Allopurinol is available in 100- and 300-mg tablets and in parenteral form. It is indicated for the treatment of gout. It is given as 100 mg/d until plasma uric acid levels subside to 6 mg/dL or less. Parenterally, it is administered as 200–400 mg/m^2/d as a single infusion or in divided infusions two, three, or four times a day.

3.2.1.2. Drug Interactions

It potentiates the effects of 6-mercaptopurine, azathioprine, dicumarol, and warfarin. It also interacts with ACE inhibitors, amoxicillin, ampicillin, chlorpropamide, cyclophosphamide, thiazide diuretics, and with vitamin C when taken in large doses.

3.2.2. Uricosuric Agents

Uricosuric agents are those agents that—at large concentrations—increase the rate of excretion of uric acid by inhibiting its reabsorption at the active anionic transport sites in the proximal renal tubules *(55)*. This results in decreased urate levels in the plasma. These agents should not be used in patients who already secret large quantities of uric acid in order to prevent the formation of uric acid calculi in the kidney. Uricosuric therapy is indicated only after several gouty attacks have occurred, evidence of tophaceous gout becomes clear, or when uric acid concentration is at a level that causes tissue damage.

It is important to note that aspirin and other salicylates are contraindicated in patients with gout because at low doses (analgesic doses) salicylates inhibit the secretory transporters of uric acid resulting in its retention *(56)*. In case other NSAIDs cannot be tolerated, aspirin can be given to patients with gout. However, it must be administered in high doses (antiinflammatory doses) because at high doses salicylates have been shown to reduce the rate of reabsorption of uric acid by active transport sites in the renal proximal tubule.

3.2.2.1. PROBENECID

Probenecid is a sulfonamide derivative. It is available in 500-mg tablets. It is indicated for the treatment of chronic gouty arthritis and hyperuricemia due to chronic gout. It is given in 250-mg dose twice a day for 1 wk, then increased to a maintenance dose of 500 mg twice a day. The dose can be increased until uric acid excretion surpasses 700 mg/d. Maximum dose should not exceed 3 g/d.

Adverse effects associated with probenecid include dizziness, headache, anorexia, vomiting, nausea, facial flushing, and rash. It is contraindicated in patients who are less than 2 yr old, are with blood dyscrasias, have renal calculi, or are hypersensitive to probenecid or its components.

3.2.2.1.1. Drug Interactions. Probenecid may increase the effects of a wide array of therapeutic agents, including acyclovir, allopurinol, antineoplastics, zidovudine, thiopental, sulfonylureas, rifampin, sulfonamides, riboflavin, aminosalicylate sodium, cephalosporins, ciprofloxacin, clofibrate, dapsone, ganciclovir, imipenem, methotrexate, nitrofurantoin, norfloxacin, penicillins, diazoxide, mecamylamine, pyrazinamide, furosemide, dyphilline, lorazepam, and NSAIDs, by slowing their normal removal via the kidney.

3.2.2.2. SULFINPYRAZONE

Sulfinpyrazone is a pyrazalone derivative. It is available in 100-mg tablets and 200-mg capsules. It is indicated for the treatment of chronic gouty arthritis. It is given as 100–200 mg/d progressing to 400 mg twice a day until plasma urate level is under control. Its adverse effects include dizziness and rash. It is contraindicated in patients with peptic ulcer disease, blood dyscrasias, or hypersensitivity to sulfinpyrazone or its components.

3.2.2.2.1. Drug Interactions. Sulfinpyrazone interacts with several therapeutic agents including acetaminophen, salicylates, antineoplastics, cefamandole, cefoperazone, cefotetan, moxalactam, plicamycin, valproic acid, diazoxide, mecamylamine, pyrazinamide, hydantoin, niacin, nitrofurantoin, NSAIDs, oral anticoagulants, antiplatelet drugs, oral antidiabetic drugs, probenecid, theophilline, and verapamil.

3.2.2.3. OXAPROZIN

Oxaprozin is a nonselective COX inhibitor that possesses mild uricosuric effects. This agent is discussed in detail under NSAIDs.

ACKNOWLEDGMENTS

This work was supported, in part, by NASA Grant NCC9-112 and NIH Grants RCRII 2P20 RR11104-08 and 5P20RR11104-7.

REFERENCES

1. Vane JR, Bakhle YS, and Botting RM. Cyclooxygenase 1 and 2. Annu Rev Pharmacol Toxicol 38:97–120 (1998).
2. Deininger MH, Weller M, Streffer J, Mittelbronn M, and Meyermann R. Patterns of cyclooxygenase-1 and -2 expression in human gliomas in vivo. Acta Neuropathol (Berl) 98:240–244 (1999).

3. Meade EA, Smith WL, and DeWitt DL. Differential inhibition of prostaglandin endoperoxide synthase (cyclooxygenase) isozymes by aspirin and other nonsteroidal anti-inflammatory drugs. J Biol Chem 268:6610–6614 (1993).
4. Mitchell JA, Akarasereenont P, Thiememann C, Flower RJ, and Vane JR. Selective of nonsteroidial antiinflammatory drugs as inhibitors of constitutive and inducible cyclooxygenase. Proc Natl Acad Sci USA 90:11693–11697 (1993).
5. Vane JR and Botting RM. New insights into the mode of action of anti-inflammatory drugs. Inflamm Res 44:1–10 (1995).
6. McAdam BF, Catella-Lawson F, Mardini IA, Kapoor S, Lawson JA, and Fitzgerald GA. Systemic biosynthesis of prostacyclin by cyclooxygenase (COX)-2: the human pharmacology of a selective inhibitor of COX-2. Proc Natl Acad Sci USA 96:272–277 (1999).
7. Bannwarth B, Demotes-Mainard F, Schaeverbeke T, Labat L, and Dehais J. Central analgesic effects of aspirin-like drugs. Fundam Clin Pharmacol 9:1–7 (1995).
8. Velo GP and Milanino R. Nongastrointestinal adverse reactions to NSAID. J Rheumatol 17(Suppl 20):42–45 (1990).
9. Gabriel SE, Jaakkimainen L, and Bombardier C. Risk for serious gastrointestinal complications related to use of nonsteriodal anti-inflammatory drugs. A meta-analysis. Ann Intern Med 115:787–796 (1991).
10. Verbeeck RK. Pharmacokinetic drug interactions with nonsteroidal anti-inflammatory drugs. Clin Pharmacokinet 19:44–66 (1990).
11. Weissmann G. Aspirin Sci Am 264:84–90 (1991).
12. Vane J. Towards a better aspirin. Nature 367:215–216 (1994).
13. Lecomte M, Lancoville O, Ji C, DeWitt DL, and Smith WL. Acetylation of human prostaglandin endoperoxide synthase-2 (cyclooxygenase-2) by aspirin. J Biochem 269:13207–13215 (1994).
14. Diaz-Gonzalez F and Sanchez-Madrid F. Inhibition of leukocyte adhesion: an alternative mechanism for action for anti-inflammatory drug. Immunol Today 19:169–172 (1998).
15. Willard JE, Lange RA, and Hillis LD. The use of aspirin in ischemic heart disease. N Engl J Med 327:175–181 (1992).
16. Patrono C. Aspirin as an antiplatelet drug. N Engl J Med 330:1287–1294 (1994).
17. Miners JO. Drug interactions involving aspirin (acetylsalicylic acid) and salicylic acid. Clin Pharmacocinet 17:327–344 (1989).
18. Svensson CI and Yaksh TL. The spinal phospholipase-cyclooxygenase-prostanoid cascade in nociceptive processing. Annu Rev Pharmacol Toxicol 42:553–583 (2002).
19. Douidar SM, Richardson J, and Snodgrass WR. Role of indomethacin in ductus closure: an update evaluation. Dev Pharmacol Ther 11:196–212 (1988).
20. Emery P, Zeidler H, Kvien TK, Guslandi M, Naudin R, Stead H, et al. Celecoxib versus diclofenac in long-term management of rheumatoid arthritis: randomized double-blind comparison. Lancet 354:2106–2111 (1999).
21. Norton ME, Merrill J, Cooper BA, Kuller JA, and Clyman RI. Neonatal complications after the administration of endomethacin for preterm labor. N Engl J Med 329:1602–1607 (1993).
22. Scott DL and Palmer RH. Safety and efficacy of nabumetone in osteoarthritis: emphasis on gastrointestinal safety. Aliment Pharmacol Ther 14:443–452 (2000).
23. Bjarnason I and Thjodleifsson B. Gastrointestinal toxicity of non-steroidal anti-inflammatory drugs: the effect of nimesulide compared with naproxen on the human gastrointestinal tract. Rheumatology (Oxford) 38(Suppl 1):24–32 (1999).
24. Turck D, Roth W, and Busch U. A review of the clinical pharmacokinetics of meloxicam. Br J Rheumatol 35(Suppl 1):13–16 (1996).
25. Rumack BH, Peterson RC, Koch GG, and Amara IA. Acetaminophen overdose. 662 cases with evaluation of oral acetylcysteine treatment. Arch Intern Med 141:380–385 (1981).

26. Linden CH and Rumack BH. Acetaminophen overdose. Emerg Med Clin North Am 2: 103–119 (1984).
27. Black M. Acetaminophen hepatotoxicity. Annu Rev Med 35:577–593 (1984).
28. Davies NM, McLachlan AJ, Day RO, and Williams KM. Clinical pharmacokinetics and pharmacodynamics of celecoxib: a selective cyclooxygenase-2 inhibitor. Clin Pharmacokinet 38:225–242 (2000).
29. Simon LS, Weaver AL, Graham DY, Kivitz AJ, Lipsky PE, Hubbard RC, et al. Anti-inflammatory and upper gastrointestinal effects of celecoxib in rheumatoid arthritis: a randomized, controlled trial. JAMA 282:1921–1928 (1999).
30. Bensen WG, Fiechtner JJ, McMillen JI, Zhao WW, Yu SS, Woods EM, et al. Treatment of osteoarthritis with celecoxib, a cyclooxygenase-2 inhibitor: a randomized controlled trial. Mayo Clin Proc 74:1095–1105 (1999).
31. Hawkey C, Laine L, Simon T, Beaulieu A, Maldonado-Cocco J, Acevedo E, et al. Comparison of the effect of rofecoxib (a cyclooxygenase-2 inhibitor), ibuprofen and placebo on the gastroduodenal mucosa of patients with osteoarthritis: a randomized, double-blind, placebo-controlled trial. The Rofecoxib Osteoarthritis Endoscopy Multinational Study Group. Arthritis Rheum 43:370–377 (2000).
32. Laine L, Harper S, Simon T, Bath R, Johanson J, Schwartz H, et al. A randomized trial comparing the effect of rofecoxib, a cyclooxygenase 2-specific inhibitor, with that of ibuprofen on the gastrointestinal mucosa of patients with osteoarthritis. Rofecoxib Osteoarthritis Endoscopy Study Group. Gastroenterology 117:776–783 (1999).
33. Morrison BW, Daniels SE, Kotey P, Cantu N, and Seidenberg B. Rofecoxib, a specific cyclooxygenase-2 inhibitor, in primary dysmenorrhea: a randomized controlled trial. Obstet Gynecol 940:504–508 (1999).
34. Schnitzer TJ, Truitt K, Fleischmann R, Dalgin P, Block J, Zeng Q, et al. The safety profile, tolerability and effective dose range of rofecoxib in the treatment of rheumatoid arthritis. Phase II Rofecoxib Rheumatoid Arthritis Study Group. Clin Ther 21:1688–1702 (1999).
35. Gierse JK, Koboldt C, Hood B, Zhang Y, Zweifel B, Kurumbail R, et al. Valdecoxib: a highly selective and potent inhibitor of COX-2. FASEB 16:A181 (Abst 168.1), 2002.
36. Green JM and Winickoff RN. Cost-conscious prescribing of nonsteroidal anti-inflammatory drugs for adults with arthritis. Arch Intern Med 152:1995–2002 (1992).
37. Arnold M, Schreiber L, and Brooks P. Immunosuppressive drugs and corticosteroids in the treatment of rheumatoid arthritis. Drugs 36:340–463 (1988).
38. Fries JF, Williams CA, Ramey D, and Bloch DA. The relative toxicity of disease-modifying antirheumatic drugs. Arthritis Rheum 36:297–306 (1993).
39. Furst DE. Rational use of disease-modifying antirheumatic drugs. Drugs 39:19–37 (1990).
40. Wolfe F, Hawley DJ, and Cathey MA. Termination of slow acting antirheumatic therapy in rheumatoid arthritis: a 14-year prospective evaluation of 1017 consecutive starts. J Rheumatol 17:994–1002 (1990).
41. Stewart CF and Evans WE. Drug–drug interactions with antirheumatic agents: review of selected clinically important interactions. J Rheumatol 17(Suppl 22):16–23 (1990).
42. Kremer JM and Phelps CT. Long-term prospective study of the use of methotrexate in the treatment of rheumatoid arthritis. Update after a mean of 90 months. Arthritis Metab 35: 138–145 (1992).
43. Arend WP and Dayer JM. Cytokines and cytokine inhibitors or antagonists in rheumatoid arthritis. Arthritis Rheum 33:305–315 (1990).
44. Faulds D, Goa KL, and Benfield P. Cyclosporin. A review of its pharmacodynamic and pharmacokinetic properties, and therapeutic use in immunoregulatory disorders. Drugs 45: 953–1040 (1993).

45. Epstein WV, Henke CJ, Yelin EH, and Katz PP. Effect of parenterally administered gold therapy on the course of adult rheumatoid arthritis. Ann Intern Med 114:437–444 (1991).
46. Harriman G, Harper LK, and Schaible TF. Summary of clinical trials in rheumatoid arthritis using infliximab, an anti-TNFα treatment. Ann Rheum Dis 58:161–164 (1999).
47. Jones RE and Moreland LW. Tumor necrosis factor inhibitors for rheumatoid arthritis. Bull Rheum Dis 48:1–4 (1999).
48. Maini RN, Breedveld FC, Kalden JR, Smolen JS, Davis D, Macfarlane JD, et al. Therapeutic efficacy of multiple intravenous infusions of anti-tumor necrosis factor α monoclonal antibody combined with low-dose weekly methotrexate in rheumatoid arthritis. Arthritis Rheum 41:1552–1563 (1998).
49. Garrison L and McDonnell ND. Etanercept: therapeutic use in patients with rheumatoid arthritis. Ann Rheum Dis 58(Suppl I):I165–I169 (1999).
50. Jarvis B and Faulds D. Etanercept: a review of its use in rheumatoid arthritis. Drugs 57: 945–966 (1999).
51. Moreland LW, Schiff MH, Baumgartner SW, Tindall EA, Fleischmann RM, Bulpitt KJ, et al. Etanercept therapy in rheumatoid arthritis. A randomized, controlled trial. Ann Intern Med 130:478–486 (1999).
52. Emmerson BT. The management of gout. N Engl J Med 334:445–451 (1996).
53. Star VL and Hochberg MC. Prevention and management of gout. Drugs 45:212–222 (1993).
54. Hande KR, Noone RM, and Stone WJ. Severe allopurinol toxicity. Description and guidelines for prevention in patients with renal insufficiency. Am J Med 76:47–56 (1984).
55. Dan T and Koga H. Uricosurics inhibit urate transporter in rat renal brush border membrane vesicles. Eur J Parmacol 187:303–312 (1990).
56. Yu TF, Dayton PG, and Gutman AB. Mutual suppression of the uricosuric effects of sulfinpyrazone and salicylate: a study in interactions between drugs. J Clin Invest 42:1330–1339 (1963).

GENERAL REFERENCES

Brenner GM. Pharmacology, 1st ed. Philadelphia: Saunders, 2000:317–328.
Brody TM, Larner J, and Minneman KP. Human pharmacology: molecular to clinical, 3rd ed. St. Louis: Mosby, 1998:249–258.
Craig CR and Stitzel RE. Modern pharmacology, 4th ed. Boston: Little, Brown, 1990:477–508.
Ellenhorn MJ, Schonwald S, Ordog G, and Wasserberger J. Ellenhorn's medical toxicology: diagnosis and treatment of human poisoning, 2nd ed. Baltimore: Williams & Wilkins, 1997:175–223.
Gold Standard Clinical Pharmacology 2000. http://cpip.gsm.com/, May 2002.
Hardman JG and Limbird LE. Goodman and Gilman's: the pharmacological basis of therapeutics, 10th ed. New York: McGraw-Hill, 2001:687–732.
Kalant H and Roschlau WH. Principles of medical pharmacology, 5th ed. New York: Oxford University Press, 1998:410–427.
Katzung BG. Basic & clinical pharmacology, 8th ed. New York: McGraw-Hill, 2001:596–623.
Klaassen CD. Casarett and Doul's toxicology: the basic science of poisons, 5th ed. New York: McGraw-Hill, 1996:969–986.
Page C, Curtis M, Sutter M, Walker M, and Hoffman B. Integrated pharmacology, 2nd ed. St. Louis: Mosby International, 2002:437–454.
Rang HP, Dale MM, Ritter JM, and Gardner P. Pharmacology, 4th ed. New York: Churchill Livingstone, 2001:229–240.
Smith CM and Reynard AM. Essentials of pharmacology, 1st ed. Philadelphia: Saunders, 1995: 147–163.
Tryniszewski C. Nurses drug looseleaf. San Francisco: Blanchard & Loeb, 2001:1–796.

PART V
Environmental and Social Pharmacology

Chapter 11

Food and Drug Interactions

Shahla M. Wunderlich, PhD, RD

1. INTRODUCTION

The relationships and interactions between foods, the nutrients they contain, and drugs are gaining recognition in the health care and medical fields. Certain foods and specific nutrients in foods, if ingested concurrently with some drugs, may affect the overall bioavailability, pharmacokinetics, pharmacodynamics, and therapeutic efficacy of the medications. Furthermore, the therapeutic efficacy of many drugs depends on the nutritional status of the individual. In other words, the presence or absence of some nutrients in the gastrointestinal tract and/or in the body's physiological system, such as in the blood, can enhance or impair the rate of drug absorption and metabolism. All of these types of interactions are considered to be nutrient–drug interactions.

There are also drug–nutrient interactions, which means that the presence of some drugs can significantly affect the food and nutrient metabolism and bioavailability in humans. Medications can alter appetite and taste, and also change the absorption and metabolism of nutrients. This can lead to impaired nutritional status, such as depletion of some minerals and vitamins from the digestive system, and sometimes weight problems. There are many clinical issues and questions regarding drug–nutrient interactions that require further research. However, there is already enough evidence to conclude that some drugs affect nutritional status, sometimes adversely, and that nutritional factors can alter the therapeutic efficacy of some drugs significantly. This chapter describes some of more common interactions between food and drugs.

2. PHARMACOLOGICAL AND NUTRITIONAL ASPECTS

In this chapter, drugs refer to the chemical formulations used to prevent or treat disease conditions, i.e., those that are prescribed or are over-the-counter medications.

From: *Handbook of Drug Interactions: A Clinical and Forensic Guide*
A. Mozayani and L. P. Raymon, eds. © Humana Press Inc., Totowa, NJ

Nutrients are considered to be the chemicals found in foods that are essential for the normal physiological functions of the human body and optimal health. Therefore, these two groups of chemicals may simply interact with each other when they are present at the same time within the human body.

As an example of how this interaction can occur, the metabolism or biotransformation of many drugs in the liver depends on enzyme systems such as the mixed-function oxidase system (MFOS), a multienzyme system responsible for the metabolism of drugs and other foreign compounds. This system includes cytochrome P450, nicotinamide-adenine-dinucleotide-phosphate (NADPH), cytochrome P450 reductase, and phosphatidylcholine among others. Microsomal cytochrome P450 monooxygenase system metabolizes many drugs by hydroxylation. Both NADH and NADPH donate reducing equivalents.

Example: $DRUG-H + O_2 + 2Fe^{2+} (P450) + 2 H^+ \rightarrow DRUG-OH + H_2O + 2Fe^{3+} (P450)^{Hydroxylase}$

Oxygen is also needed as shown in the equation. Drugs such as aminopyrine, aniline, bezphetamine bezypyrene, and morphine are metabolized by this system. Some drugs such as phenobarbital can induce the formation of microsomal enzymes and cytochrome P450.

Phosphatidylcholine, or lecithin, a phospholipid, is indirectly involved in the biotransformation of drugs or detoxification whereby the drugs are transformed from lipid-soluble molecules into water-soluble molecules. Phosphatidylcholine is a constituent of natural membranes and it participates in complex cellular signaling events for detoxification. Detoxification in the liver is divided into two phases. In phase I, cytochrome P450 enzymes act on toxins to oxidize, reduce, or hydrolyze them, after which some of them can be excreted. In phase II, conjugation enzymes covert toxins to water-soluble forms for excretion or elimination.

Many essential nutrients are required for the optimal function of this enzyme system. For example, low levels of protein, essential amino acids, ascorbic acid, retinol, tocopherol, and other nutrients in the diet and in the body's physiological system can decrease the function of this enzyme system in the liver. The presence of some drugs, with certain nutrients in food or in supplements, can lead to biochemical interactions that alter the absorption and metabolism of drugs or nutrients in this vital organ. Awareness of these interactions and provision of the appropriate interventions can optimize the effectiveness and minimize the toxicities of medications.

3. NUTRIENT–DRUG INTERACTIONS

Nutrient–drug interactions can occur in three phases, which are described in this section.

3.1. Pharmaceutical Phase: The Initial Phase of Drug Dissolution and Disintegration

Some foods and nutrients that influence the luminal pH may impact drug dissolution and disintegration and, therefore, the acidity of these foods may alter the effectiveness and solubility of certain drugs. For example, high levels of ascorbic acid (vitamin C) can change the pH of the gastrointestinal (GI) tract and therefore influence the solubility of certain medications. One drug affected by gastric pH is saquinavir, a protease inhibitor for HIV treatment. Its bioavailability increases by solubilization induced by changes in the gastric pH. Foods that raise gastric pH, on the other hand, can also prevent dissolution of some drugs such as isoniazid.

3.2. Pharmacokinetic Phase: Absorption, Transport, Distribution, Metabolism, and Excretion of Drugs

The pharmacokinetic phase, the more studied stage of nutrient–drug interactions, is the study of the absorption, distribution metabolism, and excretion of drugs. The most significant nutrient–drug interactions involve the absorption process. The intestine, a primary absorptive organ, plays an important role in drug absorption at many levels. Intestinal functions, such as motility, or the affinity of drugs to attach to intestinal carrier systems, can influence the rate and degree of drug absorption. Foods and the nutrients within foods can accelerate (Table 1) or reduce (Table 2) drug absorption and hence alter the bioavailability of drugs *(1)*.

Foods that affect the degree of ionization and solubility or chelating reaction (i.e., form an inactive complex) change the drug absorption significantly. Examples of chelating reactions are:

1. Combination of tetracycline with divalent minerals, such as calcium in milk or antacids. Calcium may affect absorption of quinolones adversely. Therefore, the ingestion of foods rich in calcium should be avoided in the presence of antimicrobial medications.
2. Reactions between iron (ferrous or ferric) and tetracycline, fluoroquinolone antibiotics, ciprofloxacin (Cipro), ofloxacin (Floxin), lomefloxacin (Maxaquin), and enoxacin (Penetrex). Furthermore, the bioavailability of ciprofloxacin and ofloxacin were reduced by 52 and 64%, respectively, in the presence of iron.
3. Zinc and fluoroquinolones may result in inactive compounds and therefore decreased absorption of drugs *(2)*.

Table 3 summarizes some important food–drug interactions.

The rate of gastric emptying is significantly influenced by the composition of the food ingested. This rate, consequently, can affect the bioavailability of the drugs. High-fiber and high-fat foods are known to normally delay the gastric emptying time. Some drugs, such as nitrofurantoin and hydralazine, are better absorbed when gastric emptying is delayed because of longer exposure to the low pH of the stomach. Other drugs, such as L-dopa, penicillin G, and digoxin, degrade and become inactive when they are exposed to the low pH of the stomach for a long time.

The sodium-restricted diet prescribed for individuals with high blood pressure can also enhance renal tubular absorption of certain drugs, such as the antipsychotic lithium, leading to toxic blood levels *(3)*. On the other hand, sodium restriction indicated for individuals with high blood pressure may interfere with the antihypertensive action of diuretics, β-blockers, and angiotensin-converting enzyme (ACE) inhibitors. This may have the opposite effect in individuals taking calcium antagonists, nifedipine and verapamil.

The full extent of drug interaction with grapefruit juice is still unclear and more scientific research is needed to clarify the effects of different components in grapefruit juice on specific drugs. Some drugs become more bioavailable when taken with grape-

Table 1
**Examples of Food (Nutrient) Interactions
That Accelerate the Absorption of Some Drugs**

Drug	Mechanism	Remarks
Carbamazepine	Increased bile production: enhanced dissolution and absorption	Take with food
Diazepam	Food enhances enterohepatic recycling of drug: increased dissolution secondary to gastric acid secretion	None
Dicumerol	Increased bile flow; delayed gastric emptying permits dissolution and absorption	Drug taken with meal
Erythromycin	Unknown	Take with food
Griseofulvin	Drug is lipid soluble, enhanced absorption	Take with high-fat foods, or suspend in corn oil unless contraindicated.
Hydralazine	Food reduces first-pass extraction and metabolism, blocks enzymatic transformation in GI tract	Take with food
Hydrochlorothiazide	Delayed gastric emptying enhances absorption from small bowel	Take with food
Labetalol	Food may reduce first-pass extraction and metabolism	Take with food
Lithium citrate	Purgative action decreases absorption	Take on full stomach
Metaprolol	Food may reduce first-pass extraction and metabolism	Take with food
Nitrofurantoin	Delayed gastric emptying permits dissolution and increased absorption	Take with food
Phenytoin	Delayed gastric emptying and increased bile production improves dissolution and absorption	Always take the same time in relation to meals
Propoxyphene	Delayed gastric emptying improves dissolution and absorption	Take with food
Propranolol	Food may reduce first-pass extraction and metabolism	Take with food
Spironolactone	Delayed gastric emptying permits dissolution and absorption; bile may solubilize	Take with food

Data from (1).

fruit juice and therefore should not be taken at the same time. The flavonoid, naringenin, in grapefruit and its mechanism of inhibiting metabolic enzymes is reported to be the key component (4). However, other components such as quercetin (also found in strawberries) and furocoumarin derivatives have also been found to inhibit some drug oxidation in humans. A more recent report indicated that constituents of grapefruit juice not only may influence intestinal drug metabolism, but also can interfere with the secretary transport system in the intestine such as P-glycoprotein (5). Another study compared the red-wine interaction with cisapride and grapefruit juice and found that the identical volume of red wine produced minor changes in cisapride pharmacokinetics

Table 2
Examples of Food (Nutrient) Interactions That Delay the Absorption of Some Drugs

Drug	Mechanism	Remarks
Acetaminophen	High pectin foods act as absorbent and protectant	Take on empty stomach if not contraindicated
Ampicillin	Reduction in stomach fluid volume	Take with water
Amoxicillin	Reduction in stomach fluid volume	Take with water
Aspirin	Direct interference; change in gastric pH	Taking on empty stomach is not advisable
Atenolol	Mechanism unknown, possibly physical barrier	Take on empty stomach if tolerated
Captopril	Mechanism unknown	Take before meals
Cephalosporins	Mechanism unknown	None
Chlorpromazine	Drug undergoes first-pass metabolism in gut: delayed gastric emptying affects bioavailability	None
Cimetadine	Mechanism unknown	May not be clinically significant
Digoxin	High-fiber, high-pectin foods bind drug	Take drug same time with relation to food; Avoid taking with high-fiber foods
Erythromycin stearate	Mechanism unknown; also impaired by water	None
Furosemide	Mechanism unknown	May not be clinically significant
Glipizide	Unknown	Affects blood glucose; more potent when taken half hour before meals
Isoniazid	Food raises gastric pH preventing dissolution and absorption; also delayed gastric emptying	Take on empty stomach if tolerated
Levodopa	Drug competes with amino acids for absorption transport	Avoid taking drug with high-protein foods
Lincomycin	Mechanism unknown	Take on empty stomach; food impairs absorption
Methyldopa	Competitive absorptions	Avoid taking with high-protein foods
Metronidazole	Mechanism unknown	None
Nafcillin	Mechanisms unknown: may be alteration of gastric fluid on pH	Take on empty stomach
Penicillamine	May form chelate with calcium or iron	Avoid taking with taking with dairy products or iron-rich foods or supplements

(continued)

Table 2 (*continued*)

Drug	Mechanism	Remarks
Penicillin G	Delayed gastric emptying; gastric acid degradation; impaired dissolution	Take on empty stomach
Penicillin VK	More rapid dissolution in gastric fluids	Take on empty stomach with full glass of water
Piroxicam	Mechanism unknown	None
Propantheline	Mechanism unknown	Evaluate take with meals directions
Quinidine	Possibly protein binding	May take with food to prevent GI upset
Rifampin	Mechanism unknown: conflicting reports	Absorption limited with dose less than 150 mg: unaffected dose greater than 700 mg
Sulfonamides	Mechanism unknown: may be physical barrier	Taking with meals may prolong gastric emptying
Tetracyclines	Binds with calcium ions or iron salts forming insoluble chelates	Take 1 h before, 2 h after meals; do not take with milk
Valproic acid	Mechanism unknown	Delayed absorption may give uniform blood levels

Data from *(1)*.

despite some inhibition of cytochrome P450 P3A4 (CY P3A4) in most individuals *(6)*. The interactions of the many compounds in grapefruit juice with cyclosporine have been studied more extensively. Drugs such as some calcium channel blockers and the antihistamine terfenadine, and some antiviral agents such as saquinavir are examples of those that are affected in the presence of grapefruit juice *(7)*. Table 4 provides some examples of drugs that have demonstrated some interaction with grapefruit *(8)*.

Drugs are eliminated from the body unchanged or as metabolites primarily by the kidneys, lungs, or GI tract via bile. The drug excretion can also be affected by dietary nutrients, such as protein and fiber, or nutrients that influence the urinary pH.

3.3. Pharmacodynamic Phase: The Physiologic and Psychological Response to Drugs

The mechanism of a drug action depends on its agonist or antagonist activities, which will enhance or inhibit the normal metabolic and physiologic functions in the human body. Drugs, therefore, can produce desirable or undesirable effects. The magnitude of these effects is influenced by the drug's absorption, distribution, biotransformation, and excretion and some nutrients can alter all these stages *(9)*. For example, the anticlotting medication warfarin (Coumadin), structurally similar to vitamin K, opposes clotting by interfering with vitamin K's action. Therefore, the warfarin dose should be

Table 3
Some Important Food–Drug Interactions

Drug	Nutrient Type	Effect of Interaction	Recommendation
Azithromycin (Zithromax)	Food	Decreased absorption of azithromycin reducing bioavailability by 43% and maximum concentration by 52%	Space drug and nutrient at least 2 h apart
Captopril (Capoten)	Food	May decrease absorption of captopril	Take drug on an empty stomach or consistently at the same time each day
Erythromycin	Food	Decreased absorption of erythromycin base or stearate	Space drug and nutrient at least 2 h apart
Fluoroquinolones	Iron, Mg++	Decreased absorption of flurouquinolones due to complextaion with divalent cations	Space drug and nutrient at least 2 h apart
Ciprofloxacin (Cipro)	Zn++, Ca++ Mg++		
Ofloxacin (Floxin) Lomefloxacin (Maxaquin) Enoxacin (Penetrex)	Zn++		
Isoniazid	Food	May delay and decrease absorption of isoniazid	Space drug and nutrient at least 2 h apart
MAOIs[a] Phenelzine (Nardil) Isocarboxazid (Marplan) Tranylcypromine (Parnate)	Food	Hypertensive crisis	Avoid foods high in protein and tyramine, including aged, fermented, pickled, or smoked foods
Oral penicillins	Food	Decreased absorption of penicillins	Space drug and nutrient at least 2 h apart
Zidovudine (Retrovir)	Food	Decreased concentration of zidovudine	Space drug and nutrient at least 2 h apart
Sucralfate (Carafate)	Food	Decreased effect of sucralfate, binding of sucralfate to protein components of food	Administer drug 1–2 h before meals
Tetracycline	Dairy or iron	Decreased absorption of tetracycline as a result of chelation	Space drug and nutrient at least 2 h a part
Theophylline Timed Release (Theo-Dur Sprinkle, Theo-24, Uniphyl)	High-fat diet	Rate of absorption can be affected, causing elevated theophylline concentrations	Avoid concomitant administration food high in fat content or medicine 1 h before eating
Warfarin, (Coumadin, Panwarfin)	Food high in Vitamin K	Vitamin K can antagonize the effect of warfarin	Maintain a balanced diet without abrupt intake of large amounts of foods rich in vitamin K

[a]MAOIs = monoamine oxidase inhibitors.
Data from (2).

Table 4
Grapefruit and Drug Interactions[a]

Drug	Interaction
Calcium channel blockers	
Amlodopine (Norvasc)	Yes
Felodopine (Plendil)	Yes
Nifedipine (Procardia)	Yes
Nimodopine (Nimotap)	Yes
Nisoldipine (Sular)	Yes
Diltiazem (Cardizem)	No
Verapamil (Calan, Isoptin)	No
HMG-CO inhibitors (statin)	
Atorvastatin (Lipitor)	Yes
Cervastatin (Baycol)	Yes
Lovastatin (Mevacor)	Yes
Simvostatin (Zocor)	Yes
Fluvastatin (Lescol)	? No
Pravastatin (Pravacol)	? No
Others	
Sildenafil (Viagra)	Yes
Diazepam (Valium)	Yes
Buspirone (Buspar)	Yes
Quinidine	No
Prednisone	No
Quinine	No
Ethenil estradiol	No

[a]This is a partial list; many other medications are being investigated.
Data from *(8)*.

high enough to counteract vitamin K. Individuals taking this medication should be consuming the same amount of vitamin K per day as recommended. The antineoplastic drugs that heavily rely on oxidizing properties to kill tumor cells, for example, have an antagonistic relationship with high doses of vitamin C, an antioxidant. Another example is methotrexate; similar structurally to the B vitamin folate, it can cause severe folate deficiency. Figure 1 demonstrates the similarities between the chemical structures of these compounds. Aspirin can cause folate deficiency as well, when it is taken for a long period of time, because the aspirin competes with folate protein carrier. It is crucial for health care professionals to advise those who are taking this medication to provide sufficient folate either through the diet or by taking supplements.

4. DRUG–NUTRIENT INTERACTIONS

Drug–food interactions also play an important role in the nutritional status and nutrient requirements of individuals. A drug can enhance or inhibit nutrient bioavailability and, therefore, affect the nutritional status of individuals. Individuals, such as

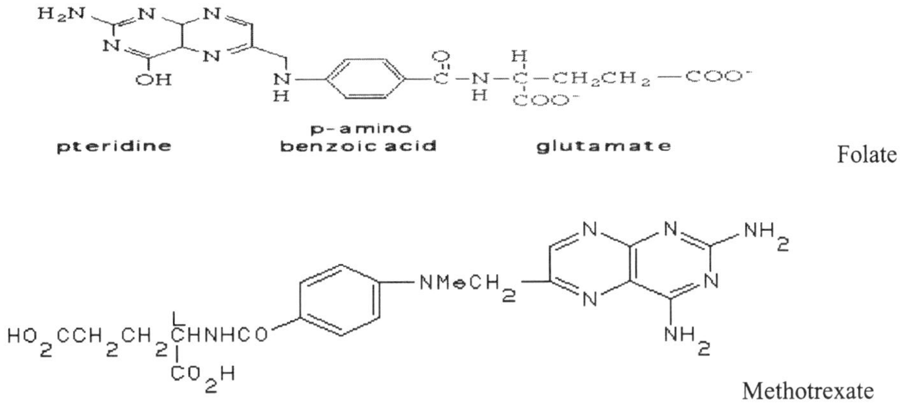

Fig. 1. The chemical structures of methotrexate and folate.

the elderly, who are taking multiple medications for a long period of time are often found to be deficient in one or more nutrients *(10)*. Other age groups, such as young children and adolescents, are also particularly at risk. There is a potential problem with drug–nutrient interactions in adolescents because their nutrient needs are higher than those of adults. Pregnant women and infants are the other groups also at particular risk. The magnitude of these deficiencies depends not only on the chemical reactions between drugs and nutrients, such as vitamins and minerals, but also on the dose and duration of treatment/exposure to the drug. Drugs can interfere with nutrient utilizations at several sites starting from the ingestion of the food to the final stage of excretion. Some of the nutrients that can be affected by common drugs are the B vitamins folacin and pyridoxine, Vitamin C, fat-soluble vitamins A and D, and minerals such as calcium and zinc. Drugs such as aspirin, barbiturates, primidone, ethinyl estradiol, cycloserine, and methotrexate are reported to affect vitamin B folate metabolism *(11,12)*.

Phenytoin (and possibly carbamazepine) interferes with the intestinal conjugase allowing folate absorption and results in teratogenicity secondary to folate deficiency and megaloblastic anemia. Another example is isoniazid, which uses B6, the vitamin required for the heme synthesis via delta-ALA synthetase, for its metabolism and therefore can cause sideroblastic anemia. The supplementation of B6 in these conditions is recommended.

4.1. Food Intake

Many drugs can cause anorexia, alter taste and smell, cause nausea and vomiting, and ultimately affect overall food intake. For example, medications such as methylphenidate (Ritalin), which influences the central nervous system, may reduce appetite. This medication is often prescribed for hyperactive young children who are in their rapid growth phase. Long-term use of this drug may cause growth retardation in these children. Therefore, when this drug is prescribed to young children, their food intake must be monitored. On the other hand, some anorectic drugs are used for weight loss and to treat obesity by reducing appetite. Examples are adrenergic and serotoninergic agents, which cause satiety, reduce appetite, and increase energy expenditure leading

**Table 5
Examples of Drugs That Change Taste Perception**

Acetyl sulfasalicylic acid	Griseofulvin
Allopurinol	Lidocaine
Amphetamines	Lithium carbonate
Amphotericin B	Meprobamate
Ampicillin	Methicillin sodium
Amylocaine	Methylthiouracil
Benzocaine	Metronidazole
Captopril	Nifedipine
Chlorpheniramine maleate	D-Penicillamine
Clofibrate	Phenindione
Diltiazem	Phenytoin
Dinitrophenol	Probucol
5-Fluorouracil	Sulfasalazine
Flurazepam (Dalmane)	Triazolam (Halcion)

Data from *(9)*.

to weight loss. Amphetamines are good examples of adrenergic drugs that stimulate secretion of norepinephrine and reduce food intake *(13)*. Serotoninergic drugs, such as fenfluramine and dexfenfluramine, inhibit the reuptake of serotonin, stimulate satiety, and therefore reduce food intake. However, these drugs were found to have adverse effects on the cardiovascular system and were withdrawn from the market in the United States in 1997. There are other drugs for treating obesity, such as the appetite suppressant, sibutramine (also as antidepressant), and orlistat (lipase inhibitor), and some new biological compounds such as bombesin and neuropeptide Y, which also affect satiety.

Taste and smell are very important factors that influence food intake and can subsequently affect the nutritional status of individuals. Taste alteration (dysgeusia or hypogeusia) due to medications is very common. Some hypoglycemic agents such as glipizide, the antimicrobials amphotericin B, ampicillin, and antiepileptic phenytoin are among the medications that alter taste perception. Other examples are given in Table 5 *(9)*.

Cisplatin and other cytotoxic agents commonly used in the treatment of cancer cause nausea and vomiting, which reduces food intake as a result. Using diet modifications, such as colorless, odorless meals for cancer patients, to decrease nausea and vomiting should be considered in order to increase the food intake in these patients.

4.2. Weight Gain

Several groups of drugs such as anticonvulsants (caramazepine and valproic acid), antihistamines (cyproheptadine hydrochloride-Periactin), psychotropic drugs (chlordiazepoxide hydrochloride-Librium, diazepam-Valium, chloromazine hydrochloride-Thorazine, meprobamate-Equanil), and corticosteroids (cortisone, prednisone) may increase appetite and consequently lead to weight gain. Antidepressant drugs such as monoamine oxidase inhibitors (MAOIs) cause less bodywt change than the tricyclic drugs *(14)*. A synthetic derivative of progesterone, medroxyprogesterone acetate or megestrol acetate, used for the treatment of hormone-sensitive breast and endometrial cancer, may increase appetite, food intake, and weight gain.

The formulation of drugs in lipid emulsion (e.g., in 10% soybean), such as propofol, contributes to a significant amount of additional energy (kilocalories) intake. Other drugs such as lorazepam, morphine, and pancuronium may change the bodywt by decreasing the body's energy expenditure *(15)*.

Weight gain could be therapeutically favorable in some cases such as in cancer and acquired immunodeficiency syndromes (AIDS)-related cachexia. Anabolic steroids, such as mandrolone, corticosteroids, cyproheptadine, hydrazine sulfate, megestrol acetate, dronabinol and oxandrolone, are prescribed in some cases to promote weight gain.

4.3. Nutrient Absorption

Several mechanisms may affect nutrient absorption due to the presence of drugs. Drugs can damage the intestinal absorptive surfaces including villi, microvilli, brush border enzymes, and the transport system. Drugs can also influence the absorption of nutrients by changing the GI transit time or the overall GI chemical environment, like the pH of the stomach. Absorption of micronutrients, vitamins and minerals, as well as macronutrients, protein and fat, are affected by the type, dosage, and strength of some drugs.

GI damage can come from over-the-counter drugs such as aspirin and other acidic drugs, or from antibiotic neomycin or laxatives. The resulting changes in the mucosal lining interfere with optimum absorption of nutrients such as iron, calcium, fat (including some fat-soluble vitamins), protein, sodium, and potassium. Colchicines, antiinflammatory drugs, *para*-aminosalicylic acid, antituberculosis, trimethoprim, antibacterial, and sulfasalazine, antiinflammatory (antiarthritic) drugs *are* known to interfere with the intestinal transport mechanisms. They can impair the absorption of the B vitamins, B12 and folacin.

Many laxatives, mineral oil, and cathartic agents reduce transit time in the GI tract and may cause steatorrhea and loss of fat-soluble vitamins, A and E, and possibly calcium and potassium. Drugs containing sorbitol, such as theophyline solutions, may induce osmotic diarrhea and therefore shorten the transit time. Antacids change the pH of the stomach and cause chelating with some minerals, consequently reducing their absorption. Higher pH in the stomach reduces the absorption of iron, calcium, zinc, and magnesium.

4.4. Nutrient Metabolism

Some of the important functions of vitamins and several minerals are their roles as coenzymes/cofactors in metabolic processes in the human body. Therefore, certain drugs are targeted to these coenzymes (antivitamins) in order to reduce the activity of some enzymes in related metabolic reactions. Good examples of these drugs are methotrexate (MTX) for treating leukemia and rheumatoid arthritis; trimethoprim, used with sulfa for *Pneumocystis carinii* pneumonia; and aminopterin and pyrimethamine, used for treating malaria and ocular toxoplasmosis. Vitamin folate is a cofactor for the enzyme dihydrofolate reductase, which is necessary for nucleic acid biosynthesis and cell replication. This vitamin will be excreted because the drugs displace it from dihydrofolate reductase to reduce cell replication. Prescription for supplements for these patients should be cautioned and monitored. Another example is the anticoagulant drug, coumarin, which is a vitamin K antagonist. Dietary vitamin K can interact with anticoagulant drugs; it also changes the safety and therapeutic efficacy of these drugs *(16)*. Therefore, many patients are advised to avoid foods, such as vegetables, high in vitamin K. Patient nutrition education is necessary in order to include some vegetables in their daily diets without changing the efficacy of these drugs.

Bile, an emulsifier, is required for the metabolism of fat and also as an aid in the absorption of fat-soluble vitamins such as A, D, E, and K. Some bile-sequestering resins such as cholestyramine, therefore, interfere with the fat metabolism and absorption and may result in deficiency of the essential fatty acid linoleic acid and impair the synthesis of arachidonic acid. Lipids are important components of cell membrane structure. Individuals who are taking these types of medications should therefore be monitored for any deficiencies of essential fatty acids or fat soluble vitamins.

MAOIs, diamine oxidase inhibitors such as a group of antidepressant drugs, antimicrobials, and antineoplastic drugs interact with the biologically active pressor amines in foods very strongly. These reactions result in blood vessel constriction and, consequently, high blood pressure, tachycardia, chest pain, and severe headache. Patients taking these medications are encouraged to avoid foods high in tyramine (vasoactive amine) such as hard cheeses, smoked or pickled fish, broad beans, Chianti or vermouth wines, meat and yeast extracts, dry sausage, and beer and ale. The amines in these foods usually deaminate very rapidly by monoamine and diamine oxidases and therefore they cause no adverse effects. However, in the presence of the inhibiting drugs, the blood levels of these amines will elevate and in severe cases can cause intracranial hemorrhage, cardiac arrhythmias, and cardiac failure. Table 6 lists the foods that one should monitor while taking the MAOIs *(17)*.

4.5. Nutrient Excretion

Competitive binding and altered reabsorption are the two recognized mechanisms that may cause drugs to induce nutrient excretion. D-Penicillamine chelates with intended toxic metals, but it may also bind with other metals such as zinc, eliminating it via urine. Ethylenediaminetetra-acetic acid (EDTA) has been shown to cause urinary excretion of zinc. Some diuretics, such as furosemide, ethacrynic acid, and triamterene, reduce the reabsorption of electrolytes and minerals such as potassium, magnesium, zinc, and calcium and increase renal excretion of these elements. Sodium loss in the urine is common with thiazide and loop diuretics. Potassium-sparing diuretics spare potassium and magnesium loss but augment urinary sodium loss *(18)*. Depletion of magnesium is associated with chemotherapeutic agents such as cisplatin. Therefore, magnesium supplement often is recommended between the chemotherapy treatments for these patients.

5. CONCLUSIONS

Many nutrient–drug and drug–nutrient interactions, and the impact of these interactions on overall health have been identified and many more are being investigated. Health care professionals need to keep abreast of the new findings in this area and recognize that these interactions do occur, especially when a drug is used over a long period of time. Nutrient interactions are not unique to prescription drugs. Over-the-counter drugs, because of their increasing availability, are used by many older adults and may impair nutritional status by interfering with bioavailability of many critical nutrients.

Table 6
The Tyramine-Restricted Diet

Foods High in Tyramine Must Be Avoided	Foods Should Be Used With Caution	Foods Low in Tyramine No Restriction
Cheese	Avocado	Fresh fish
Smoked or pickled fish	Raspberries	Canned figs
Nonfresh meats, livers	Soy sauce	Mushrooms
Chianti and vermouth wines	Chocolate	Cucumber
Broad beans	Red and white wines, port wines	Sweet corn
Banana peels		Fresh pineapple
Meat extracts	Distilled spirits	Worcestershire sauce
Yeast extracts/brewers yeast	Peanuts	Salad dressings
Dry sausage	Yogurt and cream from unpasteurized milk	Yeast bread
Sauerkraut		Raisins
Beer and ale		Tomato juice
		Curry powder
		Beet root
		Junket
		Boiled egg
		Coca Cola
		Cookies (English biscuits)
		Cottage cheese
		Cream cheese

Data from (17).

Clients should consult with physicians about potential interactions, with pharmacists for instructions on taking drugs, and with registered dietitians to assess nutritional status while taking medications. Food is essential for good health as are medications that enable people to enjoy better health, but they also bring side effects and risks that need to be addressed.

REFERENCES

1. Thomas JA. Drug–nutrient interactions. Nutr Rev 53:271–282 (1995).
2. Kirk JK. Significant drug–nutrient interactions. Am Family Physician 51:1175–1182 (1995).
3. Bennett WM. Drug interactions and consequences of sodium restriction. Am J Clin Nutr 65(Suppl 2):678S–681S (1997).
4. Ameer B and Weintraub RA. Drug interaction with grapefruit juice. Clin Pharmacokine 33:103–121 (1997).
5. Wagner D, Spahn-Langguth H, Hanafy A, and Langguth P. Intestinal drug efflux: formulation and food effects. Adv Drug Deliv Review 50(Suppl 1):513–531 (2001).
6. Offman EM, Freeman DJ, Dresser GK, Munoz C, Bend JR, and Bailey DG. Red wine-cisapride interaction: comparison with grapefruit juice. Clin Pharmacol Therpy 70(1):17–23 (2001).
7. Feldman EB. How grapefruit juice potentiates drug bioavailability. Nutr Rev 55:398–400 (1997).
8. Karpman HL. Is grapefruit juice harmful? Internal Medicine Alert 23:1–4 (2001).
9. Haken V. Interactions between drugs and nutrients. In: Mahan LK and Escott-Stump S, eds. Krause's food, nutrition, and diet therapy. Philadelphia: Saunders, 2000:399–414.

10. Lamy PP. Effects of diet and nutrition on drug therapy. J Am Geriatr Soc 30:S99–S112 (1982).
11. Roe DA. Effects of drugs on nutrition. Life Science 15:1219–1234 (1974).
12. Thomas JA and Markovac J. Aspects of neural tube defects: a mini review. Toxic Substances J 13:303–312(1994).
13. Atkinson RL. Use of drugs in the treatment of obesity. Ann Rev Nutr 17:383–404 (1997).
14. Pijl H and Meinders AE. Bodyweight change as an adverse effect of drug treatment. Drug Safety 14(5):329–342 (1996).
15. Mirenda J and Broyles G. Propofol as used for sedation in the ICU. Chest 108:539–548 (1995).
16. Couris RR, Tataronis GR, Dallal GE, Blumberg JB, and Dwyer JT. Assessment of healthcare professionals' knowledge about warfarin–vitamin K drug–nutrient interactions. J Am Coll Nutr 19:439–445 (2000).
17. Simpson GM and Gratz SS. Comparison of the pressor effect of tyramine after treatment with phenelzine and moclobemide in healthy volunteer. Clin Pharmacol Therap 52:286–291 (1992).
18. Nicholls MG. Interaction of diuretics and electrolytes in congestive heart failure. Am J Cardiol 65:17E–21E (1990).

Related Websites

Lambrechtk JE. Review of herb–drug interactions; documented and theoretical U.S. Pharmacist 25(8):42–53 (2000). http://www.uspharmacist.com/NewLook/DisplayArticle.cfm?item_num=566

IBIS Guide to drug–herb and drug–nutrient interactions, October 12, 1999. http://www.IBIS medical.com/announcinter.html

FDA Public Health Advisory of possible interaction between *Hypericum perforatum* (St. John's wort) and Indinavir, a protease inhibitor used to treat HIV infection. http://www.fda.gov/cder/drug/advisory/stjwort.htm

AHealthyMe.com-Theophylline Learn how to take the asthma treatment drug properly and explore its side effects and interactions with medications and foods. http://www.ahealthyme.com/topic/topic100592224

Clinical Pharmacology Online-Doxercalciferol Patient's guide to this synthetic form of vitamin D profiles its mode of action, proper dosage, and interactions with foods and other medications. http://www.lifeclinic.com/scripts/fullmono/showinfo_f.pl?mononum=568&drugidx=1&infotype=5

MedicineNet-Etidronate (Didronel) Learn how the medication works to strengthen bone and explore its dosage, side effects, and interactions with food and other medicines.
 http://www.FocusOnMedications.com/script/main/art.asp?articlekey=738

MDAdvice.com-Cholestyramine Description of the antihyperlipidemic agent's uses, dosage, and side effects includes details about its interactions with foods and medications. http://www.mdadvice.com/library/drug/drug113html

Food Medication Interactions Find a table of contents and sample page of HIV Medications-Food Interactions Handbook. Resource offers information on food and drug interactions. http://www.foodmedinteractions.com/

Clinical Reference Systems-Paricalcitol (Zemplar) Patient education leaflet describes how the drug works and lists its potential side effects. Find advice on food and medication interactions. http://www.patienteducation.com/paricalcitol.html

11. Food and Drug Interactions

FDA Food and Drug Interactions From the U.S. Food and Drug Administration with information that explains how certain foods may interact with some groups of medications. http//vm.cfsan.fda.gov/~lrd/fdinter.html

InteliHealth-Phenelzine Sulfate (Nardil) Discover how the medication works to relieve depression and investigate its food, drug, and disease interactions. http://www.intelihealth.com/IH/ihtIH/WSIHW000/19689/11728/214201.html?rbrand=Nardil

Thyroid Drugs: Food, Drug and Supplement Interactions Discover which foods, supplements, and drugs interact with thyroid medications. http://www.thyroid-info.com/articles/thyroid-drug-faq.htm

Chapter 12

Alcohol and Drug Interactions

A. Wayne Jones, PhD, DSc

1. Introduction

Drug interactions involving alcohol[1] constitute a major problem in clinical and forensic medicine owing to the widespread use and abuse of alcoholic beverages throughout adult life *(1–3)*. The combined effects of alcohol and other drugs acting on the central nervous system (CNS) are particularly dangerous and have accounted for many fatal poisonings both accidental and through deliberate suicide attempts *(4–8)*. Adverse drug interactions are a constant concern for the pharmaceutical industry whenever a new drug is marketed and such possibilities need to be carefully explored in both human and animal studies *(9,10)*.

Most people drink alcohol in moderation but for about 10–15% of the population, especially among men, ethanol is a major drug of abuse and is responsible for considerable morbidity and mortality worldwide *(11–14)*. Alcohol has been called the Jekyll and Hyde of the drug world because when taken in moderation it is relatively harmless, whereas overconsumption and abuse wrecks people's lives and costs the health care system billions of dollars annually *(15)*. Alcohol is a legal drug and, although a minimum drinking age has been set at 18 yr in most countries (21 yr in the United States), teenage drinking is a fact of life and is virtually impossible to control. The combined effects of alcohol and drugs whether licit or illicit represent a serious public health problem not least in connection with traffic safety and deaths on the roads caused by impaired drivers *(16,17)*. The ready availability of alcohol and the increasing popularity and use of recreational drugs underscores the need to consider very carefully the risks associated with drug–alcohol interactions *(18)*.

---

[1] The words *alcohol* and *ethanol* are used interchangeably in this article.

From: *Handbook of Drug Interactions: A Clinical and Forensic Guide*
A. Mozayani and L. P. Raymon, eds. © Humana Press Inc., Totowa, NJ

The concentration of alcohol in a person's blood has important ramifications in forensic science as reflected in the setting of punishable limits of blood alcohol concentration (BAC) for driving, such as 0.08 or 0.10 g/100 mL in most US states *(19,20)*. Lower statutory limits, e.g., 0.02 and 0.05 g/100 mL, apply in other countries and also for novice drivers and those engaged with safety-sensitive work. For a 70-kg man with a BAC of 0.1 g/100 mL, a simple calculation shows that there is about 50 g of ethanol distributed in all body fluids and tissues. This amount vastly exceeds by several orders of magnitude the normal dose of any prescription drug, e.g., 10 mg diazepam or 500 mg aspirin *(21)*. Whether a certain prescription drug taken together with a moderate dose of alcohol increases a person's BAC above that expected without the drug is often a much discussed question in legal proceedings concerned with driving under the influence of alcohol *(22)*.

Investigations into drug–alcohol interactions are complex owing to the different timing of administration of alcohol relative to the drug and vice versa as well as the particular dosages administered. Experiments designed to evaluate drug–alcohol interactions differ depending on whether a single dose of alcohol and or drug was administered or whether long-term treatment had developed such as in heavy drinkers or alcoholics, or after multiple doses of a drug resulting in steady-state plasma drug concentration before the alcohol was consumed *(23–25)*.

Drug–alcohol interactions can be subdivided into four broad categories:

- The effect of acute or chronic consumption of alcohol on the absorption, distribution, metabolism, and excretion of a particular drug.
- The effect of acute or chronic consumption of alcohol on the dynamics of drug action, that is, the action of the drug particularly in the CNS including drug-receptor binding and synaptic functioning.
- The effect of a particular drug or other chemical agent after single or multiple doses on absorption, distribution, metabolism, and excretion of ethanol and the resulting tissue concentrations.
- The effect of a drug or other chemical substance after single or multiple doses on the behavioral effects produced by ethanol including impairment of performance of skilled tasks and signs and symptoms of inebriation and toxicity.

A schematic diagram showing possible sites of interaction between drugs and ethanol after combined oral administration is shown in Fig. 1. This diagram illustrates absorption from the gastrointestinal canal *(26)*, metabolism in the liver by phase I and phase II enzymes as well as first-pass metabolism *(27,28)*, and also the excretory mechanisms in the kidney and lung *(29)*. The intensity and duration of drug–action is determined to a large extent by the rate of metabolic breakdown of the active substance, which in turn is linked to the availability of various metabolizing enzymes *(27,28)*.

When considering drug interactions with ethanol one needs to distinguish between pharmacokinetic and pharmacodynamic interactions *(30,31)*. Because most drugs undergo metabolism in the liver the competition between ethanol and the drug for enzyme-binding sites is a key consideration *(32)*. Various metabolic interactions might result from altered intermediary metabolism during the breakdown (oxidation) of alcohol in the liver *(33,34)*. Those who suffer from liver dysfunction, often caused by heavy drinking or even cirrhosis, are likely to show an impaired metabolic clearance of many drugs including alcohol *(35–37)*.

12. Alcohol and Drug Interactions 397

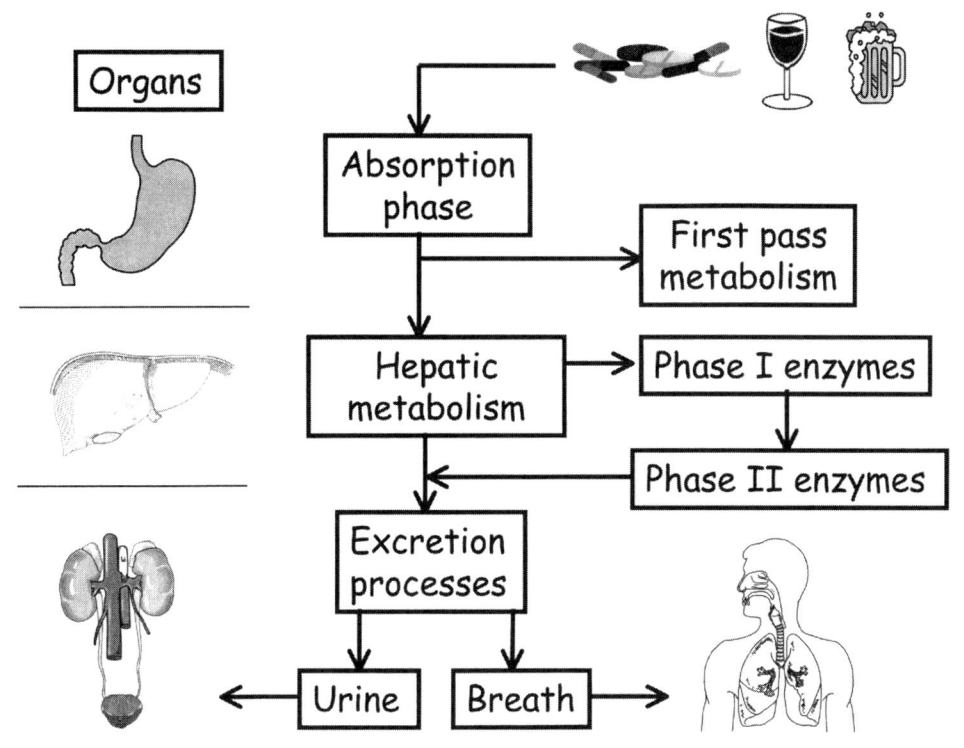

Fig. 1. Schematic diagram of the fate of alcohol and drugs in the body. Phase I enzymes introduce or remove functional groups and phase II enzymes synthesize compounds that are more soluble in water and can be excreted into the urine.

How alcohol and drugs work in the brain is crucial for understanding pharmacodynamic interactions and the resulting effects on performance and behavior of the individual *(38)*. The impairing effects of alcohol depend on prior drinking experience (tolerance development) and the concentration of the drug reaching specific receptor sites in the brain *(39,40)*. Changes in the absorption, distribution, or elimination of ethanol impacts on the amount of drug that reaches the systemic circulation (bioavailability), which in turn increases or decreases the risk of organ and tissue damage *(41–43)*. Table 1 lists some of the possible mechanisms for drug–alcohol interaction.

An enormous literature base exists under the rubric "drug–alcohol interactions" including both human and animal studies. Several monographs have been devoted to the subject of drug interactions with ethanol; the first of these appeared in 1968 *(44)* and another in 1978 *(45)*. The vast majority of studies have dealt with interactions of alcohol and drugs on driving skills and the risk of causing a traffic crash *(46–49)*. These reviews often take the form of systematic compilations of different drug categories (antidepressants, antihistamines, anticonvulsants, antipsychotics, opiates and sedative hypnotics, etc.) and provide details of the experimental protocols and the degree of impairment of body functions and performance and behavior of the test subjects *(50)*.

Lane et al. *(51)* presented a comprehensive review of the effects of ethanol on drug and metabolite kinetics and distinguished between short-term and long-term administration of many psychoactive substances. In a more recent survey, Fraser *(52)* focused

Table 1
**Examples of Sites and Mechanisms
of Pharmacokinetic and Pharmacodynamic
Interaction Between Alcohol and Drugs**

Pharmacokinetic Interactions

Absorption
  Gastric motility
  Gastric pH
  First-pass metabolism
  Hepatic blood flow
Distribution
  Blood flow to tissue mass
  Protein binding
  Body composition (adiposity)
Metabolism
  Induction of drug metabolizing enzymes
  Inhibition of drug metabolizing enzyme
Excretion
  Enhanced or diminished diuresis
  Altered urinary pH

Pharmacodynamic Interactions

Synaptic activity, receptor binding and ion channels
  Altered behavioral effects
  Enhanced or diminished impairment
  Enhanced or diminished toxicity

attention on various examples of pharmacokinetic interactions between alcohol and drugs, particularly the notion of a significant first-pass metabolism (FPM) of ethanol. Other investigators have looked more closely at alcohol's interaction with over-the-counter (OTC) medications and various food products *(53)*. Weathermon and Crabb *(54)* recently presented a comprehensive review of drug–alcohol interactions, which included OTC drugs and prescription medication. They discussed the risk for adverse effects mediated by changes in disposition kinetics and the combined effects of alcohol and drugs on the brain via receptor binding. Morland et al. *(55)* looked at a wide range of metabolic interactions between ethanol and other drugs with the main focus on detoxification mechanisms, both phase I and phase II reactions. Havier *(56)* presented a recent review of drug–alcohol interactions in one of the forensic science journals.

In this chapter only selected topics will be covered, mainly those drug–alcohol interactions with direct relevance in forensic medicine and toxicology *(57)*. Moreover, general principles and mechanisms of drug–alcohol interaction will be dealt with more so than a systematic review of drug after drug and their effects if any on changing a person's performance and behavior *(58)*. Indeed, some studies report conflicting results and much seems to depend on the experimental design, especially the demographics and selection of subjects, and also the timing of ethanol and drug administration in relation to food intake.

Most investigations of drug–alcohol interactions are seemingly prompted by interest in the combined effect on impairment of human performance in relation to driving a motor vehicle *(59)*. Studies of this kind usually employ a battery of cognitive and psychomotor tests whereby a subject performs various tasks before and after treatment with a psychoactive drug either alone or together with alcohol *(60,61)*. The testing is repeated at fixed times after drinking ends and performance scores are compared with the results obtained predosing *(62)*. If the aim of the study is to investigate hangover or residual effects of alcohol and/or medication, then the test battery is also run the following morning after an overnight sleep *(63)*. Experiments of this kind should be done double blind with crossover design and with a suitable placebo substituting for the active drug *(64)*. However, a good placebo for alcohol does not exist and the usual approach is to give an alcohol-free beverage such as orange juice or a soft drink.

Typical drug and alcohol effects monitored in such studies include heart rate, blood pressure, various kinds of eye movements, mental arithmetic, word recall, body sway, simple and choice reaction time, and various tracking tasks and divided-attention situations, the latter being particularly sensitive to impairing effects of alcohol and drugs *(65)*. The test battery is usually carried out before treatment with the drug to establish baseline values and then at various times postdosing. More recently, computer-driven performance tests have been designed to measure impairment of performance and behavior during drug–alcohol interaction studies *(66,67)*. Other protocols make use of driving simulators of various dignity *(68)* and a few studies even looked at on-the-road driving maneuvers with and without prior drug treatment *(69)*.

The International Council on Alcohol, Drugs and Traffic Safety (ICADTS) arrange meetings in which drug effects on driving skills and drug–alcohol interactions are a major part of the program. The published proceedings from these conferences (e.g., most recently, Stockholm 2000 and Montreal 2002) are available for those who require an in-depth coverage of the effects of alcohol and drugs on human performance testing in a traffic safety context. Noteworthy is a recent special edition of the publication *Forensic Science Review (70)*, which contained a number of comprehensive review articles dealing with the effects of licit and illicit drugs on human performance and behavior including the benzodiazepines, cannabis, γ-hydroxybutyrate, ketamine and methamphetamine. However, the topic of drug–alcohol interactions was not one of the things covered.

The present review looks at interactions between the legal drug ethanol and various illicit and prescription drugs with main emphasis on mechanisms of interaction and toxicity. Drug-induced changes in the absorption, distribution, and metabolism of ethanol are of interest in traffic-law enforcement when statutory alcohol limits for driving are enforced *(19,20)*. The high prevalence of alcohol in drug-related deaths makes drug–alcohol interactions a major concern in forensic medicine and toxicology.

2. Fate of Alcohol in the Body

The fate of ethanol in the body is usually considered in terms of absorption, distribution, metabolism and excretion processes (Fig. 1). Alcohol (ethanol) is a small neutral molecule with low chemical activity and after absorption into the blood it mixes completely with the body water without binding to plasma protein *(71,72)*. What happens

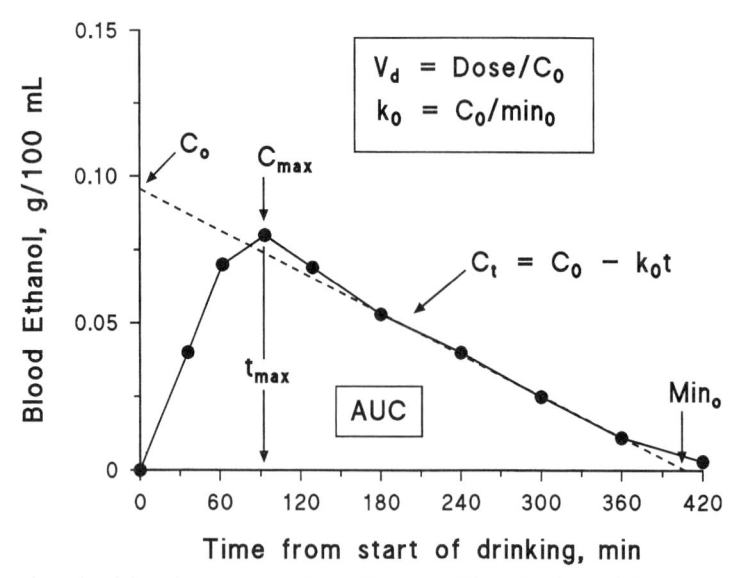

Fig. 2. Example of a blood-concentration time profile of ethanol in one male subject who drank 0.68 g ethanol per kg body wt on an empty stomach. Kinetic parameters are defined on this graph; C_{max} and t_{max} are the peak blood concentration and the time of its occurrence; C_o is the theoretical extrapolated concentration in blood at the time of starting to drink; min_o is the extrapolated time for all the alcohol to be eliminated from the bloodstream; AUC is area under the concentration-time profile; k_o is the rate of alcohol disappearance from blood.

to alcohol in the body after drinking beer, wine, or liquor is usually illustrated by plotting the concentration of ethanol in blood as a function of sampling time after the start of drinking. The shape of the BAC curve, which represents an interplay between absorption, distribution, and elimination processes, is a good starting point for discussions of drug–alcohol interactions. The characteristic features of the BAC time profile are usually described by a set of parameters (73), which have proven useful in pharmacokinetic analysis of drug–alcohol interaction (Fig. 2).

2.1. Absorption

Alcohol is absorbed rapidly from the gastrointestinal tract and, unlike most other drugs, this process starts already in the stomach. The absorption occurs by a passive diffusion process according to Fick's law (74). However, when the stomach contents empty into the duodenum alcohol is taken up into the portal venous blood almost immediately, so the rate of gastric emptying plays a pivotal role in determining the resulting C_{max} and t_{max} for ethanol (75). The absorption of ethanol from the gut depends on many variable factors including the time of day and the drinking pattern, e.g., bolus intake or drinking smaller amounts repeatedly over several hours (76,77). The dosage form (beer, wine, or spirits) and the concentration of ethanol in the beverage also impinge on the rate of absorption of ethanol and the peak blood concentration reached (78–80).

The presence of food in the stomach before drinking is probably the single most significant factor influencing gastric emptying and consequently the resulting C_{max}

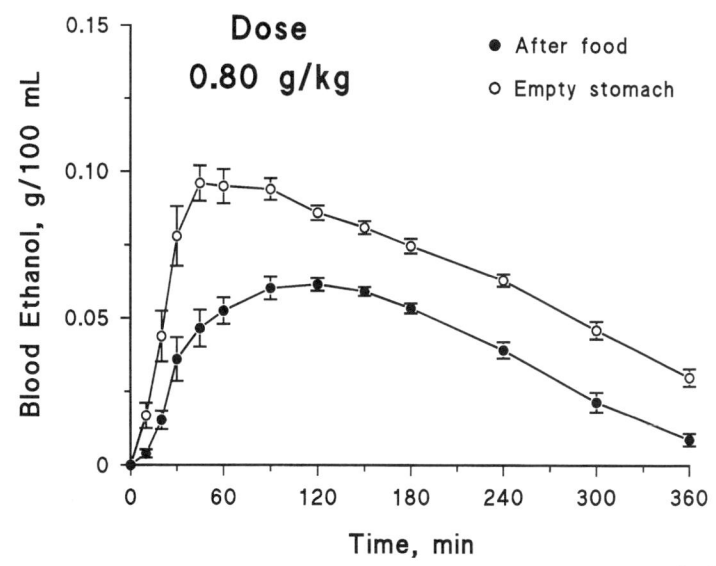

Fig. 3. Effect of eating a meal on the blood-concentration time curves of ethanol. Mean curves are shown for subjects after they drank 0.8 g ethanol per kg either after an overnight fast (empty stomach) or immediately after eating a standardized breakfast.

and t_{max} for ethanol *(81–84)*. In one study into the effects of eating a meal on the rate of ethanol absorption, the stomach and duodenal contents were sampled and the concentration of ethanol remaining was determined at various times postdosing *(85)*. The results showed that a substantial amount of the ethanol remained in the stomach for several hours after dosing, probably being bound to constituents of the meal *(85)*.

Figure 3 shows average BAC profiles derived from a drinking experiment with nine healthy men under fed and fasted conditions. The peak concentration in blood is lowered by about 40% when alcohol is ingested after eating food *(86)*. In this respect, the composition of the food in terms of protein, fat, and carbohydrate content was less important then the amount eaten and the timing of the meal relative to drinking the alcohol *(87,88)*. The effect of food is not simply to slow the rate of absorption, because alcohol seems to be eliminated from the body faster in the fed state judging by a shorter time (1–2 h) required to reach a specified low BAC (e.g., 0.03 g/100 mL) *(89)*. The rate of disposal of ethanol is seemingly boosted in the well-nourished state when there is food in the stomach. This points to either a more effective enzymatic metabolism in well-nourished individuals, e.g., owing to more effective enzymes and/or enhanced hepatic blood flow after eating a meal *(90)*. In this respect, carbohydrates seem to be more effective then protein or fat *(91,92)*. Another possibility is that part of the dose of alcohol is metabolized in the liver or stomach or both organs before the blood reaches the systemic circulation, and this process is called first-pass metabolism.

Many studies have verified a large interindividual variation in the rate of absorption of ethanol even under standardized drinking conditions *(93–95)*. In theory, a more concentrated alcoholic drink, such as vodka or whisky (40% v/v), should be absorbed faster then a weaker one (beer or wine, 5–10% v/v) but this is not always the case *(80)*.

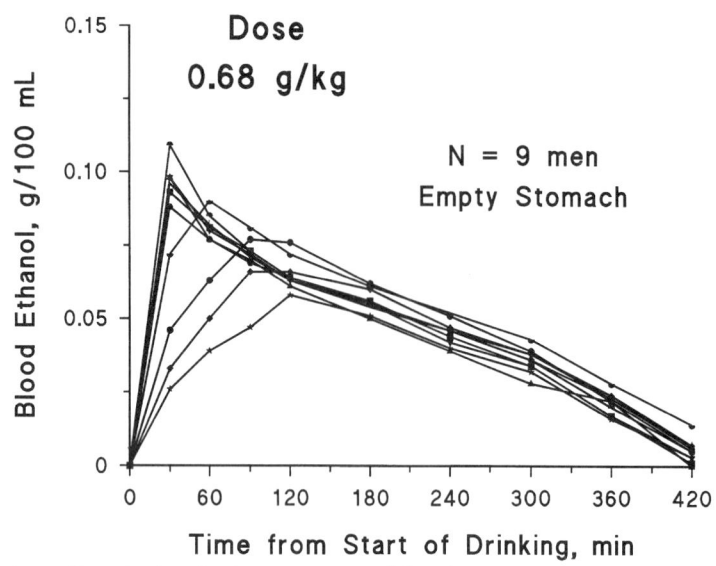

Fig. 4. Examples of interindividual variations in blood-concentration time profiles of ethanol in nine healthy men after they drank 0.68 g/kg after an overnight fast. Note the wide variation in C_{max} and t_{max} parameters even under these standardized conditions without any drug treatment.

Intake of neat spirits (40–50 vol%) might irritate the gastric surfaces and provoke a pyloric spasm *(96)*. This leads to a retardation of stomach emptying so that alcohol is absorbed more slowly, sometimes over several hours, resulting in both lower C_{max} and later t_{max} compared with drinking weaker beverages *(96)*.

Figure 4 gives an example of the magnitude of interindividual variations in absorption kinetics of ethanol in experiments done under standardized conditions in nine healthy men who drank 0.68 g ethanol per kg body wt as neat whisky in 20 min after an overnight fast *(96)*. Note the large differences in C_{max} (0.06–0.109 g/100 mL) and the time of occurrence of t_{max} (10–110 min) after end of drinking. This large interindividual variation even without any drug treatment underscores the need for large numbers of subjects to give sufficient statistical power to detect an effect of a drug treatment on the absorption kinetics of alcohol.

When alcohol is ingested on an empty stomach (overnight fast) this sometimes results in a very rapid absorption and the concentration-time profiles resemble those seen when alcohol is given by intravenous (iv) infusion *(97)*. Figure 5 compares BAC profiles after a subject drank 0.4 g/kg alcohol in 15 min and another subject received the same dose by iv infusion over 30 min. After parenteral administration, the peak BAC coincided with stopping the infusion and this was followed by an abrupt drop in BAC (the diffusion plunge) during which time the alcohol in the central blood compartment becomes distributed into all body fluids. After oral administration the peak BAC was reached 45 min after the end of drinking.

The absorption rate of alcohol including C_{max} and t_{max} seems to be more reproducible in the same individual than between different individuals. This suggests that, in

12. Alcohol and Drug Interactions

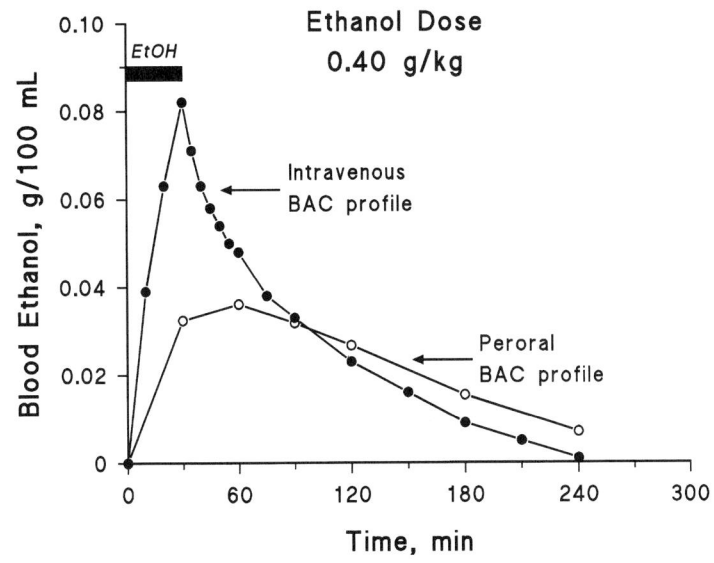

Fig. 5. Examples of blood-concentration time profiles of ethanol after oral and intravenous administration of the same ethanol dose (0.4 g/kg) in two different male subjects. The drinking time was 15 min starting ~2 h or more after eating and the time for infusion of ethanol was 30 min.

studies of drug–alcohol interaction, a randomized crossover design should be used and results evaluated by comparing intraindividual differences in the test variables *(98,99)*. Many environmental factors, such as time of day *(100)*, smoking cigarettes *(101)*, etc., influence gastric emptying and the speed of absorption of ethanol from the gut *(102,103)*. It seems that gastric emptying is faster in the morning before eating breakfast because blood glucose is low at this time *(104,105)*. Hypoglycemia increases the gastric emptying rate in healthy subjects *(105)*.

2.2. Distribution

Alcohol is completely miscible with water and binding to plasma protein or other endogenous structures is seemingly negligible, which means that alcohol should not participate in displacement reactions with highly protein-bound drugs *(106)*. Accordingly, absorbed alcohol distributes into the total body water and, when equilibrium distribution is complete, the concentration determined in all body fluids and tissue will be proportional to their water content *(73)*. Because body water content in women represents 50–55% of body wt compared with 55–62% in men, there will be gender-related differences in volume of distribution (V_d) for ethanol *(107)*. The average values of V_d for ethanol are 0.7 L/kg for men and 0.6 L/kg for women, but there is considerable variation within and between genders depending on a person's age and the relative proportions of fat to lean tissues *(108–110)*. If the dose of alcohol is given per kg body wt and not according to body water or lean body mass, after equilibrium of ethanol is complete in all body fluids and tissues the BAC for women will be roughly 10% higher than for men. It has been suggested that the phase of the menstrual cycle and also the use of oral contraceptive steroids might influence some pharmacokinetic parameters of ethanol but opinion on this topic remains divided *(111,113)*.

In forensic science and toxicology, ethanol is usually determined in specimens of whole blood instead of plasma or serum, which are the specimens mostly used in clinical pharmacology studies. Because whole blood contains 78–80% w/w water and plasma and serum are 91–93% water, the concentration of alcohol will not be the same *(114)*. Studies have shown that the plasma/whole blood ratio of ethanol is 1.10–1.15:1 or about 10–15% more alcohol in the plasma fraction *(115)*. This uneven distribution of ethanol between plasma and erythrocytes has implications when the distribution volume is determined from the ratio dose/C_o as illustrated in Fig. 2. If the graph had been constructed from the analysis of serial samples of plasma or serum, C_o would be 10–15% higher and V_d correspondingly lower by the same amount. These same bioanalytical considerations also apply to other drugs that might bind strongly to plasma proteins or be highly concentrated in the red cells, so the distribution of a substance between plasma, erythrocytes, and whole blood cannot be neglected.

In elderly individuals, the total body water per kilogram body wt is diminished and, therefore, when the dose of alcohol is administered according to total body wt, elder individuals attain a slightly larger dose/kg lean body mass *(116–118)*. This leads to increased C_{max} and lower V_d and the BAC time profile runs on a higher level with larger area under the curve (AUC) in the elderly. Several studies have shown that total body water can be estimated by evaluating concentration-time profiles of ethanol in the fasting state or after iv administration. The results obtained by ethanol dilution compared well with independent methods such as isotope dilution techniques *(119,120)*.

During the absorption of ethanol from the gut, the BAC depends in part on the sampling site, that is, whether arterial or venous blood was taken for analysis *(121,122)*. Organs with a low ratio of blood flow to tissue mass, such as the skeletal muscles, will show the largest arterial-venous difference. When the absorption of ethanol is complete and the BAC curve enters the postabsorptive phase, the arterial and venous blood concentration is much smaller *(123)*. Thereafter, the concentration of alcohol in venous blood draining the muscle tissues and returning to the heart will hold a slightly higher concentration of ethanol compared with arterial blood leaving the heart owing to metabolism in the liver during each circulation of the blood. The slope of the BAC decline will be slightly steeper for arterial-blood samples compared with venous-blood samples *(123)*.

Besides gender-related differences in body composition (e.g., the ratio of fat to lean tissue), which are obviously important for the distribution volume of ethanol *(124, 125)*, some have suggested that efficacy of gastric FPM is different for men and women. Women tend to have lower gastric alcohol dehydrogenase (ADH) activity and hence diminished ability for presystemic oxidation of ethanol in the stomach *(126)*. This explanation was offered to account for women reaching higher BACs compared with men when the same dose of ethanol was given per kg body wt *(126)*. However, the importance of gastric ADH in FPM of ethanol has since been strongly challenged (see later).

2.3. Elimination

Between 95 and 98% of the dose of ethanol taken into the body is metabolized mainly in the liver and the remaining 2–5% is excreted unchanged in breath, urine,

12. Alcohol and Drug Interactions 405

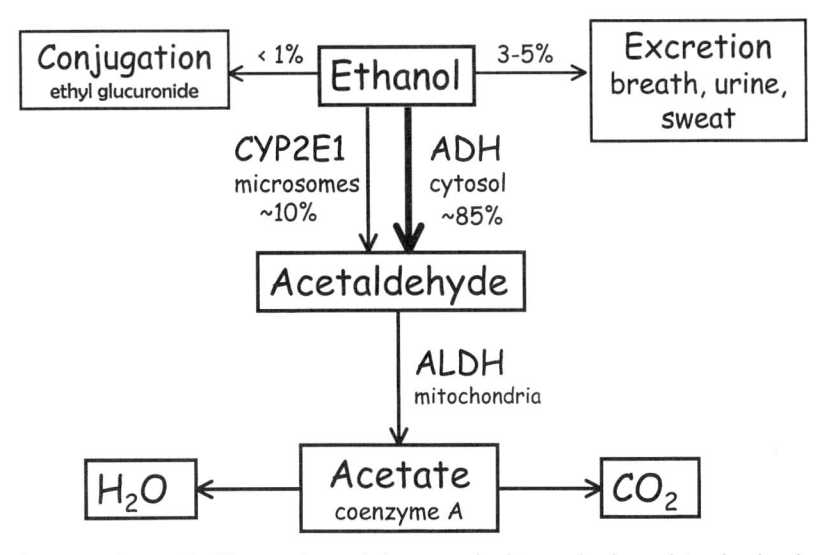

Fig. 6. Schematic illustration of the metabolism of ethanol in the body.

and sweat, and a small fraction (<1%) undergoes conjugation with glucuronic acid and becomes excreted in urine *(127–129)*. Increasing the output of urine by drinking water or taking osmotic diuretics is not a very effective way to speed up the elimination of ethanol from the body, owing to the relatively small amount that leaves via the kidney *(130)*.

Two enzyme systems are primarily responsible for in vivo oxidation of ethanol and these are located in different subcellular fractions of the liver, ADH in the cytosol and CYP2E1 in the endoplasmic reticulum *(41,42,131)*. Regardless of the enzyme involved, the first product of metabolism is acetaldehyde and this toxic substance is rapidly converted into acetate through the action of low k_m aldehyde dehydrogense (ALDH) found in the mitochondria *(132,133)*. The acetate produced undergoes further oxidation through acetyl coenzyme A, which takes place mainly in peripheral tissues. The end products of ethanol metabolism are carbon dioxide and water *(71)*. A schematic illustration of the fate of ethanol in the body is shown in Fig. 6.

Speeding up the metabolism of ethanol might find applications in clinical medicine as a way to treat heavily intoxicated individuals so that ethanol becomes eliminated from the body faster. Many attempts have been made to develop drugs that assist in sobering up faster but so far without much success. The magnitude of various kinetic parameters of ethanol metabolism based on experience from conducting hundreds of human-dosing studies is given in Table 2.

3. ALCOHOL-METABOLIZING ENZYMES

If two drugs compete for binding sites on the same enzyme, this obviously creates potential for a metabolic interaction between them. Table 3 gives examples of drugs and other chemical substances known to compete with ethanol for binding to the major alcohol-metabolizing enzymes. Note that some substances, such as disulfiram, might bind to two different enzymes (e.g., ALDH and CYP2E1).

Table 2
**Typical Pharmacokinetic Parameters
of Ethanol Derived from Controlled Drinking Experiments**

Parameter	Symbol	Normal Values	Comments
Peak concentration in blood	C_{max}	Dose of 1 g/kg gives ~0.15 g/100 mL	Depends on dose administered, gender and speed of gastric emptying.
Time of reaching the peak	t_{max}	5–120 min post drinking in most instances (median 60)	Depends on gastric emptying and whether ethanol was consumed on an empty stomach or together with food.
Rate of blood alcohol concentration decline	β or k_o	0.009–0.025 g/100 mL/h for most people	Depends on fed–fasting state and genetic factors. Values are low in malnutrition and protein deficiency and high in binge drinkers. The BAC clearance rate is slightly faster in women compared with men.
Distribution volume (Widmark's rho factor)	r or V_d	Women 0.6–0.7 L/kg Men 0.7–0.8 L/kg	Depends on age, gender, body composition (fat:lean tissue) and the ratio of water in body to water in blood.
Elimination rate from whole body per hour	B_{60}	0.08–0.15 g/kg/h	This parameter does not depend on gender but is directly proportional to k_o and V_d.

3.1. Alcohol Dehydrogenase (ADH)

The main enzyme responsible for the oxidation of ethanol, as well as other low-molecular weight alcohols, is Class I ADH, which is located in the cytosol fraction of the hepatocyte *(134)*. Human ADH occurs as various isozymes with different substrate specificity and V_{max} and k_m values for ethanol *(135)*. Indeed, a high k_m variant called Class IV ADH is located in the mucous membranes of the gut and the role this enzyme plays in gastric FPM has attracted considerable interest *(126)*. The Class I ADH occurs in three molecular forms denoted ADH1, ADH2, and ADH3, and the latter two alleles exhibit polymorphism encoding three ADH2 peptides and two ADH3 peptides *(134,136)*.

The class I isozymes of liver ADH have a k_m of 0.005–0.01 g/100 mL and therefore quickly become saturated with substrate after just a few drinks *(136)*. For forensic science purposes, the metabolism and elimination kinetics of ethanol are described by zero-order kinetics, which means that the rate of decline in the BAC occurs at a constant rate for most of the postabsorptive elimination period *(72,75,136)*. When BAC drops to approximately 0.015 g/100 mL, the Class I ADH is no longer saturated with substrate and the velocity of the enzymatic reaction drops appreciably and starts to follow first-order elimination kinetics *(136)*. A more accurate description of the entire elimination phase of the BAC profile is provided by Michaelis-Menten (M-M) saturation-type kinetics rather than a sudden change from zero-order to first-order at low BAC *(133)*. As

Table 3
Examples of Drugs That Undergo Pharmacokinetic Interaction with Ethanol Via the Major Alcohol-Metabolizing Enzymes

Alcohol Dehydrogenase (ADH)	Aldehyde Dehydrogenase (ALDH)	Microsomal P450 Enzymes (CYP2E1)
Pyrazole	Disulfiram (Antabuse®)	Acetaminophen
Fomepizole (4-methyl pyrazole)	Cyanamide (calcium carbimide) Temposil®	Acetone
Cimetidine (Tagamet®)	Coprine, contained in inky-cap mushroom	Phenobarbital (Luminal®) and other barbuiturates
Ranitidine (Zantac®)	Metronidazole (Flagyl®)	Meprobamate (Miltown®)
Acetylsalicylic acid (Aspirin®)	Chlorpropamide (Diabinese®)	Disulfiram (Antabuse®)
Methanol and other aliphatic alcohols	Tolbutamide (Orinase®)	Phenylbutazone
Ethylene glycol	Nitroglycerine	Anesthetic gases (enflurane. halothane etc.)
Trichloroethanol (metabolite of chloral hydrate)	Nitrefazole (Altimol®)	Chlorocarbons (CCl$_4$ CHCl$_3$, CH$_3$CCl$_3$)
2,3-butanediol	Cephalosporin antibiotica, e.g., cefamandole and cefoperazone	Organic solvents (aniline, benzene, toluene, xylene)

expected with saturation kinetics, the shape of the entire postabsorptive elimination phase looks more like a hockey stick rather than a straight line *(136)*.

A number of other pharmacokinetic models have been used to describe the elimination kinetics of ethanol such as multicompartment models with M-M elimination kinetics *(137,138)*. The operation of M-M equation or saturation kinetics was first demonstrated by Lundqvist and Wolthers *(139)* and expanded upon by Wagner and his associates *(139,140)*. The operation of M-M elimination kinetics helps to explain the large variability in BAC profiles after volunteers drink small doses of ethanol (<0.3 g/kg) for the following reasons. First, the nature of saturation kinetics means that the AUC increases more than proportionally with increase in dose administered *(141)*. Second, the slower the rate of absorption, the smaller is the AUC for a given dose and conversely the swifter the rate of absorption the greater the AUC *(142)*. Third, the speed by which ethanol molecules reach the hepatic enzymes becomes a major determinant of systemic availability and FPM. In this connection, gastric emptying rate and liver blood flow are important variables for the C_{max} and t_{max} observed in drinking experiments especially when small doses (<0.3 g/kg) of ethanol are taken after food *(143)*.

3.1.1. Drugs Interacting with ADH

Trace amounts of ethanol and methanol (<0.0001 g/100 mL) are naturally present in body fluids and tissues owing to fermentation reactions in the gut and possibly also as a result of other metabolic reactions. The clearance of these endogenous alcohols during the passage of portal venous blood through the liver is one of the physiological functions of ADH.

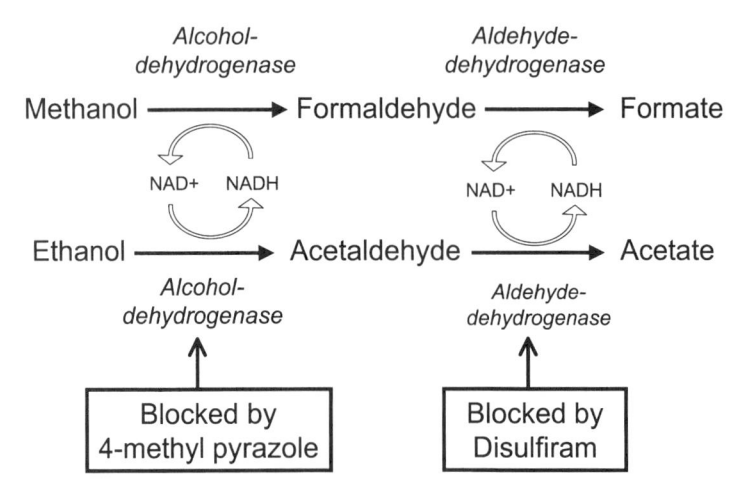

```
                  Alcohol-                      Aldehyde-
              dehydrogenase                  dehydrogenase
  Methanol ──────────────▶ Formaldehyde ──────────────▶ Formate
              ⤵       ⤴                    ⤵       ⤴
            NAD+    NADH                 NAD+    NADH
              ⤴       ⤵                    ⤴       ⤵
  Ethanol ──────────────▶ Acetaldehyde ──────────────▶ Acetate
                  Alcohol-                      Aldehyde-
              dehydrogenase                  dehydrogenase
                     ▲                              ▲
              ┌──────────────┐              ┌──────────────┐
              │  Blocked by  │              │  Blocked by  │
              │4-methyl pyrazole│           │  Disulfiram  │
              └──────────────┘              └──────────────┘
```

Fig. 7. Metabolic interaction between ethanol and methanol showing competition for oxidation with ADH, where NAD+ and NADH are oxidized and reduced forms of the coenzyme nicotinamide-adenine dinucleotide, respectively. Examples of drugs that block ADH (4-methyl pyrazole) and ALDH (disulfiram) are shown.

Accordingly, other aliphatic alcohols such as methanol, n-propanol, isopropanol, as well as toxic diols like ethylene glycol are candidates for metabolic interaction with ethanol via the ADH pathway *(144–147)*. The solvent 1,4-butanediol, which is a metabolic precursor of the abused drug γ-hydroxybutyrate (GHB), also interacts with ethanol for binding sites on ADH *(147,148)*. Indeed, the competitive inhibition between aliphatic alcohols for ADH has a long-established clinical application in the treatment of methanol poisoning *(149)*. Studies have shown that the substrate specificity of class I isozymes of ADH is about 10:1 in favor of ethanol oxidation *(150)*. Accordingly, if a person happens to drink methanol, by either accident or intent, ADH converts this alcohol into highly toxic metabolites, namely formaldehyde and formic acid. If untreated, the resulting metabolic acidosis proves fatal *(144)*. Figure 7 schematically illustrates the interaction between ethanol and methanol, both of which are oxidized by ADH.

The first-aid treatment for methanol poisoning is administration of ethanol to reach a steady-state concentration in blood between 0.10 and 0.12 g/100 mL *(149)*. This effectively blocks the oxidation of methanol into its toxic metabolites and allows time for the more dangerous alcohol to be excreted unchanged in breath and urine *(150,151)*. In severe cases of methanol or ethylene glycol poisoning, the unmetabolized alcohols and their toxic metabolites must be removed from the blood by hemodialysis *(152,153)*. Treatment with bicarbonate is recommended to counteract any metabolic acidosis that might have developed *(154,155)*.

During chronic drinking the concentration of endogenous methanol in blood increases owing to competitive inhibition of ADH from ethanol *(156–158)*. Figure 8 gives an example of the elimination kinetics of ethanol from blood in an alcoholic during detoxification *(159)*. Note this person's very high starting BAC of 0.45 g/100 mL and the ethanol elimination rate was only 0.017 g/100 mL/h, not particularly fast for a chronic heavy drinker *(159)*. The blood methanol concentration in this person was 10 mg/L and, although this is by no means toxic, the metabolism is obviously blocked

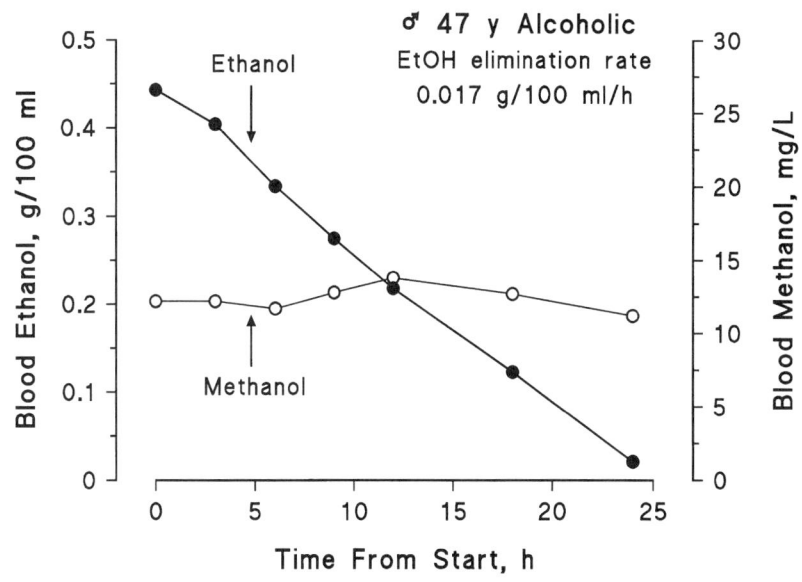

Fig. 8. Example of metabolic interaction between ethanol and methanol in an alcoholic subject with initial BAC of 0.45 g/100 mL. Note that the concentration of methanol in blood (~10 mg/L), which is by no means toxic, remains constant during the 24-h period of detoxification.

during the 24-h period when ethanol was being oxidized and removed from the bloodstream *(160)*. Methanol starts to be eliminated according to first-order kinetics (half-life 3–5 h) only after the BAC drops below 0.02 g/100 mL, that is, when ADH is no longer saturated with its preferred substrate *(161,162)*.

The drug fomepizole (4-methyl pyrazole, 4-MP) is a competitive inhibitor of the class I ADH enzyme and can be used in treatment of methanol and ethylene glycol poisoning instead of ethanol *(163–165)*. In some situations it might be less appropriate to administer ethanol, e.g., to children, alcoholics, and patients with impaired liver function. This stimulated the production and marketing of fomepizole for use in emergency clinics when patients arrive poisoned with methanol or ethylene glycol *(166)*. The fomepizole effectively blocks ADH to prevent the oxidation and formation of toxic metabolites of these alcohols thus minimizing the risk for metabolic acidosis and renal failure that would eventually cause death. The drug fomepizole has also been approved by the US Food and Drug Administration (FDA) for treatment of methanol and ethylene glycol poisoning and is sold under the trade name Antizol® *(167)*. Interestingly, giving 4-MP to human subjects increased the concentrations of endogenous ethanol and methanol in peripheral blood furnishing a neat proof that these simple alcohols are normal products of metabolism *(168)*.

One of the oldest sedative hypnotic drugs is chloral hydrate (2,2,2-trichlorethane-1-1-diol) and this substance undergoes both kinetic and dynamic interaction with ethanol *(169)*. After intake, the drug is rapidly reduced to its pharmacologically active metabolite 2,2,2-trichloroethanol *(170)*. The excess NADH (nicotinamide adenine dinucleotide) in the hepatocytes during metabolism of ethanol facilitates the reduction of chloral hydrate into trichloroethanol *(171)*. The trichloroethanol either becomes conjugated with glucuronic acid and then excreted in urine or is oxidized by ADH to an inactive metabolite trichloroacetic acid. This latter ADH reaction is inhibited in the presence of ethanol, which competes for binding sites on the enzyme so the effects of trichloroethanol on the individual are more intense and prolonged *(170)*.

3.2. Aldehyde Dehydrogenase (ALDH)

Acetaldehyde is the proximate metabolite of ethanol by all known pathways *(172)*. Unlike ethanol, the aldehyde group (–CHO) is a highly reactive chemical entity that can bind to proteins as well as many other endogenous chemicals and undergo condensation reactions with neurotransmitters like dopamine and serotonin *(173)*. Moreover, elevated levels of blood acetaldehyde cause vasodilatation, increased skin temperature, facial flushing, bronchoconstriction, lowered blood pressure, and general nausea and headache *(174)*. These adverse effects seem to be mediated through such diverse biologically active species as catecholamines, opiate peptides, histamine, and prostaglandins *(175)*. Not surprisingly, the body is equipped with an effective enzyme system to remove this toxic metabolite of ethanol from the bloodstream.

Two main isoenzymes of ALDH exist to control the concentrations of acetaldehyde passing into the peripheral circulation. The most important form of ALDH is the low-k_m variant located in the mitochondria (ALDH-2), and there is also a high-k_m variant in the cytoplasm (ALDH-1) *(176)*. ALDH enzymes are also present in erythrocytes of whole blood, various brain regions, as well as the gut and other organs and tissue *(175)*. Two main factors regulate the concentrations of acetaldehyde produced in the liver during ethanol oxidation. One is the inherent activity of hepatic ADH isozymes because the slowest step in the overall oxidation reaction is conversion of ethanol to acetaldehyde, so the faster this occurs, the more acetaldehyde is produced *(177)*. Those equipped with the ADH2*2 or ADH3*1 alleles are more likely to generate higher concentrations of acetaldehyde during hepatic oxidation of ethanol *(175)*. The second factor is the rate of oxidation of acetaldehyde to acetate by ALDH isozymes, so the affinity of the enzyme for substrate is important in this connection *(178)*.

The alcohol flush reaction exhibited by many Japanese and other Orientals when they drink alcoholic beverages is a direct consequence of acetaldehyde accumulation in the blood *(177,178)*. These individuals inherit a defective form of ALDH and are therefore genetically prone to react strongly after drinking small amounts of alcohol; in short they are equipped with a natural aversion to this drug. The isoenzyme pattern of ADH and ALDH are inherited and this is particularly apparent when different racial groups are compared *(175,176)*. The genetic polymorphism of ALDH2 is therefore crucial for control of drinking behavior, especially in Asians and perhaps also other ethnic groups. Inheriting the ALDH2*2 allele makes people especially sensitive to acetaldehyde, protecting them from developing drinking problems and other deviant behavior associated with overconsumption of alcohol *(175)*.

This pharmacogenetic trait exhibited by 40–50% of Japanese and other Asians if they consume alcohol has useful social–medical consequences because arrests for drunkenness, driving under the influence of alcohol, hospital treatment for alcoholism, liver cirrhosis, and other problems with alcohol are rare in these alcohol-sensitive individuals *(179)*. The pharmacokinetic profile of acetaldehyde is completely different when

12. Alcohol and Drug Interactions

ALDH is defective or blocked by drugs, and a number of deaths have been reported after consumption of large amounts of alcohol *(180)*.

3.2.1. Drugs Interacting with ALDH

Acetaldehyde has been incriminated in many of the untoward effects of heavy drinking including organ and tissue damage and indirectly also in alcohol dependence *(182)*. The low-k_m ALDH located in mitochondria has high affinity for substrate and ensures that blood acetaldehyde after drinking ethanol is vanishingly small. Studies have shown that the concentration of free acetaldehyde in peripheral blood when people with normal ALDH activity drink alcohol is close to the limits of detection for methods of analysis such as headspace gas chromatography *(175)*. Reports of finding high concentrations of acetaldehyde in forensic blood samples are probably artifacts caused by spontaneous oxidation of ethanol in vitro after the blood is sampled *(183)*.

The biochemistry and enzymology of ALDH has been extensively studied for two principal reasons. First, the high sensitivity of Asians to small amounts of ethanol is a good example of a genetic or inherited trait. This phenomenon has attracted considerable interest among those working in biomedical alcohol research because alcohol-sensitive individuals rarely become dependent on alcohol *(174,175)*. Second, drugs that block the action of low-k_m ALDH have proven useful as a pharmacological treatment for alcoholism known as aversion therapy *(184)*.

The alcohol-sensitizing drug disulfiram (tetraethylthiuram disulfide) is sold under the trade name Antabuse® and is the most well studied inhibitor of ALDH. This drug was discovered by accident when workers exposed to the substance at their place of work complained of strange and unpleasant feelings after drinking a couple of beers *(184)*. This observation was exploited in the 1950s, leading to development of the drug called disulfiram (Antabuse®), which was marketed as a novel treatment for alcoholism *(185)*. Those who drink alcohol after taking this drug are exposed to significantly higher concentrations of acetaldehyde, which triggers a range of unpleasant effects. Other drugs with similar properties, e.g., cyanamide or calcium carbimide (Temposil®) has also been used for treatment of alcoholism in the United States and elsewhere *(186)*. Such treatments are generally known as aversion therapy, that is, causing an aversion to drinking alcohol *(186)*. When the inky-cap mushroom was mistakenly eaten along with ingestion of alcohol, this resulted in an antabuse-like reaction owing to the presence of the chemical called coprine, which is a naturally occurring inhibitor of hepatic ALDH.

Figure 9 shows the plasma concentrations of acetaldehyde, estimated indirectly from the analysis of breath in two test situations *(187)*. A male subject drank the same small dose of ethanol (0.25 g/kg) with or without taking the ALDH inhibitor calcium carbimide (50 mg) about 60 min earlier. After the placebo control treatment, the concentrations of acetaldehyde in plasma were barely measurable, whereas after blocking ALDH the concentrations were 50 times higher and remained higher for several hours. The subjects flushed in the face and neck and experienced nausea, headache, tachycardia, and difficulties in breathing. These symptoms lasted for several hours after end of drinking *(188)*.

The abnormally high concentrations of acetaldehyde in the liver and peripheral blood after inhibition of ALDH with disulfiram accounts for the unpleasant cardiovascular effects including reduced blood pressure and increased heart rate *(188)*. This

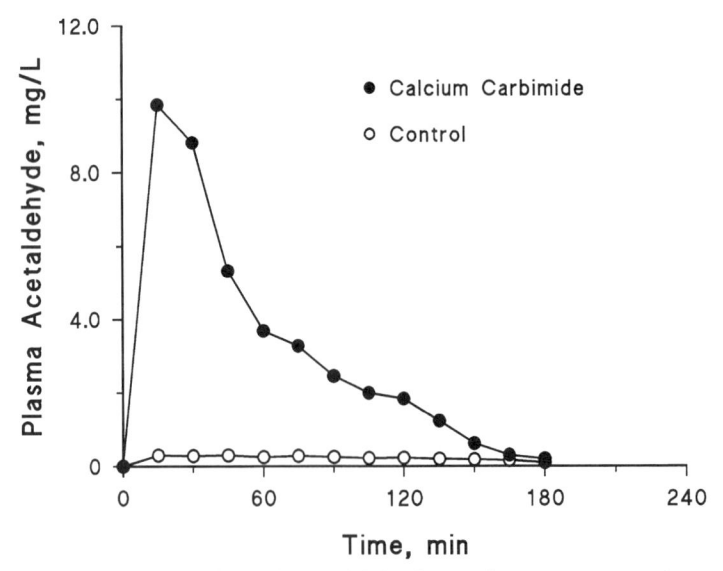

Fig. 9. Concentration-time profiles of acetaldehyde in plasma in one subject who drank 0.25 g ethanol per kg body wt in a control situation (placebo treatment) or after taking a drug (calcium carbimide) that blocked the action of low-k_m aldehyde dehydrogenase.

was confirmed experimentally when 4MP was used to treat alcoholics who had consumed alcohol despite being treated with antabuse *(189)*. The dangerous cardiovascular effects immediately subsided after the subjects were given 4-MP and the blood acetaldehyde concentration also dropped abruptly *(189)*. The use of aversion therapy with drugs like antabuse for treatment of alcohol dependence is controversial because a number of deaths have been reported in people who, despite taking their medication, also drank a large amount of alcohol *(190)*. A fatality was also reported in a Japanese with ALDH2*2 genotype owing to abnormally high concentrations of acetaldehyde in blood after consumption of ethanol and associated adverse physiological effects *(191)*.

Certain prescription drugs interfere with the metabolism of acetaldehyde by blocking ALDH to cause antabuse-like reactions, albeit less intense than after taking more potent inhibitors of ALDH *(54)*. For example, oral hypoglycemic agents such as chlorpropamide and tolbutamide, which are used for treatment of adult-onset Type 2 diabetes, interact with the low-k_m ALDH enzyme *(192)*. People taking this medication should be warned about drinking alcohol. These sulfonylurea derivatives compete with acetaldehyde for binding sites on ALDH and the concentration of acetaldehyde in blood is higher after taking this medication together with alcohol. This causes facial flushing, nausea, etc., although the response is milder then that observed during an antabuse reaction *(193,194)*. The classic drug for treating angina and heart failure, namely nitroglycerine, functions as a substrate for ALDH and this enzymatic reaction is regarded as the mechanism triggering release of free nitric oxide, which relaxes vascular smooth muscle *(195)*.

Metronidazole (Flagyl®), an effective agent for treating anaerobic bacterial infections, has been considered unsafe to use together with ethanol, owing to a purported antabuse-like reaction that occurs *(196)*. This undesirable effect was attributed to metronidazole inhibiting hepatic ALDH so that the concentration of acetaldehyde in blood during oxidation of ethanol was higher then expected. A number of case reports support this example of an adverse drug–alcohol interaction and one death was apparently caused by combined influences of ethanol and metronidazole *(197)*.

Notwithstanding these reports, a seemingly faultless study was just published that cast doubt on the existence of interaction between metronidazole and ethanol *(198)*. In a carefully controlled double-blind study, 12 healthy men drank ethanol (0.4 g/kg) after treatment with metronidazole or a placebo for 5 d. No measurable blood acetaldehyde concentration was seen in either the test or control groups and the blood ethanol profiles were also similar. Moreover, objective evidence of an alcohol–antabuse reaction (e.g., skin temperature, blood pressure, and heart rate) was absent. Neither did the volunteers experience any untoward subjective feelings of nausea compared with the placebo treatment. The authors question whether metronidazole functions as an inhibitor of ALDH and instead suggested that special subgroups of people might be allergic to this drug and respond differently after drinking alcohol *(196,198)*.

3.3. Cytochrome P450 Enzymes

The primary means for detoxification or removal of drugs from the body is oxidative metabolism by an important group of hepatic enzymes located within the endoplasmic reticulum structure, particular the microsomal fraction *(199–204)*. The cytochrome P450 enzymes constitute a broad family of proteins that catalyze the oxidation, reduction, and hydroxylation of many drugs and xenobiotics, including ethanol *(205–207)*. Besides oxidation by ADH, ethanol is metabolized to acetaldehyde by a microsomal enzyme denoted cytochrome P4502E1 (CYP2E1) *(199,200)*. The contribution of the CYP2E1 pathway to overall ethanol metabolism depends on the underlying BAC and therefore the dose of alcohol ingested *(72)*. After low to moderate doses the hepatic Class I ADH is the dominant pathway for oxidation of ethanol, but as the BAC increases to exceed 0.08 g/100 mL the CYP2E1 starts to make a greater contribution *(199)*. The k_m of this enzyme for ethanol as substrate is usually given as 8–13 mM (0.04–0.06 g/100 mL) *(200)*. Because cytochrome P450 enzymes are involved in oxidative metabolism of a wide range of endogenous and exogenous substances, including therapeutic agents, an important mechanism for drug–alcohol interaction will involve either an inhibition or induction of P4502E1 enzymes *(208–212)*.

Drinking a large acute dose of ethanol will compete for CYP450 enzymes and therefore temporarily prevent the metabolism of another drug that utilizes the same oxidative enzyme for detoxification *(213)*. Alternatively, drinking a large amount of alcohol daily causes induction of the CYP450 system and alcoholics therefore acquire an enhanced capacity for drug metabolism *(214)*. These people often require a higher dose of the drug to achieve the desired therapeutic effect because the substance is more rapidly metabolized owing to hyperactive P450 enzymes *(215,216)*. The fact that alcoholics often exhibit more rapid rates of BAC clearance, sometimes exceeding 0.025 g/100 mL/h is also attributable to contribution of CYP2E1 enzymes *(215)*. However, this enhanced oxidative activity is not long lasting because after end of drinking and sobering up for a few days the person's capacity for faster disposal of ethanol via CYP2E1 disappears, owing to a rapid turnover or resynthesis of the enzyme *(217)*. Alcoholics with liver disease may show a slower rate of ethanol and drug metabolism if tissue necrosis is advanced *(218)*.

3.3.1. Drugs Interacting with CYP2E1

The hepatic cytochrome P450 enzymes constitute the body's main defense against chemical attack, and a vast number of xenobiotics that might enter the organism with the air we breathe, or the food we eat are made less dangerous by the P450 enzymes. The CYP450 enzymes also accomplish the oxidative metabolism of a multitude of endogenous compounds (steroids, bile acids, fat-soluble vitamins, prostaglandins, and fatty acids) as well as many exogenous substances including medicines, organic solvents, and environmental carcinogens *(219,220)*.

The particular isoform of P450 that oxidizes ethanol is denoted CYP2E1 and this enzyme is also involved, at least in part, with the detoxification of many organic solvents, anesthetic gases, prescription medications, and endogenous compounds *(221)*. The P450 mediated oxidation of a substrate involves the reaction of molecular oxygen with the coenzyme nicotinamide adenine dinucleotide phosphate (NADPH) to give one molecule of water and the other oxygen atom is introduced into the drug molecule causing an oxidation reaction *(30)*:

$$\text{Drug} + \text{NADPH} + \text{H}^+ + \text{O}_2 \xrightarrow{\text{P450 enzymes}} \text{NADP} + \text{H}_2\text{O} + \text{Drug-OH}$$

Some recent work indicates that besides CYP2E1 other P450 enzymes might play a role in the oxidation of ethanol (e.g., CYP3A4 and CYP1A2), which suggests that ethanol treatment can interfere with metabolism of drugs that utilize other P450 systems besides CYP2E1 *(222)*.

The interaction between ethanol and drugs via the CYP2E1 pathway depends on whether a single acute dose of ethanol is administered after taking the drug or whether the drug was administered after a period of binge drinking so that CYP2E1 enzymes were hyperactive. These two situations are illustrated in Fig. 10. Drinking a large amount of alcohol by a person who has not recently been exposed to alcohol results in competition with other drugs for oxidation by CYP2E1 and accordingly a more prolonged therapeutic effect of the medication. By contrast, if the drug is given to a person with enhanced microsomal enzyme activity (e.g., chronic heavy drinkers), the drug is more effectively converted into its metabolites resulting in a diminished therapeutic response *(216)*. This latter scenario creates a problem if the drug metabolites are highly reactive or toxic as in the case of acetaminophen and many organic solvents encountered in the workplace.

3.3.1.1. ACETAMINOPHEN

An example of a dangerous drug–ethanol interaction involving CYP2E1 enzymes is seen with the OTC analgesic and antipyretic acetaminophen (*N*-acetyl-*p*-aminophenol). This ubiquitous nonprescription drug, known as paracetamol in Europe, has been available for more then a century and is used by all age groups for treatment of headache, fever, muscle pain, and other ailments *(223–225)*. Acetaminophen is the most commonly used substance for self-poisoning in both the UK and the United States, and an extensive literature pertaining to toxicity and emergency treatment procedures exists

12. Alcohol and Drug Interactions

Moderate Drinker

Drug

CYP450 + EtOH ✗

↓ Drug Metabolites

Prolonged Therapeutic Effect of the Drug

Heavy Drinker

Drug

Activated CYP450

↑ Drug Metabolites ✗

Diminished Therapeutic Effect of the Drug

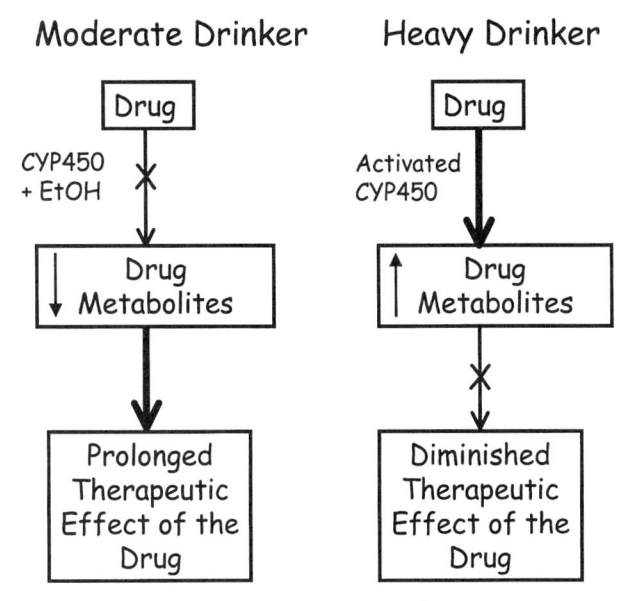

Fig. 10. Schematic illustration of metabolic drug–alcohol interaction via the cytochrome P450 enzyme leading to either diminished or prolonged effect of the drug depending on the activity of CYP2E1. The left diagram shows a moderate drinker after coingestion of drug and alcohol and the right diagram a heavy drinker or alcoholic with zero blood ethanol but immediately after a period of heavy drinking, which activates CYP2E1 enzymes.

(226,227). When taken in overdose acetaminophen is an extremely dangerous drug causing irreversible hepatotoxicity with end-stage liver failure and eventually death *(228)*.

Acetaminophen is metabolized in the liver primarily via phase II conjugation reactions with glucuronic acid (60%) and sulfate (35%) and a small fraction (5%) also undergoes oxidation with P450 enzymes including CYP2E1 to produce a reactive intermediate known as *N*-acetyl-*p*-benzoquinone imine (NAPQI) *(229)*. Under normal circumstances the NAPQI metabolite is either reduced back to acetaminophen or is rapidly inactivated by conjugation with the free-radical scavenger, the tripeptide glutathione, and eventually excreted in urine after undergoing other phase II reactions to produce cysteine and mercapturic acid conjugates *(230)*. The metabolism of acetaminophen in the body is illustrated schematically in Fig. 11.

When huge doses of acetaminophen are taken, the hepatic glutathione stores soon become depleted and the reactive NAPQI intermediate starts to accumulate in the blood and liver *(231)*. This highly reactive intermediate undergoes covalent binding to vital cell constituents, causing impairment of calcium homeostasis, oxidative stress, and cell death, particularly in the liver where this toxin is produced *(232)*. The toxicity of acetaminophen is enhanced by factors that activate the CYP2E1 enzymes thus producing more NAPQI. Conditions such as prolonged fasting, protein deficiency, and binge drinking make alcoholics more prone to hepatotoxicity, owing to their activated CYP2E1 detoxification enzymes *(233)*. Alcoholics should be cautious about taking ace-

```
            ┌─────────────┐          ┌──────────────┐
            │   Sulfate   │          │  Glucuronide │
            │  conjugate  │◄── Acetaminophene ──►│   conjugate  │
            │    ~35%     │          │     ~60%     │
            └─────────────┘          └──────────────┘
                        CYP2E1 │ Induced by alcohol,
                         ~5%   │ fasting, protein deficiency
                               ▼
                    ┌──────────────────┐
                    │ N-acetyl-p-benzo-│        Reactive
                    │   quinone imine  │      intermediate
                    │      (NAPQI)     │
                    └──────────────────┘
          Glutathione  │           │
          inactivation │           │
                       ▼           ▼
            ┌─────────────┐   ┌────────────────────┐
            │ Glutathione │   │ Covalent binding to│
            │  conjugate  │   │ tissues – cell death│
            └─────────────┘   └────────────────────┘
                                    Hepatotoxicity
```

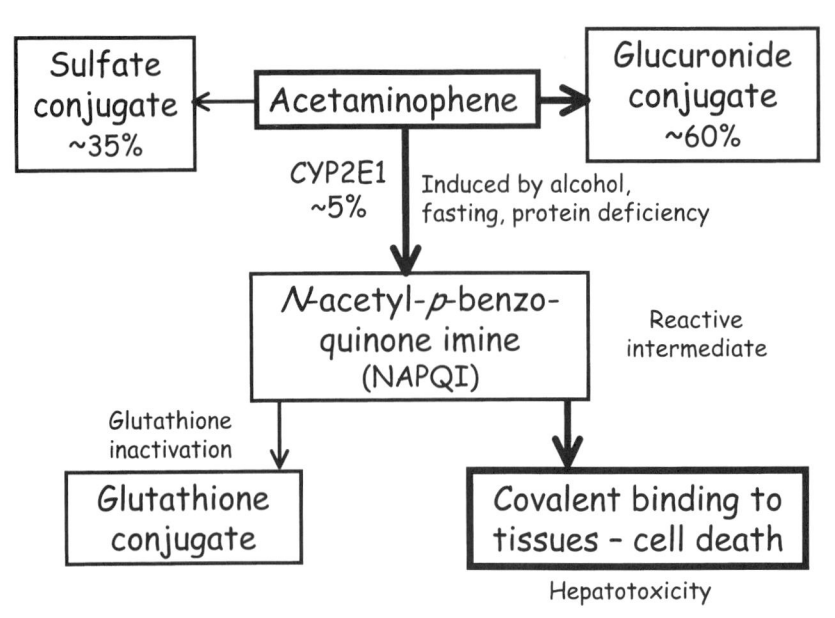

Fig. 11. Scheme for metabolism of the OTC analgesic drug acetaminophen (paracetamol) showing formation of inactive conjugates (glucuronide, sulfate, and glutathione) and a toxic metabolite (N-acetyl-p-benzoquinone imine), which causes necrosis and cell death mainly in the liver.

taminophen even in moderate amounts, owing to the added risk of drug toxicity *(234)*. Another consequence of long-term abuse of alcohol is a lower antioxidative capacity of the liver because glutathione stores are depleted, thus making alcoholics even more susceptible to acetaminophen toxicity *(235)*. Moreover, many alcoholics suffer from hypoglycemia because they neglect to eat properly during a drinking binge and carbohydrate metabolism is also disturbed during the hepatic oxidation of ethanol *(236)*. Hypoglycemia and fasting are predisposing factors in the toxicity of acetaminophen because glucuronidation of drugs is less effective under these circumstances *(237)*.

Effective treatment of acetaminophen poisoning depends on how much time elapses after the drug was taken, so it is important to obtain a rapid and specific determination of the plasma concentration of this analgesic *(237,238)*. Shortly after overdose, gastric lavage or induction of emesis is effective or administration of activated charcoal can help to bind the drug and prevent further absorption *(238)*. If the elapsed time after taking the drug overdose is unknown, the recommended treatment is to give the antioxidant N-acetylcysteine, which replenishes glutathione stores and helps in detoxification of NAPQI *(237)*. If all else fails, the only available life-saving treatment is to perform a liver transplant *(238)*.

The enzymes involved in the biotransformation of ethanol (ADH, ALDH, and CYP2E1) are nonspecific and interact with a wide variety of drugs and chemicals (Table 3), which might result in altered rates of metabolism of ethanol and/or the drugs and their metabolites. These kinds of drug–alcohol interactions are therefore referred to as metabolic or pharmacokinetic interactions.

4. First-Pass Metabolism of Ethanol

First-pass metabolism (FPM) refers to the metabolism of an orally administered drug during its first passage through the gut and liver before reaching the peripheral circulation *(239)*. Accordingly, FPM occurs in the stomach and intestine or when the portal venous blood passes through the liver for the first time *(240)*. Moreover, any loss of the drug, whether by oxidation or excretion, in the lungs might also be considered presystemic elimination. FPM lowers the bioavailability of a drug and, as might be expected, the therapeutic effect is also diminished because less of the active substance reaches target organs via the blood circulation *(240)*.

The notion of a substantial FPM of ethanol occurring in the stomach attracted considerable attention among investigators in biomedical alcohol research during the past 15 yr *(241,242)*. This interest was initiated after publication of several articles in prestigious medical journals such as the *New England Journal of Medicine* and the *Journal of the American Medical Association (JAMA) (243,244)*. Although some earlier studies showed that ADH was located in the gastric mucosa, it was not considered to have much practical importance in the overall oxidation and elimination of ethanol from the body *(245)*.

This metabolic oxidation of ethanol in the stomach was attributed to a special form of ADH called the Class IV isozyme, located in gastric mucosa and having a higher k_m for ethanol oxidation compared with the major hepatic ADH or Class I enzyme *(246, 247)*. This meant that gastric ADH was appropriate for oxidative metabolism when the concentration of ethanol was highest, such as in the stomach after drinking alcoholic beverages. Another study showed that gastric metabolism of ethanol was eliminated in subjects who had undergone gastrectomy *(248)*.

Interest in FPM was fueled appreciably when it was reported that some widely prescribed drugs such as Aspirin®, Tagamet®, and Zantac® blocked the action of gastric ADH *(244,249)*. This meant that more of the alcohol a person consumed was available to reach the peripheral circulation, because gastric ADH was prevented from participating in FPM by the drug taken. Much speculation arose about the consequences of reaching a higher C_{max} and greater AUC in individuals lacking gastric ADH and these individuals were therefore considered predisposed to the toxic effects of drinking ethanol *(250,251)*. The activity of gastric ADH was found to be less in women compared with men and also less in alcoholics compared with moderate drinkers, making these groups more vulnerable to the negative effects of alcohol on health *(243,250)*.

Much debate erupted about the significance of gastric ADH and the effects of various commonly prescribed drugs, their interaction with ethanol and what that meant for health risks associated with moderate alcohol consumption *(243)*. Dr. Charles Lieber and his research team from New York were the strongest proponents of the role played by gastric ADH as a protective barrier against many of the dangers of long-term consumption of alcohol and they published extensively on this topic *(251–253)*. However, many of the conclusions were challenged because of the experimental design used, the analytical methodology, and the way that FPM of ethanol was calculated from BAC profiles *(254,255)*. Moreover, gastric FPM of ethanol appeared to be greatest after subjects drank very small doses of ethanol (0.15–0.30 g/kg) although under these conditions the resulting BAC profiles were highly variable and not easy to interpret *(256,257)*.

Some recent studies of gastric FPM of ethanol noted a greater influence if the alcohol was consumed in divided doses over several hours rather then as a single bolus dose *(258,259)*. Such a slower drinking pattern is more in keeping with real-world conditions. However, the general opinion appears to be that FPM is strongly dose-dependent and seemingly more pronounced when very small doses (0.15 g/kg), corresponding to just one glass of wine, are consumed after a meal *(256,257)*. Other studies have shown that C_{max} for ethanol as well as AUC are highly dependent on gastric emptying, so the residence time of ethanol in the stomach also has importance for exposure to gastric ADH and effectiveness of FPM *(260,261)*.

M-M elimination kinetics of ethanol is important to consider when calculating the amount of FPM and whether this is predominantly gastric or hepatic. After small doses of ethanol and especially when stomach emptying is delayed and intermittent, the hepatic Class 1 ADH does not become saturated with substrate. The ethanol molecules in the portal venous blood entering the liver are more easily cleared via hepatic FPM, not necessarily gastric FPM *(257)*. If the dose of ethanol consumed is plotted against area under the BAC time profile (AUC), a nonlinear relationship is obtained as one consequence of the saturation-type kinetics of ethanol in the liver *(142,143)*.

The efficacy of FPM of ethanol is highly variable and depends on many factors, particularly the dose taken and the speed of gastric emptying *(260)*. The emptying of the stomach shows large inter- and intrasubject variations depending on a person's age, gender, anatomy of the gut, any disease states, time of day, blood sugar level, and not least the kind of medication being used *(262–268)*. A particularly convincing study of FPM in men and women concluded that only a small fraction (<6%) of the dose of 0.3 g/kg occurred by presystemic metabolism in either the gut or liver or both organs and that gender-related differences were minor *(269)*. Some maintain that there is little doubt that the liver is the predominant site for FPM of ethanol for the simple reason that ADH activity in the liver vastly exceeds that in the gastric mucosa *(254–257)*.

4.1. Drugs Influencing FPM

Gastric emptying is an important determinant of the absorption rate and FPM of ethanol, so drugs and medication that delay or accelerate stomach emptying are important to consider *(270,271)*. If gastric emptying is delayed, as often occurs after eating a meal, this allows more time for oxidation of ethanol by gastric ADH. According to this theory, when ethanol is retained in the stomach for a longer time, e.g., because of delayed gastric emptying, a small fraction of the dose never actually reaches the liver or systemic circulation and the resulting BAC time curve gives the impression that a smaller dose of ethanol was taken *(241,242)*.

Drugs that speed up or delay gastric emptying can dramatically alter the shape of the BAC profile, which means that great care is needed to resolve the effect of drug treatment on gastric emptying from an effect on the rate of metabolism of ethanol, which is not always easy. Many articles claiming to find an effect of drug treatment on the rate of ethanol metabolism can instead be explained by a drug-induced effect on gastric emptying.

One way to resolve the relative importance of gastric emptying is to give the test drug orally and the ethanol intravenously so that the confounding influence of stomach emptying on the rate of absorption of ethanol is avoided *(272)*. Another approach is

12. Alcohol and Drug Interactions

called breath-clamping, which involves measuring breath alcohol concentration at 5-min intervals. The ethanol is given by intravenous infusion to reach a plateau concentration in blood as monitored by the analysis of breath *(273)*. The test drug or treatment is then applied, e.g., eating a meal or taking some medication, and over the next few hours the infusion rate of ethanol is adjusted to keep the same steady-state breath alcohol concentration as before the treatment. With this study design, Ranchandani et al. *(88)* found that alcohol was eliminated faster after eating a meal regardless of the protein, fat, and carbohydrate composition *(88)*. It was speculated that food either enhanced the activity of alcohol-metabolizing enzymes or increased liver blood flow or both, leading to a more effective hepatic oxidation of ethanol *(274)*.

4.1.1. Aspirin

Aspirin® (acetylsalicylic acid) is a well-known in vitro inhibitor of gastric ADH *(275)* and this drug might theoretically increase the bioavailability of ethanol in vivo. Roine et al. *(249)* reported that 1.0 g aspirin taken before drinking ethanol (0.3 g/kg body wt) at 1 h after eating a standard breakfast gave higher blood alcohol curves as reflected in C_{max} and AUC. However, inspection of the BAC profiles in the aspirin and control groups showed that in reality the major influence of the drug treatment centered on the absorption phase of ethanol kinetics and not FPM. Melander et al. *(276)* failed to confirm any influence of the same dose of drug and alcohol on C_{max}, t_{max}, or AUC, despite the fact that the experimental conditions were almost identical. However, in this latter study, women were included among the volunteer subjects and some claimed that this skewed the results. Another study showed that women, owing to lower gastric ADH activity, ordinarily have less FPM of ethanol than do men *(277)*. The mechanism was attributed to inhibition of gastric ADH by aspirin thus preventing FPM of ethanol in men rather than speeding up gastric emptying *(277)*.

Kechagias et al. *(278)* investigated the effect of low-dose aspirin (75 mg once daily) on the pharmacokinetics of ethanol in a crossover design study. This small dose of acetylsalicylic acid is widely prescribed for common conditions such as ischaemic heart disease and cerebrovascular disease. It was found that drug treatment delayed the absorption of ethanol into the blood as reflected in a lowered peak BAC compared with the no-drug arm of the study *(278)*. Figure 12 (upper trace) shows the mean BAC profiles from this study. Note that after treatment with aspirin, the rate of rise in BAC was slower but the two curves met by 90 min postdosing and thereafter overlapped. This supports an effect of the drug on the rate of absorption of ethanol with no differences in presystemic metabolism. If there had been a higher degree of FPM in the control group not given aspirin, one would expect the BAC time profile to run on a lower level for the duration of blood sampling. The aspirin treatment caused a slower absorption by delaying gastric emptying as confirmed by monitoring the absorption kinetics of acetaminophen, a drug that is only taken up from the small intestine *(278)*.

The nonsteroidal antiinflammatory drug ibuprofen, a prostaglandin synthetase inhibitor, had no effect on the pharmacokinetic profile of ethanol in a human study that utilized a crossover design *(279)*. The concentrations of ethanol in blood were estimated indirectly from analysis of breath and neither C_{max} (0.095 ± 0.026 vs 0.095 ± 0.033 g/100 mL) nor rate of blood ethanol clearance (0.018 ± 0.006 g/100 mL/h vs 0.017 ± 0.007 g/100 mL/h) showed any significant differences. In another study with eight volunteer

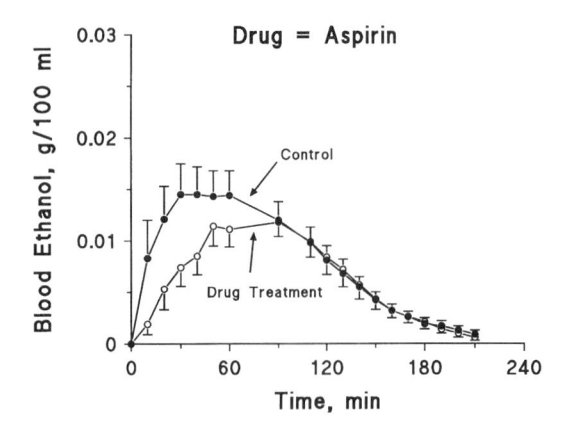

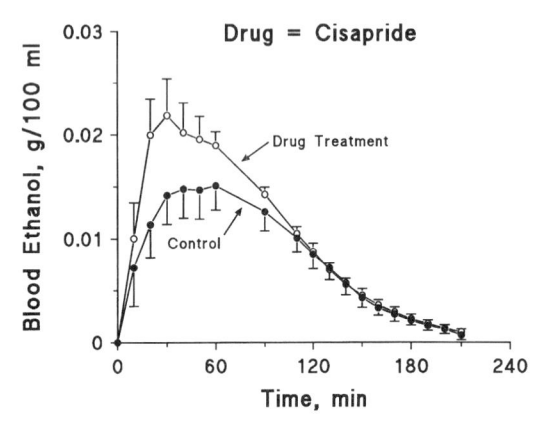

Fig. 12. Effect of pretreatment with commonly prescribed drugs on concentration-time profiles of ethanol after subjects drank 0.3 g ethanol per kg body wt in a crossover design study. Ethanol was given as a bolus dose 1 h after subjects had eaten breakfast. The upper plot (mean ± SD, n = 10 male subjects) shows the effect of pretreatment with aspirin (75 mg once daily for 7 d), which tends to delay stomach emptying, and the bottom plot shows cisapride pretreatment (10 mg three times daily for 4 d), which tends to stimulate gastric emptying.

subjects using another breath alcohol analyzer, it was reported that the rate of ethanol elimination from blood was decreased by 10% after treatment with ibuprofen. The investigators also looked at the effect of this drug–alcohol interaction on various cognitive tasks and found a worsened performance when ibuprofen was combined with alcohol compared with a placebo control treatment *(280)*.

4.1.2. Cisapride

Drugs used in the treatment of gastroduodenal diseases are likely to influence gastric emptying and alter the rate of absorption of ethanol into the bloodstream *(281, 282)*. Cisapride is a prokinetic drug that accelerates gastric emptying and increases gastrointestinal motility by indirectly facilitating cholinergic transmission in the myenteric plexus *(283,284)*. The absorption of ethanol (0.5 g/kg body wt) in five healthy volunteers was tested with or without taking 10 mg cisapride. Both C_{max} and $AUC_{0-4\,h}$

were higher after treatment with cisapride when subjects drank ethanol (0.5 g/kg body wt) on an empty stomach but not when the same dose was ingested together with food *(285)*. However, the volunteer subjects took only two tablets of cisapride before drinking the ethanol and plasma concentrations of the medication were not reported.

Kechagias et al. *(286)* gave 10 male subjects cisapride for 4 d (10 mg, three times daily before meals) to establish steady-state plasma concentrations of the drug and to mimic clinical conditions. Ethanol (0.3 g/kg body wt) was ingested 1 h after a meal and the mean peak BAC rose 43% after cisapride compared with the no-drug control session (Fig. 12 bottom trace). However, the increase in absolute units was only 0.01 g/100 mL ($p < 0.05$). In this study, gastric emptying was measured by the acetaminophen absorption test and the serum curves of this marker mirrored the changes in BAC, which proves that the higher C_{max} after the cisapride was largely the result of an accelerated gastric emptying *(286)*.

4.1.3. Verapamil

The calcium channel blocker verapamil (Verelan®) is widely used for the treatment of angina, control of arrhythmias, and other cardiovascular problems such as hypertension *(287)*. Because ion channels and calcium transport might be related to ethanol's effects on the brain, it seemed reasonable to investigate a likely interaction with ethanol. Drugs that block calcium transport (verapamil and nifedipine) were evaluated for potential interaction with ethanol *(287)*. One study reported a significant pharmacokinetic interaction between ethanol and verapamil *(288)*, in particular a higher C_{max} after drug treatment (0.124 ± 0.024 vs 0.106 ± 0.021 g/100 mL). However, the concentration-time profiles of ethanol in this study were not presented in the article to allow detailed evaluation *(288)*. The higher C_{max} and AUC after verapamil treatment might have been caused by drug effects on absorption of ethanol from the stomach and not a faster rate of metabolism or FPM as speculated upon in the article *(288)*.

A later study compared verapamil, nifedipine, and placebo but failed to find any difference between treatments on the shape of the blood alcohol curves or on subjective feelings of inebriation including various psychomotor performance tests *(289)*. Thus the effect of verapamil on pharmacokinetics of ethanol remains an open question.

4.1.4. Erythromycin

The widely used antibiotic erythromycin appears to increase the rate of gastric emptying and if this drug is taken with ethanol one can expect a higher C_{max} and AUC *(290)*. Erythromycin is believed to function as an agonist of the gastrointestinal peptide motilin and thereby modulating gastric motility *(291)*. When erythromycin was given as an intravenous dose (3 mg/kg body wt) to eight subjects, this treatment increased the absorption of ethanol (0.5 g/kg body wt) ingested immediately after a solid meal *(292)*. The mean C_{max} increased from 0.055 ± 0.004 (± standard error) to 0.077 ± 0.004 g/100 mL ($p < 0.05$) and the mean $AUC_{0-330\ min}$ increased from 6.6 ± 0.27 to 7.6 ± 0.35 g/100 mL × min ($p < 0.05$).

4.1.5. Ranitidine

Adverse drug interactions involving H_2-receptor antagonists such as ranitidine (Zantac®), cimetidine (Tagamet®), famotidine (Pepcid®), and nizatidine (Axid®) became a concern when this kind of medication for stomach ailments was made available OTC in several countries. In particular, the risk for interaction with ethanol was of concern because over consumption of ethanol is often a cause of stomach problems (e.g., gastritis). Interest in histamine-2 antagonists and alcohol attracted worldwide attention when it was shown in vitro that gastric ADH was blocked by this kind of medication.

A paper in *JAMA* attracted considerable attention *(244)* when it was claimed that, because ranitidine inhibited gastric ADH, the bioavailability of ethanol was increased. Those regularly taking this drug along with alcohol were therefore more prone to ethanol-induced damage to organs and tissue. This drug–alcohol interaction also meant a greater risk for accidents of various kinds owing to the higher C_{max} for ethanol when ranitidine and ethanol were taken together. In the *JAMA* study, the doses of ethanol were very low (0.15–0.3 g/kg) and were administered 1 h after a small number of subjects had eaten a fat-rich breakfast *(244)*. The C_{max} for ethanol was highly variable and low (0.01–0.15 g/100 mL) so that small absolute increases in BAC in themselves not remarkable gave large percentage changes.

Amir et al. *(293)* recently confirmed that ranitidine (300 mg every evening for 1 wk) increased bioavailability of ethanol and attributed this to accelerated gastric emptying. The shorter residence time of ethanol in the stomach after drug treatment gave less opportunity for metabolism of ethanol to occur via gastric ADH. In many of these studies, the investigators fail to separate the contribution of hepatic ADH from that of gastric ADH in FPM.

Attempts to replicate the *JAMA* study were unsuccessful even under similar test conditions with many more volunteer subjects and varying the dose of ethanol from 0.15 to 0.3 and 0.6 g/kg *(295)*. An influence of drug treatment if any was seen after the smallest dose (0.15 g/kg) but the investigators warned that the finding might also be explained by large intersubject variability in absorption kinetics of ethanol *(295)*. In a particularly good experiment, a small dose of ethanol (0.3 g/kg) was administered in the morning, at midday, and in the evening in a well-designed randomized crossover study *(296)*. The treatment with ranitidine was optimal to achieve therapeutic concentrations in blood before each dose of ethanol was administered *(296)*. The median BAC time profiles were remarkably similar regardless of drug treatment or the time of day when the alcohol was consumed.

Several other studies into this same drug–alcohol interaction failed to support the conclusions in the *JAMA* article, namely that ranitidine has any marked effect on C_{max} or increases the bioavailability of ethanol *(297,298)*.

4.1.6. Cimetidine

The first H_2-receptor blocker was cimetidine (Tagamet®) and this drug received considerable attention regarding potential for interaction with ethanol *(299–301)*. Cimetidine was shown to inhibit gastric ADH activity in vitro using gastric biopsy specimens. Indeed, the chemical structure of cimetidine includes a five-membered imidazole ring, which resembles that of pyrazole and its derivatives, which are well-known inhibitors of hepatic ADH *(302)*.

A large body of literature has appeared dealing with the interaction between cimetidine and the pharmacokinetics of ethanol with special reference to FPM. The current opinion appears to be that the effect of this drug is negligible and can be largely explained

12. Alcohol and Drug Interactions

by the large interindividual variations in gastric emptying *(303–306)*. One of the few studies in patients suffering from duodenal ulcers and normally taking this medication also failed to confirm an effect of cimetidine on pharmacokinetics of ethanol *(307)*. Some older reports failed to show that this drug altered the pharmacokinetic parameters of ethanol such as C_{max} and t_{max} or AUC compared with a placebo control treatment. Other studies reported that the peak BAC after cimetidine was higher compared with a control treatment but no attempt was made to resolve confounding effects of the drug on gastric emptying *(308)*.

The effect of cimetidine on ethanol pharmacokinetics, if any, seems to center on the absorption process and probably involves factors that control gastric emptying. In most studies of this drug–alcohol interaction, a bolus dose of ethanol is usually administered 1 h after subjects are given a standardized breakfast *(309)*. Drinking after a meal is known to influence rate and extent of ethanol absorption in an unpredictable manner and C_{max} is usually decreased compared with intake of alcohol on an empty stomach. Seitz et al. *(310)* reported that the peak concentration of ethanol in plasma was 0.086 g/100 mL for cimetidine treatment compared with 0.078 g/100 mL for placebo, a small absolute difference. Seitz et al. *(311)* also gave ethanol by intravenous infusion and found no difference in the rate of blood alcohol decline after pretreatment with cimetidine compared with placebo, which supports the lack of any metabolic interaction between ethanol and cimetidine.

Feely and Wood *(312)* studied six male subjects to assess the effect of cimetidine on pharmacokinetics of ethanol and at the same time also recorded subjective feelings of ethanol-induced inebriation. The peak plasma alcohol concentrations (PAC) were within the range expected for the dose and conditions of drinking. After cimetidine treatment the C_{max} was higher compared with placebo (0.146 g/100 mL vs 0.163 g/100 mL) and AUC was increased, although these findings might reflect a faster absorption of ethanol after drug treatment. The subjective intoxication scores were maximum at or near the C_{max} as expected.

Webster et al. *(313)* reported a negligible effect of cimetidine on ethanol absorption, distribution, and elimination in the body. These workers employed a breath alcohol analyzer to map the BAC profile in four men and three women who were given cimetidine (200 mg three times daily), ranitidine (150 mg twice daily), or placebo for 2 d. The peak BAC and AUC were slightly higher after ranitidine but not after pretreatment with cimetidine or placebo. Dobrilla et al. *(314)* also failed to find any significant effect of cimetidine treatment on the pharmacokinetics of ethanol in a human study that also included measurements of ethanol-induced impairment.

The results of a carefully controlled study by Jönsson et al. *(314)* into the effect of H_2-antagonists on the metabolism and pharmacokinetics of ethanol are shown in Table 4. Because the same subjects participated in each arm of the study, this kind of experimental design has a high power to detect any differences between treatments. However, neither pretreatment with cimetidine, ranitidine, nor an alternative drug for stomach ailments (the proton-pump inhibitor omeprazole) seemed to influence C_{max}, t_{max}, rate of elimination from blood (k_0), or AUC for ethanol. No significant differences were observed compared with a control no-drug treatment, thus failing to support an interaction between H_2-receptor antagonists and the kinetics of ethanol. However, the study by Jönsson et al. *(314)* used a higher dose of ethanol (0.8 g/kg) and this was

Table 4
Effect of Cimetidine, Ranitidine, Omeprazole, and a No-Drug Control Treatment on the Peak Blood Alcohol Concentration (C_{max}), the Time to Reach the Maximum (t_{max}), the Rate of Elimination of Alcohol From Blood (k_0), and the Area Under the Curve (AUC)

Treatment	C_{max} g/100 mL mean (range)	t_{max} min median (range)	k_0 g/100 mL/h mean (range)	AUC g x h/100 mL mean (range)
Cimetidine	0.101 (0.094–0.108)	70 (52–88)	0.015 (0.014–0.016)	0.414 (0.376–0.451)
Ranitidine	0.103 (0.092–0.113)	64 (51–77)	0.014 (0.013–0.015)	0.436 (0.395–0.478)
Omeprazole	0.102 (0.091–0.113)	69 (53–84)	0.014 (0.013–0.015)	0.433 (0.380–0.487)
Control (no drug)	0.105 (0.092–0.118)	70 (49–91)	0.014 (0.013–0.015)	0.443 (0.387–0.500)

Twelve healthy men participated in a randomized crossover study.

consumed on an empty stomach instead of 1 h after subjects had eaten breakfast. The studies reporting an increased area under the BAC time curve after cimetidine or ranitidine treatment involved the use of smaller doses of ethanol (0.15–0.3 g/kg). None of these studies actually resolved the relative importance of the stomach and the liver as the site for FPM of ethanol. These discrepancies underscore the dangers of drawing false conclusions from drug interaction studies because of differences in experimental protocol might lead to quite different results and conclusions.

Fraser *(315)* presented a balanced review of studies dealing with the interaction of ethanol and H_2-receptor antagonists. He came to the conclusion that except for very special circumstances such as drinking small doses of ethanol (0.15 g/kg) after eating a meal there was no evidence to support that this class of drug altered the absorption, distribution, or elimination of ethanol. The results after a very low dose of ethanol (0.15 g/kg) seemingly approached significance, but this could just as well be accounted for by the large intersubject variability in C_{max} and AUC, making it virtually impossible to draw any firm conclusion about how this kind of drug treatment alters the disposition kinetics of ethanol. The major confounding factors are stomach-emptying rate and food-induced alteration of blood flow to the liver as well as the amount and composition of food ingested before drinking the ethanol. This example of drug–alcohol interaction has been referred to as "much ado about nothing" or mountain or molehill *(316)*.

5. Pharmacodynamic Aspects of Ethanol

Ethanol is unique among drugs of abuse in exhibiting two completely different actions on the body, one being metabolic and nutritional and the other depression of the CNS leading to tolerance and dependence after chronic exposure *(45)*. The combustion of ethanol liberates substantial amounts of energy, actually 7 kcal per gram, making it intermediate as an energy source between fats (9 kcal per gram) and carbohydrates and proteins (4 kcal per gram). Alcoholics can derive much of their daily energy needs from the large amounts of alcohol they drink. However, the energy derived from alcohol cannot be stored in other forms for use when needed as glucose is stored as glycogen. Moreover, alcoholic drinks lack the important micronutrients (vitamins and minerals) contained in ordinary foodstuffs *(41–43)*. Accordingly, when the liver is metabolizing ethanol it cannot conduct its normal metabolic functions such as taking care of fats, carbohydrates, and proteins. The metabolic disturbances associated with hepatic oxidation of ethanol are related to a shift in the redox state of the liver toward a more reduced potential (higher NADH/NAD$^+$ ratio). Many physiological NAD-dependent reactions are offset during ethanol oxidation, resulting in among other things an increase in lactate-to-pyruvate ratio and thereafter metabolic acidosis, accumulation of fatty deposits, hypoglycemia, and other untoward effects *(41)*.

5.1. Ethanol-Induced Impairment

Ethanol must be considered a relatively weak psychoactive substance compared with most other drugs of abuse considering the much larger doses and higher blood concentrations necessary to alter a person's mood and behavior and cause inebriation *(71)*. The way ethanol acts on the brain and CNS was long considered to involve nonspecific interaction with cell membrane lipids, similar to the action of organic solvents (e.g., ether and chloroform) and general anesthetic gases (e.g., N$_2$O, enflurane, and halothane). It is well established that lipid solubility determines the potency of anesthetic agents according to the Meyer-Overton theory, which would therefore make ethanol a weak narcotic agent *(317,318)*.

Like all other drugs, the effect of ethanol on the body is dose-dependent and, as the amounts consumed increase, molecules of ethanol penetrate neuronal membrane lipids making then more fluid *(319)*. This structural change disrupts the functioning of receptor proteins embedded in the membrane lipids, which in turn offsets electrical signaling in the neurons. However, in vitro studies showed that the amounts of ethanol necessary to bring about fluidization of membrane lipids were considerably higher than those normally associated with intoxication and altered behavior. Furthermore, a pure narcotic action on neuronal membranes was not in line with the wide spectrum of ethanol's pharmacological effects including euphoria, impaired motor coordination, arousal, and cognition *(319)*. This led to the search for other mechanisms to explain the effects of ethanol on mood and behavior, such as specific receptor proteins that regulate synaptic activity and neurotransmission *(320)*.

The best candidate for a brain receptor for ethanol's intoxicating effect is that used by the major inhibitory neurotransmitter γ-aminobutyric acid (GABA), in particular the GABA$_A$ receptor *(321–324)*. A diverse range of compounds bring about sedation and anesthesia and these work by enhancing the effects of GABA *(317,318)*. This receptor complex is made up of a number of subunits arranged symmetrically to form an ion-channel (Fig. 13). When the receptor is activated (e.g., by a GABA agonist) the ion channel opens and chloride ions flow into the cell, which starts a chain of molecular events that eventually produces a pharmacological response. GABA binds to the β-subunit of the receptor and the presence of ethanol potentiates the agonist action of the neurotransmitter *(321)*.

Yet another site for the action of ethanol in the brain is the receptor for glutamate, which is the dominant excitatory neurotransmitter *(319)*. Ethanol seems to antagonize the NMDA (*N*-methyl-D-aspartate) glutamate receptor, which can also account for some of the diverse effects associated with overconsumption of ethanol. This occurs not by blocking the binding of glutamate but by mechanisms that are more complex involving the flux of sodium and calcium ions through the receptor channel to trigger

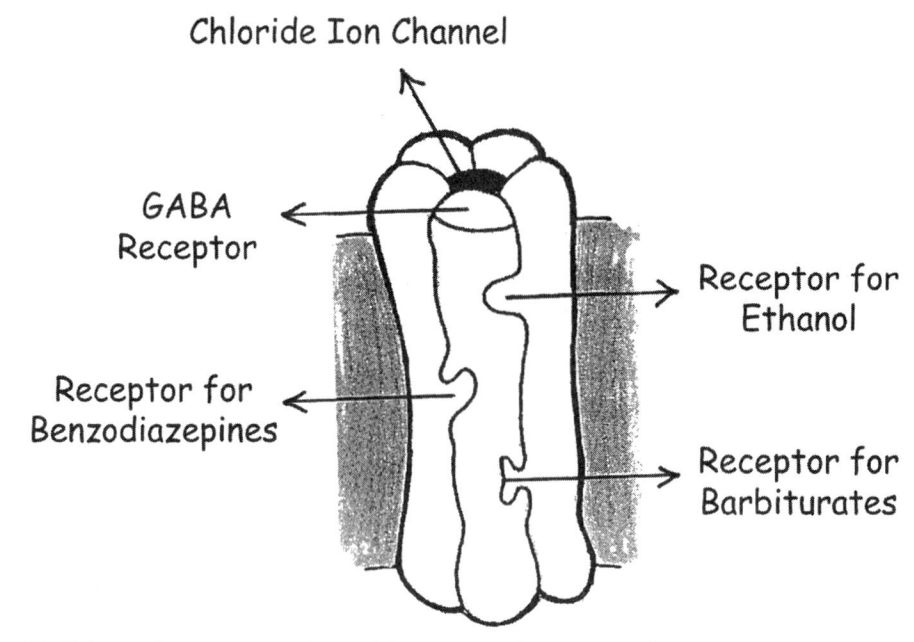

Fig. 13. Schematic representation of the γ-aminobutyric acid receptor (GABA$_A$) showing its ion channel for chloride and the different binding sites for GABA, benzodiazepines, barbiturates, and ethanol. When activated chloride ions flow into the cell, a chain of events is triggered, ending in a pharmacological response.

the action of second messengers. Activation of NMDA receptors was also suggested as a mechanism to explain some of the antisocial and aggressive behaviors seen in drunken people *(324)*.

Both during and after drinking ethanol, the drug distributes rapidly with the bloodstream to reach all parts of the body. Ethanol passes the blood–brain barrier with ease. After a single drink people experience feelings of mild euphoria, indicating that ethanol molecules have already entered the brain and started to interfere with neurochemical transmission. Ethanol, like other low-mol wt alcohols, is classified as a CNS depressant, which means that other CNS depressant drugs (e.g., barbiturates and benzodiazepines) are obvious candidates for pharmacodynamic interaction *(325–328)*. Drug-induced effects on the brain depend on the dose taken, the route of administration, lipid solubility, and the degree of tolerance development in the individual.

When BAC is relatively low (<0.03 g/100 mL) most people experience mild euphoria with a loss of inhibitions and some become more sociable and talkative *(325)*. As drinking continues and the BAC rises to 0.05–0.10 g/100 mL, judgment is impaired and some people become emotionally unstable, showing diminished attention and control. At even higher BAC (0.15–0.20 g/100 mL) speech is slurred and incoherent, balance is seriously impaired, and reaction time is slowed appreciably, especially in choice situations. However, moderate drinkers rarely reach such high BACs owing to the ill effects and nausea they experience, especially after rapid drinking when vomiting also frequently occurs. For those who continue to drink and tolerate higher BACs, the impairment of body function becomes progressively worse with pronounced ataxia and balance disturbances and some people cannot walk or stand upright without support. At still higher BAC (>0.3 g/100 mL), the narcotic action of ethanol becomes evident with deep sedation and stupor with a general loss of consciousness, and impaired circulation. A profound depression of the respiratory center in the brain stem occurs when BAC is between 0.4 and 0.5 g/100 mL and, depending on circumstances, many deaths occur owing to respiratory failure *(329,330)*.

5.2. Tolerance Development

Large variation in individual response and sensitivity to ethanol exists in a population of drinkers, and the BAC necessary to cause death in one person might be well tolerated by another depending on, among other things, their experience with alcohol and duration of exposure to this drug *(329,330)*. Tolerance is the diminution of the effect of a drug as a result of a prolonged or heavy use *(40)*. If a person's BAC rises rapidly after drinking to pass 0.15 g/100 mL, this often triggers a vomit reflex, which has doubtless saved the lives of many inexperienced drinkers. On the other hand, many people die through asphyxia by aspiration of stomach contents when they vomit in a deeply comatose state. Moreover, certain drugs might block the vomit reflex or, if alcohol is consumed in divided doses over several hours and the BAC rises more slowly to pass 0.15 g/100 mL, the person might not necessarily vomit.

After intake of a single intoxicating dose of ethanol when distribution of the drug into all body fluids and tissues is complete, there is a marked recovery from the initial impairment effects *(331)*. This phenomenon of adaptation is called the "Mellanby effect" after the British pharmacologist who first made the observation during experiments with dogs *(332)*. The animals regained their ability to stand on four legs and walk and react to orders several hours postdosing despite the fact that BAC was the same or even higher then it was when they first became incapacitated on the rising limb of the BAC curve *(332)*.

The Mellanby effect is also called acute tolerance, that is, the tolerance that develops during a single exposure to the drug. This condition is distinct from chronic tolerance, which develops after long-term administration of high doses of the drug *(39,40, 331)*. Ethanol also exhibits cross-tolerance with other sedative-hypnotic drugs and CNS depressants such as barbiturates and benzodiazepines, via adaptation at the cellular level via the $GABA_A$ receptor complex *(40)*. Yet another kind of tolerance is metabolic or dispositional tolerance, which is the ability of a person to dispose of the drug more effectively after a period of continuous heavy drinking *(40,331)*. The mechanism underlying metabolic tolerance is related to an increased capacity of microsomal enzymes (e.g., CYP2E1) to oxidize ethanol after continuous heavy drinking or taking other CNS depressants for prolonged periods *(28,32)*.

Reports of some impaired drivers with BAC above 0.4 g% and a few even exceeding 0.5 g% seem hard to rationalize when some authorities maintain that a median BAC of 0.35 g% or thereabouts is sufficient to cause death *(333)*. This introduces the need to consider development of chronic tolerance and its time course whenever toxicity of ethanol and drug–ethanol interactions are considered. After people consume large amounts of ethanol daily for several weeks or months, they develop chronic tolerance and the brain somehow manages to adapt to its alcoholic environment. The individual

Table 5
Number of Individuals Considered Under the Influence
of Alcohol as a Function of Blood Alcohol Concentration Based
on a Clinical Examination and Questionnaire by One and the Same Physician

Blood Alcohol, g/100 mL	N	Not Under Influence of Alcohol	Mild Signs and Symptoms	Moderate Signs and Symptoms	Severe Signs and Symptoms
0.00–0.049	29	3	26	–	–
0.05–0.099	39	2	37	–	–
0.10–0.149	54	2	41	10	1
0.15–0.199	47	1	24	17	5
0.20–0.249	47	–	20	22	5
0.25–0.299	25	–	7	11	7
0.30–0.359	3	–	1	1	1

The people examined (N = 244) were suspected of driving under the influence of alcohol in Sweden.

learns to walk and talk and function well enough to attempt to drive and can perform other skilled tasks albeit with difficulty. These very high BACs of 0.4 g% or more are seemingly tolerated without the need for emergency hospital treatment (334). By contrast, starting from a zero BAC and drinking sufficient quantities of alcohol during a single evening to reach 0.4 g% would result in gross intoxication, stupor with loss of consciousness, coma, and perhaps death by termination of the breathing reflex located in the medulla oblongata. Death may occur at considerably lower BACs if the person suffocates by inhalation of vomit, e.g., when in a comatose state and when arousal is severely impaired.

Table 5 gives an example of individual tolerance development to alcohol in apprehended drinking drivers (N = 244), each of whom was examined by the same physician without knowledge of their actual BAC. Using a questionnaire and checklist for clinical signs and symptoms normally associated with drunkenness, the physician formed an opinion whether the suspects were not under the influence of alcohol, or showed mild, moderate, or severe symptoms of alcohol influence. Very different conclusions were reached within each 0.05 g/100 mL BAC range and widely different BAC were noted for the same diagnosis (mild, moderate, or severe). This example illustrates development of both acute and chronic alcohol tolerance. Because the same person examined all suspects, the differences noted cannot be attributed to the experience of the physician. Furthermore, some people have the ability to pull themselves together when under pressure or they find themselves in a critical situation.

5.3. Toxicity of Ethanol

Ethanol should really be considered a dangerous drug considering the small difference between a harmless social drink and a fatal dose. This ratio of lethal dose (LD_{50}) to social dose (ED_{50}) is only about 10:1 corresponding to the amount necessary to cause mild euphoria (0.05 g%) and to cause death (0.5 g%). However, the question of the BAC necessary to cause death is not easy to answer and widely different opinions exist among specialists in forensic toxicology and legal medicine (329,330). One problem stems from the fact that the BAC determined at autopsy is not always a reliable reflection of the total amount of alcohol the person consumed or even the highest BAC reached before death.

Also the sampling site used to obtain blood for toxicological analysis needs to be carefully considered to minimize the risk of postmortem artifacts compromising the results *(335)*. The phenomenon of postmortem redistribution of alcohol and drugs has been discussed in detail elsewhere *(335)*. The blood-sampling site recommended for toxicological analysis is the femoral vein after clamping off the vein prior to drawing blood. The metabolism of alcohol commences immediately at the start of drinking and in the vast majority of people the rate of elimination from blood is between 0.01 and 0.025 g%/h. In those with metabolic tolerance, which is not uncommon in alcoholics and heavy drinkers prone to die of alcohol toxicity, the rate of elimination might be 0.03 g%/h or more *(159)*. What this means is that the BAC at autopsy gives a conservative estimate of the amount of alcohol consumed or the BAC prevailing several hours before death. Depending on the circumstances, the BAC at autopsy might need to be adjusted for the metabolism of ethanol that occurs between the start of drinking and time of death *(335)*.

After death BAC continues to decreases somewhat as the body cools and enzyme activity terminates. Also water content of autopsy blood is somewhat less then for fresh blood and because ethanol distributes into the water fraction, some feel that this difference should be considered. So besides measuring BAC, the blood water content should also be determined by desiccation and BAC then adjusted to a blood water content of 80% w/w *(335)*. Another problem in postmortem alcohol analysis is the risk for production of ethanol after death by microbes utilizing glucose and other substrates. This problem is not trivial especially if the body is decomposed and putrefaction processes have started. To some extent the validity of the BAC can be controlled and verified by sampling and analysis of ethanol in other body fluids, such as urine or vitreous humor *(335)*.

One of the effects of drinking a large dose of ethanol is to lower body temperature by upsetting the central regulatory mechanisms in the brain *(336,337)*. This effect is exaggerated when the environmental temperature is also unusually low *(337)*. Accordingly, a very drunk person exposed to the cold, such as a skid row alcoholic sleeping outdoors in the winter, is likely to be found dead with a BAC that otherwise he or she would have easily tolerated *(338,339)*. Hypothermia-related deaths might be important to consider when the toxicity of alcohol is evaluated *(340)*. One study reported a BAC at death of 0.36 ± 0.08 g/100 mL (range 0.21–0.70) in alcoholics ($N = 116$) not exposed to cold compared with 0.17 ± 0.09 g/100 mL (range 0–0.32) in another group ($N = 35$), which were classified as hypothermic deaths *(341)*.

An oft-times overlooked factor in alcohol-related deaths is positional asphyxia, particularly if the person is lying facedown with partial obstruction of the airway. Most heavy drinkers are also heavy smokers, and impaired lung functioning and breathing difficulties as a result of long-term use of cigarettes might be another factor to consider in addition to respiratory depression. If a person in a stupor or alcoholic coma is placed in a compromising position so that the breathing becomes restricted, this could result in death. Also, heavy cigarette smokers (which most heavy drinkers are) have higher carbon monoxide levels and lower oxygen tension in blood supply to the brain and in extreme cases this can lead to tissue hypoxia.

Finally, the role of ketoacidosis as a cause of death in alcoholics is just beginning to be better understood *(342,343)*. Alcoholics not only drink a lot of alcohol; they also neglect to eat properly and glycogen stores quickly become depleted. The combined influence of a hypoglycemic state and other metabolic disturbances make alcoholics a risk group for ketoacidosis and this might have accounted for their demise *(343)*. This diagnosis is thought to be applicable when an alcoholic is discovered dead at home with zero or low BAC and nothing more remarkable found at autopsy apart from an enlarged and fatty liver *(344)*. The determination of ketone bodies (acetone, acetoacetate, and β-hydroxybutyrate) in postmortem blood was suggested as a useful biochemical test to support a diagnosis of ketoacidosis death *(344,345)*.

Another major factor influencing toxicity of ethanol is concomitant use of other drugs, especially sedative-hypnotics like barbiturates and benzodiazepines that share similar mechanism of action via GABA neurotransmission *(346–349)*. Thus the BAC necessary to cause death might be substantially lower in a person who also had a high concentration of a barbiturate or a benzodiazepine in the blood *(329,330,346)*.

5.4. Toxicity of Drug–Ethanol Interactions

Many drugs that interact with ethanol at the cellular level can produce unexpected reactions, sometimes adding to or even potentiating the pharmacological effects expected from either drug alone *(350–352)*. Drugs such as heroin, morphine, methadone, as well as other opiates have multiple actions depending on where in the body the target receptors are located. So besides the relief of pain, opiate-like drugs also depresses respiration making them particular dangerous when taken together with a large dose of ethanol, which also functions as a respiratory depressant *(325,353)*.

5.4.1. Propoxyphene

Propoxyphene (called dextropropoxyphene in Europe) was synthesized in 1953 and in terms of chemical structure and pharmacology is similar to methadone *(325)*. Propoxyphene ($t_{1/2}$ 8–24 h) is prescribed for treatment of mild to moderate pain, but the drug also causes sedation and is often available in tablets together with aspirin or acetaminophen (paracetamol). Shortly after propoxyphene became widely prescribed (~1957) a number of overdose fatalities were reported and one common finding in these deaths was the high prevalence of ethanol *(354–358)*. Deaths associated with propoxyphene use continue unabated and the drug is no longer registered in some countries (e.g., Denmark). The ratio between lethal and therapeutic concentrations for propoxyphene is fairly narrow *(359)*. Moreover, the toxicity of propoxyphene is enhanced in alcohol abusers and binge drinkers. Although the mechanism of interaction with ethanol is not completely understood, it seems to be related to synaptic activity at GABA and opiate receptors with additive effects on the depression of respiration *(356,358)*.

5.4.2. Sedative-Hypnotic Drugs

Sedative-hypnotic drugs have diverse chemical and pharmacological properties and are prescribed to calm anxious patients and to produce drowsiness, sedation, and sleep by depressing the activity of the nervous system *(325–327)*. These drugs are widely prescribed and are obvious candidates for interaction with ethanol, owing to the similar mechanism and sites of action in the brain, namely the GABA receptor complex

Table 6
**Examples of Sedative-Hypnotic Drugs
with Strong Potential for Pharmacodynamic Interaction with Ethanol**

Barbiturates (Trade Name) and Half-Life	Benzodizepines (Trade Name) and Half-Life	Other CNS Depressants (Trade Name) and Half-Life
Amobarbital (Amytal®) 15–40 h	Alprazolam (Xanax®) 6–22 h	Chlormethiazole (Heminevrin®) 3–5 h
Aprobarbital (Alurate®) 14–34 h	Chlordizepoxide (Librium®) 6–27 h	Chloral hydrate (Noctec®) 6–10 h
Butabarbital (Butisol®) 34–42 h	Diazepam (Valium®) 21–37 h	Ethchlorvynol (Placidyl®) 19–32 h
Hexobarbital (Sombulex®) 3–7 h	Flunitrazepam (Rohypnol®) 9–25 h	Glutethimide (Doriden®) 7–15 h
Mephobarbital (Mebaral®) 10–70 h	Flurazepam (Dalmane®) 1–3 h	γ-hyroxybuyrate GHB 0.3–1.0 h
Methohexital (Brevital®) 3–5 h	Lorazepam (Ativan®) 9–16 h	Meprobamate (Miltown®) 6–17 h
Pentobarbital (Nembutal®) 20–30 h	Midazolam (Versed®) 1–4 h	Methaqualone (Sopor®) 20–60 h
Phenobarbital (Luminal®) 48–120 h	Nitrazepam (Mogadon®) 17–48 h	Methyprylon (Noludar®) 7–11 h
Probarbital (Ipral®) 15–40 h	Oxazepam (Serax®) 4–11 h	Paraldehyde (Paral®) 3–10 h
Secobarbital (Seconal®) 15–40 h	Temazepam (Restoril®) 5–15 h	Zolpidem (Ambien®) 1.4–4.5 h
Thiopental (Pentothal®) 6–46 h	Triazolam (Halcion®) 2–4 h	Zopiclone (Imovane®) 0.5–6.5 h

The sedative-hypnotic drugs' trade names (US), and elimination half-lives are given *(325,469)*.

(360). Alcohol use should be avoided when taking this kind of medication because of the risk of additive or supra-additive effects leading to more pronounced sedation *(361, 362)*. Besides a worsened behavioral impairment and judgment when ethanol and other CNS depressants are combined, there is a heightened risk for acute toxicity *(363)*, as evidenced by the many barbiturate–ethanol poisonings documented over the years with many fatalities *(364)*.

Examples of sedative hypnotics drugs exerting a pharmacodynamic interaction with ethanol including barbiturates, benzodiazepines, and miscellaneous substances are given in Table 6.

5.4.2.1. Barbiturates

Among the oldest sedative-hypnotic drugs are derivatives of barbituric acid, which was prepared in 1863 as a condensation product between urea and malonic acid *(325, 366)*. Many alkyl derivatives of barbituric acid were synthesized and these found wide use in therapeutics as sedative-hypnotic agents *(325)*. Barbiturates were classified as very short acting (anesthetics), short to medium acting (sleeping pills or hypnotics),

Table 7
Concentrations of Some Sedative-Hypnotic Drugs in Postmortem
Blood in Drug-Related Deaths with and Without the Presence of Alcohol

Drug	N[a]	Conc. Without Alcohol Mean (Range) mg/L	N[a]	Conc. with Alcohol Mean (Range) mg/L	Blood Alcohol Conc. Mean (Range) g/100 mL
Phenobarbital	11	93 (51–183)	4	69 (46–90)	0.11 (0.05–0.23)
Pentobarbital	11	26 (9–59)	11	21 (6–51)	0.11 (0.02–0.21)
Secobarbital	6	25 (0.7–47)	10	15 (2–66)	0.12 (0.01–0.30)
Meprobamate	12	112 (34–258)	18	99 (39–220)	0.14 (0.02–0.25)

Data from *(341)*.
[a]Number of cases.

and long acting (sedatives and anticonvulsants). Barbiturates became the most common drugs found in cases of accidental or fatal self-poisoning *(326,327)*. They were notoriously dangerous in overdose owing to a narrow therapeutic index, and tens of thousands of deaths have been caused by inadvertent use of these drugs either by accident or for purposes of suicide *(367)*. The barbiturates were commonly prescribed to relieve anxiety, cause sedation and sleep, and also as antiepeleptic medication. Certain very short-acting barbiturates were used as premedication before general anesthesia (e.g., thiopental).

The major clinical feature of barbiturate overdose was deep depression of the CNS, and this was made worse when taken together with a large dose of alcohol *(367)*. Table 7 shows the concentrations of various barbiturates and meprobamate in blood in a number of fatal poisonings with and without the presence of alcohol. Note that the blood concentrations of these sedative-hypnotics are lower when the victim also had an elevated BAC *(341)*.

Chronic use of barbiturates causes induction of CYP450 enzymes including CYP2E1, which results in faster metabolism of many other psychoactive drugs and medications as well as of ethanol *(41–43)*. Similarly, chronic intake of ethanol induces CYP enzymes so that barbiturates are more rapidly metabolized in heavy drinkers and alcoholics *(32,199)*. Without any doubt, the most serious interaction between barbiturates and ethanol was their combined action in the brain via voltage and ligand-gated ion channels that control neuronal activity. The major site for interaction is the receptor for the inhibitory neurotransmitter GABA. The risk for toxicity and high abuse potential of barbiturates has meant that they are not prescribed much today. Instead, much safer anxiolytic drugs such as the benzodiazepines and more recently the pyrazolopyrimidine hypnotics are available, such as zolpidem and zopiclone *(368,369)*.

5.4.2.2. BENZODIAZEPINES

The first benzodiazepines (chlordiazepoxide and diazepam) became available in the early 1960 and swiftly dominated the market as a class of sedative-hypnotic drugs. As a group they possess a much wider safety margin and are less toxic in overdose then barbiturates *(370–373)*. The benzodiazepines were and still are widely prescribed for the treatment of such conditions as anxiety, muscle spasm, alcohol withdrawal, epilep-

12. Alcohol and Drug Interactions

tic seizures, and insomnia *(325,375)*. These drugs dominated the market as mild tranquilizers, especially for treating anxiety and sleep disorders *(325)*. However, their potential for toxicity should not be underestimated, especially the swifter acting hypnotics midazolam, triazolam, and flunitrazepam *(374,375)*. These substances have been incriminated in many deaths both alone and especially together with other CNS depressants such as opiates and ethanol *(376–379)*.

Although much safer then barbiturates, the class of drugs they replaced, the generous prescribing of benzodiazepines along with their potential for abuse and dependence make them dangerous, especially when taken together with a large amount of alcohol *(379–383)*. Most of the benzodiazepine group of drugs have low hepatic clearance and are highly bound to plasma proteins making them less susceptible to metabolic interaction with ethanol via CYP450 enzymes *(384)*. The interaction with ethanol is predominantly pharmacodynamic *(385)*.

Benzodiazepines are absorbed rapidly and on reaching the brain they function by binding to a specific type of receptor, which is widely distributed in those parts of the brain that control anxiety, memory, sedation, and coordination *(385–387)*. The endogenous brain chemical that normally activates these same receptors is GABA, the most important inhibitory neurotransmitter. The binding site for benzodiazepines is distinct from the GABA receptor site, which in turn is distinct from the binding site for barbiturates *(321–323)*.

Figure 13 gives a schematic representation of the GABA receptor complex showing the binding sites for ethanol, barbiturates, and benzodiazepines. Drugs of the benzodiazepine and barbiturate families act as agonists and therefore enhance the effects of GABA, leading to a diminished brain activity and a tranquilizing effect *(321)*. Ethanol also facilitates GABA neurotransmission and, depending on the dose and the concentration reaching the receptor, elicits anxiolytic, anticonvulsive, and anaesthetic properties. The $GABA_A$ receptors are considered the molecular targets for the action of benzodiazepines, barbiturates, and ethanol *(323)*.

Diazepam is a GABAergic agonist that binds tightly to specific sites on the $GABA_A$ receptor to open an ion channel allowing chloride ions to flow into the cell *(324)*. Ethanol also acts on the $GABA_A$ receptor but at a different binding site from diazepam, and when taken together with diazepam these drugs interact in an additive way to reduce nerve activity in the brain leading to, among other things, deeper sedation. Also, the many other sedative-hypnotic drugs listed in Table 5 are thought to act in one way or another via the $GABA_A$ or $GABA_B$ receptors and thus have potential for interaction with ethanol.

The combined effect of ethanol and chloral hydrate, the oldest sedative-hypnotic drug, gained the reputation of having devastating effects on the individual in terms of sedation *(169–171)*. This drug combination became known as knock-out drops or a Mickey Finn and was the mixture of choice for quickly putting people to sleep. However, there is not much scientific evidence that the ethanol-chloral mixture is any more effective than chloral hydrate alone. After ingesting chloral hydrate, the drug is rapidly hydrolyzed ($t_{1/2}$ = ~4 min) to form trichlorethanol, which is a pharmacologically active metabolite having a longer half-life than the parent drug. Detoxification of trichlorethanol occurs via conjugation reactions with glucuronic acid or oxidation via the ADH pathway to produce an inactive metabolite trichloroacetic acid *(171)*. Chloral hydrate furnishes an example of a sedative-hypnotic drug exerting both a metabolic as well as a pharmacodynamic interaction with ethanol.

5.4.3. Illicit Drugs

Any drug or chemical agent with psychoactive properties, that is, having its site of action in the CNS, has the potential for pharmacodynamic interaction with ethanol, thus altering a person's mood and behavior. The entire range of abused drugs including CNS stimulants such as cocaine, amphetamine, and methamphetamine, the opiates (heroin and morphine), cannabis and marijuana, as well as hallucinogens like LSD are candidates for interaction with ethanol at the cellular level. Also commonly prescribed medications such as antidepressants and antihistamines that modulate the uptake and/or release of neurotransmitters are also strong candidates for pharmacodynamic interaction with ethanol *(390–392)*.

Polydrug use is widespread among drug-dependent individuals and coabuse of the legal drug ethanol is no exception. An interesting example of the combined influence of an illicit drug and a legal drug is the interaction between cocaine and ethanol, which leads to the synthesis of a new psychoactive substance called cocaethylene *(393)*.

5.4.3.1. COCAETHYLENE

The epidemic of crack cocaine abuse in the United States meant that coingestion of cocaine and alcohol became one of the most commonly encountered drug combinations in many abusers. Indeed, the use of alcohol and cocaine became popular in some circles because it allegedly gave more intense feelings of high *(394)*. Cocaine also seemed to antagonize some of the learning deficits and the impairment of psychomotor performance after drinking ethanol *(395)*. Interestingly, it was observed that when cocaine and ethanol were used together, a new pharmacologically active substance was produced called cocaethylene *(396)*. This compound was biosynthesized during the metabolism of cocaine in individuals with elevated BAC *(397)*. Cocaine undergoes rapid hydrolysis by various carboxyl esterases to produce its major metabolite benzoylecgonine and simultaneously also cocaethylene *(398)*. Cocaethylene was shown to pass the blood–brain barrier and to exert its pharmacological effects through the dopamine receptor thus enhancing the feelings of euphoria *(399)*. Moreover, the elimination half-life of cocaethylene is longer than for cocaine, which helps to maintain and prolong the effects of the stimulant drug on the individual. Several studies suggested that when cocaine was taken together with ethanol the risk for cardiotoxicity was increased *(400,401)*.

6. DRUGS USED IN THE TREATMENT OF ALCOHOLISM

Alcohol abuse and alcoholism create enormous costs for the individual and society, and much research effort has focused on early detection of problem drinkers by use of various questionnaires and clinical tests searching for so-called biochemical markers *(402)*. The development of pharmacological treatments for addiction to alcohol and other drugs is a major goal for the pharmaceutical industry *(403–405)*. The ideal agent should reduce craving for alcohol, and also block the reinforcing or pleasurable effects associated with consumption of alcohol. The medication should also be free from side effects and not interact with other medication the patient might be using. In recent

Table 8
Drugs Used in the Treatment of Alcoholism and Their Mechanism of Action

Drug	Mechanism of Action
Disulfiram (Antabuse®)	This drug blocks the low-k_m enzyme of aldehyde dehydrogenase and makes the patient more sensitive to effects of alcohol. The concentrations of acetaldehyde in blood increase and this causes unpleasant effects, including facial flushing, nausea, headache, palpitations, tachycardia, etc., and hence the name of this treatment is aversion therapy.
Diazepam/Lorazepam (Valium®/Ativan®)	These benzodiazepines are given to patients who are undergoing detoxification after long-term heavy drinking to counteract the potentially dangerous withdrawal signs and symptoms associated with alcohol abstinence including cramps, convulsions, and deliriums.
γ-hydroxybutyrate (GHB)	A sedative-hypnotic drug, GHB interacts with the receptor for GABA and can counteract some alcohol withdrawal symptoms and seems also to reduce alcohol consumption and craving.
Naltrexone (ReVia®)	This orally active opiate antagonist decreases craving during long-term abstinence thus reducing the risk for relapse and the desire to start drinking alcohol again. This treatment should be used together with a program of social and psychological counseling.
Acamprosate (Campral®)	This drug is a specific antagonist of the excitatory neurotransmitter glutamate acting via the *N*-methyl-D-aspartate (NMDA) receptor. Blocking the receptor reduces the intensity of craving for alcohol and patients remain abstinent for longer. Again, a program of psychological intervention is needed.
Ondansetron (Zofran®)	This drug is one of the new serotonin ($5HT_3$) antagonists and helps to diminish the rewarding effect of drinking ethanol by blocking activity at the dopamine receptor.

years considerable progress has been made in the search for effective drug therapy to treat alcoholism but there is still a long way to go *(403–405)*.

Table 8 lists some of the drugs currently used for treatment of alcoholics during the early detoxification period after stopping drinking and during the protracted abstinence period months later. Efforts to discover effective pharmacotherapy for treating addiction to cocaine and opiates is also well underway and the various strategies used were the subject of a recent review *(405)*.

The first pharmacotherapy for abuse of alcohol utilized the disulfiram–alcohol interaction, which was discussed earlier under the section dealing with ALDH inhibitors *(406,407)*. The underlying mechanism was interference with the second stage of ethanol metabolism to cause an excess of the toxic metabolite acetaldehyde in the blood *(175)*. This precipitated a wide range of unpleasant effects such as flushing of the face and upper arms, palpitations, headache, and breathing difficulties severe enough to scare the person into stopping drinking. Another treatment strategy made use of subcutaneous implants of antabuse tablets so responsibility for taking the medication was not with the patient. However, the efficacy of this mode of treatment is questionable because the concentration of acetaldehyde in blood was not increased in those subjects with antabuse implants after they drank alcohol compared with a placebo control implant *(407)*.

The alcohol withdrawal phase that commences after a period of chronic heavy drinking can become particularly dangerous and has sometimes resulted in death *(406)*. To alleviate the life-threatening episodes of seizures, convulsions, and delirium, the patient is treated with various drugs. In the early phase of withdrawal, to help counteract mild to severe anxiety, agitation, and tremor, benzodiazepine agonists such as lorazepam or diazepam are prescribed and the latter drug is sometimes referred to as "dry alcohol," indicating close similarity to ethanol in mode of action. Such $GABA_A$ agonists have proved useful for management of the early alcohol withdrawal phase but are not effective for treating dependence on ethanol and protracted abstinence. Indeed, these drugs are themselves dependence producing so care is needed not to replace one addictive drug (alcohol) with another (diazepam). The seizures and hallucinations often associated with severe withdrawal from alcohol can be treated with phenytoin and haloperidol respectively *(406)*.

Newer pharmacological adjuncts for treatment of alcoholism include the opiate antagonist naltrexone (ReVia®) *(408)*. The mechanism by which this opiate works against alcohol addiction is not clear but it seems to stop craving and the desire to continue drinking particularly during the rehabilitation phase. It is known that opioid peptides stimulate dopamine release in the brain, so blocking these receptors with naltrexone helps to eliminate some of the reinforcing effects of ethanol. However, a number of randomized controlled studies aimed at evaluating the effectiveness of naltrexone gave conflicting results. It seems that besides drug therapy an important element in the treatment is psychological and social intervention, and without these the results were not so impressive *(408,409)*.

The medication acamprosate (Campral®) has been approved in several European countries for treating alcohol dependence, and this drug seems to prolong the time for relapse in abstinent alcoholics *(410)*. The drug works via the $GABA_A$ and NMDA receptors by modulating their activity and somehow reducing the unpleasant feelings of abstinence from alcohol therefore helping to reduce craving and relapse.

Besides being a dangerous drug of abuse the GABA analog GHB, which has sedative-hypnotic properties, has been shown to alleviate withdrawal symptoms associated with alcohol abstinence. However, great care is needed in finding the optimal dose of GHB for effective therapy *(411)*. This drug apparently interacts with the $GABA_B$ receptor *(412)*.

One of the most recent drugs to emerge for pharmacological treatment of alcoholism is Ondansetron (Zofran®), which blocks the serotonergic $5HT_3$ receptor *(413,414)*. Taking this drug seems to regulate the release of dopamine into the nucleus accumbens thereby lowering the lust to continue drinking alcohol. In a placebo-controlled trial with mildly alcohol-dependent male outpatients, the drug helped to reduce alcohol consumption *(413)*.

Many other substances with their mode of action in the brain have been proposed or tested in the quest to find an effective pharmacological treatment for alcohol dependence. Substances such as lithium, the drug of choice in mania, to newer antidepressants such as the serotonin selective reuptake inhibitors (SSRIs), e.g., citalopram or anxiolytic agents, buspirone, and ritanserin, as well as antipsychotic drugs like the dopamine antagonist haloperidol, have been investigated but without much success *(406,414)*.

7. SOBERING-UP DRUGS

Many attempts have been made to develop a drug that would prove effective in sobering up heavily intoxicated or comatose patients *(415)*. One such line of research looked at the possibility of accelerating the rate of hepatic oxidation of ethanol and thus reducing the time needed to clear ethanol from the blood and bring the person below some threshold BAC such as the legal alcohol limit for driving *(416)*. Another approach was directed toward finding a specific alcohol antagonist that would counteract alcohol-induced impairment but without necessarily speeding up the rate of elimination of ethanol from the bloodstream. A substance that initially showed promise as an effective antagonist of some of ethanol's CNS effects was a novel benzodiazepine derivative denoted Ro15-4513 *(417)*. Administering this drug to rats made immobile by a large dose of ethanol ameliorated some of the untoward behavioral and neuropharmacological effects of the depressant drug *(320)*. Also the $GABA_B$ receptor antagonist phaclofen proved useful in modifying some of the behavioral effects of ethanol, at least for a short time after administration *(418)*.

Sobering-up drugs are known as amethystic agents, being derived from the Greek word *amethystos* meaning a remedy against drunkenness *(406,416)*. The availability of an effective sobering agent might have clinical applications for the treatment of highly inebriated or comatose patients in a similar fashion to naloxone, which is the drug of choice for reversing the effects of heroin or opiate overdose. An OTC sobering-up pill would obviously find a market among those who drink and drive to bring them below some critical threshold value in a shorter time, e.g., the legal alcohol limit for driving *(415)*. The ideal sobering-up agent should (a) antagonize ethanol without itself altering physiology or behavior; (b) have no adverse or toxic effects; (c) have a rapid onset of action lasting long enough to eliminate ethanol from the body; and (d) not have any of its own dependence-producing properties *(419)*.

Various carbohydrates such as sucrose, glucose, and fructose have been extensively studied in attempts to speed up the elimination of ethanol. In some countries, small packets of fructose were made available at pubs and bars as a sobering remedy but their effectiveness has been difficult to verify in controlled human studies *(419)*. Along the same lines, much interest was shown in developing a "hangover pill" that would alleviate some of the unpleasant after effects of an evening's heavy drinking *(420)*. Such a hangover remedy might involve taking a mixture of various vitamins or salt solutions to correct the water and electrolyte imbalance resulting from an evening's heavy drinking. Once again, no proper validation of such a hangover cure has been published to my knowledge *(420)*.

Testing the effectiveness of a sobering-up agent is not easy owing to the many variables that need to be considered, and the particular experimental design makes correct interpretation of the results difficult *(421–423)*. When fructose is ingested before or together with ethanol, the sugar treatment also delays stomach emptying so absorption of ethanol is slower, resulting in low C_{max} and later t_{max} *(424)*. This complicates evaluation of the fructose effect because eating a meal before drinking also slows absorption of ethanol and lowers C_{max}. Moreover, large doses of sugar might have an osmotic effect, which slows intestinal absorption of ethanol, and hypertonic sugar solutions could retain water and ethanol in the gastrointestinal tract for longer periods compared with intake of isotonic fluids. Great care is needed not to confuse the influence of the sugars on the rate of absorption of ethanol from an influence of carbohydrate on the rate of hepatic clearance of ethanol. Novel experimental designs are necessary for obtaining unambiguous results *(423)*.

The mechanism of the fructose effect is considered to involve a swifter reoxidation of the reduced coenzyme NADH back to NAD+ necessary for further oxidation of ethanol via the ADH pathway *(425,426)*. However in a healthy, well-nourished individual, fructose treatment was not very effective in accelerating the elimination of ethanol although some beneficial effect might be seen in fasted or malnourished individuals *(427)*. Some reports warned about giving large amounts of fructose because of the risk of gastrointestinal pains, lactic acidosis, and hyperuricemia owing to metabolic shifts in the hepatic redox state of the liver *(428)*.

When fasted or malnourished subjects were treatment with fructose, the rate of ethanol oxidation was increased by 25–100% compared with a placebo treatment *(427)*. Some investigators administered fructose orally and gave the ethanol intravenously, thus sidestepping the confounding influence of sugars on absorption of ethanol from the gut *(429)*. In some of these studies, 25–30% increases in the rate of ethanol elimination from the blood were reported. The clinical usefulness of fructose in acute alcoholic intoxication was questioned, however, because of possible side effects such as upper abdominal pains, nausea, and diarrhea *(428)*.

8. MISCELLANEOUS SUBSTANCES

Hundreds of papers can be found describing interaction studies between ethanol and other coadministered drugs, and a large bibliography on this subject was prepared in 1970 *(430)*. A plethora of agents were tested, ranging from inert substances such as sodium chloride *(431)* to oxygenated water *(432)* to the artificial sweetener xylitol *(433)* to vitamin mixtures *(434,435)*, ascorbic acid *(436,437)*, hormones and peptides *(438)*, as well as herbal medicines of various kinds *(439–441)*. Examples of central stimulants such as the legal drugs caffeine *(442,443)* and nicotine from smoking cigarettes *(444)* to illicit drugs such as methamphetamine *(445)* and cocaine *(394)* have all been tested for their interaction with ethanol in human studies. Medications with drugs acting on the CNS, such as antihistamines *(446)* and the SSRI drugs *(447,448)* have all been investigated for their potential adverse interactions with ethanol. Many substances have been tested without any prior theoretical basis for expecting an interaction with ethanol, via metabolic pathways or through pharmacodynamic CNS effects *(449–453)*. The marginal effects reported in some studies could be ascribed to the limited number of subjects used or other experimental design features such as demographics of the participants or their smoking, drinking, and dietary habits. The results from many quarters make it much more likely that coadministration of ethanol will have a much greater influence on the absorption, distribution, and elimination characteristics of the drug or medication, rather then vice versa *(454)*.

9. CONCLUDING REMARKS

This chapter has presented an overview of various drug–alcohol interactions and the underlying mechanisms involved. The main focus was on drugs of interest in forensic medicine and toxicology. No attempt was made to review the hundreds of studies describing the effects of alcohol and drugs on psychomotor skills relevant to driving; these are dealt with elsewhere *(24,31,38,48)*. Instead, the major focus was placed on the underlying mechanisms of drug–alcohol interaction, whether involving inhibition or induction of drug-metabolizing enzymes or behavioral effects caused by altered synaptic activity in the brain.

The legal drug ethanol is a leading candidate for interacting with prescription drugs and OTC medications and clear warnings should be given by the physician and pharmacist when these preparations are used *(53,54,454)*. Drugs that can increase a person's BAC, by whatever mechanism, are much discussed and debated in legal proceedings relating to driving under the influence of alcohol *(22)*. The question of intent to commit a drunk-driving offense becomes an issue if evidence can be mustered that use of a prescription or OTC drug raised the BAC or slowed down the rate of removal of ethanol from the blood. In this connection it is worth keeping in mind that some OTC and prescription medications contain alcohol as one of the ingredients. For example, many cough syrups (e.g., Nyquil ~25% v/v ethanol) and the opiate antitussive medication ethylmorphine are dispensed mixed with ethanol (10% v/v). Also many mouthwashes, vitamin tonics, and pick-me-up drinks are available containing 10–20% v/v ethanol, so like any alcoholic beverage, drinking these in excess can certainly raise a person's BAC *(54,455,456)*.

Sudden deaths resulting from the combined use of large doses of alcohol and sedative-hypnotic sleeping pills such as barbiturates are classic in the annals of toxicology *(326,327)*. There is always a risk of toxicity when ethanol is combined with CNS depressants owing to similar mode of action in the brain and a high potentially for dangerous respiratory depression and circulatory arrest *(454)*. This needs to be considered when cause of death is decided in medical examiner cases. Furthermore, the concomitant use of alcohol and CNS depressants results in diminished performance of skilled tasks and risk of accidents at home, at work, and on the roads is increased *(457)*.

Table 9 lists the drugs most commonly encountered in femoral venous blood samples from medical examiner cases in Sweden *(458)*. For comparison, the most common drugs found in blood of drug-impaired drivers are also listed. In medical examiner cases mostly licit drugs were identified, whereas in impaired drivers illicit drugs dominated with amphetamine and tetrahydrocannabinol topping the list. Alcohol is the number one drug in both lists and is either present alone or together with other psychoactive substances, both licit and illicit drugs. The drugs identified in the medical examiner cases are not necessarily the cause of death but instead reflect the frequency of use of these substances in this population of individuals. Moreover, diazepam (rank 4) has a very long half-life (20–50 h), which means that this substance and its metabolite (nordiazepam) might be detected in blood for up to a week after last use *(372,373)*.

The behavioral effects of ethanol and drugs depend on dose, route of administration, and the concentration of the substances reaching the brain, which in turn depends on many genetic and environmental factors *(459)*. Susceptibility to become addicted

Table 9
Top 10 Drugs Identified in Medical Examiner Cases and in Impaired Drivers in Sweden

Rank	Medical Examiner Cases[a]	Impaired Drivers[b]
1	Ethanol	Ethanol
2	Acetaminophen	Amphetamine
3	Diazepam + nordiazepam	Tetrahydrocannabinol
4	Propoxyphene	Diazepam + nordiazepam
5	Morphine[c]	Flunitrazepam + 7-amino flunitrazepam
6	Citalopram	Morphine[c]
7	Codeine	Methamphetamine
8	Propiomazine	Codeine
9	Carbon monoxide	Acetaminophen
10	Zopiklone	MDMA (Ecstacy)

Many of these substances occur in combination with ethanol, the number one drug in both lists.
[a]Femoral venous blood.
[b]Cubital venous blood.
[c]Metabolite of heroin and codeine.

to drugs also includes a strong genetic component *(460)*. There are marked racial and ethnic differences in phase I drug-metabolizing enzymes, and CYP2D6, CYP2C9, and CYP2C19 show polymorphism, which not only influences the rate of metabolism of drugs but also helps explain the large variability in plasma concentrations and therapeutic response of the particular medication *(461–465)*. The subject of pharmacogenetics of drug action and interaction has emerged as a hot research topic and the notion of manufacturing tailor-made drugs based on genetic profiling of the individual is something for the future *(466,467)*. If this becomes a reality, perhaps adverse effects of drugs and undesirable drug–alcohol interactions could be avoided *(466)*. The alcohol flush reaction seen in many Asians when they drink alcohol is a direct result of the inactive form of ALDH they inherit that makes them highly sensitive to acetaldehyde produced during metabolism of ethanol. This adverse reaction protects them from becoming heavy drinkers and alcoholics and is a good example of a pharmacogenetic trait *(468)*.

Much of the variability in pharmacokinetics of ethanol can be explained by a combination of genetic and environmental factors as well as the experimental design of the studies *(469)*. Such things as the route and timing of administration of ethanol and drugs and the selection and allotment of subjects to test and control groups will influence outcome of the study. More work is needed to investigate variability in pharmacokinetics and pharmacodynamics of ethanol and drug–alcohol interactions in real-world drinking situations with repeated intake of different kinds of alcoholic beverages without reference to body wt or previous exposure to drugs.

Confusion and controversy exist regarding the reality of certain drug–alcohol interactions. Animal studies are often not very helpful in elucidating the problem and such articles have not been cited or considered in this review. Many older studies purporting to find a significant metabolic or CNS interaction between ethanol and a particular drug have not always withstood a careful scrutiny or reevaluation applying modern experimental and statistical techniques. Some reports suggested that the antibacterial drug metronidazole interacted with alcohol to produce an antabuse-like reaction but this could not be confirmed in a recent study *(198)*. Another experimental design issue is the fact that most studies of drug–alcohol interactions are done with young healthy volunteers and not with hospital patients or those people suffering from the ailment that the medication is intended to treat.

It is hard to envisage a drug interacting with the absorption of ethanol to increase a person's BAC above that expected from drinking the same dose on an empty stomach. Inhibition of the hepatic breakdown of ethanol is possible through a metabolic interaction with 4MP (fomepizole) *(152)*. The acute phase of alcohol intoxication depends on the dose taken, the speed of drinking, as well as many factors that influence gastric emptying, particularly the presence of food in the stomach *(24,25)*. Interaction between ethanol and psychoactive substances often leads to exaggerated impairment of body function or enhanced toxicity compared with the effect of either drug taken alone. The effect of ethanol and prescription drugs such as barbiturates or benzodiazepines represents a particularly dangerous combination owing to the common sites and mechanisms of action in the brain, namely via $GABA_A$ receptors.

References

1. Dhossche DM, Rich CL, and Isacsson G. Psychoactice substances in suicides: comparison of toxicologic findings in two samples. Am J Forens Med Pathol 22:239–243 (2001).
2. Heninger MM. Commonly encountered prescription medications in medical-legal death investigations: a guide for death investigators and medical examiners. Am J Forens Med Pathol 21:287–299 (2000).
3. Alsén M, Ekedahl A, Löwenhielm P, Niméus A, Regnell G, and Träskman-Bendz L. Medicine self-poisoning and the sources of drugs in Lund, Sweden. Acta Psychiat Scand 89: 255–261 (1994).
4. Prescott LF and Highley MS. Drugs prescribed for self-poisoners. Br Med J 290:1633–1636 (1985).
5. Lazarou J, Pomeranz BH, and Corey PN. Incidence of adverse drug reactions in hospitalized patients. JAMA 279:1200–1205 (1998).
6. Buajordet I, Ebbesen J, Erikssen J, Brors O, and Hilberg T. Fatal adverse drug events: the paradox of drug treatment. J Intern Med 250:327–341 (2001).
7. Osselton MD, Blackmore RC, King LA, and Moffat AC. Poisoning associated deaths for England and Wales between 1973–1980. Hum Toxicol 3:201–221 (1984).
8. Rivara FP, Mueller BA, Somes G, Menoza CT, Rushforth NB, and Kellermann AL. Alcohol and illicit drug abuse and the risk of violent death in the home. JAMA 278:569–575 (1997).
9. Edwards IR and Aronson JK. Adverse drug reactions: definitions, diagnosis and management. Lancet 356:1255–1259 (2000).
10. Lasser KE, Allen PD, Woodhandler SJ, Himmelstein DU, Wolfe SM, and Bor DH. Timing of new black box warnings and withdrawals for prescription medications. JAMA 287:2215–2220 (2002).
11. Sjögren H, Eriksson A, and Ahlm K. Role of alcohol in unnatural deaths: a study of all deaths in Sweden. Alcohol Clin Exp Res 24:1050–1056 (2000).
12. Cox DE, Sadler DW, and Pounder DJ. Alcohol estimation at necropsy: epidemiology, economics, and the elderly. J Clin Pathol 50:197–201 (1997).

13. Pentilla A, Karhunen PJ, and Vuori E. Blood alcohol in sudden and unexpected deaths. Forens Sci Intern 43:96–102 (1989).
14. Roche AM, Watt K, McClure R, Purdi DM, and Green D. Injury and alcohol: a hospital emergency department study. Drug & Alc Rev 20:155–166 (2001).
15. White IR, Altmann DR, and Nanchahal K. Alcohol consumption and mortality: modelling risks for men and women at different ages. Br Med J 325:191–194 (2002).
16. Neutel CI. Risk of traffic accidents injury after a prescription for a benzodiazepine. Ann Epidemiol 5:239–244 (1995).
17. Skurtveit S, Abotnes B, and Christophersen AS. Drugged drivers in Norway with benzodiazepine detection. Forens Sci Intern 125:75–82 (2002).
18. Ropero-Miller JD and Goldberger BA. Recreational drugs—current trends in the 90s. Clin Lab Med 18:727–746 (1998).
19. Jones AW. Enforcement of drink-driving laws by use of "per se" legal alcohol limits: blood and/or breath concentration as evidence of impairment. Alc Drugs Driving 4:99–112 (1988).
20. Jones AW. Medicolegal alcohol determinations—Blood- or breath-alcohol concentration? Forens Sci Rev 12:23–48, 2000.
21. Ferner RE. Forensic pharmacology: medicines, mayhem and malpractice. Oxford, England: Oxford University Press, 1996:1–236.
22. Jones AW. Top-ten defense challenges among drinking drivers in Sweden. Med Sci Law 31:429–439 (1991).
23. Ito K, Iwatsubo T, Kanamitsu S, Ueda K, Suzuki H, and Sugiyama Y. Prediction of pharmacokinetic alterations caused by drug–drug interactions: metabolic interactions in the liver. Pharmacol Rev 50:335–492 (1998).
24. Seppala T, Linnoila M, and Mattila MJ. Drugs, alcohol and driving. Drugs 17:389–408 (1979).
25. Sellers EM and Holloway MR. Drug kinetics and alcohol ingestion. Clin Pharmacokinet 3:440–452 (1978).
26. Griffin JP. Drug interactions occurring during absorption from the gastrointestinal tract. Pharmacol Ther 15:79–88 (1981).
27. Sitar DS. Human drug metabolism in vivo. Pharmacol Ther 43:363–375 (1989).
28. Mezey E. Ethanol metabolism and ethanol–drug interactions. Biochem Pharmacol 25:869–874 (1976).
29. Offerhaus L. Drug interactions at excretory mechanisms. Pharmacol Ther 15:69–78 (1981).
30. Orrenius S. Alcohol and drug interactions; basic concepts. In: Lieber CS, ed. Recent advances in the biology of alcoholism, Vol. 1, New York: Haworth, 1981:25–40.
31. Linnoila M, Mattila MJ, and Kitchell BS. Drug interactions with alcohol. Drugs 18:299–311 (1979).
32. Lieber CS. Interaction of alcohol with other drugs and nutrients: implications for the therapy of alcoholic liver disease. Drugs 40(Suppl 3):23–44 (1990).
33. Bloor JH, Mapoles JE, and Simon FR. Alcoholic liver disease: new concepts of pathogenesis and treatment. Adv Intern Med 39:49–92 (1994).
34. Hoyumpa AM and Schenker S. Major drug interactions: effect of liver disease, alcohol, and malnutrition. Ann Rev Med 33:113–149 (1982).
35. Howden CW, Birnie GG, and Brodie MJ. Drug metabolism in liver disease. Pharmacol Ther 40:439–474 (1989).
36. McLean AJ and Morgan DJ. Clinical pharmacokinetics in patients with liver disease. Clin Pharmacokinet 231:42–69 (1991).
37. Sonne J. Drug metabolism in liver disease. Implications for therapeutic drug monitoring. Therap Drug Monitor 18:397–401 (1996).

38. Mattila MJ. Alcohol and drug interactions. Ann Med 22:363–369 (1990).
39. Kalant H, LeBlanc SE, and Gibbins RJ. Tolerance to and dependence on some non-opiate psychotropic drugs. Pharmacol Rev 23:135–191 (1971).
40. Chesher G and Greeley J. Tolerance to the effects of alcohol. Alc Drugs Driving 8:93–106 (1992).
41. Lieber CS. Biochemical and molecular basis of alcohol-induced injury to liver and other tissues. N Engl J Med 319:1639–1650 (1988).
42. Lieber CS. Mechanism of ethanol induced hepatic injury. Pharmacol Ther 46:1–41 (1990).
43. Lieber CS. Hepatic, metabolic and nutritional disorders of alcoholism: from pathogenesis to therapy. Crit Rev Clin Lab Sci 37:551–584 (2000).
44. Forney RB and Hughes FW. Combined effects of alcohol and other drugs. Springfield, IL: Charles C. Thomas Publisher, 1968.
45. Pirola RC. Drug metabolism and alcohol. Baltimore: University Park Press, 1978.
46. Milner G. Drugs and driving. Basel, Switzerland: S. Karger, 1972.
47. Mattila MJ, ed. Alcohol, drugs and driving. Basel, Switzerland: S. Karger, 1976.
48. Morland J. Driving under the influence of non-alcohol drugs. Forensic Sci Rev 12:79–105 (2000).
49. Hemmelgaran B, Suissa S, Huang A, Boivin J-F, and Pinard G. Benzodiazepine use and the risk of motor vehicle crashes in the eldery. JAMA 278:27–31 (1997).
50. Sands BE, Knapp CM, and Ciraulo A. Medical consequences of alcohol–drug interactions. Alc Health Res World 17:316–320 (1993).
51. Lane EA, Guthrie S, and Linnoila M. Effects of ethanol on drug metabolite pharmacokinetics. Clin Pharmacokinet 10:228–247 (1985).
52. Fraser AG. Pharmacokinetic interactions between alcohol and other drugs. Clin Pharmacokinet 33:79–90 (1997).
53. Monroe ML and Doering PL. Effect of common over-the-counter medications on blood alcohol levels. Ann Pharmacother 35:918–924 (2001).
54. Weathermon R and Crabb DW. Alcohol and medication interactions. Alc Res Health 23:40–54 (1999).
55. Morland J, Bodd E, and Gadeholt G. Interaction of ethanol and drug metabolism. In: Crow KE and Batt RT, eds. Human metabolism of alcohol, Vol III. Boca Raton, FL: CRC Press, 1982:141–160.
56. Havier RG. The interaction of ethanol with drugs. Forensic Sci Rev 3:41–56 (1991).
57. Drummer OH and Odell M. Forensic pharmacology of drugs of abuse. London: Arnold, 2001.
58. Sands BF, Knapp CM, and Ciraulo DA. Interaction of alcohol with therapeutic drugs and drugs of abuse. Chapter 19 In: Kranzler HR, ed. The pharmacology of alcohol abuse. Berlin: Springer Verlag, 1995:475–512.
59. Baselt RC. Drug effects on psychomotor performance. Foster City, CA: Biomedical Publications, 2001.
60. Starmer GA and Bird KD. Investigating drug–alcohol interactions. Br J Clin Pharmacol 18:27S–35S (1984).
61. Kelly TH, Foltin RW, Emurian CS, and Fischman MW. Performance-based testing for drugs of abuse: dose and time profiles of marijuana, amphetamine, alcohol and diazepam. J Anal Toxicol 17:264–272 (1993).
62. Irving A and Jones W. Methods for testing impairment of driving due to drugs. Eur J Clin Pharmacol 43:61–66 (1992).
63. Kelly M, Myrsten AL, Neri A, and Rydberg U. Effects and after-effects of alcohol on psychological and physiological functions in man. Blutalkohol 7:422–436 (1970).

64. Hrobjartsson A and Gotzsche PC. Is the placebo powerless? An analysis of clinical trials comparing placebo with no treatment. N Engl J Med 344:1594–1602 (2001).
65. Moskowitz H and Fiorentino D. A review of the scientific literature regarding the effects of alcohol on driving-related behavior at blood alcohol concentrations of 0.08 grams per deciliter and lower. Washington, DC: U.S. Department of Transportation, National Highway Traffic Safety Administration, 2000.
66. Kennedy RS, Turnage JJ, Wilkes RL, and Dunlap WP. Effects of graded dosages of alcohol on nine computerized repeated-measures tests. Ergonomics 36:1195–1222 (1993).
67. Kunsman GW, Manno JE, Manno BR, Kunsman CM, and Przekop MA. The use of microcomputer-based psychomotor tests for the evaluation of benzodiazepine effects on human performance: a review with emphasisi on temazepine. Br J Clin Pharmacol 34:289–301 (1992).
68. Törnros J, Viklander B, Ahlner J, and Jönsson K-Å. Simulated driving performance of benzodiazepine users. J Traffic Med 29:4–15 (2001).
69. Robbe HWJ and O'Hanlon JF. Marijuana, alcohol and actual driving performance. Washington, DC: U.S. Department of Transportation, National Highway Traffic Safety Administration, DOT HS 808 939, 1999.
70. Farrell L and Logan BK, eds. The effects of drugs on human performance. Forensic Sci Rev 14:1–151 (2002).
71. Kalant H. Pharmacokinetics of ethanol: absorption, distribution, and elimination. In: Begleiter H and Kissin B, eds. The pharmacology of alcohol and alcohol dependence. Oxford & New York: Oxford University Press, 1996:15–58.
72. Ramchandani VA, Bosron WF, and Li T-K. Research advances in ethanol metabolism. Pathol Biol 49:676–682 (2001).
73. Widmark EMP. Principles and applications of medicolegal alcohol determination. Davis, CA: Biomedical Publications, 1981.
74. Berggren SM and Goldberg L. The absorption of ethyl alcohol from the gastrointestinal tract as a diffusion process. Acta Physiol Scand 1:245–270 (1940).
75. Holt S. Observations on the relation between alcohol absorption and the rate of gastric emptying. Can Med Assoc J 124:267–277 (1981).
76. Winek CL, Wahba WW, and Dowdell JL. Determinatiuon of absorption time of ethanol in social drinkers. Forens Sci Intern 77:169–177 (1996).
77. Jones AW, Jönsson KÅ, and Neri A. Peak blood-ethanol concentration and the time of its occurrence after rapid drinking on an empty stomach. J Forensic Sci 36:376–385 (1991).
78. Schwartz JG, Salman UA, McMahan CA, and Phillips WT. Gastric emptying of beer in Mexican-Americans compared with non-Hispanic whites. Metabolism 45:1174–1178 (1996).
79. Roine RP, Gentry RT, Lim RT, Baraona E, and Lieber CS. Effect of concentration of ingested ethanol on blood alcohol levels. Alcohol Clin Exp Res 15:734–738 (1991).
80. Roine RP, Gentry RT, Lim RT, Heikkonen E, Salaspuro M, and Lieber CS. Comparison of blood alcohol concentration after beer and whiskey. Alcohol Clin Exp Res 17:709–711 (1993).
81. Welling PG. Effects of food on drug absorption. Ann Rev Nutr 16:383–415 (1996).
82. Welling PG. Pharmacokinetics of alcohol following single low doses to fasted and nonfasted subjects. J Clin Pharmacol 17:199–206 (1977).
83. Singh BN. Effects of food on clinical pharmacokinetics. Clin Pharmacokinet 37:213–255 (1999).
84. Schultz J, Weiner H, and Wetscott J. Retardation of ethanol absorption by food in the stomach. J Stud Alcohol 41:861–870 (1980).

12. Alcohol and Drug Interactions

85. Cortot A, Jobin G, Ducrot F, Aymes C, Giraudeaux V, and Modigliani R. Gastric emptying and gastrointestinal absorption of alcohol ingested with a meal. Dig Dis Sci 31:343–348 (1986).
86. Jones AW and Jönsson KÅ. Food-induced lowering of blood-ethanol profiles and increased rate of elimination immediately after a meal. J Forensic Sci 39:1084–1093 (1994).
87. Jones AW, Jönsson K-Å, and Kechagias S. Effect of high-fat, high-protein and high-carbohydrate meals on the pharmacokinetics of a small dose of alcohol. Br J Clin Pharmacol 44:521–526 (1997).
88. Ramchandani VA, Kwo PY, and Li T-K. Effect of food and food composition on alcohol elimination rates in healthy men and women. J Clin Pharmacol 41:1345–1350 (2001).
89. Sedman AJ, Wilkinson PK, Sakmar DJ, Weidler DJ, and Wagner JG. Food effects on absorption and metabolism of alcohol. J Stud Alcohol 37:1197–1214 (1976).
90. Pikaar NA, Wedel M, and Heemus RJJ. Influence of several factors on blood alcohol concentrations after drinking alcohol. Alc Alcohol 23:289–297 (1988).
91. McFarlane A, Pooley L, Welch IML, Rumsey RDE, and Read NW. How does dietary lipid lower blood alcohol concentrations? Gut 27:15–18 (1986).
92. Rogers JO, Smith J, Starmer GA, and Whitfield J. Differing effects of carbohydrate fat and protein on the rate of ethanol metabolism. Alc Alcohol 22:345–353 (1987).
93. Wagner JG and Patel JA. Variations in absorption and elimination rates of ethyl alcohol in a single subject. Res Comm Chem Pathol Pharmacol 4:61–76 (1972).
94. O'Neill B, Williams AF, and Dubowski KM. Variability in blood alcohol concentration: implications for estimating individual results. J Stud Alcohol 44:222–230 (1983).
95. Friel PN, Baer JS, and Logan BK. Variability of ethanol absorption and breath concentrations during a large scale alcohol administration study. Alcohol Clin Exp Res 19:1055–1060 (1995).
96. Jones AW. Inter-individual variations in the disposition and metabolism of ethanol in healthy men. Alcohol 1:385–391 (1984).
97. Hahn RG, Norberg Å, and Jones AW. Over-shoot of ethanol in the blood after drinking on an empty stomach. Alc Alcohol 32:501–505 (1997).
98. Jones AW and Jönsson K-Å. Between subject and within subject variations in the pharmacokinetics of ethanol. Br J Clin Pharmacol 37:427–431 (1994).
99. Passananti GT, Wolff CA, and Vesell ES. Reproducibility of individual rates of ethanol metabolism in fasting subjects. Clin Pharmacol Ther 47:389–396 (1990).
100. Lotterle J, Husslein EM, Bolt J, and Wirtz PM. Tageszeitliche Unterschiede der Alkoholresorption. Blutalkohol 26:369–375 (1989).
101. Dawson GW and Vestal RE. Smoking and drug metabolism. Pharmacol Ther 15:207–221 (1981).
102. Johnson RD, Horowitz M, Maddox AF, Wishart JM, and Shearman DJC. Cigarette smoking and rate of gastric emptying—effect on alcohol absorption. Br Med J 302:20–23 (1991).
103. Scott AM, Kellow JE, Shuter B, Nolan JM, Hoschl R, and Jones MP. Effects of cigarette smoking on solid and liquid intragastric distribution and gastric emptying. Gastroenterology 104:410–416 (1993).
104. Rose EF. Factors influencing gastric emptying. J Forensic Sci 24:200–206 (1979).
105. Schvarcz E, Palmer M, Åman J, and Berne C. Hypoglycemia increases the gastric emptying rate in healthy subjects. Diabet Care 18:674–676 (1993).
106. Bailey DN. Effect of coadministered drugs and ethanol on the binding of therapeutic drugs to human serum in-vitro. Therap Drug Monitor 23:71–74 (2001).
107. Edelman IS and Leibman J. Anatomy of body water and electrolytes. Am J Med 27:256–277 (1959).

108. Lucey MR, Hill E, Young JP, Demo-Dananberg L, and Beresford TP. The influence of age and gender on blood ethanol concentrations in healthy humans. J Stud Alcohol 60: 103–110 (1999).
109. Kwo PY, Ramchandani VA, O'Connor S, Amann D, Carr LG, Sandrasegaran K, et al. Gender differences in alcohol metabolism: relationship to liver volume and effect of adjusting for body mass. Gastroenterology 115:1552–1557 (1998).
110. Mumenthaler MS, Taylor JL, and Yesavage JA. Ethanol pharmacokinetics in white women: nonlinear model fitting versus zero-order elimination analysis. Alcohol Clin Exp Res 24: 1353–1362 (2000).
111. Mumenthaler MS, O'Hara R, Taylor JL, Friedman L, and Yesavage JA. Influence of menstrual cycle on flight simulator performance after alcohol ingestion. J Stud Alcohol 62: 422–433 (2001).
112. Hobbes J, Boutagy J, and Shenfield GM. Interaction between ethanol and oral contraceptive steroids. Clin Pharmacol Ther 38:157–163 (1987).
113. Marshall AW, Kingstone D, Boss M, and Morgan MY. Ethanol elimination in males and females: relationship to menstrual cycle and body composition. Hepatology 5:701–706 (1983).
114. Winek CL and Carlagna M. Comparison of plasma, serum and whole blood ethanol concentrations. J Anal Toxicol 6:267–268 (1987).
115. Jones AW, Hahn RG, and Stalberg H. Distribution of ethanol and water between plasma and whole blood: inter- and intra-individual variations after administration of ethanol by intravenous infusion. Scand J Clin Lab Invest 50:775–780 (1990).
116. Wang MQ, Nicholson ME, Jones CS, Fitzhugh EC, and Westerfield CR. Acute alcohol intoxication, body composition, and pharmacokinetics. Pharm Biochem Behav 43:641–643 (1992).
117. Jones AW and Neri A. (1985). Age-related changes in blood-alcohol parameters and subjective feelings of intoxication in healthy men. Alc Alcohol 20:45–52 (1985).
118. Vestal RE, McGuire EA, Tobin NA, Andrea R, Norris AH, and Mezey E. Aging and ethanol metabolism. Clin Pharmacol Ther 21:343–354 (1977).
119. Endres HG and Gruner O. Comparison of D_2O and ethanol dilutions in total body water measurements in humans. Clin Investig 72:830–837 (1994).
120. Jones AW, Hahn RG, and Stalberg HP. Pharmacokinetics of ethanol in plasma and whole blood: estimation of total body water by the dilution principle. Eur J Clin Pharmacol 42: 445–448 (1992).
121. Chiou WL. The phenomenon and rationale of marked dependence of drug concentration on blood sampling site; implications in pharmacokinetics, pharmacodynamics, toxicology and therapeutics. Clin Pharmacokinet 17:175–199 (1989).
122. Mather LE. Anatomical-physiological approaches in pharmacokinetics and pharmacodynamics. Clin Pharmacokinet 40:707–722 (2001).
123. Jones AW, Norberg Å, and Hahn RG. Concentration-time profiles of ethanol in arterial and venous blood and end-expired breath during and after intravenous infusion. J Forensic Sci 42:1088–1094 (1997).
124. Meibohm B, Beierle I, and Derendorf H. How important are gender differences in pharmacokinetics? Clin Pharmacokinet 21:329–342 (2002).
125. Cheymol G. Effects of obesity on pharmacokinetics: implications for drug therapy. Clin Pharmacokinet 39:215–231 (2000).
126. Baraona E, Abittan CS, Dohmen K, Moretti M, Pozzato G, Chayes ZW, et al. Gender differences in pharmacokinetics of alcohol. Alcohol Clin Exp Res 25:502–507 (2001).
127. Wartburg Von J-P. Pharmacokinetics of alcohol. In: Batt RC and Crow KE, eds. Human metabolism of alcohol, Vol. 1: pharmacokinetics, medicolegal and general interests. Boca Raton, FL: CRC Press, 1989:9–22.

128. Droenmer P, Schmitt G, Aderjan R, and Zimmer H. A kinetic model describing the pharmacokinetics of ethyl glucuronide in humans. Forens Sci Intern 126:24–29 (2002).
129. Seidl S, Wurst FM, and Alt A. Ethyl glucuronide: a biological marker for recent alcohol consumption. Addict Biol 6:205–212 (2001).
130. Jones AW. Excretion of alcohol in urine and diuresis in healthy men in relation to their age, the dose administered and the time after drinking. Forens Sci Intern 45:217–224 (1990).
131. Matsumoto H and Fujui Y. Pharmacokinetics of ethanol a review of the methodology. Addict Biol 7:5–14 (2002).
132. Ehring T, Bosron WJ, and Li T-K. Alcohol and aldehyde dehydrogenase. Alc Alcohol 25:105–116 (1990).
133. Jörnvall H, Höög J-O, Persson B, and Pares X. Pharmacogenetics of the alcohol dehydrogenase system. Pharmacology 61:184–191 (2000).
134. Pettersson G. Liver alcohol dehydrogenase. CRC Critical Rev Biochem 21:349–389 (1987).
135. Jörnvall H and Höög JO. Nomenclature of alcohol dehydrogenase. Alc. Alcohol 30:153–161 (1995).
136. Holford NGH. Clinical pharmacokinetics of ethanol. Clin Pharmacokinet 13:273–292 (1987).
137. Wedel M, Pieters JE, Pikaar NA, and Ockhuizen T. Application of a three-compartment model to a study of the effects of sex, alcohol dose and concentration, exercise and food consumption on the pharmacokinetics of ethanol in healthy volunteers. Alc Alcohol 26:329–336 (1991).
138. Norberg Å, Jones AW, Hahn RG, and Gabrielsson J. Role of variability in explaining ethanol pharmacokinetics. Clin Pharmacokinet 42:1–31 (2003).
139. Lundquist F and Wolthers H. The kinetics of alcohol elimination in man. Acta Pharmacol Toxicol 14:265–289 (1958).
140. Wilkinson PK, Sedman AJ, Sakmar E, Kay DR, and Wagner JG. Pharmacokinetics of ethanol after oral administration in the fasting state. J Pharmacokinet Biopharm 5:207–224 (1977).
141. Wagner JG, Wilkinson PK, and Games DA. Parameters of V_{max} and k_m for elimination of alcohol in young male subjects following low doses of alcohol. Alc Alcohol 24:555–564 (1989).
142. Wilkinson PK. Pharmacokinetics of ethanol—a review. Alcohol Clin Exp Res 4:6–21 (1980).
143. Wagner JG. Lack of first-pass metabolism of ethanol at blood concentrations in the social drinking range. Life Sci 39:407–414 (1986).
144. Jacobsen D and McMartin KE. Methanol and ethylene glycol poisonings mechanism of toxicity clinical course diagnosis and treatment. Med Toxicol 1:309–334 (1986).
145. Eder AF, McGrath CM, Dowdy YG, Tomaszewski JE, Rosenberg FM, et al. Ethylene glycol poisoning: toxicokinetics and analytical factors affecting laboratory diagnosis. Clin Chem 44:168–177 (1998).
146. Karlson-Stibler C and Persson H. Ethylene glycol poisoning: experiences from an epidemic in Sweden. J Toxicol Clin Tox 30:565–574 (1992).
147. Zvosec DL, Smith SW, McCutcheon JR, Spillane J, Hall BJ, and Peacock EA. Adverse events, including death, associated with the use of 1,4-butanediol. N Engl J Med 344:87–94 (2002).
148. Nicholson KL and Balster RL. GHB: a new and novel drug of abuse. Drug Alc Dep 63:1–22 (2001).
149. Röe O. The metabolism and toxicity of methanol. Pharmacol Rev 7:399–412 (1955).
150. Mani JC, Pietruszko R, and Theorell H. Methanol activity of alcohol dehydrogenase from human liver, horse liver and yeast. Arch Biochem Biophys 140:52–59 (1970).

151. Fraser AD. Clinical toxicologic implications of ethylene glycol and glycolic acid poisoning. Therap Drug Monitor 24:232–238 (2002).
152. Jacobsen D and McMartin KE. Antidotes for methanol and ethylene glycol poisoning. J Toxicol Clin Tox 35:127–143 (1997).
153. Burkhart K. Methanol and ethylene glycol toxicity. J Toxicol Clin Tox 35:149–150 (1997).
154. Barceloux DG, Krenzelok EP, Olson K, and Watson WW. American academy of clinical toxicology practice guidelines on the treatment of ethylene glycol poisoning. J Toxicol Clin Tox 37:537–560 (1999).
155. Wiener HL and Richardson KE. The metabolism and toxicity of ethylene glycol. Res Commun Sub Abuse 9:77–87 (1988).
156. Majchrowicz E and Mendelson JH. Blood methanol concentrations during experimental induced ethanol intoxications in alcoholics. J Pharmacol Exp Ther 179:293–300 (1971).
157. Jones AW, Skaggerberg S, Yonekura A, and Sato A. Metabolic interaction between endogenous methanol and exogenous ethanol studied in human volunteers by analysis of breath. Pharmacol Toxicol 65:48–53 (1990).
158. Haffner H-T, Banger M, Graw M, Besserer K, and Brink T. The kinetics of methanol elimination in alcoholics and the influence of ethanol. Forens Sci Intern 89:129–136 (1997).
159. Jones AW and Sternebring B. Kinetics of ethanol and methanol in alcoholics during detoxication. Alc Alcohol 27:641–647 (1992).
160. Graw M, Haffner H-T, Althaus L, Besserer K, and Voges S. Invasion and distribution of ethanol. Arch Toxicol 74:313–321 (2000).
161. Haffner H-T, Besserer K, Graw M, and Voges S. Methanol elimination in non-alcoholics. Inter- and intra-individual variation. Forens Sci Intern 86:69–76 (1997).
162. Jones AW. Elimination half-life of methanol during hangover. Pharmacol Toxicol 60:217–220 (1987).
163. Blomstrand R, Ostling-Wintzell H, Lof A, McMartin K, Tolf BR, and Hedstrom KG. Pyrazoles as inhibitors of alcohol oxidation and as important tools in alcohol research: an approach to therapy against methanol poisoning. Proc Natl Acad Sci USA 76:3499–503 (1979).
164. Baud FJ, Galliot M, Astier A, VuBien D, Garnier R, Likforman J, et al. Treatment of ethylene glycol poisoning with intravenous 4-methylpyrazole. N Engl J Med 319:97–100 (1988).
165. Jobard E, Harry P, Turcant A, Roy PM, and Alain P. 4-methylpyrazole and hemodialysis in ethylene glycol poisoning. J Toxicol Clin Tox 34:373–377 (1996).
166. Bekka R, Borron SW, Astier A, Sandouk P, Bismuth C, and Baud FJ. Treatment of methanol and isopropanol poisoning with intravenous fomepizole. J Toxicol Clin Tox 39:59–67 (2001).
167. Brent J, McMartin K, Phillips S, Aaron C, and Kulig K. Fomepizole for the treatment of methanol poisoning. N Engl J Med 344:424–429 (2001).
168. Sarkola T and Eriksson CJP. Effect of 4-methyl pyrazole on endogenous plasma ethanol and methanol levels in humans. Alcohol Clin Exp Res 25:513–516 (2001).
169. Kaplan HL, Forney RB, Hughes FW, and Jain NC. Chloral hydrate and alcohol metabolism in human subjects. J Forensic Sci 12:295–304 (1967).
170. Sellers EM, Lang M, Koch-Weser J, LeBlanc E, and Kalant H. Interaction of chloral hydrate and ethanol in man. 1. Metabolism. Clin Pharmacol Ther 13:37–49 (1972).
171. Heller PF, Goldberger BA, and Caplan YH. Chloral hydrate overdose: trichloroethanol detection by gas chromatography-mass spectrometry. Forens Sci Intern 52:231–234 (1992).
172. Hawkins RD and Kalant H. The metabolism of ethanol and its metabolic effects. Pharmacol Rev 24:67–157 (1972).

173. Wartburg von JP and Bühler R. Biology of disease—alcoholism and aldehydism: new biomedical concepts. Lab Invest 50:5–15 (1984).
174. Crabbe DW, Edenberg HJ, Bosron WH, and Li T-K. Genotypes for aldehyde dehydrogenase deficiency and alcohol sensitivity. J Clin Invest 83;314–316 (1989).
175. Eriksson CJP. The role of acetaldehyde in the actions of alcohol (update 2000). Alcohol Clin Exp Res 25:15S–32S (2001).
176. Mizoi Y, Tatsuno T, Adachi J, Kogame M, Fukunaga T, Fujiwara S, et al. Alcohol sensitivity related to polymorphism of alcohol metabolizing enzymes in Japanese. Pharm Biochem Behav 18(Suppl 1):127–133 (1983).
177. Harada S, Agarwal DP, Normura F, and Higuchi S. Metabolic and ethnic determinants of alcohol drinking habits and vulnerability to alcohol-related disorders. Alcohol Clin Exp Res 25:71S–75S (2001).
178. Harada S, Agarwal DP, and Goedde HW. Aldehyde dehydrogenase deficiency as cause of facial flushing reaction to alcohol in Japanese. Lancet 2:982 (1981).
179. Bosron WF and Li T-K. Genetic polymorphism of human liver alcohol and aldehyde dehydrogenases and their relationship to alcohol metabolism and alcoholism. Hepatology 6: 502–510 (1986).
180. Goedde HW, Agarwal DP, and Harada S. Pharmacogenetics of alcohol sensitivity. Pharma-col Biochem Behav 18(Suppl 1):161–166 (1983).
181. Peachey JE and Sellers EM. The disulfiram and calcium carbimide acetaldehyde mediated ethanol reaction. Pharmacol Ther 15:89–97 (1981).
182. McBride WJ, Li T-K, Deitrich RA, Zimatkin S, Smith BR, and Rodd-Henricks ZA. Involvement of acetaldehyde in alcohol addiction. Alcohol Clin Exp Res 26:114–119 (2002).
183. Lindros KO. Human blood acetaldehyde levels. With improved methods a clearer picture emerges. Alcohol Clin Exp Res 7:70–75 (1983).
184. Hald J and Jacobsen E. A drug sensitizing the organism to ethyl alcohol. Lancet 2:1001–1004 (1948).
185. Yoshida A. Genetic polymorphisms of alcohol metabolizing enzymes related to alcohol sensitivity and alcoholic disease. Alc Alcohol 29:693–696 (1994).
186. Park CW and Riggio S. Disulfiram-ethanol induced delirium. Ann Pharmacother 35:32–35 (2001).
187. Jones AW, Neiman J, and Hillbom M. Concentration-time profiles of ethanol and acetaldehyde in human volunteers treated with the alcohol-sensitizing drug, calcium carbimide. Br J Clin Pharmacol 25:213–221 (1988).
188. Jones AW. Drug-alcohol flush reaction and breath-acetaldehyde concentration: no interference with an infrared breath-alcohol analyzer. J Anal Toxicol 10:98–101 (1986).
189. Lindros KO, Stowell A, Pikkarainen P, and Salaspuro M. The disulfiram (antabus) alcohol reaction in male alcoholics: its efficient management by 4-methyl pyrazole. Alcohol Clin Exp Res 5:528–530 (1981).
190. Heath MJ, Pachar JV, Perez-Martinez AL, and Toseland PA. An exceptional case of lethal disulfiram alcohol reaction. Forens Sci Int 56:45–50 (1992).
191. Yamamoto H, Tangegashima A, Hosoe H, and Fukunaga T. Fatal acute alcohol intoxication in an ALDH2 heterozygote: a case report. Forens Sci Intern 112:201–207 (2000).
192. Jerntorp P. The chlorpropamide alcohol flush test in diabetes mellitus: methods for objective evaluation. Scand J Clin Lab Invest 43:249–254 (1984).
193. Groop L, Eriksson CJP, Boll-Wåhlin E, and Melander A. Chlorpropamide-alcohol flush: significance of body weight, sex, and serum chlorpropamide level. Eur J Clin Pharmacol 26:723–725 (1984).

194. Jerntorp P, Ohlin H, Sundkvist G, and Almer LO. Effects of chlorpropamide and alcohol on aldehyde dehydrogenase activity and blood acetaldehyde concentration. Diabetes Res 3:369–372 (1986).
195. Chen Z, Zhang J, and Stamler JS. Identification of the enzymatic mechanism of nitroglycerine bioactivation. Proc Natl Acad Sci USA 99:8306–8311 (2002).
196. Williams CS and Woodcock KR. Do ethanol and metronidazole interact to produce a disulfiram-like reaction? Ann Pharmacother 34:255–257 (2000).
197. Cina SJ, Russell RA, and Conradi SE. Sudden death due to metronidazole–ethanol interaction. Am J Forens Med Pathol 17:343–346 (1996).
198. Visapää J-P, Tillonen JS, Kalhovaara PS, and Salaspuro MP. Lack of disulfiram-like reaction with metronidazole and ethanol. Ann Pharmacother 36:971–974 (2002).
199. Lieber CS. Cytochrome P4502E1: its physiological and pathological role. Physiol Rev 77: 517–544 (1997).
200. Lieber CS. Microsomal ethanol-oxidizing system (MEOS): the first 30 years (1958–1998) —a review. Alcohol Clin Exp Res 23:991–1007 (1999).
201. Spatzenegger M and Jaeger W. Clinical importance of hepatic cytochrome P450 in drug metabolism. Drug Metab Rev 27:397–417 (1995).
202. Bertilsson L, Dahl M-L, Dalen P, and Al-Shurbaji A. Molecular genetics of CYP2D6: clinical relevance with focus on psychotropic drugs. Br J Clin Pharmacol 53:111–122 (2001).
203. Cho AK, Narimatsu S, and Kumagai Y. Metabolism of drugs of abuse by cytochromes P450. Addict Biol 4:283–301 (1999).
204. Gonzalez FJ. The molecular biology of cytochrome P450s. Pharmacol Rev 40:243–288 (1989).
205. Teschke R and Gellert J. Hepatic microsomal ethanol-oxidizing system (MEOS): metabolic aspects and clinical implications. Alcohol Clin Exp Res 10:20S–32S (1986).
206. Guengerich EP. Cytochrome P450 enzymes. Am Sci 81:440–447 (1993).
207. Landrum-Michalets E. Update: clinically significant cytochrome P-450 drug interactions. Pharmacotherapy 18:84–112 (1998).
208. Barry M and Feely J. Enzyme induction and inhibition. Pharmacol Ther 48:71–94 (1990).
209. Lin JH and Lu AYH. Inhibition and induction of cytochrome P450 and the clinical implications. Clin Pharmacokinet 35:361–390 (1998).
210. Lin JH and Lu AYH. Interindividual variability in inhibition and induction of cytochrome P450 enzymes. Ann Rev Pharmacol 41:535–567 (2001).
211. Murray M and Reidy GF. Selectivity in the inhibition of mammalian cytochromes P-450 by chemical agents. Pharmacol Rev 42:85–101 (1990).
212. Park BK, Pirmohamed M, and Kitteringham NR. The role of cytochrome P450 enzymes in hepatic and extrahepatic human drug toxicity. Pharmacol Ther 58:385–424 (1995).
213. Park BK, Kitteringham NR, Pirmohamed M, and Tucker GT. Relevance of induction of human drug-metabolizing enzymes: pharmacological and toxicological implications. Br J Clin Pharmacol 41:477–491 (1996).
214. Park DV, Ioannides C, and Lewis DFV. The role of the cytochrome P450 in the detoxication and activation of drugs and other chemicals. Can J Physiol Pharmacol 69:537–549 (1991).
215. Oneta CM, Lieber AS, Li J, Rüttimann S, Schmid B, Lattmann J, et al. Dynamics of cytochrome P4502E1 activity in man: induction by ethanol and disappearance during withdrawal phase. J Hepatol 36:47–52 (2002).
216. Pelkonen O and Sotaniemi E. Drug metabolism in alcoholics. Pharmacol Ther 16:261–268 (1982).

12. Alcohol and Drug Interactions

217. Keiding S, Christensen NJ, Damgaard SE, Dejgård A, Iversen HL, Jacobsen A, et al. Ethanol metabolism in heavy drinkers after massive and moderate alcohol intake. Biochem Pharmacol 32:3097–3102 (1983).
218. Morgon DJ and McLean AJ. Clinical pharmacokinetics and pharmacodynamic considerations in patients with liver disease: an update. Clin Pharmacokinet 29:370–391 (1995).
219. Tanaka E, Terada M, and Misawa S. Cytochrome P450 2E1: its clinical and toxicological role. J Clin Pharm Therap 25:165–175 (2000).
220. Klotz U and Ammon E. Clinical and toxicological consequences of the inductive potential of ethanol. Eur J Clin Pharmacol 54:7–12 (1998).
221. Nakajima T. Cytochrome P450 isoforms and the metabolism of volatile hydrocarbons of low relative molecular mass. J Occup Health 99:83–91 (1997).
222. Salmela KS, Kessova IG, Tsyrlov IB, and Lieber CS. Respective roles of human cytochrome P4502E1 1A2 and 3A4 in the hepatic microsomal oxidizing system. Alcohol Clin Exp Res 22:2125–2132 (1998).
223. Slattery JT, Nelson SD, and Thummel KE. The complex interaction between ethanol and acetaminophen. Clin Pharmacol Ther 60:241–246 (1996).
224. Prescott LF. Paracetamol, alcohol and the liver. Br J Clin Pharmacol 49:291–301 (2000).
225. Makin AJ and Williams R. Acetaminophen-induced hepatotoxicity: predisposing factors and treatments. Adv Intern Med 42:3433–3483 (1997).
226. Schmidt LE and Dalhoff K. Concomitant overdosing of other drugs in patients with paracetamol poisoning. Br J Clin Pharmacol 53:535–541 (2002).
227. Riordan SM and Williams R. Alcohol exposure and paracetamol-induced hepatotoxicity. Addict Biol 7:191–206 (2002).
228. Thomas SHL. Paracetamol (acetaminophen) poisoning. Pharmacol Ther 60:91–120 (1993).
229. Vale JA and Proundfoot AT. Paracetamol (acetaminophen) poisoning. Lancet 346:547–552 (1995).
230. Zimmerman HJ and Maddrey WC. Acetaminophene (paracetamol) hepatotoxicity with regular intake of alcohol: analysis of instances of therapeutic misadventure. Hepatology 22: 767–773 (1995).
231. Seeff LB, Cuccherini BA, Zimmerman HJ, Adler E, and Benjamin SB. Acetaminophene hepatotoxicity in alcoholics. Ann Intern Med 104:399–404 (1986).
232. Rumack BH. Acetaminophen hepatotoxicity: the first 35 years. Clin Toxicol 40:3–20 (2002).
233. Makin AJ, Wendon J, and Williams R. A 7-year experience of severe acetaminophene-induced hepatotoxicity (1987–1993). Gastroenterology 109:1907–1916 (1995).
234. Jones AL. Mechanism of action and value of N-acetylcysteine in the treatment of early and late acetaminophene poisoning: a critical review. J Toxicol Clin Toxicol 36:277–285 (1998).
235. Whitcomb DC and Block GD. Association of acetaminophen hepatotoxicity with fasting and ethanol use. JAMA 272:1845–1850 (1994).
236. Thummel KE, Slattery JT, Ro H, Chien JY, Nelson SD, Lown KE, and Watkins PB. Ethanol and production of the hepatoxic metabolite of acetaminophene in healthy adults. Clin Pharmacol Ther 67:591–599 (2000).
237. Janes J and Routledge PA. Recent developments in the management of paracetamol (acetaminophene) poisoning. Drug Safety 7:170–177 (1992).
238. Jones AL. Recent advances in the management of poisoning. Therap Drug Monitor 24: 150–155 (2002).
239. Pond SM and Tozer TN. First-pass elimination; basic concepts and clinical consequences. Clin Pharmacokinet 9:1–25 (1984).

240. Lin JH, Chiba M, and Baillie TA. Is the role of the small intestine in first-pass metabolism overemphasized? Pharmacol Rev 51:135–157 (1999).
241. Baraona E, Gentry RT, and Lieber CS. Bioavailability of alcohol: role of gastric metabolism and its interaction with other drugs. Dig Dis 12:351–367 (1994).
242. Julkunen RJK, Dipadova C, and Lieber CS. First pass metabolism of ethanol—a gastrointestinal barrier against the systemic toxicity of ethanol. Life Sci 37:567–573 (1985).
243. Frezza M, Dipadova C, Pozzato G, Terpin M, Baraona E, and Lieber CS. High blood alcohol levels in women—the role of decreased gastric alcohol dehydrogenase activity and first-pass metabolism. N Engl J Med 322:95–99 (1990).
244. DiPadova C, Roine R, Frezza M, Gentry RT, Baraona E, and Lieber CS. Effects of ranitidine on blood alcohol levels after ethanol ingestion. Comparison with other H2-receptor antagonists. JAMA 267:83–86 (1992).
245. Hempel JD and Pietruszko R. Human stomach alcohol dehydrogenase: isoenzyme composition and catalytic properties. Alcohol Clin Exp Res 3:95–98 (1979).
246. Gentry RT, Baraona E, and Lieber CS. Gastric first pass metabolism of alcohol. J Lab Clin Med 123:21–26 (1994).
247. Lieber CS, Gentry RT, and Barana E. First pass metabolism of ethanol. Alc Alcohol Suppl 2:163–169 (1994).
248. Caballeria J, Frezza M, Hernandez-Munoz R, Dipadova C, Korsten MA, Baraona E, and Lieber CS. Gastric origin of the first-pass metabolism of ethanol in humans: effect of gastrectomy. Gastroenterology 97:1205–1209 (1989).
249. Roine R, Gentry RT, Hernandez-Munoz R, Baraona E, and Lieber CS. Aspirin increases blood alcohol concentrations in humans after ingestion of ethanol. JAMA 264:2406–2408 (1990).
250. DiPadova C, Worner TM, Julkunen RJK, and Lieber CS. Effects of fasting and chronic alcohol consumption on the first-pass metabolism of ethanol. Gastroenterology 92:1169–1173 (1987).
251. Julkunen RJK, Tannenbaum L, Baraona E, and Lieber CS. First-pass metabolism of ethanol: an important determinant of blood levels after alcohol consumption. Alcohol 2:437–441 (1985).
252. Lim RT, Gentry RT, Ito D, Yokoyarna H, Baraona E, and Lieber CS. First-pass metabolism of ethanol is predominantly gastric. Alcohol Clin Exp Res 17:1337–1344 (1993).
253. Lieber CS. Gastritis in the alcoholic, relationship to gastric alcohol metabolism and helicobacter pylori. Add Biol 3:423–434 (1998).
254. Levitt MD. Do histamine-2 receptor antagonists influence the metabolism of ethanol. Ann Intern Med 118:564–565 (1993).
255. Levitt MD. The case against first-pass metabolism of ethanol in the stomach. J Lab Clin Med 123:28–31 (1994).
256. Levitt MD and Levitt DG. The critical role of the rate of ethanol absorption in the interpretation of studies purporting to demonstrate gastric metabolism of ethanol. J Pharmacol Exp Ther 269:297–304 (1994).
257. Levitt MD and Levitt DG. Appropriate use and misuse of blood concentration measurements to quantitate first-pass metabolism. J Lab Clin Med 136:275–280 (2000).
258. Gupta AM, Baraona E, and Lieber CS. Significant increase of blood alcohol by cimetidine after repetitive drinking of small alcohol doses. Alcohol Clin Exp Res 19:1083–1087 (1995).
259. Arora S, Baraona E, and Lieber CS. Alcohol levels are increased in social drinkers receiving ranitidine. Am J Gastroenterol 95:208–213 (2000).
260. Oneta CM, Simanowski UA, Martinez M, Allali-Hassani A, Pares X, Homann N, et al. First pass metabolism of ethanol is strikingly influenced by the speed of gastric emptying. Gut 43:612–619 (1998).

12. Alcohol and Drug Interactions

261. Horowitz M, Maddox A, Bochner M, Wishart J, Bratasuik K, Collins P, et al. Relationship between gastric emptying of solid and caloric liquid meals and alcohol absorption. Am J Physiol 257:G291–G298 (1989).
262. Mattila MJ and Venho VMK. Drug absorption from abnormal gastrointestinal tract. Prog Pharmacol 2:63–86 (1979).
263. Petring OU and Flachs H. Intersubject and intrasubject variability of gastric emptying in healthy volunteers measured by scintigraphy and paracetamol absorption. Br J Clin Pharmacol 29:703–708 (1990).
264. Lartigue S, Bizais Y, Desvarannes SB, Murat A, Pouliquen B, and Galmiche JP. Inter- and intrasubject variability of solid and liquid gastric emptying parameters—a scintigraphic study in healthy subjects and diabetic patients. Dig Dis Sci 39:109–115 (1994).
265. Elashoff JD, Reedy TJ, and Meyer JH. Analysis of gastric emptying data. Gastroenterology 83:1306–1312 (1982).
266. Madsen JL. Effects of gender, age, and body mass index on gastrointestinal transit times. Dig Dis Sci 37:1548–1553 (1992).
267. Goo RH, Moore JG, Greenberg E, and Alazraki NP. Circadian variations in gastric emptying of meals in humans. Gastroenterology 93:515–518 (1987).
268. Hunt JN and Stubbs DF. The volume and energy content of meals as determinants of gastric emptying. J Physiol 245:209–225 (1975).
269. Ammon E, Schäfer C, Hoffmann U, and Klotz U. Disposition and first pass metabolism of ethanol in humans: is it gastric or hepatic and does it depend on gender? Clin Pharmacol Ther 59:503–513 (1996).
270. Rinetti M, Ugolotti G, Calbiani B, Colombi-Zinelli L, Cisternino M, and Papa N. Anti-inflammatory drugs and gastric emptying. A comparison between acetylsalicylic acid and carprofen. Arzneimittelforschung 32:1561–1563 (1982).
271. Pfeiffer A, Högl B, and Kaess H. Effect of ethanol and commonly ingested alcoholic beverages on gastric emptying and gastrointestinal transit. Clin Investig 70:487–491 (1992).
272. Mascord D, Smith J, Starmer G, and Whitfield J. Effect of increasing the alcohol metabolism rate on plasma acetate concentration. Alc Alcohol 27:25–28 (1992).
273. O'Conner S, Morzorati S, Christian J, and Li K. Clamping breath alcohol concentration reduces experimental variance: application to the study of acute tolerance to alcohol and alcohol elimination rate. Alcohol Clin Exp Res 22:202–210 (1998).
274. Svensson CK, Edwards DJ, Mauriello PM, Barde SH, Foster AC, Lanc RA, et al. Effect of food on hepatic blood flow. Implications in the "food effect" phenomenon. Clin Pharmacol Ther 34:316–323 (1983).
275. Palmer RH, Frank WO, Nambi P, Wetherington JD, and Fox MJ. Effects of various concomitant medications on gastric alcohol dehydrogenase and the first-pass metabolism of ethanol. Am J Gastroenterol 86:1749–1755 (1991).
276. Melander O, Liden A, and Melander A. Pharmacokinetic interactions of alcohol and acetylsalicylic acid. Eur J Clin Pharmacol 48:151–153 (1995).
277. Gentry RT, Baraona E, Amir I, Roine R, Chayes ZW, Sharma R, and Lieber CS. Mechanism of the aspirin-induced rise in blood alcohol levels. Life Sci 65:2505–2512 (1999).
278. Kechagias S, Jönsson K-Å, Norlander B, Carlsson B, and Jones AW. Low-dose aspirin decreases blood alcohol concentrations by delaying gastric emptying. Eur J Clin Pharmacol 53:241–246 (1997).
279. Barron SE, Perry JR, and Ferslew KE. The effect of ibuprofen on ethanol concentration and elimination rate. J Forensic Sci 37:432–435 (1992).
280. Minocha A, Barth JT, Herold DA, Gideon DA, and Spyker DA. Modulation of ethanol-induced central nervous system depression by ibuprofen. Clin Pharmacol Ther 39:123–127 (1986).

281. Greiff JMC and Rowbotham D. Pharmacokinetic drug interactions with gastrointestinal motility modifying agents. Clin Pharmacokinet 27:447–461 (1994).
282. Griffiths GH, Owen GM, Campbell H, and Shields R. Gastric emptying in health and in gastroduodenal disease. Gastroenterology 54:1–7 (1968).
283. Madsen JL. Effects of cisapride on gastrointestinal transit in healthy humans. Dig Dis Sci 35:1500–1504 (1990).
284. McCallum RW, Prakash C, Campoli-Richards DM, and Goa KL. Cisapride. A preliminary review of its pharmacodynamic and pharmacokinetic properties, and therapeutic use as a prokinetic agent in gastrointestinal motility disorders. Drugs 36:652–681 (1988).
285. Dziekan G, Contesse J, Werth B, Schwarzer G, and Reinhart WH. Cisapride increases peak plasma and saliva ethanol levels under fasting conditions. J Intern Med 242:479–482 (1997).
286. Kechagias S, Jönsson KÅ, and Jones AW. Impact of gastric emptying on the pharmacokinetics of ethanol as influenced by cisapride. Br J Clin Pharmacol 48:728–732 (1999).
287. Deponti F, Giaroni C, Cosentino M, Lecchini S, and Frigo G. Calcium-channel blockers and gastrointestinal motility—basic and clinical aspects. Pharmacol Ther 60:121–148 (1993).
288. Bauer LA, Schumock G, Horn J, and Opheim K. Verapamil inhibits ethanol elimination and prolongs the perception of intoxication. Clin Pharmacol Ther 52:6–10 (1992).
289. Perez-Reyes M, White WR, and Hicks RE. Interaction between ethanol and calcium channel blockers in humans. Alcohol Clin Exp Res 16:769–775 (1992).
290. Edelbroek MAL, Horowitz M, Wishart JM, and Akkermans LMA. Effects of erythromycin on gastric emptying, alcohol absorption and small intestinal transit in normal subjects. J Nucl Med 34:582–588 (1993).
291. Peeters T, Matthijs G, Depoortere I, Cachet T, Hoogmartens J, and Vantrappen G. Erythromycin is a motilin receptor agonist. Am J Physiol 257:G470–G474 (1989).
292. Urbain JL, Vantrappen G, Janssens J, Van Cutsem E, Peeters T, and De Roo M. Intravenous erythromycin dramatically accelerates gastric emptying in gastroparesis diabeticorum and normals and abolishes the emptying discrimination between solids and liquids. J Nucl Med 31:1490–1493 (1990).
293. Smith SR and Kendall MJ. Ranitidine and cimetidine: a comparison of their potential to cause clinically important drug interactions. Clin Pharmacokinet 15:44–56 (1988).
294. Amir I, Anwar N, Baraona E, and Lieber CS. Ranitidine increases the bioavailability of imbibed alcohol by accelerating gastric emptying. Life Sci 58:511–518 (1996).
295. Bye A, Lacey LF, Gupta S, and Powell JR. Effect of ranitidine hydrochloride (150 mg twice daily) on the pharmacokinetics of increasing doses of ethanol (0.15, 0.3, 0.6 g kg^{-1}). Br J Clin Pharmacol 41:129–133 (1996).
296. Toon S, Khan AZ, Holt BI, Mullins FG, Langley SJ, and Rowland MM. Absence of effect of ranitidine on blood alcohol concentrations when taken morning, midday, or evening with or without food. Clin Pharmacol Ther 55:385–391 (1994).
297. Raufman JP, Notarfrancesco V, Raffaniello RD, and Straus EW. Histamine-2 receptor antagonists do not alter serum ethanol levels in fed, non-alcoholic men. Ann Intern Med 118:488–494 (1993).
298. Tanaka E and Nakamura K. Effects of H-2 receptor antagonists on ethanol metabolism in Japanese volunteers. Br J Clin Pharmacol 26:96–99 (1988).
299. Somogyi A and Muirhead M. Pharmacokinetic interactions of cimetidine. Clin Pharmacokinet 12:321–366 (1987).
300. Hernandez-Munoz R, Caballeria J, Baraona E, Uppal R, Greenstein R, and Lieber CS. Human gastric alcohol dehydrogenase—its inhibition by H$_2$-receptor antagonists, and its effect on the bioavailability of ethanol. Alcohol Clin Exp Res 14:946–950 (1990).

12. Alcohol and Drug Interactions

301. Caballeria J, Baraona E, Rodamilans M, and Lieber CS. Effects of cimetidine on gastric alcohol dehydrogenase activity and blood ethanol levels. Gastroenterology 96:388–392 (1989).
302. Stone CL, Hurley TD, Peggs CF, Kedishvili NY, Davis GJ, Thomasson HR, et al. Cimetidine inhibition of human gastric and liver alcohol dehydrogenase isoenzymes: identification of inhibitor complexes by kinetics and molecular modeling. Biochemistry 34: 4008–4014 (1995).
303. Dauncey H, Chesher GB, and Palmer RH. Cimetidine and ranitidine: lack of effect on the pharmacokinetics of an acute ethanol dose. J Clin Gastroenterol 17:189–194 (1993).
304. Fraser AG, Hudson M, Sawyerr AM, Smith M, Rosalki SB, and Pounder RE. Ranitidine, cimetidine, famotidine have no effect on post-prandial absorption of ethanol 0.8 g/kg taken after an evening meal. Aliment Pharmacol Therapeut 6:693–700 (1992).
305. Fraser AG, Prewett EJ, Hudson M, Sawyerr AM, Rosalki SB, and Pounder RE. The effect of ranitidine, cimetidine or famotidine on low-dose post-prandial alcohol absorption. Aliment Pharmacol Therapeut 5:263–272 (1991).
306. Clemmesen JO, Ott P, and Sestoft L. The effect of cimetidine on ethanol concentrations in fasting women and men after two different doses of alcohol. Scand J Gasteroenterol 32:217–220 (1997).
307. Casini A, Pizzigallo AM, Mari F, Bertol E, and Surrenti C. Prolonged bedtime treatment with H_2-receptor antagonists (ranitidine and famotidine) dose not affect blood alcohol levels after ethanol ingestion in male patients with duodenal ulcer. Am J Gastroenterol 89: 745–749 (1994).
308. Sharma R, Gentry RT, Lim RT, and Lieber CS. First-pass metabolism of ethanol: absence of diurnal variation and its inhibition by cimetidine after evening meal. Dig Dis Sci 40: 2091–2097 (1995).
309. Seitz HK, Bösche J, Czygan P, Veith S, Simon B, and Kommerell B. Increased blood ethanol levels following cimetidine but not ranitidine. Lancet 1:760 (1983).
310. Seitz HK, Veith S, Czygan P, Bösche J, Simon B, Gugler R, and Kommerell B. In-vivo interactions between H2-receptor antagonists and ethanol metabolism in man and in rats. Hepatology 4:1231–1233 (1984).
311. Feely J and Wood AJJ. Effects of cimetidine on the elimination and actions of ethanol. JAMA 247:2819–2821 (1982).
312. Webster LK, Jones BD, and Smallwood RA. Influence of cimetidine and ranitidine on ethanol pharmacokinetics. Austr NZ J Med 15:359–360 (1985).
313. Dobrilla G, de Pretis G, Piazzi L, et al. Is ethanol metabolism affected by oral administration of cimetidine and ranitidine at therapeutic doses? Hepatogastroenterology 31:35–37 (1984).
314. Jönsson K-Å, Jones AW, Boström KL, and Andersson T. Lack of effect of omeprazole, cimetidine and ranitidine on the pharmacokinetics of ethanol in fasting male volunteers. Eur J Clin Pharmacol 42:209–212 (1992).
315. Fraser AG. Is there an interaction between H_2-antagonists and alcohol? Drug Metabol Drug Interactions 14:123–145 (1998).
316. Crabbe DW. First-pass metabolism of ethanol; Gastric or hepatic: mountain or molehill. Gasterenterology 25:1292–1294 (1997).
317. Antkowiak B. How do general anaesthetic work? Naturwissenschaften 88:201–213 (2001).
318. Urban BW and Bleckween M. Concepts and correlations relevant to general anaesthesia. Br J Anesth 89:3–16 (2002).
319. Little HJ. Mechanisms that may underlie the behavioural effects of ethanol. Prog Neurbiol 36:171–194 (1991).

320. Lüddens H, Pritchett DB, Köhler M, Killisch I, et al. Cerebellar GABA$_A$ receptor selective for a behavioural alcohol antagonist. Nature 346:648–651 (1990).
321. Bormann J. The ABC of GABA receptors. Trends Pharmacol Sci 21:16–19 (2000).
322. Pritchett DB, Sontheimer H, Shivers BD, Ymer S, et al. Importance of a novel GABA$_A$ receptor subunit for benzodiazepine pharmacology. Nature 338:582–585 (1989).
323. Meheta AK and Ticku MK. An update on GABA$_A$ receptors. Brain Res Bull 29:196–217 (1999).
324. Rudolph U, Crestani F, and Möhler H. GABA$_A$ receptor subtypes: dissecting their pharmacological functions. Trends Pharmacol Sci 22:188–194 (2001).
325. Hobbs WR, Rall TW, and Verdoorn TA. Hypnotics and sedatives; ethanol. In: Goodman & Gilman's The pharmacological basis of therapeutics, 9th ed. New York: McGraw-Hill, 1996:361–396.
326. Byatt C and Volans G. ABC of poisoning: sedative and hypnotic drugs. Br Med J 289:1214–1217 (1984).
327. Gary NE and Tresznewsky O. Barbiturates and a potpourri of other sedative, hypnotics, and tranquilizers. Heart & Lung 12:122–127 (1983).
328. Bailey L, Ward M, and Musa MN. Clinical pharmacokinetics of benzodiazepines. J Clin Pharmacol 34:804–911 (1994).
329. Johnson HRM. At what blood levels does alcohol kill? Med Sci Law 25:127–130 (1985).
330. Odesanmi WO. The fatal blood alcohol level in acute poisoning. Med Sci Law 23:25–30 (1983).
331. Kalant H. Research on tolerance: what can we learn from history. Alcohol Clin Exp Res 22:67–76 (1998).
332. Mellanby E. Alcohol: its absorption into and disappearance from the blood under different conditions. Special report, Series No. 31, London: National Safety Council 1919.
333. Jones AW. The drunkest drinking driver in Sweden; blood alcohol concentration 0.545 % w/v. J Studies Alc 60:400–406 (1999).
334. Urso T, Gavaler JS, and Van Thiel DH. Blood ethanol levels in sober alcohol users seen in an emergency room. Life Sci 28:1053–1056 (1985).
335. Jones AW. Alcohol; post-mortem. In: Encyclopedia of forensic sciences. London: Academic Press, 2000:112–126.
336. Ward ME and Cowley AR. Hypothermia: a natural cause of death. Am J Forens Med Pathol 20:383–386 (1999).
337. Gallaher MM, Fleming DW, Berger LR, and Sewell CM. Pedestrian and hypothermia deaths among native Americans in New Mexico. JAMA 267:1345–2348 (1992).
338. Kortelainen ML. Drugs and alcohol in hyporthermia and hypethermia related deaths. A retrospective study. J Forensic Sci 32:1704–1712 (1987).
339. Kalant H and Le AD. Effects of ethanol on thermoregulation. Pharmacol Ther 23:313–364 (1984).
340. Larach MG. Accidental hypothermia. Lancet 345:493–498 (1995).
341. Teige B and Fleischer E. Blodkonsentrasjoner ved akutte forgiftningsdodsfall. Tidsskr Nor Laegeforen 103:679–685 (1983).
342. Thomsen JL, Theilade P, Felby S, and Nielsen E. Alcoholic ketoacidosis as a cause of death in forensic cases. Forens Sci Intern 75:163–171 (1995).
343. Thomsen JL. Various mechanisms of death and their possible association with alcoholism. Forens Sci Intern 79:199–204 (1996).
344. Pounder DJ, Stevenson RJ, and Taylor KK. Alcoholic ketoacidosis at autopsy. J Forensic Sci 43:812–816 (1998).
345. Brinkmann B, Fechner G, Karger B, and DuChesne A. Ketoacidosis and lactic acidosis—frequent causes of death in chronic alcoholics? Int J Leg Med 111:115–119 (1998).

12. Alcohol and Drug Interactions

346. Lahti RA and Vuori E. Fatal alcohol poisoning: medico-legal practices and mortality statistics. Forens Sci Intern 126:203–209 (2002).
347. Höjer J, Baehrendtz S, and Gustafsson L. Benzodiazepine poisoning: experience of 702 admissions to an intensive care unit during a 14-year period. J Intern Med 226:117–122 (1989).
348. Buckley NA, Dawson AH, Whyte IM, and O'Connell DL. Relative toxicity of benzodiazepines in overdose. Br Med J 310:219–221 (1995).
349. Serfaty M and Masterton G. Fatal poisonings attributed to benzodiazepines in Britain during the 1980s. Br J Psyciatr 163:383–393 (1993).
350. Drummer OH and Ranson DL. Sudden death and benzodiazepines. Am J Forens Med Pathol 7:336–342 (1996).
351. Druid H, Holmgreen P, and Ahlner J. Flunitrazepam: an evaluation of use, abuse and toxicity. Forens Sci Intern 122:136–141 (2001).
352. Tanaka E. Toxicological interactions between alcohol and benzodiazepines. J Toxicol Clin Toxicol 40:69–75 (2002).
353. Caplan YH, Ottinger WE, and Crooke CR. Therapeutic and toxic drug concentrations in post mortem. A six year study in the state of Maryland. J Anal Toxicol 7:225–230 (1983).
354. Jonasson B, Jonasson U, and Saldeen T. The manner of death among fatalities where dextropropoxyphene caused or contributed to death. Forens Sci Intern 96:181–187 (1998).
355. Jonasson U, Jonasson B, Holmgren P, and Saldeen T. The prevalence of dextropropoxyphene in autopsy blood samples. Forens Sci Intern 96:135–142 (1998).
356. Sturner WQ and Garriott JC. Deaths involving propoxyphene: a study of 41 cases over a two-year period. JAMA 223:1125–1130 (1973).
357. Buckley BM and Vale JA. Dextropropoxyphene poisoning: problems with interpretation of analytical data. Hum Toxicol 3:95–101 (1984).
358. Young RJ. Dextropropoxyphene overdosage: pharmacological considerations and clinical management. Drugs 26:70–79 (1983).
359. Finkle BS, Caplan YH, Garriott JC, Montforte JR, Shaw RF, and Sonsalla PK. Propoxyphene in postmortem toxicology 1976–1978. J Forensic Sci 26:739–757 (1981).
360. Finkle BS. Self-poisoning with dextropropoxyphene and dextropropoxyphene compounds. Hum Toxicol Supp 115S–134S (1984).
361. Tallman JF, Paul SM, Skolnick P, and Gallager DW. Receptors for the age of anxiety: pharmacology of the benzodiazepines. Science 207:274–281 (1980).
362. Koski A, Ojanperä I, and Vuori E. Alcohol and benzodiazepines in fatal poisonings. Alcohol Clin Exp Res 26:956–959 (2002).
363. Drummer OK, Syrjanen ML, and Cordner SM. Deaths involving the benzodiazepine flunitrazepam. Am J Forens Med Pathol 14:238–243 (1993).
364. Carmen Del Rio M, Prada C, and Alvarez FJ. Do Spanish patients drink alcohol while undergoing treatment with benzodiazepines? Alcohol 26:31–34 (2002).
365. Fraser AD. Use and abuse of the benzodiazepines. Therap Drug Monitor 20:481–489 (1998).
366. Stead AH and Moffatt AC. Quantification of the interaction between barbiturates and alcohol at different concentrations. Hum Toxicol 2:5–14 (1983).
367. Stead AH, Allan AR, Ardrey RE, Bal TS, Callaghan TM, Gill R, et al. Drug misuse—the barbiturate problem. J Forens Sci Soc 21:41–53 (1981).
368. Möhler H, Fritschy JM, and Rudolph U. A new benzodiazepine pharmacology. J Pharmacol Exp Therap 300:2–9 (2002).
369. George CFP. Pyrazolopyrimidines. Lancet 358:1623–1626 (2001).
370. Laurijssens BE and Greenblatt DJ. Pharmacokinetic–pharmacodynamic relationships for benzodiazepines. Clin Pharmacokinet 30:52–76 (1996).

371. Mandelli M, Tognono G, and Gerattini S. Clinical pharmacokinetics of diazepam. Clin Pharmacokinet 3:72–91 (1978).
372. Greenblatt DJ, Harmatz JS, Friedman H, Locnisker A, and Shader RI. A large sample study of diazepam pharmacokinetics. Therap Drug Monitor 11:652–657 (1989).
373. Greenblatt DJ, Laughren TP, Allen MD, Harmatz JS, and Shader RI. Plasma diazepam and desmethyldiazepam concentrations during long term diazepam therapy. Br J Clin Pharmacol 1:35–40 (1981).
374. Joynt BP. Triazolam blood concentrations in forensic cases in Canada. J Anal Toxicol 17: 171–177 (1993).
375. Edwards JG. Medicolegal aspects of benzodiazepine dependence: duties and responsibilities of doctors. Med J Aust 156:733–737 (1992).
376. Steentoft A, Teige B, Ceder G, Vuori E, Kristinsson E, Kaa J, et al. Fatal poisoning in drug addicts in the Nordic countries. Forens Sci Intern 123:63–69 (2001).
377. Steentoft A and Worm K. Cases of fatal triazolam poisoning. J Forensic Sci Soc 33:45–48 (1993).
378. Sunter JP, Bal TS, and Cowan WK. Three cases of fatal triazolam poisoning. Br Med J 297: 719 (1998).
379. Finkle BS, McCloskey KL, and Goodman LS. Diazepam and drug-associated deaths. JAMA 242:429–434 (1979).
380. Costa E and Guidotti A. Benzodiazepines on trial: a research strategy for their rehabilitation. Trends Pharmacol Sci 17:192–200 (1996).
381. Garretty DJ, Wolff K, Hay AWM, and Raistrick D. Benzodiazepine misuse by drug addicts. Ann Clin Biochem 34:68–73 (1997).
382. Woods JH, Katz JL, and Winger G. Abuse liability of benzodiazepines. Pharmacol Rev 39: 251–419 (1987).
383. Woods JH, Katz JL, and Winger G. Benzodiazepines: use, abuse and consequences. Pharmacol Rev 44:151–347 (1992).
384. Woods JH and Wingler G. Abuse liability of flunitrazepam. J Clin Psychopharmacol 17: 1S–57S (1997).
385. Bertilsson L, Baillie TA, and Reviriego J. Factors influencing the metabolism of diazepam. Pharmacol Ther 45:85–91 (1990).
386. Laisi U, Linnoila M, Seppälä T, Himberg I-J, and Mattila MJ. Pharmacokinetic and pharmacodynamic interactions of diazepam with different alcoholic beverages. Eur J Clin Pharmacol 16:263–270 (1979).
387. Friedman H, Greenblatt DJ, Peters GR, Metzler CM, Charlton MD, Marmatz JS, et al. Pharmacokinetics and pharmacodynamics of oral diazepam: effect of dose, plasma concentration, and time. Clin Pharmacol Ther 52:139–150 (1992).
388. Greenblatt DJ, Allen MD, Harmatz JS, and Shader RI. Diazepam disposition determinants. Clin Pharmacol Ther 27:301–312 (1980).
389. Jonasson B and Saldeen T. Citalopram in fatal poisoning cases. Forens Sci Intern 126:1–6 (2002).
390. Worm K, Dragsholt C, Simonsen K, and Kringsholm B. Citalopram concentrations in samples from autopsies and living persons. Int J Legal Med 111:188–190 (1998).
391. Bailey DN and Shaw RF. Interpretation of blood and tissue concentrations in fatal self-poisoning overdoses involving amitriptyline: an update 1978–1979. J Anal Toxicol 4:232–236.
392. Gruchalla RS. Clinical assessment of drug-induced disease. Lancet 356:1505–1511 (2000).
393. Pennings EJM, Leccese AP, and de Wolff FA. Effects of concurrent use of alcohol and cocaine. Addiction 97:773–779 (2002).

12. Alcohol and Drug Interactions

394. Farre M, de la Torre R, Gonzalez ML, Teran MT, Roset PN, Menoyo E, and Cami J. Cocaine and alcohol interactions in humans: neuroendocrine effects and cocaethylene metabolism. J Pharmacol Exp Therap 283:164–176 (1997).
395. Hearn WL, Rose S, Wagner J, Ciarleglio A, and Mash DC. Cocatheylene is more potent than cocaine in mediating lethality. Pharmacol Biochem Behav 39:531–533 (1991).
396. McCance EF, Price LH, Kosten TR, and Jatlow P. Cocaethylene: pharmacology, physiology and behavioral effects in humans. J Pharmacol Exp Therap 274:215–223 (1995).
397. Andrews P. Cocaethylene toxicity. J Addict Dis 16:75–84 (1997).
398. Bailey DN. Serial plasma concentrations of cocoethylene, cocaine, and ethanol in trauma victims. J Anal Toxicol 17:79–83 (1993).
399. Bailey DN. Comprehensive review of cocaethylene and cocaine concentrations in patients. Am J Clin Pathol 106:701–704 (1996).
400. Jatlow P. Cocaethylene. Pharmacologic activity and clinical significance. Therap Drug Monitor 15:533–536 (1993).
401. Jatlow P, McChance EF, Bradberry CW, Elsworth JD, Taylor JR, and Roth RH. Alcohol plus cocaine: the whole is more than the sum of its parts. Therap Drug Monitor 18:460–464 (1996).
402. Sharpe PC. Biochemical detection and monitoring of alcohol abuse and abstinence. Ann Clin Biochem 38:652–664 (2001).
403. Johnson BA and Ait-Daoud N. Medications to treat alcoholism. Alc Res Health 23:99–105 (1999).
404. Garbutt JC, West SL, Carey TS, Lohr KN, and Crews FT. Pharmacological treatment of alcohol dependence: a review of the evidence. JAMA 281:1318–1325 (1999).
405. Kreek MJ, LaForge KS, and Butelman E. Pharmacotherapy of addictions. Nature Rev Drug Disc 1:710–726 (2002).
406. Sellers EM and Kalant H. Alcohol intoxication and withdrawal. N Engl J Med 294:757–762 (1976).
407. Johnsen J, Stowell A, Stensrud T, Ripel A, and Morland J. A double-blind placebo controlled study of healthy volunteers given a subcutaneous disulfiram implantation. Pharmacol Toxicol 66:227–230 (1990).
408. Swift RM. Effect of naltrexone on human alcohol consumption. J Clin Psychiatry 56(Suppl 7):24–29 (1995).
409. Krystal JH, Cramer JA, Krol WF, Kirk GF, and Rosenheck RA. Naltrexone in the treatment of alcohol dependence. N Engl J Med 345:1734–1739 (2001).
410. Swift RM. Medications and alcohol craving. Alc Res Health 23:207–213 (1999b).
411. Ferrara SD, Zotti S, Tedeschi L, Frison G, Castagna F, Gallimberti L, et al. Pharmacokinetics of gamma-hydroxybutyrate in alcohol dependent patients after single and repeated oral doses. Br J Clin Pharmacol 34:231–235 (1992).
412. Carai MAM, Colombo G, Reali R, Serra S, et al. Central effects of 1,4 butanediol are mediated by $GABA_B$ receptors via its conversion into γ-hydroxybutyric acid. Eur J Pharmacol 441:157–163 (2002).
413. Swift RM, Davidson D, Whelihan W, and Kuznetsov O. Ondansetron alters human alcohol metabolism. Biol Psychiatry 15:514–521 (1996).
414. Swift RM. Drug therapy for alcohol dependence. N Engl J Med 340:1482–1490 (1999a).
415. Schneble H. Ernüchterungsmittel—nüchtern betrachtet. Blutalkohol 25:18–65 (1988).
416. Linnoila M and Mattila MJ. How to antagonize ethanol-induced inebrieation. Pharmacol Ther 15:99–109 (1981).
417. Lister R and Nutt DJ. Is RO 15-4513 a specific alcohol antagonist? Trends Neur Sci 10:223–225 (1987).

418. Allan AN and Harris RA. A new alcohol antagonist: phaclofen. Life Sci 45:1771–1779 (1989).
419. Jones AW. Forensic science aspects of ethanol metabolism. Forens Sci Prog 5:33–90 (1991).
420. Wiese JG, Shlipak MG, and Browner WS. The alcohol hangover. Ann Intern Med 132:897–902 (2000).
421. Mascord D, Smith J, Starmer GA, and Whitfield JB. Effect of oral glucose on the rate of metabolism of ethanol in humans. Alc Alcohol 23:365–370 (1988).
422. Mascord D, Smith J, Starmer GA, and Whitfield JB. The effect of fructose on alcohol metabolism and on the lactate/pyruvate ratio in man. Alc Alcohol 26:53–59 (1991).
423. Rogers J, Smith J, Starmer GA, and Whitfield JB. Differing effects of carbohydrates, fat and protein on the rate of ethanol metabolism. Alc Alcohol 22:345–353 (1987).
424. Clark ER, Hughes IE, and Letley E. The effect of oral administration of various sugars on blood ethanol concentration in man. J Pharm Pharmacol 25:309–323 (1973).
425. Ylikahri RH, Leino T, Huttunen MO, Poso AR, Eriksson CJ, and Nikkila EA. Effects of fructose and glucose on ethanol-induced metabolic changes and on the intensity of alcohol intoxication and hangover. Eur J Clin Invest 6:93–102 (1976).
426. Crow KE, Newland KM, and Batt RD. The fructose effect. NZ Med J 93:232–234 (1981).
427. Bode C. The metabolism of alcohol: physiological and pathological aspects. J Roy Coll Phys 12:122–135 (1978).
428. Cohen RD. Effect of fructose on blood alcohol level. Lancet 2:1086 (1972).
429. Soterakis J and Iber FL. Increased rate of alcohol removal from blood with oral fructose and sucrose. Am J Clin Nut 28:254–257 (1975).
430. Polacsek P. Interaction of alcohol and other drugs an annotated bibliography. Toronto: Addiction Research Foundation, 1970:1–535.
431. Li J, Mills T, and Erato R. Intravenous saline has no effect on blood ethanol clearance. J Emerg Med 17:1–5 (1999).
432. Hyvärinen J, Laakso M, Sippel H, Roine R, et al. Alcohol detoxification accelerated by oxygenated drinking water. Life Sci 22:553–560 (1978).
433. Ylikahri R and Leino T. Metabolic interactions of xylitol and ethanol in healthy males. Metabolism 28:25–29 (1979).
434. Alkana RL, Parker ES, Cohen HB, Birch H, and Nobel EP. Interaction of sted-eze, nikethamide, pipradrol, or ammonium chloride with ethanol in human males. Alcohol Clin Exp Res 4:84–92 (1980).
435. Kelly M, Myrsten AL, and Goldberg L. Intravenous vitamins in acute alcoholic intoxication: effects on physiological and psychological functions. Br J Addict 66:19–30 (1971).
436. Chen MF, Boyce Worth H, and Hsu JM. Effect of ascorbic acid on alcohol clearance. J Am Coll Nutrit 9:185–189 (1990).
437. Susick RL and Zannoni VG. Effect of ascorbic acid on the consequences of acute alcohol consumption in humans. Clin Pharmacol Ther 41:502–509 (1987).
438. Linnoila M, Mattila MJ, Karhunen P, Nuotto E, and Seppälä T. Failure of TRH and ORG 2766 hexapeptide to counteract alcoholiic inebriation in man. Eur J Clin Pharmacol 21:27–32 (1981).
439. Kraemer R, Mallach HJ, Raff G, and Schulz H. Influence of mobiletten on the effect of alcohol drinking in man. Int J Clin Pharmacol 15:301–309 (1977).
440. Mallach HJ, Raff G, and Kraemer R. On the influence of mobiletten on the effect of alcohol in the human. Int J Clin Pharmacol 15:576–580 (1977).
441. Miller LG. Herbal medicines: selected clinical considerations focusing on known or potential drug–herb interactions. Arch Intern Med 158:2200–2211 (1998).

442. Azcona O, Barbanol MJ, Torrent J, and Jane F. Evaluation of the central effects of alcohol and caffeine interaction. Br J Clin Pharmacol 40:393–400 (1993).
443. Liguori A and Robinson JH. Caffeine antagonism of alcohol-induced driving impairment. Drug Alc Depend 63:123–129 (2001).
444. Shoaf SE and Linnoila M. Interaction of ethanol and smoking on the pharmacokinetics and pharmacodynamics of psychotropic medications. Psychopharm Bull 27:577–594 (1991).
445. Mendelson J, Jones RT, Upton R, and Jacob P. Methamphetamine and ethanol interactions in humans. Clin Pharmacol Ther 57:559–568 (1995).
446. Mattila MJ, Kuitunen T, and Pletan Y. Lack of pharmacodynamic and pharmacokinetic interactions of the antihistamine ebastine with ethanol in healthy subjects. Eur J Clin Pharmacol 43:179–184 (1992).
447. Lader M, Melhuish A, Frcka G, Fredricson Overo K, and Christensen V. The effects of citalopram in single and repeated doses and with alcohol on physiological and psychological measures in healthy subjects. Eur J Clin Pharmacol 31:183–190 (1986).
448. Van Harten J, Stevens LA, Raghoebar M, Holland RL, et al. Fluvoxamine does not interact with alcohol or potentiate alcohol-related impairment of cognitive function. Clin Pharmacol Ther 52:427–435 (1992).
449. Naranjo CA, Sullivan JT, Kadlec KE, Woodley-Remus DV, Kennedy G, and Sellers EM. Differential effects of viqualine on alcohol intake and other consummatory behaviors. Clin Pharmacol Ther 46:301–309 (1989).
450. Anton R, Paladino JA, Morton A, and Thomas RW. Effect of acute alcohol consumption on lithium kinetics. Clin Pharmacol Ther 38:52–55 (1985).
451. Dole VP, Fishman J, Goldfrank L, Khanna J, and McGivern RF. Arousal of ethanol-intoxicated comatose patients with naloxone. Alcohol Clin Exp Res 6:275–279 (1982).
452. Bodd E, Beylich M, Christophersen A, and Morland J. Oral administration of codeine in the presence of ethanol: a pharmacokinetic study in man. Pharmacol Toxicol 61:297–300 (1987).
453. Donnelly B, Balkon J, Lasher C, DePaul Lynch V, et al. Evaluation of the methadone–alcohol interaction. 1. Alterations of plasma concentration kinetics. J Anal Toxicol 7:246–248 (1983).
454. Griffin JP, D'Arcy PF, and Speirs CJ. A manual of adverse drug interactions, 4th ed. London: Wright, 1988.
455. Logan BK and Distefano S. Ethanol content of various foods and soft drinks and their potential for interference with a breath-alcohol test. J Anal Tox 22:181–183 (1998).
456. Baum CR, Shannon MW, and Woolf A. Breath and blood ethanol following use of a cough-cold preparation. J Tox Clin Tox 35:643–644 (1997).
457. Barbone F, McMahon AD, Davey PG, Morris AD, Reid IC, McDevitt DG, and MacDonald TM. Association of road-traffic accidents with benzodiazepine use. Lancet 352:1331–1336 (1998).
458. Druid H and Holmgren P. A compilation of fatal and control concentrations of drugs in postmortem femoral blood. J Forensic Sci 42:79–87 (1997).
459. Li T-K. Pharmacogenetics of responses to alcohol and genes that influence alcohol drinking. J Studies Alc 61:5–12 (2000).
460. Nestler EJ. Genes and addiction. Nature Med 26:277–281 (2000).
461. Kalow W. Pharmacogenetics in biological perspective. Pharmacol Rev 49:369–379 (1997).
462. Ingelman-Sundberg M. Genetic variability in susceptibility and response to toxicants. Toxicol Lett 120:259–268 (2001).
463. Knowles SR, Uetrecht J, and Shear NH. Idiosyncratic drug reactions: the reactive metabolite syndrome. Lancet 356:1587–1591 (2000).

464. Pirmohamed M and Park BK. Genetic susceptibility to adverse drug reactions. Trends Pharmacol Sci 22:298–305 (2001).
465. Nebert DW. Drug-metabolizing enzymes, polymorphisms and interindividual response to environmental toxicants. Clin Chem Lab Med 38:857–861 (2000).
466. Meyer UA. Pharmacogenetics and adverse drug reactions. Lancet 359:1667–1671 (2000).
467. Ingelman-Sundberg M. Pharmacogenetics: an opportunity for a safer and more efficient pharmacotherapy. J Intern Med 250:186–200 (2001).
468. Li T-K, Yin SJ, Crabb DW, O'Connor S, and Ramchandani VA. Genetic and environmental influences on alcohol metabolism in humans. Alcohol Clin Exp Res 25:136–144 (2001).
469. Vesell ES, Page JG, and Passananti GT. Genetic and environmental factors affecting ethanol metabolism in man. Clin Pharmacol Ther 12:192–201 (1971).
470. Baselt RC and Cravey RH. Disposition of toxic drugs and chemicals in man, 4th ed. Foster City, CA: Chemical Toxicology Institute, 1995.

Chapter 13

Nicotine and Tobacco

Edward J. Cone, PhD, Reginald V. Fant, PhD, and Jack E. Henningfield, PhD

1. INTRODUCTION

1.1. Forms of Nicotine Replacement Therapy and Prevalence of Use

1.1.1. Forms of Nicotine Replacement Therapy

The first nicotine replacement therapy (NRT) that was made available to consumers was transmucosally delivered nicotine polacrilex ("nicotine gum"). The 2-mg-containing formulation of nicotine gum was first marketed in the United States in 1984 as a prescription medication. The 4-mg form was marketed in 1992 to enable heavier-smoking patients the replacement levels that they required for successful smoking cessation. In 1996, both the 2- and 4-mg forms were marketed as over-the-counter (OTC) medications in the United States, which has made the products much more widely available to consumers. In 1999, a mint-flavored gum was marketed in the United States in an effort to increase compliance with use instructions among patients who found the original ("peppery") flavor to be unpalatable. About 50% of the nicotine in gum is absorbed, most via the buccal mucosa and a small portion through the stomach due to swallowed saliva *(1)*. Thus, when nicotine gum is chewed on a fixed schedule of 10 pieces per day, a smoker receives about 10 mg or 20 mg of nicotine per day using the 2-mg or 4-mg gum formulations, respectively. The average systemic intake of nicotine from cigarettes is about 30 mg/d *(2)*. Thus, most gum chewers do not match daily the nicotine levels achieved through the smoking of a cigarette. Furthermore, because of the relatively slow absorption of nicotine from gum compared to smoke inhalation, individual doses do not produce the extremely high arterial levels of nicotine produced by smoke inhalation *(3)*.

From: *Handbook of Drug Interactions: A Clinical and Forensic Guide*
A. Mozayani and L. P. Raymon, eds. © Humana Press Inc., Totowa, NJ

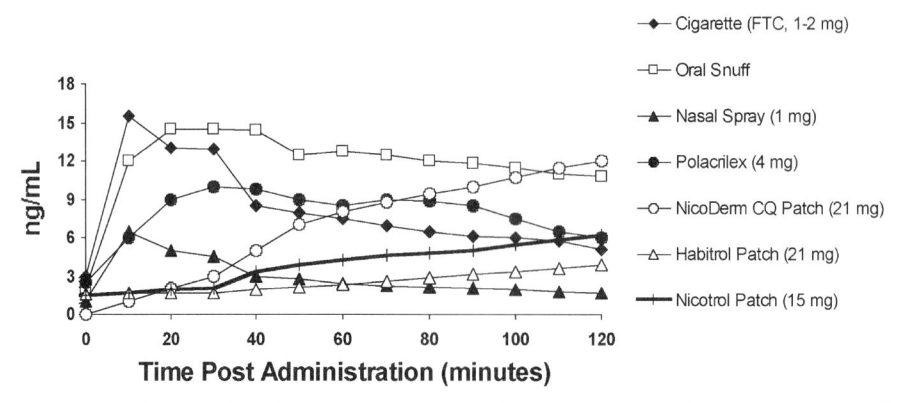

Fig. 1. Venous plasma nicotine concentrations in nanograms of nicotine per milliliter of blood as a function of time for various nicotine delivery systems. Data adapted from *(156–158)*.

In the United States, prescription-only marketing of four transdermal-delivery ("nicotine patch") systems began in late 1991 and 1992. In 1996, two brands of nicotine patches were marketed as OTC medications to increase availability to consumers. The transdermal patch delivers nicotine throughout the day. Compliance is based on whether or not the patient places the patch on the body in the morning, rather than actively using a product throughout the day, as is the case with the gum. As shown in Fig. 1, the nicotine patch delivers nicotine more slowly to the bloodstream than the gum does, although nicotine plasma concentrations can get higher during the day with patch use than with gum use, especially if the patient uses fewer pieces of gum than recommended. The highest dose of all patch brands deliver an average of 0.9 mg nicotine per hour although, as shown in Fig. 1, the within-day kinetics varies considerably across the brands. The maximum plasma concentrations range from 13 to 23 ng/mL and the times taken to reach maximum plasma concentration range from 4 to 9 h *(4)*.

Nicotine nasal spray was first marketed in the United States as a prescription smoking cessation medication in 1997. The nasal spray was designed to deliver doses of nicotine to the smoker more rapidly than was possible with use of the gum or patch. The device currently available to consumers is a multidose bottle with a pump mechanism fitted to a nozzle that delivers 0.5 mg of nicotine per 50-µL spray. Each dose consists of two sprays, one to each nostril. As shown in Fig. 1, nicotine nasal spray is absorbed into the blood rapidly relative to gum and patch. Whereas the rate of plasma nicotine absorption with the spray approaches that of cigarettes and oral snuff, the magnitude of the increase in plasma nicotine concentrations is lower. According to labeling, the dose of nasal spray should be individualized for each patient based on the patient's level of nicotine dependence and the occurrence of adverse effects resulting from nicotine excess. Patients should be started with 1 or 2 doses per hour, which may be increased up to the maximum of 40 doses per day. One dose of nasal spray per hour (1-mg nicotine) for 10 h produces average plasma concentrations of 8 ng/mL. The nasal spray is the only nicotine replacement product documented to provide rapid enough delivery to produce an arterial blood level spike. Although not achieving the 10-fold arterial to venous ratio sometimes produced by cigarettes *(5)*, it can produce a twofold arterial bolus *(6)*.

The nicotine vapor inhaler, which consists of a mouthpiece and a plastic cartridge containing nicotine, was first marketed in the United States in 1998 as a prescription smoking cessation medication. The vapor inhaler was designed to satisfy behavioral aspects of smoking, namely, the hand-to-mouth ritual, while delivering nicotine to combat physiological withdrawal symptoms produced by tobacco withdrawal. Each inhaler cartridge contains 10 mg nicotine, of which 4 mg can be delivered, and 2 mg can be absorbed by inhaling approximately 80 times per inhaler *(7)*. Because extraction of nicotine from the mouthpiece is influenced by ambient air temperature and the difficulty of many people in taking 80 inhalations per hour that would be required to provide 2-mg doses, typical absorption levels are probably substantially lower than 2 mg/h *(8)*. The majority of nicotine is delivered into the oral cavity (36%) and in the esophagus and stomach (36%) *(9)*. Very little nicotine is delivered to the lung (4%). Because absorption is primarily through the oral mucosa, the rate of absorption is similar to that of nicotine gum. Patients may self-titrate with the inhaler to the level of nicotine they require. However, as with nicotine gum, success is largely dependent on the number of doses taken per day. In clinical trials, most smokers who successfully abstained from smoking used between 6 and 16 cartridges per day.

1.1.2. Prevalence of Use of Nicotine Replacement Therapy

According to the Centers for Disease Control, in 1998, there were about 8.5 million pharmacologically assisted quit attempts *(10)* by smokers. The nicotine patch accounted for 49% of pharmacologically assisted quit attempts and nicotine gum accounted for 28%. Twenty-one percent of pharmaceutically assisted cessation attempts were made using bupropion (Zyban). The nicotine inhaler and nasal spray accounted for less than 3%.

1.2. Forms of Tobacco and Prevalence of Use

1.2.1. Forms of Tobacco

Tobacco is available in a variety of forms for human consumption. The most common form today is the cigarette. Although cigarettes come in many forms, there are specific definitions for their composition. According to section 26 U.S.C. 5702(b) of the Bureau of Alcohol, Tobacco, and Firearms (BATF), a cigarette is defined as follows: (a) any roll of tobacco wrapped in paper or in any substance not containing tobacco, and (b) any roll of tobacco wrapped in any substance containing tobacco, which, because of its appearance, the type of tobacco used in the filter, or its packaging and labeling, is likely to be offered to, or purchased by, consumers as a cigarette. The Food and Drug Administration (FDA) further clarified the definition of a cigarette for purposes of regulation in section 897.3 of 21 CRF Part 801 as follows: any product (including components, accessories, or parts) that contains or delivers nicotine, and is intended to be burned under ordinary conditions of use *(11)*. Cigarette tobacco is flue cured; i.e., it is rapidly dried over smokeless heat, resulting in an acidic smoke when the product is burned *(12)*. Because of the acidity of the smoke, there is little resulting nicotine absorption via the oral mucosa. However, pulmonary absorption of nicotine from the inhaled smoke is rapid and almost complete.

Cigars, in contrast, consist of tobacco that is air cured, then wrapped in tobacco leaf or reconstituted paper made of tobacco plant material. The resulting smoke of air-cured tobacco is much more basic than flue-cured tobacco *(12)*. Nicotine from this smoke is readily absorbed through the oral mucosa, as well as the lung. Nicotine can also be absorbed directly from the tobacco if the cigar is held in the mouth. Unlike cigarettes, which are fairly consistent in their tobacco weight and size, cigars vary greatly. Henningfield et al. *(13)* studied a variety of cigar types and found that the weight of the cigars ranged from 0.77 to 22 g, lengths ranged from 68 to 214 mm, and diameter ranged from 8 to 21 mm. In addition, the total nicotine content of these cigars ranged from 10.1 to 444 mg, and the pH values of the tobacco ranged from 6.2 to 8.2.

The tobacco from pipes can be air cured, fire cured, sun cured, or flue cured, depending on the quality of the tobacco *(12)*. The tobacco is not wrapped for smoking. Because of these differences in curing methods, the resulting smoke can vary widely in its pH, in turn resulting in wide variability of nicotine absorption through the oral mucosa.

Chewing tobacco and oral snuff are made from air-cured tobacco, resulting in a tobacco that has a basic pH, which is ideal for buccal absorption *(12)*. However, there is wide variability between products on the nicotine concentration of the tobacco as well as the pH of the tobacco in solution, resulting in large differences in rate of nicotine absorption and peak plasma levels *(14)*.

1.2.2. Prevalence of Use

The 2000 National Health Survey on Drug Abuse *(15)*, conducted by the Substance Abuse and Mental Health Services Administration, is the most recent source of national data on rates of tobacco use. The latest survey estimated that in 2000, 65.5 million Americans aged 12 and older (29.3%) reported current use of a tobacco product. An estimated 55.7 million (24.9%) smoked cigarettes, 10.7 million (4.8%) smoked cigars, 7.6 million (3.4%) used smokeless tobacco, and 2.1 million (1.0%) smoked tobacco in pipes.

The majority of current adult cigarette smokers smoke at least a pack of cigarettes on a daily basis. Of the 55.7 million current smokers in 2000, 64.6% (35.9 million) reported smoking every day in the past 30 d and 55.2% of all daily smokers aged 12 and older smoked a pack or more a day. Younger smokers tend to smoke less, and with less regularity, because of parental and societal constraints, lack of financial means, and lower tolerance to nicotine's effects than long-term smokers. Among smokers aged 12 to 17, only 31.8% were daily smokers and only 24.1% of youth daily smokers reported smoking a pack or more a day.

In 2000, males were more likely than females to report past month use of any tobacco product. In 2000, 35.2% of males aged 12 and older were current users of any tobacco product compared to 23.9% of females. Males were 10 times more likely than their female counterparts to report current use of smokeless tobacco in 2000 (6.5% of males aged 12 and older compared with 0.5% of females). As seen for smokeless tobacco, males were more likely than females to report past-month cigar use. Specifically, males were five times more likely than females to report the past-month use of cigars (8.4% compared to 1.5%).

Passive smoking also delivers nicotine to nonsmokers. Passive smoking is exposure to tobacco smoke that occurs when a nonsmoker is exposed to the sidestream smoke of a cigarette. Drug interactions may occur in nonsmokers, particularly infants and children, exposed to tobacco smoke in the home. The proportion of infants exposed to tobacco smoke varies across the United States. In 2000, the percentage of homes with at least one smoker ranged from 21% in Colorado to 39.2% in West Virginia *(16)*. Smoking in the workplace also varies widely. The proportion of indoor workplaces with no smoking policies ranged from 61.4% in Mississippi to 83.9% in Montana.

1.3. Components of Nicotine Replacement Therapy and Tobacco

NRTs essentially contain nicotine, and ingredients required for the specific formulations to operate as intended, e.g., stabilizing ingredients, buffering compounds, and flavors. Nicotine is generally the only compound in these products of interest in determining drug interactions.

In contrast to NRTs, ingredients included in cigarette tobacco may be any combination from a list of approximately 600 provided at the Philip Morris website (http://www.philipmorrisusa.com). Brown & Williamson, according to their website (*see* http://www.bw.com/index_sub2.cfm?Page=/SHC/Index.cfm%3FID%3D4%26Sect%3D4), in 2000, used 299 ingredients in the manufacture of their tobacco products. These include: ammonium compounds that have been shown to enhance the delivery of nicotine, glycerol to which nicotine binds for effective lung delivery, and flavorings such as chocolate and cinnamon. Although the website states that these ingredients "…are either a food, a beverage, an approved food additive, an approved tobacco product additive, or affirmed to be acceptable for addition to foods by an Expert Body such as the FDA, the Flavor and Extract Manufacturers Association (FEMA) or the Council of Europe (COE)," none of them have been specifically approved by any regulatory agency as safe for use in conditions in which they are subjected to pyrolysis and combustion since that process can radically alter their chemistry and toxicity. In addition, the process of generating cigarette smoke produces more than 4000 compounds together with those contained in tobacco *(17,18)*. Thus, identifying all of the potential drug interactions with individual compounds in tobacco smoke is not possible. Nonetheless, several major influences on drug disposition and several important interactions have been documented as discussed further on in this review.

1.4. Nicotine and Tobacco Pharmacology

Two medical disorders are now widely recognized elements of what is more generally referred to as "tobacco addiction" or "tobacco dependence." The first is nicotine dependence, which is characterized by the maladaptive and persistent use of tobacco products. The second is nicotine withdrawal, which is characterized by a constellation of symptoms that accompany abstinence from tobacco use *(19)*. These withdrawal symptoms include: dysphoric or depressed mood, insomnia, irritability, frustration or anger, anxiety, difficulty in concentrating, restlessness, decreased heart rate, and increased appetite or weight gain. Tobacco craving is also common and can be persistent. These signs and symptoms make it difficult if not impossible for the vast majority of cigarette smokers to sustain abstinence for more than a few days *(17)*.

Tobacco dependence and withdrawal are associated with a number of changes in the structure and function of the nervous and endocrine system, which lead the individual to feel "normal" and perform optimally while receiving daily doses of nicotine, and to feel dysfunctional when abstinent. Many of these symptomatic feelings correspond to objectively measurable changes in electroencephalogram (EEG), regional cerebral glucose metabolism, and performance on cognitive test batteries *(20,21)*. These changes in the structure and function of the body, and the fact that the tobacco industry engineered its products to ensure that their use could cause such effects, led the FDA to conclude that nicotine in cigarettes and smokeless tobacco is a drug and that these products are drug delivery systems *(22)*.

Even though most nicotine clears the body within 1–2 d of abstinence (its half-life is about 2 h), the mental dysfunction and other signs of withdrawal can persist for weeks and powerful cravings can resurge for months and years. Individuals vary widely in the severity and course of these symptoms. In part, the persistence of these symptoms can be attributed to changes in the body from which it may take many months to fully recover. However, the addictive process is more than altered physiology, but rather is related to psychological and behavioral factors as well.

1.5. Nicotine and Tobacco Toxicity

The toxicity of nicotine is generally related to its pharmacological activity at the high dosages delivered by cigarettes, though rarely achieved by nicotine replacement medications. For example, nicotine delivered by cigarettes can produce striking levels of heart rate acceleration and sympathetic hormone release that can be mimicked by rapid intravenous infusions but rarely by nicotine medication use *(6,23)*. Similarly, cigarette smoking readily produces plasma nicotine levels associated with increased fetal risk during pregnancy, but nicotine medications do not reliably produce such levels *(24)*. Nicotine has well-documented effects on cardiovascular physiology *(23)*. It increases blood pressure and force of contraction of the heart. Nicotine poisoning, as has occurred after exposure to nicotine-containing insecticides, can produce cardiovascular collapse and death. Rapid delivery of high doses of nicotine, as in cigarette smoking, produces more intense cardiovascular effects than does more gradual dosing with products such as nicotine gum or transdermal nicotine patches *(25)*.

Nicotine has also been shown to be potentially harmful to the gastrointestinal mucosa because it increases acid and pepsin secretions, gastric motility, and gastric reflux of bile salts *(26)*. Nausea and vomiting are the most common symptoms of acute nicotine poisoning in man. In animals, vomiting and diarrhea have also been observed. Such responses are caused by both the central and peripheral actions of nicotine.

1.5.1. Single-Dose Nicotine Toxicity

In experimental animals, the dose of nicotine that is lethal to 50% of animals (LD_{50}) varies widely, depending on the route of administration and the species tested. Intravenous LD_{50} doses of nicotine in mice range between 0.3 and 1.8 mg/kg body wt. The intraperitoneal LD_{50} values for nicotine bitartrate in mice and rats have been found to be 13 and 83 mg/kg body wt, respectively, whereas the values for five inbred hamster strains varied between 125 to 320 mg/kg body wt. The lethal oral dose of nicotine in adult humans has been estimated to be 40–60 mg *(27,28)*.

Lethal doses of nicotine cause peripheral curare-like paralysis of the respiratory muscles *(29)*. Extremely high doses of nicotine can cause transient stimulation fol-

13. Nicotine

lowed by depression and paralysis of the central nervous system (CNS). Such doses also affect peripheral autonomic nervous system ganglia and nerve endings on skeletal muscles. Death usually occurs within a short period and is most often due to paralysis of respiratory muscles. Excessive doses of nicotine may also produce tremors followed by convulsions.

1.5.2. Smoking and Cardiovascular Disease Risk

Smoking has firmly been linked to increased risks of cardiovascular diseases including coronary heart disease, arteriosclerotic vascular disease, and stroke *(30)*. There are a number of mechanisms by which smoking may increase the risk of cardiovascular disease *(31)*. Nicotine and carbon monoxide acutely affect myocardial performance and cause tachycardia, hypertension, and vasoconstriction. Components of cigarette smoke injure the walls of blood vessels by destroying endothelial cells. Smoking produces metabolic and biochemical changes including elevations in plasma-free fatty acids, and vasopressin. Smoking causes an inhibition of cyclooxygenase, which decreases levels of prostacyclin and increase levels of thromboxane A2. Chronic smoking leads to arteriosclerosis by increasing serum cholesterol and reducing high-density lipoprotein. In addition, smokers have increased platelet adhesiveness and aggregability that may lead to increased risk of thrombosis.

Many toxins are believed to contribute to smoking-related cardiovascular disease, including carbon monoxide, polycyclic aromatic hydrocarbons, glycoproteins, and nicotine. Some but not all of the characteristics of tobacco-related disease seem to be nicotine related. Nicotine increases CNS sympathetic outflow, adrenal release of catecholamines, and local release of catecholamines from vascular nerve endings *(26)*. The net result is heart rate acceleration, increased myocardial contractility, constriction of some blood vessels, and a small increase in blood pressure. Nicotine can precipitate or aggravate acute coronary ischemic events by increasing myocardial work, and therefore nutrient demand, while reducing nutrient supply through coronary vasoconstriction. Catecholamine release may also precipitate or aggravate ischemia-induced arrhythmias, leading to sudden arrhythmic death. Other possible adverse effects of nicotine include injury to endothelial cells, induction of atherogenic lipid profile, and promotion of thrombosis *(17)*.

1.5.3. Smoking and Cancer Risk

Several forms of cancer have been shown to be associated with smoking including cancers of the lung, lip and oral cavity, esophagus, pancreas, larynx, uterine cervix, bladder, and kidney *(30)*. Cigarette smoke is known to contain more than 4000 compounds including over 40 carcinogens that include polyaromatic hydrocarbons, heterocyclic hydrocarbons, N-nitrosamines, aromatic amines, aldehydes, volatile carcinogens, inorganic compounds, and radioactive elements *(30)*. Carcinogenesis can be divided into two phases: initiation, in which DNA is damaged by the bonding of the carcinogen, and promotion, in which initiated cells become malignant. Compounds found in the particulate matter of cigarette smoke ("tar") have been shown to be major tumor initiators in laboratory animals *(30)*. There are data suggesting that nicotine could theoretically play some role as a cancer promoter *(32)*; however, the majority of the effects of tobacco on cancer appear related to nonnicotine components of tobacco smoke and the risk of nicotine-related cancer, if any, is small or insignificant in smokers who are exposed to a high concentration of many carcinogens *(32)*.

1.5.4. Smoking and Pulmonary Disease Risk

Pulmonary problems associated with tobacco smoking include chronic obstructive pulmonary disease (COPD), asthma, pneumonia, influenza, bronchitis, and emphysema *(30)*. Several mechanisms have been identified by which smoking may contribute to the development of these pulmonary problems *(33,34)*. These include smoking-induced alterations of central and peripheral airways, alveoli and capillaries, and immune function. Changes in the central airways include loss of cilia, mucus gland hyperplasia, increased number of goblet cells, and histological changes. These histological changes include regression of normal pseudostratified ciliated epithelium to squamous metaplasia, carcinoma *in situ*, and eventually invasive bronchogenic permeability. Changes in peripheral airways include inflammation and atrophy of the airways, goblet cell metaplasia, mucus plugging, smooth muscle hypertrophy, and peribronchiolar fibrosis. Changes in alveoli and capillaries include destruction of peribronchiolar alveoli, reduction in the number of small arteries, bronchoalveolar lavage fluid abnormalities, elevated levels of IgA and IgG, and increased percentages of activated macrophages. Regarding immune function, smoking produces higher peripheral leukocyte cell counts, elevations in peripheral eosinophils, increased levels of serum IgE, lower allergy skin test reactivity, and reduced immune response to inhaled antigens. None of these effects appear to be related to nicotine delivery, but rather to other constituents of tobacco smoke.

1.5.5. Summary of Toxicity

The foregoing discussion of the health effects of nicotine and tobacco suggests that most of the adverse health effects of tobacco are related to nonnicotine components of tobacco smoke, rather than from the delivery of nicotine *per se*. Further, the vast majority of smokers who use nicotine replacement medications obtain lower doses of nicotine than when they were smoking. Thus, to the extent that diseases demonstrate a dose response to nicotine, persons on NRT have lower risk of these diseases.

2. MECHANISMS OF INTERACTIONS WITH NICOTINE AND TOBACCO

2.1. Pharmacokinetic Mechanisms

Pharmacokinetic interactions of nicotine and tobacco with other drugs can take place through direct drug–drug interactions or via indirect mechanisms. Kinetic alterations can result from changes in absorption, distribution, metabolism, and elimination. Changes in absorption can occur through delayed gastric emptying. Changes in distribution can occur through displacement of drug binding to plasma protein by nicotine or tobacco constituents. When a highly protein-bound drug is displaced from binding, a sharp increase in free-drug concentration may occur, leading to changes in distribution, and possible toxic effects. Drug metabolic alterations can occur through multiple mechanisms. Most drugs are metabolized by oxidation, reduction, hydrolysis, and conjugation reactions. The resultant metabolite(s) usually is less active than the parent compound, but occasionally metabolism results in conversion of drug to a species with increased pharmacological activity and increased potential for toxicity. Metabolism also generally results in production of molecules that are more amenable to excretion. Changes in the level or activity of metabolic processes can substantially increase or reduce drug and tissue levels leading to either enhanced or diminished effects or even toxic effects. Enzyme inhibition is the most commonly encountered form of drug–drug interaction, and perhaps is the most common mechanism responsible for development of toxic drug levels. Enzyme induction generally lowers effective drug levels and reduces therapeutic effects. Changes in elimination rate could potentially be produced by an alteration in excretory processes.

Nicotine and tobacco constituents may influence metabolic rates by induction or inhibition of enzyme systems. Nicotine is mainly metabolized in the liver via multiple pathways. Inhibition of one or more of these pathways could lead to increased nicotine plasma levels. For example, 70–80% of nicotine is metabolized to cotinine by the enzyme CYP2A6. Sellers et al. *(35)* showed that inhibition of the CYP2A6 enzyme with the selective inhibitor, methoxsalen, significantly increased plasma levels of oral nicotine. In addition, studies have shown that individuals carrying defective CYP2A6 alleles are underrepresented in the tobacco-dependent population, and that smokers with deficient nicotine metabolism smoked fewer cigarettes *(36,37)*. It was postulated that individuals with genetically deficient CYP2A6 nicotine metabolism are at lower risk to become smokers and that CYP2A6 inhibitors could play an important role in smoking cessation therapy.

Nicotine also has been reported to induce its own metabolism, but smokers have been shown to have a lower clearance of nicotine compared to nonsmokers *(38)*. Cigarette smoke contains literally thousands of compounds, among which polycyclic aromatic hydrocarbons (PAHs) are primarily responsible for its enzyme-inducing characteristics. PAHs have been shown to induce primarily three cytochrome P450 enzymes (e.g., CYP1A1, CYP1A2, and CYP2E1) as well as glucuronosyltransferases *(39)*. CYP1A2 and CYP2E1 are primarily associated with the liver but have been found in lung and other tissues and in the placenta of mothers who smoke. CYP1A1 levels are low in hepatic microsomes, but are found in lung, intestine, skin, lymphocytes, and placenta.

2.2. Pharmacodynamic Mechanisms

Pharmacodynamic interactions can occur through receptor site competition, by alteration of receptors, and through additive or opposing pharmacological effects. Nicotine is the major alkaloid in tobacco and exerts prominent effects including catecholamine release, peripheral and coronary vasoconstriction, decreased skin temperature, tachycardia, and elevated blood pressure *(40)*. Acute tolerance develops rapidly. Depending upon the drug, interactions may occur by additive, synergistic, or opposing effects.

3. NICOTINE INTERACTIONS

3.1. Interactions

3.1.1. Alcohol

Nicotine (spray, 20 µg/kg) administered together with alcohol to abstinent smokers generally produced additive subjective effects ("head rush" and dizziness) and cardiovascular effects, although nicotine tended to attenuate fatigue and intoxication *(41)*. Some differences were noted between men and women in subjective responses from combined administration. For men, nicotine combined with alcohol attenuated measures of dizzy, relaxed and tension, whereas effects were enhanced in women. In a study of female smokers and nonsmokers who chewed nicotine gum (2 mg), memory and motor function were facilitated by nicotine, and the debilitating effects of alcohol were antagonized *(42)*. In animal studies, intragastric administration of nicotine was shown to lower peak blood alcohol concentrations in neonatal rats *(43)*. Soderpalm et al. *(44)* reported that subchronic intermittent pretreatment with nicotine enhanced the dopamine-activating and -reinforcing properties of ethanol in rats. Another study in dogs showed that nicotine administration after alcohol produced significant increases in cardiovascular measures, but when alcohol was administered after nicotine, all excitatory effects were attenuated *(45)*.

Ethanol administration also has effects on nicotine metabolism. When administered acutely to laboratory animals, ethanol retards rates of nicotine metabolism, whereas chronic ethanol pretreatment generally accelerates metabolic rates of nicotine *(46)*.

3.1.2. Antidepressants

Pretreatment of rats with amitriptyline produced a significant increase in the hypothermic response to nicotine *(47)*. Supersensitivity persisted from 7 to 14 d. The findings indicate that tricyclic antidepressants alter a nicotinic mechanism in mammalian species.

3.1.3. Antihistamines

In rats, nicotine in combination with tripelennamine produced supra-additive toxicity *(48)*. The interaction of nicotine with diphenhydramine was more complicated; supra-additive toxicity was observed at some doses, but antagonism occurred at other doses.

3.1.4. Antipsychotics

Nicotine has been widely shown to stimulate the release of dopamine. Given the disturbances of dopamine systems in schizophrenics, it has been speculated that schizophrenics may smoke as a form of self-medication. The interactions of haloperidol and nicotine (patch, 7 and 14 mg/d) on cognitive performance in a group of schizophrenics were studied by Levin et al. *(49)*. Nicotine administration was found to produce a dose-related reversal of impairments in memory and complex reaction times induced by haloperidol. In addition, nicotine gum *(50,51)* and transdermal nicotine patch *(52)* are reported to ameliorate symptoms of Tourette's syndrome in haloperidol-treated adolescents. In rats, nicotine has been shown to potentiate the catalepsy produced by haloperidol *(53,54)*. Neither cotinine nor nornicotine, the principal pharmacologically active metabolites of nicotine, produced potentiation. Although the mechanism remains unclear, it was suggested that nicotine's effect is related to striatal D2 receptor mechanisms.

3.1.5. Barbiturates

Nicotine potentiated sodium pentobarbital sleep time in a dose-dependent manner in mice *(55)*. At the highest tested dose of nicotine (5 mg/kg), an increase of 52% in sleep time was observed. Atropine reduced sleep time, but did not change the nicotine effect. Pretreatment with mecamylamine, a nicotine receptor antagonist, normalized sleep time.

Phenobarbital is a model-inducing agent for numerous drug-metabolizing enzyme systems. Phenobarbital pretreatment of laboratory animals has been shown to induce the metabolism of nicotine and its metabolites, primarily through increased expression of CYP enzymes *(46)*. Phenobarbital induces not only the metabolism of nicotine, but also its metabolite, cotinine. Nicotine also has effects on phenobarbital disposition. A study in rats showed that acute pretreatment of rats with nicotine significantly reduced phenobarbital concentrations in serum, brain, and cerebrospinal fluid (CSF) at the onset of the righting reflex, but acute or chronic pretreatment with nicotine had no effect on the elimination kinetics of phenobarbital *(56)*.

3.1.6. Benzodiazepines

The combination of nicotine and diazepam in rats responding to a fixed-interval schedule of liquid food reinforcement produced rate-increasing effects of nicotine at low diazepam doses *(57)*. At higher diazepam doses, the interaction between nicotine and diazepam was complex and was determined by the doses of drug and the aspect of behavior studied.

3.1.7. Caffeine

Nicotine and caffeine are among the most widely self-administered licit substances. Anecdotal evidence suggests that a pharmacological interaction may occur between these substances *(58)*. Recently, Tanda and Goldberg *(59)* reviewed the pharmacologic effects of combining caffeine and nicotine. They indicated that the rewarding and subjective properties of nicotine can be changed by chronic caffeine exposure and concluded that caffeine exposure may be an important environmental factor in shaping and maintaining tobacco smoking. In particular, chronic exposure to caffeine in drinking water potentiated nicotine self-administration. Acute administration of nicotine (gum, 2 mg) combined with caffeine (250 mg) has been shown to facilitate memory and motor function of female smokers and nonsmokers *(42)*. In addition, a study in 10 healthy volunteers (5 men and 5 women) showed that nicotine (gum, 4 mg) combined with intravenous caffeine (250 mg) produced additive effects on cardiovascular parameters *(60)*. In dogs, caffeine and nicotine combination produced significant synergistic excitatory effects *(61)*.

3.1.8. Carbon Tetrachloride

The effects of nicotine on the liver were studied in both the presence and absence of carbon tetrachloride, a known hepatotoxic solvent *(62)*. Nicotine alone, when given to rats at a concentration of 54 µmol/L, produced slight hepatotoxic effects, but when coadministered with carbon tetrachloride, the result was significant confluent necrosis compared to the control group and to the group receiving only carbon tetrachloride. Treatment with a higher dose of nicotine, 108 µmol/L, alone also showed significant pathological changes. These levels of nicotine were indicated to be comparable to those found in chronic smokers. It was also reported that pregnant rats were more resistant to the hepatotoxicity produced by nicotine and carbon tetrachloride suggesting that pregnancy somehow protects animals from the hepatotoxicity of nicotine and carbon tetrachloride.

3.1.9. Cimetidine

Cimetidine produces a variety of drug–drug interactions by inhibition of oxidative metabolism. In humans, cimetidine has been shown to increase plasma area under the curve (AUC) of nicotine and half-life by 48% and 45%, respectively *(63)*. A similar effect by cimetidine has also been demonstrated in stumptailed macaques *(64)*.

3.1.10. Cocaine

Nicotine treatment (two transdermal patches containing 22 mg) produced enhanced cue-induced cocaine craving and anxiety in patients with a history of crack cocaine abuse *(65)*. In contrast, nicotine treatment (transdermal patch containing 14 mg) of seven male tobacco smokers who used cocaine occasionally attenuated cocaine-induced increases of "high" and "stimulated," but did not alter cocaine's cardiovascular effects or plasma concentrations of cocaine and its metabolites *(66)*.

3.1.11. Nitrites

The presence of nitrosamines in tobacco has been conclusively established. Additional amounts of nitrosamines could be formed endogenously by interaction between nicotine and sodium nitrite. Carmella et al. *(67)* identified N'-nitrosonornicotine (NNN), a known carcinogen, in the urine of rats treated with nicotine and sodium nitrite. The authors hypothesized that NNN formation could have occurred by direct reaction of nicotine with sodium nitrite in the acidic environs of the stomach, or by nitrosation of nornicotine produced metabolically from nicotine. Interestingly, Du et al. *(68)* found that penetration of NNN across porcine oral mucosa was significantly increased in the presence of nicotine and ethanol. The authors suggested that the synergy between tobacco and alcohol in the etiology of oral cancer could be explained by the permeabilizing effects of alcohol on the penetration of tobacco-specific carcinogens across the oral mucosa.

3.1.12. Opioids

In self-administration studies with methadone-maintained patients, nicotine administration (gum, 2 and 4 mg) produced a significant increase in methadone consumption as compared to when subjects were nicotine abstinent *(69)*. It was suggested that nicotine enhanced methadone consumption either by potentiating the reinforcing effects of methadone or by serving as a conditioned or discriminative stimulus.

3.1.13. Phencyclidine

In mice, nicotine blocked phencyclidine-induced behavioral toxicity (circular movements, side-to-side head movements, and hyperactivity) at high doses (12.3 and 30.8 µmol/kg), but at low doses (1.5 µmol/kg) significantly potentiated phencyclidine-induced convulsions *(70)*. In rats treated chronically with saline or nicotine (1 mg/kg twice daily for 11 d), there were no significant differences in the disposition of phencyclidine *(71)*. These results suggested that the interactions of phencyclidine and nicotine occurred through central nicotinic and muscarinic acetylcholine receptors.

3.2. Tobacco Interactions

3.2.1. Alcohol

It is well known that heavy drinkers tend to be heavy smokers and that consumption of alcohol is correlated with cigarette smoking. It has also been suggested that tobacco smoking could serve to attenuate the sedating effects of alcohol consumption *(72)*. Both drugs appear to operate through common neurologic systems. Behavioral reinforcement by either nicotine or ethanol is associated with the release of dopamine from mesolimbic dopaminergic terminals located in the nucleus accumbens *(73)*. Accordingly, it has been hypothesized that tobacco may decrease the risk of drinking for abstinent alcoholics. However, the role of smoking in the alcohol relapse process is controversial. If alcohol craving involves depletion of dopamine or endogenous opiates, the stimulatory effects of smoking on these systems may decrease craving. On the other hand, tobacco use may stimulate common neurological mechanisms, thereby increasing craving. It seems doubtful at this point that any favorable effects of smoking on alcohol recovery would outweigh the long-term harmful effects produced by smoking *(73)*.

3.2.2. Analgesic/Antipyretics

The inductive effect of smoking on the metabolism of phenacetin was first reported by Pantuck et al. *(74)*. Oral doses of 900 mg of phenacetin resulted in significantly lower plasma phenacetin concentrations in smokers compared to nonsmokers. Peak plasma levels of phenacetin at 2 h were 2.24 µg/mL in nonsmokers and 0.48 µg/mL in smokers. Recovery of N-acetyl-p-aminophenol (APAP) in urine indicated that similar drug absorption had occurred in both groups leading to the presumption that smoking had induced increased metabolism during the "first pass" through the liver *(75)*. Subsequent studies in animals exposed to cigarette smoke confirmed this assumption *(76)*. The effects of smoking on the disposition of acetaminophen have not been as consistent *(77)*. Miller *(78)* concluded that because of the large therapeutic index of acetaminophen, it is not likely that an increase in its metabolism would be clinically important.

The metabolism of nonsteroidal antiinflammatory drugs (NSAIDs) may be affected by smoking. For example, Garg and Ravi *(79)* administered a single oral dose of 6 mg phenylbutazone/kg to seven cigarette smokers and to seven nonsmokers. Plasma phenylbutazone half-life was shortened significantly in the cigarette smokers as compared to the nonsmoker control group. Phenylbutazone was cleared from the blood significantly faster in the smoking group than in the nonsmoking group. This difference in metabolism was attributed to liver enzyme induction. However, there are no studies reporting similar effects with other NSAIDs including aspirin, ibuprofen, naproxen, and indomethacin. Further, there are no data indicating a decreased analgesic efficacy or higher dose requirements of these medications among smokers compared to nonsmokers.

There is an indication that smokers may be more susceptible to the antiaggregatory effects of aspirin. Aspirin has been recommended as an adjuvant therapy in the prevention of cardiovascular event. Smoking causes atherosclerosis, and smokers have increased thromboxane A2 (TXA2) formation *(30)*. The effect of smoking on TXA2 appears to be related to a nonnicotine component of tobacco smoke. In a study comparing the effects of smoking compared to nicotine patch, Benowitz et al. *(80)* found that smoking produced significantly greater increases in TXA2 metabolite excretion than with nicotine patch treatment, despite comparable levels of nicotine.

Weber et al. *(81)* investigated the effects of aspirin (100 mg every second day for 14 d) on platelet function in nine healthy nonsmokers and in nine healthy habitual smokers. There was a significantly stronger inhibition of collagen- and (adenosine 5'-diphosphate) ADP-induced platelet aggregation by aspirin in smokers as compared to nonsmokers. This difference occurred in the presence of an almost complete inhibition of TXA2 synthesis in both groups. The platelet capacity to generate TXA2 in vitro was significantly reduced in smokers; urinary excretion of TXA2, however, was significantly increased. Thus, the better susceptibility of smokers to antiaggregatory effects of aspirin is very likely to be related to a chronic smoking-induced alteration of platelet TXA2 system.

3.2.3. Anticoagulants

Heparin pharmacokinetics have been shown to be altered in smokers compared to nonsmokers. Smoking induced a significant decrease in heparin's elimination half-life (0.97 ± 0.28 h in nonsmokers and 0.62 ± 0.16 h in smokers), faster clearance rate, and a modest increase in dosage requirements *(82)*. Consequently, smokers may require higher heparin doses relative to nonsmokers for anticoagulant therapy.

Smoking has modest effects on the pharmacokinetics of warfarin. In a study of nine cigarette smokers who ingested an average of 0.032 mg/kg of warfarin for 2 wk while smoking and for 2 additional wk following a month of abstinence, clearance was decreased by 13% during smoking abstinence *(83)*. A concomitant 13% increase in warfarin concentration occurred, but there was no accompanying effect on prothrombin time. It was concluded that despite the apparent pharmacokinetic interaction between smoking and warfarin, the net effect on warfarin pharmacodynamics was negligible.

3.2.4. Antidepressants

There is clear evidence that smoking in patients with depression is higher than in the general population. Indications are that induction of CYP isoenzymes by smoking generally lower plasma levels of the parent antidepressant, but may or may not affect active metabolite levels. Desai et al. *(84)* recently reviewed the evidence of smoking on psychotropic medications. Serum levels of amitriptyline, nortriptyline, imipramine, clomipramine, fluvoxamine, and trazodone were found to be lower in smokers compared to nonsmokers; however, differences were not always significant. Amfebutamone (bupropion) levels do not appear to be affected by smoking. Dosage adjustments for smokers receiving amitriptyline, nortriptyline, and bupropion were not suggested, but there may be a need for higher dosages of fluvoxamine and trazodone for optimal therapy.

3.2.5. Antipsychotics

Smoking prevalence in schizophrenia is generally highest among neuropsychiatric disorders (approximately 80%) and smoking withdrawal results in worsening of schizophrenic symptoms *(85)*. Tobacco use may represent an attempt to self-medicate, relieve drug-induced adverse events, and improve cognitive deficits. The reduction in drug-induced adverse events may be caused by PAH enzyme induction with resultant reduced blood concentrations of medication *(86)*. In a review by Desai et al. *(84)*, it was reported that the frequency of drowsiness induced by chlorpromazine was lowest in heavy smokers (3%) compared to light smokers (11%) and nonsmokers (16%). Pantuck et al. *(87)* evaluated the disposition of a single 75-mg oral dose of chlorpromazine in healthy male smokers and nonsmokers. Greater sleepiness was noted in nonsmokers compared to smokers. Chlorpromazine peak levels and AUC were 24% and 36% lower, respectively, in smokers compared to nonsmokers. However the differences were not significant, probably because of the small number of subjects in the study. There was no correlation between plasma drug concentrations and either the degree of sleepiness or the degree of orthostatic hypotension in the subjects. Chetty et al. *(88)* reported higher clearance rate of chlorpromazine in smokers with chronic schizophrenia (175 L/h) compared to nonsmokers (127 L/h). It was suggested that a higher dosage may be necessary in patients who are smokers. Interestingly, cannabis smokers demonstrated even higher clearance rates (191 L/h) than tobacco smokers.

Clearance rates of tiotixene and fluphenazine have been reported to be significantly higher and resulting plasma levels lower for smokers compared to nonsmokers *(84)*. Plasma levels of haloperidol and metabolite were significantly lower in smokers in some studies *(89,90)*, but results in other studies were inconclusive *(84,91)*. No significant differences in pharmacokinetic parameters were found for patients receiving a single dose of trifluoroperazine.

Haring et al. *(92)* and Seppala et al. *(93)* reported significantly lower mean plasma clozapine concentrations in smokers compared to nonsmokers. Haseqawa et al. *(94)* also found lower plasma levels of clozapine in schizophrenic patients who were smokers, but the differences were not significant. If enzyme induction by smoking is the cause for lower clozapine plasma levels, it is reasonable to expect that smoking cessation could result in increased drug levels and incidence of adverse side effects. Meyer *(95)* reported a mean increase in clozapine levels of 71.9% upon smoking cessation in 11 patients who were on stable clozapine doses. Oyewumi *(96)* describes a case in which emergence of clozapine side effects (urinary hesitancy, constipation, and erectile and ejaculatory dysfunction) occurred in a male patient who stopped smoking. The patient had been successfully maintained on clozapine for 4 yr prior to his decision to stop smoking. Skogh et al. *(97)* describes a 35-yr-old man who had been successfully treated with clozapine at a daily dose of 700–725 mg for more than 7 consecutive years. Two weeks after cessation of smoking, he suddenly developed tonic clonic seizures followed by stupor and coma. When he recovered, clozapine therapy was reinstituted successfully at 425 mg daily.

Plasma levels of zotepine have been generally found to be lower in smokers compared with nonsmokers. In contrast, the C_{max} of olanzapine was slightly greater in smokers, but clearance rates for smokers were significantly higher (23% increase).

Fluvoxamine is a selective serotonin reuptake inhibitor metabolized partly by CYP1A2. Spigset et al. *(98)* reported that smokers had significantly lower AUCs and C_{max} serum concentrations than nonsmokers, but there was no significant difference in half-life. The authors suggested that a higher dose may be needed for smoker compared to nonsmokers.

3.2.6. Benzodiazepines

No significant differences in the pharmacokinetic parameters of smokers vs nonsmokers were found in a study of a single dose of 0.5 mg of triazolam (99). Similar findings were made in studies of 0.5 mg of triazolam and 0.8 mg alprazolam in healthy Japanese men, but the mean elimination half-life of alprazolam was significantly shorter in smokers than in nonsmokers (100). However, another study of alprazolam showed that cigarette smoking caused a 100% increase in the clearance of alprazolam compared with nonsmokers (101). The minimal differences in plasma levels found in these studies suggest that dosage adjustments would not be needed for smokers vs nonsmokers. Intravenous administration of 2 mg of lorazepam resulted in significantly shorter half-lives in smokers compared with nonsmokers, but other pharmacokinetic parameters were unchanged (102).

The incidence of drowsiness in patients receiving diazepam and chlordiazepoxide has been noted to be highest in nonsmokers, intermediate in light smokers, and lowest in heavy smokers (103). Whether the interaction between cigarette smoking and benzodiazepines is related to altered pharmacokinetics or altered end-organ response is not known. The results of pharmacokinetic studies of diazepam and desmethyldiazepam in smokers compared to nonsmokers have not been conclusive. In one study, cigarette smoking produced significantly lower clearance rates in elderly men compared to young men (104). In a study of desmethyldiazepam, the half-life was significantly shorter and C_{max} was lower in smokers than in nonsmokers. In contrast, other researchers have found no effect of smoking on the pharmacokinetics of diazepam or desmethyldiazepam (102,105,106). Chlordiazepoxide kinetics have also been shown to be unaffected by smoking (107). However, in a study of oxazepam in relation to age, gender, and cigarette smoking, the mean clearance of oxazepam in smokers was shown to be significantly higher than in nonsmokers, suggesting that smoking is a more important determinant of oxazepam clearance than age or gender (108).

3.2.7. Caffeine

The metabolism of caffeine in humans results in production of at least 17 urinary metabolites. Considerable effort has been focused on the use of caffeine as a substrate probe for CYP1A and other xenobiotic metabolizing enzymes (109). Caffeine clearance is increased by cigarette smoking (110), presumably through induction of CYP1A enzymes by polycyclic aromatic hydrocarbons. An increase in metabolism results in a shorter half-life for caffeine during smoking. Consequently, it would be reasonable to expect that smoking cessation would result in an increase in caffeine levels thereby increasing risk for caffeine toxicity. Brown et al. (111) reported that abstinence from smoking for 4 d resulted in a 46% increase in the 24-h AUC blood caffeine levels for subjects while consuming six cups of coffee per day. Oliveto et al. (112) also found abstinence increased caffeine levels; however, the effect was not statistically significant. Benowitz et al. (113) also reported that plasma caffeine concentrations increased during abstinence after people gave up smoking and remained increased for at least 6 mo. The increase in plasma caffeine levels was substantial, averaging more than 250%, whereas levels were unchanged in subjects who continued to smoke. Thus, it appears that when a person stops smoking, metabolism of caffeine slows, clearance slows, half-life lengthens, and plasma caffeine increases.

3.2.8. Carbamazepine

Carbamazepine is metabolized mainly by CYP3A4, but also by CYP1A2. Chronic dosing produces enzyme induction and an increase in its metabolism. Studies of the effects of smoking, however, have shown no influence on postinduction carbamazepine clearance *(114)*.

3.2.9. Cardiovascular Drugs

The effectiveness of β-blockers in control of blood pressure, heart rate, and prevention of end-organ damage is reduced in smokers compared with nonsmokers *(115,116)*. However, another study found no difference in benefit derived from β-blockers between smokers and nonsmokers *(117)*. The basis of this interaction may be pharmacodynamic since nicotine causes catecholamine release and increases blood pressure and heart rate.

Hitzenberger et al. *(118)* found no effect of smoking on propranolol or pindolol; however, Walle et al. *(119)* reported that cigarette smoking increased the oral clearance of propranolol in male subjects by 77%. The kinetic and metabolic effects induced by smoking were characterized by a large induction of side-chain oxidation of propranolol without an effect on aromatic-ring oxidation. Smoking also induced an increase in the glucuronidation of propranolol. The results suggest that side-chain oxidation and glucuronidation of propranolol are mediated by isoenzymes inducible by aromatic hydrocarbons found in cigarette smoke, whereas the rate of aromatic-ring oxidation was not changed by smoking.

Increased clearance of some antiarrhythmics has also been reported. Higher metabolic clearance rates and lower trough concentrations for flecainide was observed for smokers compared to nonsmokers resulting in the need for higher doses of flecainide for arrhythmia control *(120)*. Oral clearance of lidocaine *(121)* and mexiletine *(122)* has been reported to be increased in smokers. Although the mechanism is unknown, enhanced hepatic metabolism from smoking is likely responsible for the increased clearance of antiarrhythmics.

Furosemide is a potent diuretic. Lambert et al. *(123)* found that tobacco smoking in normal subjects affects the diuretic response to furosemide without modifying kinetics. Five nonsmokers and five smokers were given a single intravenous injection of 40 mg furosemide. Cumulative 8-h urinary excretion of sodium was identical for smokers and nonsmokers. However, diuresis was smaller by 800 mL (20%) in smokers than in nonsmokers. Furosemide increased endogenous creatinine clearance from 117 to 196 mL/min in nonsmokers and from 136 to 180 mL/min in smokers. The increase in free-water clearance caused by furosemide was smaller in the smoking group than in the nonsmoking group. Protein binding and distribution of furosemide were not affected by tobacco smoking. Furosemide clearance was slightly higher in smokers than in nonsmokers, which was primarily the result of a slight increase in extrarenal furosemide clearance. Whereas the foregoing suggests that higher doses of furosemide might be required in smokers to compensate for the diminished effects on diuresis, Vapaatalo et al. *(124)* report that tolerance develops to nicotine's effects on furosemide. This development of tolerance suggests that chronic smokers would not require different doses of furosemide, but that a dosage adjustment may be required among patients using furosemide who begin smoking while on the medication.

3.2.10. Insulin

Nicotine increases CNS sympathetic overflow, adrenal release of catecholamines, and local release of catecholamines from vascular nerve endings *(23)*. This results in constriction of some blood vessels, including cutaneous blood vessels. Because of decreased blood flow through cutaneous blood vessels, the rate of absorption of insulin after subcutaneous injection is reduced *(125)*. Klemp et al. *(126)* demonstrated that insulin absorption is decreased by 113% during cigarette smoking, and showed a 30% decrease 30 min after smoking *(126)*. For this reason, smokers may require more insulin compared with nonsmokers. For example, Madsbad et al. *(127)* found smokers had on the average a 15–20% higher insulin requirement compared with nonsmokers. Further, as suggested by NRT product labeling (e.g., Nicorette), a dose adjustment may be required upon smoking cessation. It should be noted that there does not seem to be a difference in glycemic control between smokers and nonsmokers. For example, Mathiesen et al. *(128)* found no significant difference between smokers and nonsmokers in glycemic control as judged from the level of stable hemoglobin A1c *(128)*.

3.2.11. Opioids

There appears to be an interaction between some component of tobacco smoke and dextropropoxyphene. For example, 10% of nonsmokers did not have an analgesic effect from dextropropoxyphene treatment compared to 20% of heavy smokers *(129, 130)*. The effect of smoking status on the analgesic effects of dextropropoxyphene may be related to lower pain tolerance among smokers. It has been shown that, at least among Caucasians, smokers have less pain tolerance than nonsmokers *(131)*. This may indicate that smokers may require higher doses of dextropropoxyphene to obtain effective analgesia.

Vaughan et al. *(132)* studied the metabolism of pentazocine among 70 male and female smokers and nonsmokers. They found an overall threefold intersubject variation in elimination. The cumulative urinary excretion of pentazocine was normally distributed in both smokers and nonsmokers. Smokers metabolized 40% more pentazocine than do nonsmokers. It was concluded that induction is principally responsible for the observed subject variability. Consistent with the lower plasma concentrations of pentazocine caused by the increased metabolism of the drug by smokers, Keeri-Szanto et al. *(133)* found that smokers required larger doses of pentazocine to achieve an analgesic effect.

Cigarette smoking has no clinically important influence on codeine absorption or disposition. Hull et al. *(134)* found no significant difference between smokers and nonsmokers in either codeine or morphine AUCs or oral bioavailability, after oral administration of codeine *(135)*. Similarly, Rogers et al. *(136)* found no differences between smokers and nonsmokers with respect to maximum plasma concentration (C_{max}) of codeine, time to attain this concentration (t_{max}), codeine plasma half-life ($t_{1/2}$), or AUCs for codeine or morphine. There was a faster, but clinically unimportant, mean apparent plasma clearance in smokers (52.8 mL/min/70 kg) than in nonsmokers (45.0 mL/min/70 kg) after intramuscular injection only. Mean oral codeine bioavailability in smokers and in nonsmokers did not differ. Cigarette smoking slightly but significantly induced the glucuronidation of codeine as shown by a decreased metabolic ratio for glucuronidation in the smokers, whereas *O*- and *N*-demethylations were not significantly changed

13. Nicotine

as indicated by the similar metabolic ratios in smokers and in nonsmokers. Increased codeine dose requirements may be required because of the differences in pain tolerance between smokers and nonsmokers.

Long-term administration of tobacco for 28 d to rats resulted in the increase in N-demethylation of meperidine by 2.5-fold and morphine by twofold (137). In humans, however, the mean total clearance rates of meperidine in smokers and nonsmokers have not been found to be different (138).

In self-administration studies with methadone-maintained patients, cigarette smoking produced a significant increase in methadone consumption as compared to when subjects were nicotine abstinent (69).

3.2.12. Steroid Hormones

Cigarette smoking provides a protective effect in women against endometrial cancer, but may lead to earlier natural menopause and increased risk of osteoporosis (139,140). This antiestrogenic effect appears to be explained by increased hepatic metabolism of estradiol to 2-hydroxy-estrogens, metabolites that are devoid of peripheral estrogenic activity. Michnovicz et al. (141) found an approximate 50% increase in 2-hydroxylation of estradiol in premenopausal women who smoked at least 15 cigarettes per day. Increased metabolism via the 2-hydroxylation pathway would lead to decreased bioavailability at estrogen target tissues.

Smoking interactions with oral contraceptives appear to be minimal. Crawford et al. (142) examined the effects of smoking on ethinyl estradiol and levonorgestrel in 311 women and concluded that smoking did not significantly affect plasma concentrations. Kanarkowski et al. (143) evaluated the pharmacokinetics of single and multiple doses of ethinyl estradiol and levonorgestrel in smoking and nonsmoking women and found a joint effect of chronic oral contraceptive use and smoking. There was a tendency toward lower ethinyl estradiol clearances after acute oral contraceptive use in smokers, but the effect was not significant. There was a significant smoking-oral contraceptive effect noted, but this effect was based on only three subjects. Importantly, Vessey et al. (144) observed no increase in failure rates of oral contraceptives in a study of nonsmokers, exsmokers, and smoking women. Miller (145) concluded that based on available evidence, that it would be premature to adjust estrogen dosages based on cigarette consumption.

3.2.13. Tacrine

Smoking significantly induces the metabolism of tacrine. Welty et al. (146) reported consistently lower plasma levels of tacrine and its hydroxy-metabolites. The AUC for tacrine was approximately 10-fold higher in nonsmokers. The AUCs for 1-hydroxytacrine and 2-hydroxytacrine were approximately threefold higher in nonsmokers. The mean tacrine elimination half-life was 2.1 h in smokers and 3.2 h in nonsmokers. It was suggested that the increased clearance in smokers was due to induction of CYP1A2 enzyme. Consequently, smokers may require higher doses of tacrine than nonsmokers (147).

3.2.14. Theophylline

Theophylline is commonly prescribed to smokers with chronic pulmonary disease. Concentrations of 10–20 µg/mL are needed to produce effective bronchodilation, but higher levels increasingly produce unacceptable adverse reactions. Higher levels may produce severe toxicities including cardiac arrhythmias and seizure. Consequently, serum theophylline monitoring is essential for careful patient management. Cigarette smoking is known to induce the metabolism of theophylline resulting in increased theophylline clearance and a shorter half-life *(148–150)*. Hunt et al. *(149)* has suggested that young patients who require theophylline and smoke would probably need daily dosages about twice those needed by nonsmokers. Abstinence from smoking would be expected to return an individual to basal levels of theophylline metabolism. Lee et al. *(151)* showed that the effects of brief abstinence (1 wk) from smoking resulted in a 37.6% decrease in theophylline clearance and a 35.8% increase in half-life, whereas nicotine gum (4 mg) had no effect. The lack of effect by nicotine indicated that accelerated metabolism of theophylline is related to the effects of polycyclic aromatic hydrocarbons or other constituents in tobacco smoke. It was suggested that theophylline-treated patients be carefully monitored during periods of abstinence or smoking cessation and that doses of theophylline be reduced by one-fourth to one-third to avoid development of theophylline toxicity.

Passive exposure to tobacco smoke may engender many of the same effects as active smoking. Mayo *(152)* investigated the effects of passive tobacco smoking on the metabolism of theophylline in a pediatric population. Total body clearance of theophylline was significantly elevated in children exposed to environmental tobacco smoke (1.36 mL/min compared to 0.90 mL/min), and steady-state serum levels were significantly lower in those exposed compared to the children without any environmental exposure to tobacco smoke.

4. ORAL TOBACCO USE AND INTERACTIONS

Drug interactions with oral tobacco have not been well studied. However, because plasma nicotine levels reach levels as high as those seen during use of smoked tobacco, one could predict similar nicotine interactions as during smoking, as discussed above. Whether or not there are nonnicotine components of oral tobacco that interact with other drugs has not been studied.

There is an indication that nicotine and alcohol interact to increase the permeability of the tobacco-specific carcinogen, NNN, across the oral mucosa *(68)*. Concentrations of ethanol of 25% and above significantly increased the permeability of the porcine oral mucosa to NNN and the presence of 0.2% nicotine significantly increased the permeability of oral mucosa to NNN. Combined use of nicotine and ethanol significantly increased the penetration of NNN across oral mucosa over that of ethanol alone until the concentration of ethanol reached 50%. This suggests that the interaction of nicotine and alcohol could increase the risk of oral cancer. In addition, because nicotine alone increased the permeability of NNN, permeability of other oral-mucosa delivered medications may increase among users of smokeless tobacco.

5. CONTRAINDICATIONS

The only contraindications listed for nicotine replacement therapies are hypersensitivity or allergy to nicotine, or to components of the specific formulations (e.g., menthol in the vapor inhaler or adhesives in the patch). There are no contraindications based upon use of other medications.

There are no contraindications for smoking based upon concomitant use of other drugs. However, as discussed below, people who smoke, or people who stop smoking, may require dosage adjustments when using some medications.

6. Precautions for Use

Labeling for all nicotine replacement medications instruct patients to stop tobacco use completely when using NRT. This is because concomitant use of NRT and smoking might produce nicotine levels higher than smoking or NRT use alone. All NRT products urge patients to discontinue use if there is a clinically significant cardiovascular or other effect attributable to nicotine. They also note, as discussed in the next section, that concomitant medications may require a dose adjustment during cessation. This is not an effect of the nicotine replacement medication, *per se*, but rather an effect of reduced exposure to nicotine compared to smoking levels during a cessation attempt.

Because tobacco is not regulated by the FDA, there are no specific precautions for use. However, smoking is known to cause a number of cancers and heart disease, cause adverse effects on fetal development, and cause physical dependence and addiction.

7. Frequent or Serious Reactions

Given that approximately 25% of the U.S. adult population smokes cigarettes and that these persons are substantially more likely than nonsmokers to have comorbid cardiovascular and psychiatric disorders *(153,154)*, there is a substantial potential that persons undergoing smoking cessation will be receiving medications for which there will be potential alterations in dosing required to avoid toxicity and/or sustain therapeutic effects. Conversely, except during adolescence when nearly all tobacco use begins *(155)*, there is only a small risk that an adult who is receiving a medication will take up smoking and virtually no risk that nicotine medications will be used. A caveat is that with the increasing occurrence of cigar smoking among persons of all ages, this form of tobacco intake should be routinely considered for its potential interactive effects with medications. As suggested by the incredible diversity of cigar dosing potential and patterns of use, relative to cigarette smoking, it would be important to carefully question persons about the size of their cigars and frequency of use in order to provide some basis for beginning to estimate the probability of an interaction of concern. Monitoring of therapeutic effects and potential adverse interactions of the sort that would be consistent with those predicted in studies currently reviewed would then be indicated.

Approximately 17 million persons attempt smoking cessation each year and even though less than 10% of these persons achieve lasting cessation success, the numbers of people who will need potential modification of their dosing regimens for other drugs is considerable. Furthermore, because of the increasing rates of attempted smoking cessation, interactions as summarized in this review could become even more commonplace than they currently are. It is clear that, although there is a scientific basis for predicting potential interactions, much more research is needed to provide useful guidance to health care professionals regarding their use of therapeutic drugs in tobacco users, nicotine medication users, and those seeking abstinence from tobacco.

Some medications may require a dose adjustment during smoking cessation. Table 1, from nicotine gum labeling, lists several drugs that may require a dose alteration upon smoking cessation, with or without use of NRT.

Table 1
Drugs That May Require Dosage Adjustments When Smokers Quit Smoking

Drug	Possible Mechanism
Drugs that may require a dose decrease upon cessation	
Acetaminophen, caffeine, imipramine, oxazepam, pentazocine, propranolol, theophylline	Deinduction of hepatic enzymes on smoking cessation
Insulin	Increase of subcutaneous insulin absorption with smoking cessation
Adrenergic antagonists (e.g., prazosin, labetalol)	Decrease in circulating catecholamines with smoking cessation
Drugs that may require an increase in dose at cessation of smoking	
Adrenergic agonists (e.g., isoproterenol, phenylephrine)	Decrease in circulating catecholamines with smoking cessation

Table 2
Drugs That Often Require Higher Doses in Smokers Compared to Nonsmokers

Drug	Possible Mechanism
Insulin	Lower subcutaneous insulin absorption during smoking
Propoxyphene	Unknown
Propranolol	Increased oral clearance
Theophylline	Enzyme induction increases clearance and reduced half-life in smokers
Clozapine	Enzyme induction

There are five medications identified that interact with tobacco use to the extent that higher dosages of these medications may be required for tobacco users compared to patients who do not use tobacco. In addition, theophylline clearance has been shown to be altered by passive smoking, and the possibility exists that other medications may also be affected by passive smoking. These medications and their possible mechanisms of action are summarized in Table 2. It should also be noted that for each of these medications, smoking cessation might require a decrease in dosage.

REFERENCES

1. Benowitz NL. Nicotine replacement therapy. What has been accomplished—can we do better? Drugs 45:157–170 (1993).
2. Benowitz NL and Jacob P. III Daily intake of nicotine during cigarette smoking. Clin Pharmacol Ther 35:499–504 (1984).
3. Henningfield JE. Nicotine medications for smoking cessation. N Engl J Med 333:1196–1203 (1995).
4. Benowitz NL. Clinical pharmacology of transdermal nicotine. Eur J Pharm Biopharm 41:168–174 (1995).

5. Henningfield JE, Stapleton JM, Benowitz NL, Grayson RF, and London ED. Higher levels of nicotine in arterial than in venous blood after cigarette smoking. Drug Alcohol Depend 33:23–29 (1993).
6. Gourlay SG and Benowitz NL. Arteriovenous differences in plasma concentration of nicotine and catecholamines and related cardiovascular effects after smoking, nicotine nasal spray, and intravenous nicotine. Clin Pharmacol Ther 62:453–463 (1997).
7. Lunell E, Molander L, and Andersson SB. Temperature dependency of the release and bioavailability of nicotine from a nicotine vapour inhaler; in vitro/ in vivo correlation. Eur J Pharmacol 52:495–500 (1997).
8. Schuh KJ, Schuh LM, Henningfield JE, and Stitzer ML. Nicotine nasal spray and vapor inhaler: abuse liability assessment. Psychopharmacology (Berl) 130:352–361 (1997).
9. Lunell E, Bergstrom M, Antoni G, Langstrom B, and Nordberg A. Nicotine deposition and body distribution from a nicotine inhaler and a cigarette studied with positron emission tomography. Clin Pharmacol Ther 59:593–594 (1996).
10. Anonymous. Use of FDA-approved pharmacologic treatments for tobacco dependence—United States, 1984–1998. MMWR 49:665–668 (2000).
11. U.S. Department of Health and Human Services and U.S. Food and Drug Administration. Regulations restricting the sale and distribution of cigarettes and smokeless tobacco to protect children and adolescents. Federal Register 61:44396–45318 (1996).
12. McKim WA. Drugs and behavior: an introduction to behavioral pharmacology. Englewood Cliffs, NJ: Prentice-Hall, 1986.
13. Henningfield JE, Hariharan M, and Kozlowski LT. Nicotine content and health risks of cigars. JAMA 276:1857–1858 (1996).
14. Fant RV, Henningfield JE, Nelson R, and Pickworth WB. Pharmacokinetics and pharmacodynamics of moist snuff in humans. Tob Control 8:387–392 (1999).
15. Summary of findings from the 2000 National Household Survey on Drug Abuse. NHSDA Series H-13. DHHS Publication No. (SMA) 01-3549. Rockville, MD: Substance Abuse and Mental Health Services Administration, 2001.
16. Anonymous. State-specific prevalence of current cigarette smoking among adults, and policies and attitudes about secondhand smoke—United States, 2000. MMWR 50:1101–1105 (2001).
17. U.S. Department of Health and Human Services. The health benefits of smoking cessation; a report of the Surgeon General, 1990. Washington, DC: U.S. Government Printing Office, 1990.
18. Hoffmann D and Hoffmann I. The changing cigarette, 1950–1995. J Toxicol Environ Health 50:307–364 (1997).
19. American Psychiatric Association. Diagnostic and statistical manual of mental disorders. Washington, DC, 1994.
20. Heishman SJ, Taylor RC, and Henningfield JE. Nicotine and smoking: a review of effects on human performance. Exp Clin Psychopharmacol 2:345–395 (1994).
21. Henningfield JE, Schuh LM, and Jarvik ME. Pathophysiology of tobacco dependence. In: Bloom FE and Kupfer DJ, eds. Psychopharmacology: the fourth generation of progress. New York: Raven, 1995:1715–1729.
22. Kessler DA, Witt AM, Barnett PS, Zeller MR, Natanblut SL, Wilkenfeld JP, et al. The Food and Drug Administration's regulation of tobacco products. N Engl J Med 335:988–994 (1996).
23. Benowitz NL. Cardiovascular toxicity of nicotine: pharmacokinetic and pharmacodynamic considerations. In: Benowitz NL, ed. Nicotine safety and toxicity. New York: Oxford University Press, 1998:19–27.

24. Oncken CA, Hardardottir H, and Smeltzer JS. Human studies of nicotine replacement during pregnancy. In: Benowitz NL, ed. Nicotine safety and toxicity. New York: Oxford University Press, 1998:107–116.
25. Porchet HC, Benowitz NL, Sheiner LB, and Copeland JR. Apparent tolerance to the acute effect of nicotine results in part from distribution kinetics. J Clin Invest 80:1466–1471 (1987).
26. Benowitz NL. Toxicity of nicotine: implications with regard to nicotine replacement therapy. Prog Clin Biol Res 261:187–217 (1988).
27. Goldfrank L, Minek M, and Blum A. Nicotine. Hospital Physician 16:22–35 (1980).
28. Larson PS, Haag HB, and Silvette H. Tobacco. Experimental and clinical studies. A comprehensive account of the world literature. Baltimore: Williams and Wilkins, 1961.
29. U.S. Department of Health and Human Services. The health consequences of smoking: nicotine addiction; a report of the Surgeon General, 1988. Washington, DC: U.S. Government Printing Office, 1988.
30. U.S. Department of Health and Human Services. Reducing the health consequences of smoking: 25 years of progress; a report of the Surgeon General, 1989, executive summary. Washington, DC: U.S. Government Printing Office, 1989.
31. Krupski WC. The peripheral vascular consequences of smoking. Ann Vasc Surg 5:291–304 (1991).
32. Benowitz NL. Summary: risks and benefits of nicotine. In: Benowitz NL, ed. Nicotine safety and toxicity. New York: Oxford University Press, 1998:185–194.
33. Sherman CB. The health consequences of cigarette smoking. Pulmonary diseases. Med Clin North Am 76:355–375 (1992).
34. U.S. Department of Health and Human Services. The health consequences of smoking: chronic obstructive lung disease; a report of the Surgeon General, 1984. Washington, DC: U.S. Government Printing Office, 1984.
35. Sellers EM, Kaplan HL, and Tyndale RF. Inhibition of cytochrome P450 2A6 increases nicotine's oral bioavailability and decreases smoking. Clin Pharmacol Ther 68:35–43 (2000).
36. Pianezza ML, Sellers EM, and Tyndale RF. Nicotine metabolism defect reduces smoking. Nature 393:750 (1998).
37. Tyndale RF and Sellers EM. Variable CYP2A6-mediated nicotine metabolism alters smoking behavior and risk. Drug Metab Dispos 29:548–552 (2001).
38. Benowitz NL and Jacob P III. Nicotine and cotinine elimination pharmacokinetics in smokers and nonsmokers. Clin Pharmacol Ther 53:316–323 (1993).
39. Zevin S and Benowitz NL. Drug interactions with tobacco smoking. An update. Clin Pharmacokinet 36:425–438 (1999).
40. Benowitz NL and Gourlay SG. Cardiovascular toxicity of nicotine: implications for nicotine replacement therapy. J Am Coll Cardiol 29:1422–1431 (1997).
41. Perkins KA, Sexton JE, DiMarco A, Grobe JE, Scierka A, and Stiller RL. Subjective and cardiovascular responses to nicotine combined with alcohol in male and female smokers. Psychopharmacology (Berl) 119:205–212 (1995).
42. Kerr JS, Sherwood N, and Hindmarch I. Separate and combined effects of the social drugs on psychomotor performance. Psychopharmacology (Berl) 104:113–119 (1991).
43. Chen WJ, Parnell SE, and West JR. Nicotine decreases blood alcohol concentration in neonatal rats. Alcohol Clin Exp Res 25:1072–1077 (2001).
44. Soderpalm B, Ericson M, Olausson P, Blomqvist O, and Engel JA. Nicotinic mechanisms involved in the dopamine activating and reinforcing properties of ethanol. Behav Brain Res 113:85–96 (2000).
45. Mehta MC, Jain AC, and Billie M. Combined effects of alcohol and nicotine on cardiovascular performance in a canine model. J Cardiovasc Pharmacol 31:930–936 (1998).

46. Seaton MJ and Vesell ES. Variables affecting nicotine metabolism. Pharmacol Ther 60: 461–500 (1993).
47. Dilsaver SC, Majchrzak MJ, and Alessi NE. Chronic treatment with amitriptyline produces supersensitivity to nicotine. Biol Psychiatry 23:169–175 (1988).
48. Sewell RG, Nanry KP, Kennedy J, Stiger TR, and Harmon RE. Supra-additive toxic interaction of nicotine with antihistamines, and enhancement by the proconvulsant pentylenetetrazole. Pharmacol Biochem Behav 22:469–477 (1985).
49. Levin ED, Wilson W, Rose JE, and McEvoy J. Nicotine-haloperidol interactions and cognitive performance in schizophrenics. Neuropsychopharmacology 15:429–436 (1996).
50. Sanberg PR, Fogelson HM, Manderscheid PZ, Parker KW, Norman AB, and McConville BJ. Nicotine gum and haloperidol in Tourette's syndrome. Lancet 1:592 (1988).
51. Sanberg PR, McConville BJ, Fogelson HM, Manderscheid PZ, Parker KW, Blythe MM, et al. Nicotine potentiates the effects of haloperidol in animals and in patients with Tourette syndrome. Biomed Pharmacother 43:19–23 (1989).
52. Silver AA and Sanberg PR. Transdermal nicotine patch and potentiation of haloperidol in Tourette's syndrome. Lancet 342:182 (1993).
53. Emerich DF, Norman AB, and Sanberg PR. Nicotine potentiates the behavioral effects of haloperidol. Psychopharmacol Bull 27:385–390 (1991).
54. Boye SM and Clarke PB. Enhancement of haloperidol-induced catalepsy by nicotine: an investigation of possible mechanisms. Can J Physiol Pharmacol 78:882–891 (2000).
55. Modak AT and Alderete BE. Nicotine potentiates sodium pentobarbital but not ethanol induced sleep. Subst Alcohol Actions Misuse 4:321–329 (1983).
56. Hisaoka M and Levy G. Kinetics of drug action in disease states XI: effect of nicotine on the pharmacodynamics and pharmacokinetics of phenobarbital and ethanol in rats. J Pharm Sci 74:412–415 (1985).
57. White JM. Behavioral interactions between nicotine and diazepam. Pharmacol Biochem Behav 32:479–482 (1989).
58. Swanson JA, Lee JW, and Hopp JW. Caffeine and nicotine: a review of their joint use and possible interactive effects in tobacco withdrawal. Addict Behav 19:229–256 (1994).
59. Tanda G and Goldberg SR. Alteration of the behavioral effects of nicotine by chronic caffeine exposure. Pharmacol Biochem Behav 66:47–64 (2000).
60. Smits P, Temme L, and Thien T. The cardiovascular interaction between caffeine and nicotine in humans. Clin Pharmacol Ther, 54:194–204 (1993).
61. Jain AC, Mehta MC, and Billie M. Combined effects of caffeine and nicotine on cardiovascular hemodynamics in canine model. J Cardiovasc Pharmacol 29:574–579 (1997).
62. Yuen ST, Gogo AR Jr, Luk IS, Cho CH, Ho JC, and Loh TT. The effect of nicotine and its interaction with carbon tetrachloride in the rat liver. Pharmacol Toxicol 77:225–230 (1995).
63. Bendayan R, Sullivan JT, Shaw C, Frecker RC, and Sellers EM. Effect of cimetidine and ranitidine on the hepatic and renal elimination of nicotine in humans. Eur J Clin Pharmacol 38:165–169 (1990).
64. Seaton M, Kyerematen GA, Morgan M, Jeszenka EV, and Vesell ES. Nicotine metabolism in stumptailed macaques, Macaca arctoides. Drug Metab Dispos 19:946–954 (1991).
65. Reid MS, Mickalian JD, Delucchi KL, Hall SM, and Berger SP. An acute dose of nicotine enhances cue-induced cocaine craving. Drug Alcohol Depend 49:95–104 (1998).
66. Kouri EM, Stull M, and Lukas SE. Nicotine alters some of cocaine's subjective effects in the absence of physiological or pharmacokinetic changes. Pharmacol Biochem Behav 69: 209–217 (2001).
67. Carmella SG, Borukhova A, Desai D, and Hecht SS. Evidence for endogenous formation of tobacco-specific nitrosamines in rats treated with tobacco alkaloids and sodium nitrite. Carcinogenesis 18:587–592 (1997).

68. Du X, Squier CA, Kremer MJ, and Wertz PW. Penetration of N-nitrosonornicotine (NNN) across oral mucosa in the presence of ethanol and nicotine. J Oral Pathol Med 29:80–85 (2000).
69. Spiga R, Schmitz J, and Day J. Effects of nicotine on methadone self-administration in humans. Drug Alcohol Depend 50:157–165 (1998).
70. Chaturvedi AK. Effects of mecamylamine, nicotine, atropine and physostigmine on the phencyclidine-induced behavioral toxicity. Pharmacol Biochem Behav 20:559–566 (1984).
71. Vadlamani NL, Pontani RB, and Misra AL. Effect of chronic nicotine pretreatment on phencyclidine (PCP) disposition in the rat. Arch Int Pharmacodyn Ther 265:4–12 (1983).
72. Zacny JP. Behavioral aspects of alcohol–tobacco interactions. Recent Dev Alcohol 8:205–219 (1990).
73. Narahashi T, Soderpalm B, Ericson M, Olausson P, Engel JA, Zhang X, et al. Mechanisms of alcohol–nicotine interactions: alcoholics versus smokers. Alcohol Clin Exp Res 25: 152S–156S (2001).
74. Pantuck EJ, Kuntzman R, and Conney AH. Decreased concentration of phenacetin in plasma of cigarette smokers. Science 175:1248–1250 (1972).
75. Pantuck EJ, Hsiao KC, Maggio A, Nakamura K, Kuntzman R, and Conney AH. Effect of cigarette smoking on phenacetin metabolism. Clin Pharmacol Ther 15:9–17 (1974).
76. Jusko WJ. Role of tobacco smoking in pharmacokinetics. J Pharmacokinet Biopharm 6: 7–39 (1978).
77. Kuntzman R, Pantuck EJ, Kaplan SA, and Conney AH. Phenacetin metabolism: effect of hydrocarbons and cigarette smoking. Clin Pharmacol Ther 22:757–764 (1977).
78. Miller LG. Cigarettes and drug therapy: pharmacokinetic and pharmacodynamic considerations. Clin Pharm 9:125–135 (1990).
79. Garg SK and Ravi Kiran TN. Effect of smoking on phenylbutazone disposition. Int J Clin Pharmacol Ther Toxicol 20:289–290 (1982).
80. Benowitz NL, Fitzgerald GA, Wilson M, and Zhang Q. Nicotine effects on eicosanoid formation and hemostatic function: comparison of transdermal nicotine and cigarette smoking. J Am Coll Cardiol 22:1159–1167 (1993).
81. Weber AA, Liesener S, Schanz A, Hohlfeld T, and Schror K. Habitual smoking causes an abnormality in platelet thromboxane A2 metabolism and results in an altered susceptibility to aspirin effects. Platelets 11:177–182 (2000).
82. Cipolle RJ, Seifert RD, Neilan BA, Zaske DE, and Haus E. Heparin kinetics: variables related to disposition and dosage. Clin Pharmacol Ther 29:387–393 (1981).
83. Bachmann K, Shapiro R, Fulton R, Carroll FT, and Sullivan TJ. Smoking and warfarin disposition. Clin Pharmacol Ther 25:309–315 (1979).
84. Desai HD, Seabolt J, and Jann MW. Smoking in patients receiving psychotropic medications: a pharmacokinetic perspective. CNS. Drugs 15:469–494 (2001).
85. Mihailescu S and Drucker-Colin R. Nicotine, brain nicotinic receptors, and neuropsychiatric disorders. Arch Med Res 31:131–144 (2000).
86. Lyon ER. A review of the effects of nicotine on schizophrenia and antipsychotic medications. Psychiatr Serv 50:1346–1350 (1999).
87. Pantuck EJ, Pantuck CB, Anderson KE, Conney AH, and Kappas A. Cigarette smoking and chlorpromazine disposition and actions. Clin Pharmacol Ther 31:533–538 (1982).
88. Chetty M, Miller R, and Moodley SV. Smoking and body weight influence the clearance of chlorpromazine. Eur J Clin Pharmacol 46:523–526 (1994).
89. Pan L, Vander SR, Rosseel MT, Berlo JA, De Schepper N, and Belpaire FM. Effects of smoking, CYP2D6 genotype, and concomitant drug intake on the steady state plasma concentrations of haloperidol and reduced haloperidol in schizophrenic inpatients. Ther Drug Monit 21:489–497 (1999).

90. Shimoda K, Someya T, Morita S, Hirokane G, Noguchi T, Yokono A, et al. Lower plasma levels of haloperidol in smoking than in nonsmoking schizophrenic patients. Ther Drug Monit 21:293–296 (1999).
91. Perry PJ, Miller DD, Arndt SV, Smith DA, and Holman TL. Haloperidol dosing requirements: the contribution of smoking and nonlinear pharmacokinetics. J Clin Psychopharmacol 13:46–51 (1993).
92. Haring C, Fleischhacker WW, Schett P, Humpel C, Barnas C, and Saria A. Influence of patient-related variables on clozapine plasma levels. Am J Psychiatry 147:1471–1475 (1990).
93. Seppala NH, Leinonen EV, Lehtonen ML, and Kivisto KT. Clozapine serum concentrations are lower in smoking than in non-smoking schizophrenic patients. Pharmacol Toxicol 85:244–246 (1999).
94. Hasegawa M, Gutierrez-Esteinou R, Way L, and Meltzer HY. Relationship between clinical efficacy and clozapine concentrations in plasma in schizophrenia: effect of smoking. J Clin Psychopharmacol 13:383–390 (1993).
95. Meyer JM. Individual changes in clozapine levels after smoking cessation: results and a predictive model. J Clin Psychopharmacol 21:569–574 (2001).
96. Oyewumi LK. Smoking cessation and clozapine side effects. Can J Psychiatry 43:748 (1998).
97. Skogh E, Bengtsson F, and Nordin C. Could discontinuing smoking be hazardous for patients administered clozapine medication? A case report. Ther Drug Monit 21:580–582 (1999).
98. Spigset O, Carleborg L, Hedenmalm K, and Dahlqvist R. Effect of cigarette smoking on fluvoxamine pharmacokinetics in humans. Clin Pharmacol Ther 58:399–403 (1995).
99. Ochs HR, Greenblatt DJ, and Burstein ES. Lack of influence of cigarette smoking on triazolam pharmacokinetics. Br J Clin Pharmacol 23:759–763 (1987).
100. Otani K, Yasui N, Furukori H, Kaneko S, Tasaki H, Ohkubo T, et al. Relationship between single oral dose pharmacokinetics of alprazolam and triazolam. Int Clin Psychopharmacol 12:153–157 (1997).
101. Hossain M, Wright E, Baweja R, Ludden T, and Miller R. Nonlinear mixed effects modeling of single dose and multiple dose data for an immediate release (IR) and a controlled release (CR) dosage form of alprazolam. Pharm Res 14:309–315 (1997).
102. Ochs HR, Greenblatt DJ, and Knuchel M. Kinetics of diazepam, midazolam, and lorazepam in cigarette smokers. Chest 87:223–226 (1985).
103. Miller RR. Effects of smoking on drug action. Clin Pharmacol Ther 22:749–756 (1977).
104. Greenblatt DJ, Allen MD, Harmatz JS, and Shader RI. Diazepam disposition determinants. Clin Pharmacol Ther 27:301–312 (1980).
105. Ochs HR, Greenblatt DJ, Locniskar A, and Weinbrenner J. Influence of propranolol coadministration or cigarette smoking on the kinetics of desmethyldiazepam following intravenous clorazepate. Klin Wochenschr 64:1217–1221 (1986).
106. Klotz U, Avant GR, Hoyumpa A, Schenker S, and Wilkinson GR. The effects of age and liver disease on the disposition and elimination of diazepam in adult man. J Clin Invest 55:347–359 (1975).
107. Desmond PV, Roberts RK, Wilkinson GR, and Schenker S. No effect of smoking on metabolism of chlordiazepoxide. N Engl J Med 300:199–200 (1979).
108. Ochs HR, Greenblatt DJ, and Otten H. Disposition of oxazepam in relation to age, sex, and cigarette smoking. Klin Wochenschr 59:899–903 (1981).
109. Rostami-Hodjegan A, Nurminen S, Jackson PR, and Tucker GT. Caffeine urinary metabolite ratios as markers of enzyme activity: a theoretical assessment. Pharmacogenetics 6:121–149 (1996).

110. Kotake AN, Schoeller DA, Lambert GH, Baker AL, Schaffer DD, and Josephs H. The caffeine CO2 breath test: dose response and route of N-demethylation in smokers and nonsmokers. Clin Pharmacol Ther 32:261–269 (1982).
111. Brown CR, Jacob P III, Wilson M, and Benowitz NL. Changes in rate and pattern of caffeine metabolism after cigarette abstinence. Clin Pharmacol Ther 43:488–491 (1988).
112. Oliveto AH, Hughes JR, Terry SY, Bickel WK, Higgins ST, Pepper SL, and Fenwick JW. Effects of caffeine on tobacco withdrawal. Clin Pharmacol Ther 50:157–164 (1991).
113. Benowitz NL, Hall SM, and Modin G. Persistent increase in caffeine concentrations in people who stop smoking. BMJ 298:1075–1076 (1989).
114. Martin ES III, Crismon ML, and Godley PJ. Postinduction carbamazepine clearance in an adult psychiatric population. Pharmacotherapy 11:296–302 (1991).
115. Buhler FR, Vesanen K, Watters JT, and Bolli P. Impact of smoking on heart attacks, strokes, blood pressure control, drug dose, and quality of life aspects in the International Prospective Primary Prevention Study in Hypertension. Am Heart J 115:282–288 (1988).
116. Bolli P, Buhler FR, and McKenzie JK. Smoking, antihypertensive treatment benefit, and comprehensive antihypertensive treatment approach: some thoughts on the results of the International Prospective Primary Prevention Study in Hypertension. J Cardiovasc Pharmacol 16(Suppl 7):S77–S80 (1990).
117. Wilhelmsen L, Berglund G, Elmfeldt D, Fitzsimons T, Holzgreve H, Hosie J, et al. Beta-blockers versus diuretics in hypertensive men: main results from the HAPPHY trial. J Hypertens 5:561–572 (1987).
118. Hitzenberger G, Fitscha P, Beveridge T, Nuesch E, and Pacha W. Effects of age and smoking on the pharmacokinetics of pindolol and propranolol. Br J Clin Pharmacol 13:217S–222S (1982).
119. Walle T, Walle UK, Cowart TD, Conradi EC, and Gaffney TE. Selective induction of propranolol metabolism by smoking: additional effects on renal clearance of metabolites. J Pharmacol Exp Ther 241:928–933 (1987).
120. Holtzman JL, Weeks CE, Kvam DC, Berry DA, Mottonen L, Ekholm BP, et al. Identification of drug interactions by meta-analysis of premarketing trials: the effect of smoking on the pharmacokinetics and dosage requirements for flecainide acetate. Clin Pharmacol Ther 46:1–8 (1989).
121. Huet PM and Lelorier J. Effects of smoking and chronic hepatitis B on lidocaine and indocyanine green kinetics. Clin Pharmacol Ther 28:208–215 (1980).
122. Grech-Belanger O, Gilbert M, Turgeon J, and LeBlanc PP. Effect of cigarette smoking on mexiletine kinetics. Clin Pharmacol Ther 37:638–643 (1985).
123. Lambert C, Larochelle P, and du Sovich P. Effects of phenobarbital and tobacco smoking on furosemide kinetics and dynamics in normal subjects. Clin Pharmacol Ther 34:170–175 (1983).
124. Vapaatalo HI, Neuvonen PJ, Tissari A, Mansner R, and Paasonen MK. Effect of cigarette smoking on diuresis induced by furosemide. Ann Clin Res 3:159–162 (1971).
125. Kolendorf K, Bojsen J, and Nielsen SL. Adipose tissue blood flow and insulin disappearance from subcutaneous tissue. Clin Pharmacol Ther 25:598–604 (1979).
126. Klemp P, Staberg B, Madsbad S, and Kolendorf K. Smoking reduces insulin absorption from subcutaneous tissue. Br Med J (Clin Res Ed) 284:237 (1982).
127. Madsbad S, McNair P, Christensen MS, Christiansen C, Faber OK, Binder C, and Transbol I. Influence of smoking on insulin requirement and metabolic status in diabetes mellitus. Diabetes Care 3:41–43 (1980).
128. Mathiesen ER, Soegaard U, and Christiansen JS. Smoking and glycaemic control in male insulin dependent (type 1) diabetics. Diabetes Res 1:155–157 (1984).

129. Boston Collaborative Drug Surveillance Program. Decreased clinical efficacy of propoxyphene in cigarette smokers. Clin Pharmacol Ther 14:259–263 (1973).
130. Jick H. Smoking and clinical drug effects. Med Clin North Am 58:1143–1149 (1974).
131. Seltzer CC, Friedman GD, Siegelaub AB, and Collen MF. Smoking habits and pain tolerance. Arch Environ Health 29:170–172 (1974).
132. Vaughan DP, Beckett AH, and Robbie DS. The influence of smoking on the intersubject variation in pentazocine elimination. Br J Clin Pharmacol 3:279–283 (1976).
133. Keeri-Szanto M and Pomeroy JR. Atmospheric pollution and pentazocine metabolism. Lancet 1:947–949 (1971).
134. Hull JH, Findlay JW, Rogers JF, Welch RM, Butz RF, and Bustrack JA. An evaluation of the effects of smoking on codeine pharmacokinetics and bioavailability in normal human volunteers. Drug Intell Clin Pharm 16:849–854 (1982).
135. Yue QY, Tomson T, and Sawe J. Carbamazepine and cigarette smoking induce differentially the metabolism of codeine in man. Pharmacogenetics 4:193–198 (1994).
136. Rogers JF, Findlay JW, Hull JH, Butz RF, Jones EC, Bustrack JA, and Welch RM. Codeine disposition in smokers and nonsmokers. Clin Pharmacol Ther 32:218–227 (1982).
137. Ali B, Kaur S, Kumar A, and Bhargava KP. Comparative evaluation of stimulatory effects of oral tobacco and nicotine consumption on hepatic microsomal N-demethylations. Biochem Pharmacol 29:3087–3092 (1980).
138. Mather LE, Tucker GT, Pflug AE, Lindop MJ, and Wilkerson C. Meperidine kinetics in man. Intravenous injection in surgical patients and volunteers. Clin Pharmacol Ther 17:21–30 (1975).
139. Lesko SM, Rosenberg L, Kaufman DW, Helmrich SP, Miller DR, Strom B, et al. Cigarette smoking and the risk of endometrial cancer. N Engl J Med 313:593–596 (1985).
140. Baron JA. Smoking and estrogen-related disease. Am J Epidemiol 119:9–22 (1984).
141. Michnovicz JJ, Hershcopf RJ, Naganuma H, Bradlow HL, and Fishman J. Increased 2-hydroxylation of estradiol as a possible mechanism for the anti-estrogenic effect of cigarette smoking. N Engl J Med 315:1305–1309 (1986).
142. Crawford FE, Back DJ, Orme ML, and Breckenridge AM. Oral contraceptive steroid plasma concentrations in smokers and non-smokers. Br Med J (Clin Res Ed) 282:1829–1830 (1981).
143. Kanarkowski R, Tornatore KM, D'Ambrosio R, Gardner MJ, and Jusko WJ. Pharmacokinetics of single and multiple doses of ethinyl estradiol and levonorgestrel in relation to smoking. Clin Pharmacol Ther 43:23–31 (1988).
144. Vessey MP, Villard-Mackintosh L, and Jacobs HS. Anti-estrogenic effect of cigarette smoking. N Engl J Med 317:769–770 (1987).
145. Miller LG. Recent developments in the study of the effects of cigarette smoking on clinical pharmacokinetics and clinical pharmacodynamics. Clin Pharmacokinet 17:90–108 (1989).
146. Welty D, Pool W, Woolf T, Posvar E, and Sedman A. The effect of smoking on the pharmacokinetics and metabolism of Cognex in healthy volunteers. Pharm Res 10:S334 (Abstract) (1993).
147. Schein JR. Cigarette smoking and clinically significant drug interactions. Ann Pharmacother 29:1139–1148 (1995).
148. Powell JR, Thiercelin JF, Vozeh S, Sansom L, and Riegelman S. The influence of cigarette smoking and sex on theophylline disposition. Am Rev Respir Dis 116:17–23 (1977).
149. Hunt SN, Jusko WJ, and Yurchak AM. Effect of smoking on theophylline disposition. Clin Pharmacol Ther 19:546–551 (1976).

150. Jusko WJ, Schentag JJ, Clark JH, Gardner M, and Yurchak AM. Enhanced biotransformation of theophylline in marihuana and tobacco smokers. Clin Pharmacol Ther 24:405–410 (1978).
151. Lee BL, Benowitz NL, and Jacob P III. Cigarette abstinence, nicotine gum, and theophylline disposition. Ann Intern Med 106:553–555 (1987).
152. Mayo PR. Effect of passive smoking on theophylline clearance in children. Ther Drug Monit 23:503–505 (2001).
153. Hughes JR. Comorbidity and smoking. Nicotine Tob Res 1:S149–S152 (1999).
154. Breslau N. Psychiatric comorbidity of smoking and nicotine dependence. Behav Genet 25:95–101 (1995).
155. U.S. Department of Health and Human Services Preventing tobacco use among young people; a report of the Surgeon General. Washington, DC: U.S. Government Printing Office, 1994.
156. Schneider NG, Lunell E, Olmstead RE, and Fagerstrom KO. Clinical pharmacokinetics of nasal nicotine delivery. A review and comparison to other nicotine systems. Clin Pharmacokinet 31:65–80 (1996).
157. Benowitz NL, Porchet H, Sheiner L, and Jacob P III. Nicotine absorption and cardiovascular effects with smokeless tobacco use: comparison with cigarettes and nicotine gum. Clin Pharmacol Ther 44:23–28 (1988).
158. Benowitz NL. Nicotine replacement therapy. What has been accomplished—can we do better? Drugs 45:157–170 (1993).

Chapter 14

Anabolic Doping Agents

Daniel A. von Deutsch, DDS, PhD, MSCR,
Imad K. Abukhalaf, PhD, and Robin R. Socci, PhD

INTRODUCTION: HISTORY OF PERFORMANCE ENHANCERS

The desire to gain an upper edge in war and athletic competition can be traced back into antiquity. The early Greeks used hallucinogenic mushrooms and the central nervous system (CNS) stimulant strychnine in order to gain an edge in battle and in Olympic competition. Gladiators were known to use stimulants to stave off fatigue during their gladiatorial battles. During the pre- to early Christian era, the Berserkers, ancient Germanic warriors, were known for their savagery and frenzied rage in battle *(1)*. Modern scholars believe that prior to battle, they would consume hallucinogenic mushrooms (Bufotein from the fungus *Amanita muscaria*) and/or massive quantities of alcohol. It was not until the end of the 16th century that Europeans learned of caffeine-containing drugs.

The use of stimulants such as strychnine, cocaine, and caffeine became more prevalent in sports during the 19th century. In 1879 during the "Six Days" races, the competitors used a wide variety of prescriptions to give them the edge they needed. French racers used mixtures of different caffeine bases, whereas Belgians preferred sugar cubes dipped in ether. Sprinters from all over the world preferred using nitroglycerine. In 1886, a French cyclist used a "speedball," a mixture of cocaine and heroin, only to become the first recorded death from the use of performance-enhancing drugs. In 1904, Olympic marathon runner Thomas Hicks nearly died when he used a mixture of brandy and strychnine to enhance his performance. In boxing around the end of the 19th century, the combination of brandy and cocaine was used along with strychnine in order to gain an edge in performance (Fig. 1; *2,3*).

From: *Handbook of Drug Interactions: A Clinical and Forensic Guide*
A. Mozayani and L. P. Raymon, eds. © Humana Press Inc., Totowa, NJ

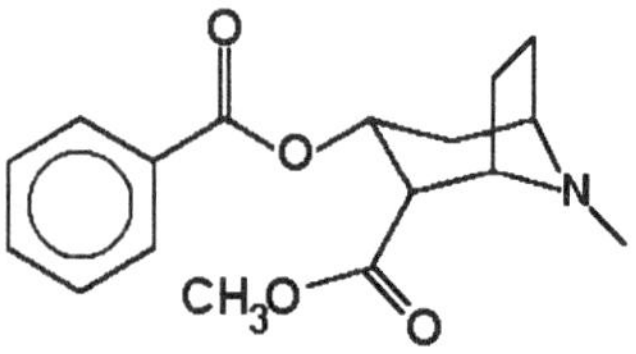

COCAINE

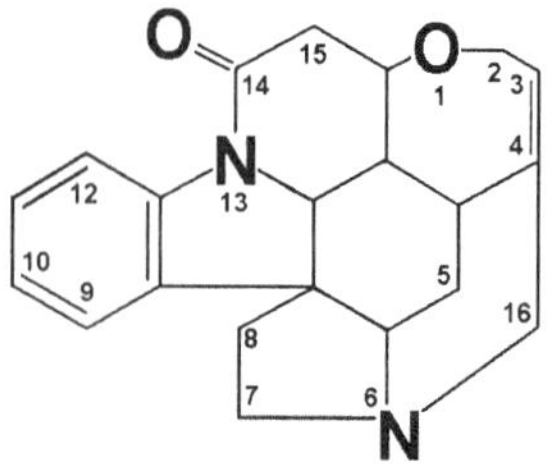

STRYCHNINE

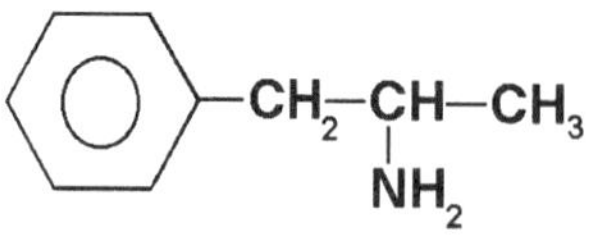

AMPHETAMINE

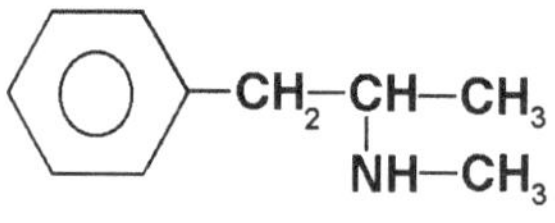

METHAMPHETAMINE

Fig. 1. Stimulants used historically to enhance performance in athletics and combat.

During the early 20th century, amphetamines as the preferred performance-enhancing drug replaced strychnine. German chemist Edeleano first synthesized amphetamine in 1887. Thirty-two years later, Japanese scientist Ogata synthesized methamphetamine, although it was not until the early 1930s that a clinical use for the amphetamine (benzedrine) was found. Increasing human performance during the Second World War was a common practice for both the Allied and Axis powers. Between 1939 and 1945, the stimulant methamphetamine (methedrine [England] and pervitine [Germany]) was used to increase a soldier's endurance on long marches or combat fatigue while conducting night flights. Although safer than strychnine, serious side effects were still associated with the use of stimulants (3,4).

The only performance enhancement drugs used by athletes or soldiers up to the 1930s were stimulants or hallucinogens. The identification of androstanediol and testosterone as anabolic and androgenic steroids and their subsequent isolation ushered in a new era with respect to performance enhancement. During the later part of the 1930s and throughout the Second World War, nations of the Axis and Allied powers sought to enhance the endurance and alertness of their armies through the use of pharmaceutical adjuvants such as amphetamines (amphetamine and methamphetamine). Stimulants enabled soldiers to function on minimal rest, endure reduced rations and long marches, or provide maximal performance during combat. Although the use of stimulants dates back to Greece and the Roman Empire, the use of anabolic steroids to "create" a more powerful warrior began in Nazi Germany. It is alleged that in an attempt to enhance the endurance, strength, and aggressiveness of his elite troops, Adolf Hitler ordered the use of the hormone testosterone. It is further alleged that Hitler administered testosterone to himself. In a move similar to Hitler's, Josef Stalin also allegedly ordered the use of anabolic steroids and stimulants for Soviet troops. In the case of Japan, it is unclear whether Tojo Hideki ordered Imperial troops to use anabolic steroids

14. Anabolic Doping Agents

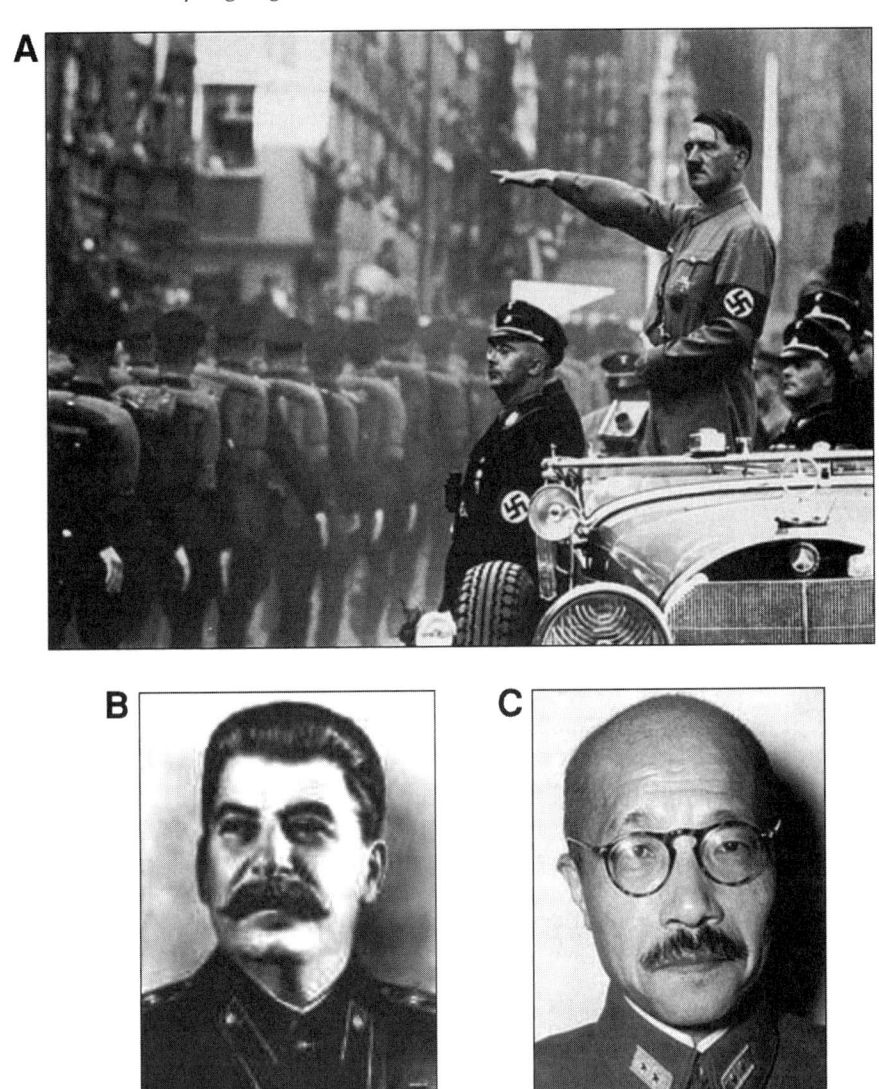

Fig. 2. **(A)** Adolf Hilter reviewing SS troops during Reich Party Day ceremonies, September 1938. **(B)** Josef Stalin, the preeminent leader of the Soviet Union from 1929 to 1953. **(C)** Tojo Hideki, military and political leader of Imperial Japan from 1938 to 1945.

and amphetamines. However, when one takes into consideration the close ties that existed between Nazi Germany and Imperial Japan, and the fact that methamphetamine was first synthesized in Japan, it seems likely that anabolic steroids were employed (Fig. 2A–C; *1*).

The unfortunate flaw in "pharmaceutically enhanced troops" is that with continual usage of amphetamines and anabolic steroids at high doses, the likelihood of a psychotic episode and violence would undoubtably increased. In times of war when adrenaline (β_1-, β_2-adrenoceptor agonist) is surging, i.e., the soldiers' "blood is up," there is little doubt that the magnitude of these violent outbursts could be horrific in nature.

The combination of steroid usage along with stimulants may have contributed to some of the excesses attributed to the SS, Soviet, and Imperial Japanese troops, as well as any others who may have used excessive amounts of stimulants and/or anabolic steroids. Although an extreme example of potential hazards that may be encountered when heavy steroid usage is coupled with frequent use of stimulants, it serves as a stern warning for those who embrace the popular fitness craze of the last decades of the 20th century.

Since the 1970s, widespread illegal use of anabolic agents among Olympic and professional athletes has been reported in the media. In particular, reports indicate that the highest frequency of steroid abuse occurs among male (95%) athletes (65%) who are usually football players, weight lifters, or heavyweight wrestlers. These users are usually attending a metropolitan school with greater than 700 students, usually a minority student, and most likely to have received the drugs via a blackmarket (60%) source *(5)*.

International Olympic Committee (IOC) List of Banned Anabolic Agents and Stimulants (6)

1. Sympathomimetic stimulants: Amfepramore, amfetamil, amphetamines (amphetamine, benzphetamine, methamphetamine), caffeine, cathine, ephedrine, cocaine, cropropamide, crothetamide, etafedrine, ethamivan, fencamfamin, fenetylline, furfenorex, mefenorex, methoxyphamine, methylephedrine, methyphenidate, morazone, nikethamide, pemoline, pentetrazol, phendimetrazine, phenmetrazine, phentermine, phenylpropanolamine, pipradol, prolintane, propylhexedrine, pyrovalerone, strychnine, and related compounds.
2. Anabolic agents: (a) anabolic steroids (androgens): bolasterone, boldenone, clostebol, dehydrochlormethyltestosterone, fluoxymesterone, mesterolone, methandienone, methenolone, methyltestosterone, nandrolone, norethandrolone, oxandrolone, oxymesterone, oxymetholone, stanozolol, testosterone, and related compounds; (b) β_2-adrenoceptor agonists: bambuterol, clenbuterol, fenoterol, formoterol*, reproterol, salbutamol*, salmeterol*, terbutaline*, ... and related substances (inhalation authorized as described in Article [I.A.]).
3. Peptide hormones, mimetics, and analogs: human chorionic gonadotropin* (HCG), pituitary and synthetic gonadotropins* (LH), corticotrophins (ACTH [adrenocorticotropic hormone], tetracosactide), human growth hormone (HGH), insulin-like growth factor (IGF-1), erythropoietin (EPO), insulin (permitted only to treat athletes with insulin-dependent diabetes), clomiphene*, cyclofenil*, tamoxifen*, aromatase inhibitors*. (*Note: Use prohibited in males).
4. β-adrenoceptor antagonists (beta-blockers): acebutolol, alprenolol, atenolol, betaxolol, bisoprolol, bunolol, carteolol, celiprolol, esmolol, labetalol, levobunolol, metipranolol, metoprolol, nadolol, oxprenolol, pindolol, propranolol, sotalol, timolol.

1. Anabolic Steroids (Androgens)

Early investigations into anabolic steroids can be dated back to the late 1700s, when John Hunter published observations on castration-induced loss of male sex accessory organs. Later studies, conducted in 1849 by Berthold, showed that transplanting a portion of testes into castrated roosters prevented the signs of castration, thus further describing the relationship between the testes and male secondary sex characteristics

(4). In an attempt to thwart the effects of aging, the physiologist Brown-Séquard (1889), prepared and self-administered extracts made from testicles. It was believed that aging was caused by failure of testicular function, and he was convinced that these injections not only reinvigorated him, but also restored his capacity to work. It was not until the 1930s that Koch and his colleagues were able to develop assays to determine androgenic activity with the growth response of the capon's comb *(4)*.

In 1931, Butenandt used Koch's activity assay to help him isolate and identify 15 mg of crystalline androsterone from 15,000 liters of male human urine. A year later, Butenandt correctly deduced the structural formula of androsterone by using only 25 mg of isolated crystal. Ruzicka finally confirmed Butenandt's work in 1934 when he successfully synthesized androsterone. Work by others showed that androsterone's activity could be enhanced significantly through the process of esterification. Furthermore, the reduction of androsterone to androstanediol was found to increase the hormone activity by two- to threefold. In 1935, David and his colleagues isolated the principal androgenic steroid, testosterone, from rat testicles and correctly elucidated its structure. Dr. Charles Kochakian, also in 1935, discovered that androstenedione possessed both androgenic and anabolic properties. These properties, however, were only significant in castrated dogs and were much weaker than the effects of testosterone *(4,7)*.

Understanding the chemistry of the anabolic steroids came about, in great part, with the development of better techniques for analytical and activity assays. Activity assays, such as the growth response of the capon's comb, provided Koch and his co-workers with a valuable approach to accurately establish the degree of anabolic activity associated with crystals derived from human male urine. Subsequent work showed that testosterone, the prototypical anabolic steroid, was produced in the greatest quantity and had the highest degree of androgenic and anabolic activity of all the endogenous steroids tested. However, later work showed that dihydrotestosterone (DHT), the active form of testosterone in tissue actually had the greatest potency while having the same affinity for the androgen receptor as testosterone *(4,7)*.

1.1. Chemistry

1.1.1. Structure

Naturally occurring steroids are generally relatively flat molecules of low molecular weight. Furthermore, they are derived from cholesterol and share a common carbon framework. The basic framework common to all steroids is the 19-carbon phenanthrene (cyclopentanoperhydrophenanthrene) nucleus formed by three hexagonal carbon rings (A, B, and C) attached to a cyclopentane ring (D). Also common to most steroids are two angular methyl groups at positions 18 and 19, and a hydrogen atom at position 5 (Fig. 3). To denote that the molecule is fully saturated the term *prehydro* is applied, where each carbon in the basic ring structure is attached to either two hydrogen atoms or a hydrogen and another carbon that is associated with an adjoining ring structure. Another common feature to the basic steroid ring structure is the presence of angular methyl groups (C18 and C19) at positions 10 and 13 of the phenanthrene nucleus. These two methyl groups serve as points of reference regarding the spacial orientation of other groups in the steroid nucleus *(8,9)*.

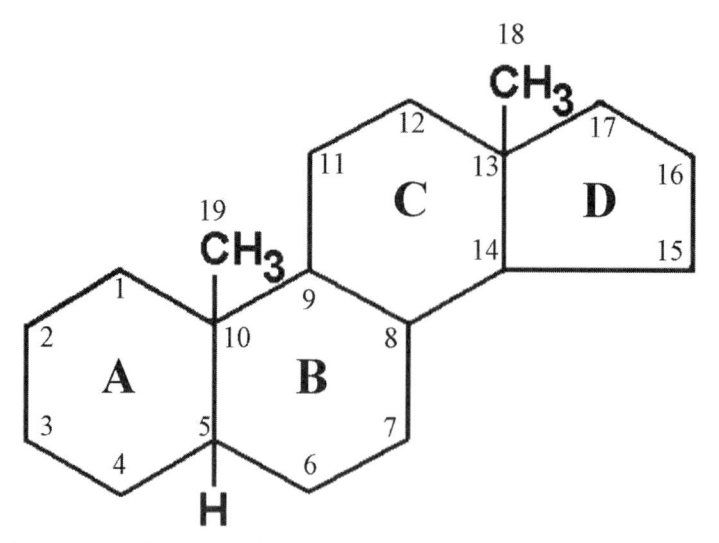

Fig. 3. 19-Carbon Phenanthrene (cyclopentanoperhydrophenanthrene, Androstane) Nucleus.

This basic structure, the phenanthrene nucleus, is found in several different naturally occurring steroidal compounds including sterols (e.g., cholesterol), bile acids (e.g., cholanic acid), corticosteroids, cardiac glycosides (e.g., digitoxigenin), and the sex hormones (estrogens and androgens). Aromatization of the phenanthrene nucleus at positions 5 and 6 on the hexagonal B ring and the addition of an alkyl side chain (carbons 20–27) at position 17 of the pentagonal carbon ring (D) yields cholesterol, the parent to all steroids. However, removal of part of the alkyl side chain at position 17 of cholesterol gives rise to C21 compounds of the pregnane series (progestins and corticosteroids). Subsequently, the total removal of the alkyl side chain produces C19 steroids of the androstane series (including the androgens), whereas the loss of the C19 angular methyl group following aromatization yields the estrane series, to which the estrogens belong *(8,9)*.

Structurally, endogenous and synthetic androgens are characterized by differences in specific functional groups (e.g., hydroxy, keto [oxo], and aldehydes) attached to the phenanthrene and cyclopentane rings. The most frequent sites for modifications of the basic ring structure occur at positions 3, 4, and 5 of ring A, and position 17 of the cyclopentane ring, whereas modifications at positions 11, 18, 20, and 21 are also common (Fig. 4). Dehydroepiandrosterone (DHEA, 3β-hydroxyandrost-5-en-17-one), a precursor to testosterone and a commonly used nutritional supplement, has hydroxyl and oxygen groups at positions 3 and 17, respectively. It is interesting to note that endogenous levels of DHEA decrease with age and possess antioxidant properties. Another nutritional supplement, androstenedione (4-androstene-3, 17-dione), has hydroxyl groups at positions 3 and 17, and a double bond at positions 4 and 5. Furthermore, the presence of hydrogen at position 5 changes testosterone (17β-hydroxy androstan-3-one) to the cellularly active form DHT (stanolone, 17β-hydroxy-5α-androstan-3-one) *(8,9)*.

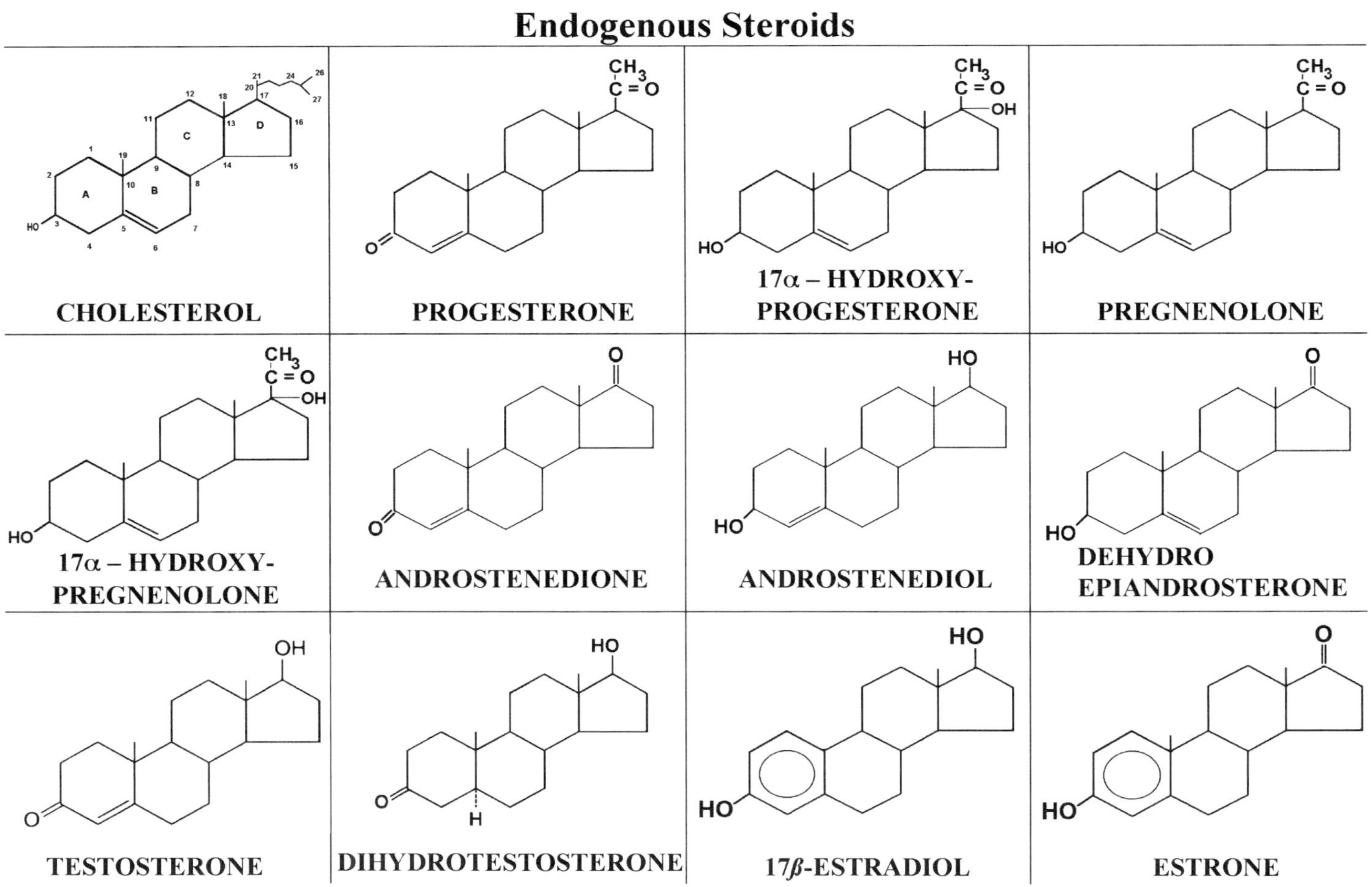

14. Anabolic Doping Agents

Endogenous Steroids

Fig. 4. The endogenous steroids commonly found in humans. (The generalized numbering scheme used for steroids is shown for cholesterol.) Data from *(12)*.

1.1.2. Stereochemistry

Of the 1850 drugs regularly prescribed by physicians, approximately 56% possess a chiral center. In contrast, approximately 99% of the naturally occurring chiral pharmaceutical compounds have a single pharmacologically active enantiomer. Enantiomers can vary greatly in their pharmacological effects upon target tissue(s) due to differences in their pharmacodynamic and/or pharmacokinetic parameters because of variations in their binding to receptors or metabolizing enzymes. Furthermore, the less active enantiomer (distomer) may interfere with the more biologically active species (eutomer) through competitive inhibition. Thus, the distomer may potentially bind to sites other than its primary receptor, thereby potentially causing adverse effects or alter the distribution and/or the activity of the eutomer, resulting in decreased or increased effect or toxicity *(9,10)*.

In general, androgens are relatively flat molecules that have functional groups that can be oriented either in equatorial or axial positions. Thus, this type of structure can potentially give rise to numerous asymmetrical sites, e.g., chiral centers, yielding molecules with the same chemical formula but different three-dimensional structures.

Groups that are in the same plane as the angular methyl groups (positions 18 and 19) are referred to being in the β-configuration and are represented by a solid line, whereas groups on the opposite side of the plane are in the α-configuration and are represented by a dashed line. Those groups that are trans to one and other are on opposite sides of the molecule whereas those that are cis are on the same side. In all naturally occurring steroid hormones, the spatial relationship between rings B/C and C/D is in the trans configuration. However, the fusion of the A and B rings into either a cis or trans conformation, can significantly increase the complexity of their stereochemistry *(8,9)*.

Research into receptor binding and binding to metabolizing enzymes has shown that a chiral preference exists. In particular, investigations into antiandrogen activity (for blocking androgen-induced prostate enlargement) with drugs such as casodex have shown a 30-fold greater effect for the (–)-R enantiomer over that of the (+)-S species *(11)*. However, chiral research into the anabolic and androgenic properties of the androgens to date has not been addressed.

1.2. Basic Physical Properties (6) (Table 1A,B)

Table 1A
Basic Physical Properties of Selected Steroids

Drug	Chemical Formula	Chemical Name	Synonym/Salt Name
Cholesterol	C27H46O	(3β)-Cholest-5-en-3-ol	
Danazol	C22H27NO2	(17alpha)-pregna-2,4-den-20-yno[2,3-d]-isoxazol-17-ol	Danocrine
Dihydrotestosterone	C19H30O2	17β-hydroxy-5alpha-androstan-3-one	DHT; Stanolone
Fluoxymesterone	C20H29FO3	(11β,17β)-9-fluoro-1,17-di-hydroxy-17-methylandrost-4-en-3-one	Oxymesterone
Methyltestosterone	C20H30O2	17-hydroxy-17-methylandrost-4-en-3-one	Androsan
Nandrolone	C18H26O2	(17β)-17-hydroxyestr-4-en-3-one	19-Nortesterone

14. Anabolic Doping Agents

Table 1A (continued)

Drug	Chemical Formula	Chemical Name	Synonym/Salt Name
Nandrolone Salts			
Cyclohexane-carboxylate	C25H36O3	19-nortestosterone hexahydrobenzoate	Norlongandron, Nor-Durandron
Cyclohexane-propionate	C27H40O3	19-nortestosteronecyclohexylpropionate	Sanabolicum
Decanoate	C28H44O3	19-nortestosteronedecanoate	Durabolin, Deca-Durabol, Retabolil
p-Hexyloxyphe-nylpropionate	C33H46O4	19-nortestosterone-3-(p-hexyloxyphenyl) proprionate	Anador, Anadur
Phenpropionate	C27H34O3	19-nortestosterone β-phenylproprionate	Activin, Durabolin, Durabol, Strabolene
Propionate	C21H30O3	19-nortestosterone proprionate	Norybol-19, Nortesto
Oxandrolone	C19H30O3	5α,17β-hydroxy-1 7-methyl-2-oxaandrostan-3-one	Anavar
Oxymetholone	C21H32O3	(5α,17β)-17-Hydroxy-2-(hydroxy-methylene)-17-met hylandrostan-3-one	Anadrol
Testosterone	C19H228O2	17β-hydroxyandrostan-3-one	
Testosterone Salts			
17-Chloral Hemiacetal	C21H29 C13O3	17β-(2,2,2-Trichoro-1-hydroxyethoxy) androst-4-en-3-one	Caprosem
17β-Cypionate	C27H40O3	17β-(3-Cyclopentyl-1-oxopropoxy) androst-4-en-3-one	Depovirin, Pertestis, Testergon
Enanthate	C26H40O3	17β-[(1-Oxoheptyl)oxyl]-androst-4-en-3-one	Testosterone Heptoate, Androtardyl
Nicotinate	C25H31NO3	17β-[(3-Pyridinylcarbonyl)oxy]androst-4-en-3-one	Bolfortan
17-Phenylacetate	C27H34O3	17β-[(Phenylactetyl)oxyl]androst-4-en	Peradren Phenylacetae
Propionate	C22H32O3	δ4-Androstene-17β-propionate-3-one	Anertan, Enarmon
Stanozolol	C21H32N2O	(5α,17β)-17-methyl-2'H-androst-2-eno[3,2-c]pyrazol-17-ol	Androstanazole

Data from *(12)*.

Table 1B
Basic Physical Properties of Selected Steroids

Drug	MW g/mol	Melting Point	Melting Point Solvent/Other	Solubility	UV Max nm
Cholesterol	386.64	149	—	Nearly insoluble in water (0.2 mg/dL), slightly soluble in alcohol, ether 0.36 g/mL, chloroform 0.22 g/mL, pyridine 0.67 g/mL.	—
Danazol	337.46	224–227	—	Insoluble in water. Soluble in alcohol, ether, chloroform, petrolium ether, oils.	—

(continued)

Table 1B (continued)

Drug	MW g/mol	Melting Point	Melting Point Solvent/Other	Solubility	UV Max nm
Dihydrotestosterone	290.43	177–179	—	Soluble in ethanol (8.0 mg/mL), acetone, ether, alcohol, and ethylacetate. Practically insoluble in water (<0.5 mg/mL).	—
Fluoxymesterone	336.45	270	—	Soluble in pyridine, slightly soluble in acetone and chloroform. Sparingly soluble in methanol and practically insoluble in water, ether, benzene, and hexanes.	240
Methyltestosterone	302.44	161–166	—	Soluble in alcohol, methanol, ether, and other organic solvents. Sparingly soluble in vegetable oil and practically insoluble in water.	—
Nandrolone	274.40	112, 124	dimorphic crystals	Soluble in alcohol, ether, and chloroform.	241
Nandrolone Salts					
Cyclohexane-carboxylate	384.56	88–89	petroleum ether	—	—
Cyclohexane-propionate	412.61		—	—	—
Decanoate	428.65	32–35	white to yellow crystals	Nandrolone decanoate is practically insoluble in water but is soluble in ethanol, ether, acetone, chloroform, and oils.	—
p-Hexyloxy-phenylpropionate	506.72	53–55	—	—	—
Phenpropionate	406.56	95–96	—	—	—
Propionate	330.47	55–60	aqueous methanol orisopropyl ether	—	240
Oxandrolone	306.45	235–238	—	—	—
Oxymetholone	332.48	178–180	ethylacetate	—	285
Testosterone	288.41	155	—	Insoluble in water. Soluble in alcohol, ether, and other organic solvents.	238
Testosterone Salts					
17-Chloral Hemiacetal	435.83	200–201	ethyl ether	—	241
17β-Cypionate	412.59	101–102	—	Soluble in oils.	—
Enanthate	400.58	36–38	—	—	—
Nicotinate	393.51	187–188	acetone	Soluble indilute HCl and other dilute mineral acids.	—
17-Phenylacetate	406.54	129–131	hexane	—	—
Propionate	344.49	118–122, 117–183	alcohol + water, methanol	Insoluble in water. Freely soluble in alcohol, ether, and other organic solvents. Soluble in vegetable oils.	—
Stanozolol	328.48	230–242	alcohol	Soluble in alcohol and chloroform.	223

Data from *(12)*.

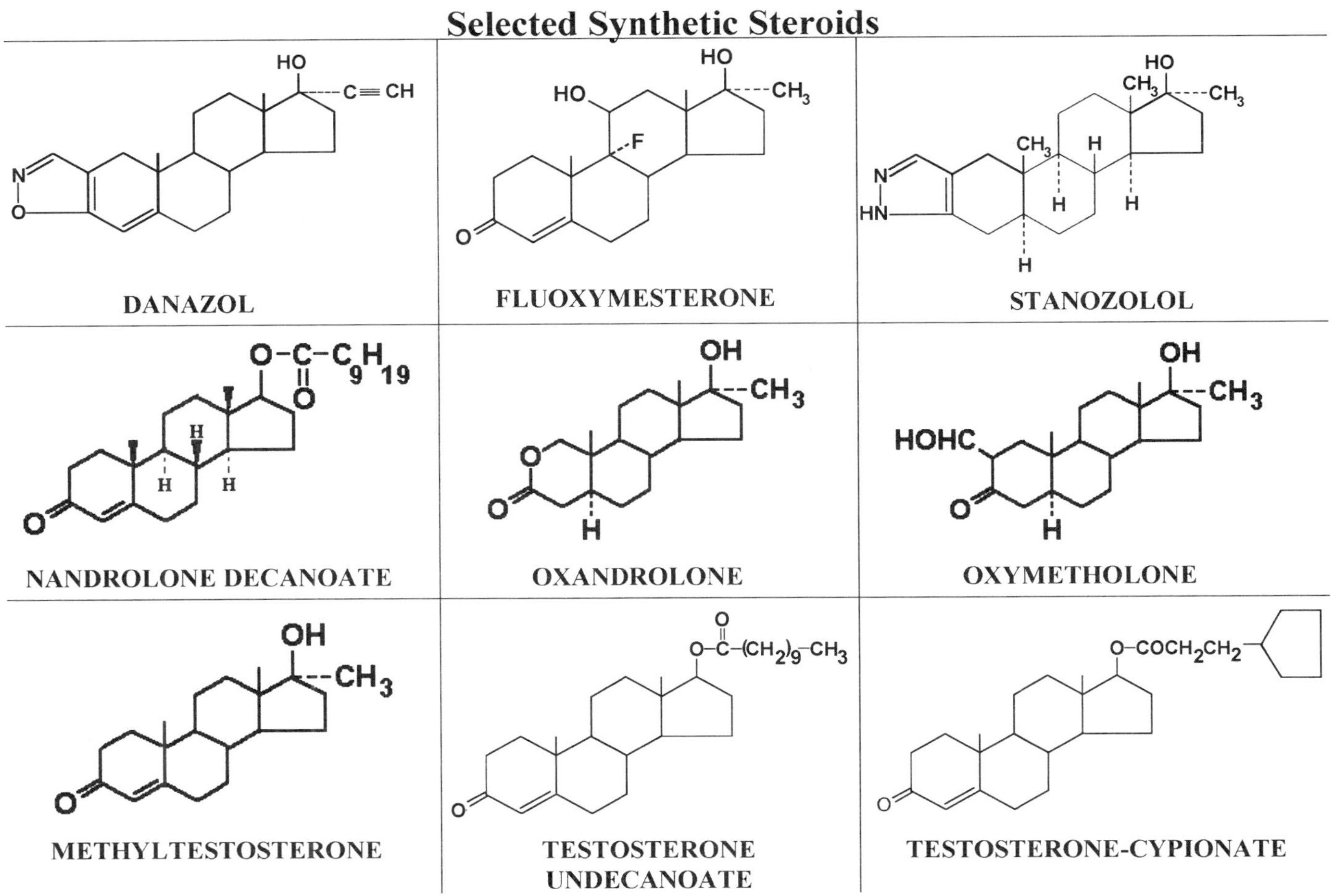

14. Anabolic Doping Agents

Selected Synthetic Steroids

Fig. 5. Modifications to the basic steroid structure have been systematically performed in order to enhance the overall anabolic properties. Please refer to Table 2 for potencies. Data from (12).

Table 2
Anabolic and Androgenic Potencies of Selected Androgens

Selected Androgen	Androgenic:Anabolic Activity
Methyltestosterone	1:1
Nandrolone decanoate	1:1
Nandrolone phenpropionate	1:1
Testosterone	1:1
Testosterone cypionate	1:1
Testosterone enanthate	1:1
Testosterone propionate	1:1
Fluoxymestrone	1:2
Metandienone	1:3
Oxymetholone	1:3
Drostanolone propionate (Dromostanolone propionate)	1:3–1:4
Stanozolol	1:3–1:6
Ethylestrenol	1:4–1:8
Oxandrolone	1:3–1:13

1.3. Pharmacology and Kinetics

1.3.1. Drug Usage: Preparations and Routes of Administration

Androgens are classified as a controlled substance under the Anabolic Steroids Control Act of 1990 and have been assigned to Schedule III. There have been no reports of acute overdosing with androgens.

Treatment with natural androgens taken both orally or by intramuscular injections is cleared rapidly by the liver and thus is not clinically effective. Modification of the position 17-hydroxyl group on testosterone by esterification renders the molecule more lipophilic. Through such modifications, variations in the aliphatic chains directly affect the solubility and rate of absorption of the androgen. Furthermore, analogs such as these are usually made up in oil and injected intramuscularly. In contrast, androgen esters are rapidly metabolized, thereby releasing the parent molecule to act at receptor site.

Esters of testosterone that are used clinically in the United States are propionate, cypionate, and enanthate and have equal potency for their androgenic and anabolic activities. However, analogs of testosterone have been synthesized to enhance the anabolic properties over that of the androgenic (Fig. 5; Table 2). In cases of hypopituitarism, androgen replacement therapy begins at puberty with a long-acting androgen, such as the enanthate ester of testosterone, in doses of 50 mg intramuscularly (im) every 4 wk. Subsequent treatments should occur every 3 and then every 2 wk, with changes taking place in 3-mo intervals. Doses are then changed to 100 mg every 2 wk until the individual is mature. For adults, the dosage is approximately 200 mg at 2-wk intervals. It should be noted that the propionate ester has a relatively short half-life and is normally not considered suitable for long-term treatment, whereas the undecanoate analog can be given orally (40 mg/d) but can give rise to liver adenomas. The use of other

14. Anabolic Doping Agents

androgen preparations for replacement therapy includes fluoxymesterone and methyltestosterone. An alternative route of administration for testosterone or its analogs is via transdermal patches or gels.

In contrast to the doses used in replacement therapy, many athletes and their coaches believe that anabolic steroids taken in megadose quantities (e.g., doses that are 10- to 200-fold greater than the normal daily production) will increase the individual's overall performance by increasing skeletal muscle mass and strength as well as their aggressiveness. In women, these anabolic effects have been observed, but in males, questions have been raised regarding the benefits gained from using anabolic steroids. Earlier versions of pharmacology texts such as Katzung's *Basic and Clinical Pharmacology (13)* and Goodman and Gilman's *The Pharmacological Basis of Therapeutics (15)* have argued that the benefits gained, if any, from using anabolic steroids are far outweighed by the risk of adverse effects. Furthermore, it was argued at that time that the use of anabolic steroids in megadose quantities do not cause an increase in skeletal muscle mass, strength, or performance, and that the weight gain observed was the result of fluid retention. However, subsequent research utilizing proper controls showed that significant increases in skeletal muscle mass and strength could be achieved in healthy male subjects (18–35 yr) when treated weekly with testosterone enanthate at levels greater than 125 mg (125, 300, or 600 mg) per week. This was especially true for individuals who were combining strength exercises along with receiving testosterone treatment *(15,23)*. Additionally, testosterone's effects on lean body mass (decreased fat content and increased muscle mass) and muscle strength were found to be dose dependent. Treatments of 25, 50, 125, 300, or 600 mg of testosterone enanthate in the presence of a gonadotropin-releasing hormone (to suppress endogenous testosterone secretions) over a period of 20 wk resulted in plasma testosterone levels of 2.5, 3.1, 5.4, 13.5, and 23.7 ng/mL. Thus, it was observed that a positive correlation exists between the dose response and plasma testosterone levels with respect to the overall anabolic effects. Furthermore, results from these studies show that higher plasma testosterone levels (>5.4 ng/mL) were required to render an anabolic effect in males. However, with the higher plasma testosterone levels that are necessary to gain the desired anabolic effects, there comes the risk of detection (Table 3).

In hormone replacement therapy, for example, with testosterone enanthate, a dose of 75–100 mg/wk would be sufficient for treating a hypogonadal man, whereas a dose of 200–250 mg/wk has been used in trial studies as a male contraceptive. However, for those abusing anabolic steroids, doses ranging up to 1000 mg/wk over a cycle of 6 wk to 7 yr (continuous usage) for power lifters have been reported. Androgens such as oxandrolone, oxymetholone, methandrostenolone, and stanozolol (orally active) and testosterone enanthate and nandrolone decanoate (parenterally administered) are commonly abused whereas mesterolone, testerone undecanoate, and methenolone thus far appear to be of lesser significance with respect to androgen abuse *(16–18)*.

Since anabolic steroids are not routinely included in drug of abuse (DAU) screens, the chances for an individual who is not actively competing in athletic events to be caught are significantly less than if they were abusing cannabis (pot), amphetamines (speed), or cocaine (crack, etc.) *(19)*. However, those individuals who routinely use anabolic steroids and compete in athletic events risk detection. This is especially true when

Table 3
Routes of Administration for Selected Anabolic Agents

Drugs: Oral Use	No. of Reported Cases	No. of Reported Cases (%)
Methandrostenolone	79	35.3
Oxandrolone	55	24.6
Stanozolol[a]	43	19.2
Oxymetholone	18	8.0
Ethylestrenol	8	3.6
Methyltestosterone	7	3.1
Methenolone acetate[a]	7	3.1
Fluoxymesterone	3	1.3
Other	4	1.8
Total Number of Cases:	224	100

Drugs: Parenteral Use	No. of Reported Cases	No. of Reported Cases (%)
Testosterone esters	88	±4 40.9
Nandrolone esters	77	±5 35.8
Methenolone esters[a]	14	6.5
Stanozolol*	15	7.0
Testosterone (aqueous)	6	2.8
Boldenone udecylenate	4	1.9
Methandriol dipropionate	7	3.3
Other	4	1.9
Total Number of Cases:	215	100

Other Drugs: Nonsteroidal	Relative Frequency of Use	
Chorionic gonadotropin	4	25.0
Growth hormone	3	18.8
Diuretics	3	18.8
Thyroid hormones	2	12.5
Testolactone/tamoxifen	1	6.3
Others	3	18.8
Total Number of Cases:	16	100

[a]Route used not clearly established.
Steroids may be stacked in varying combinations (see Table 4 for Stacking Schedule). Total number of users = 175. Data are from (5).

considering that the limit of detection (LOD) for testosterone and testosterone metabolites is significantly less than the plasma levels necessary to render an anabolic effect (19,20). In an attempt to avoid detection and to maximize the anabolic activity of androgens, the use of multiple androgens simultaneously (stacking) has been employed. In an epidemiological study focused the frequency and nature of androgen abuse, results indicated that 38.3% used injectable androgens (61.7% did not) and 43.7% used a stacked androgen regiment. Furthermore, their results indicated that a direct correlation existed between the number of cycles of androgen usage with both an increasing frequency of stacking and use of injectable androgens (21).

Table 4
Example of a Recommended Stacking Schedule Using a Combination of Transdermal- and Oral-Dosing Regimens Using Dermagain, Equibolan, and Maxeron

Cycle Week	Transdermal Application (Norandrostene & Androstene)	Oral Drug 1 (1,4-androstadienedione)	Oral Drug 2 (5α-androstanediol)
Week 1	4 mL/d		
Week 2	4 mL/d		
Week 3	4 mL/d	6 pills/d	
Week 4	4 mL/d	6 pills/d	
Week 5		6 pills/d	6 pills/d
Week 6		6 pills/d	6 pills/d
Week 7			6 pills/d
Week 8			6 pills/d

1.3.1.1. STACKING SCHEDULES (22)

Another point of variation amongst androgen users was the length of cycles. In the previously mentioned epidemiological study, it was shown that the length of cycles generally varied from 6 to greater than 13 wk. The study also showed that with greater usage, cycle lengths increased. From a user point of view, the stacking of similar drugs together in order to achieve a desired anabolic effect can have several advantages over that of a single drug. These advantages may include:

1. The use of lower doses, thereby reducing the risk of adverse side effects associated with high doses of a single drug.
2. The ability to select aspects of desired effects of one drug to offset the less desirable effects of another while maintaining sufficient combined levels to achieve an effective dose.
3. To avoid or lessen the chance of being caught using anabolic agents by keeping detectable drug levels less than the limit of detection.

For an anabolic stacking regimen to work effectively, dosing should be conducted in staggered cycles. Normal dosing cycles are usually 4 or 8 wk in length, but cycles 12 wk in length are occasionally used. When employing the different dosing cycles, breaks (drug abstinence) of 2, 4, or 6 wk, respectively, are strongly recommended in order to allow the body's endocrine system to recover (Table 4).

1.3.1.2. DRUG USAGE: PREPARATIONS AND ROUTES OF ADMINISTRATION OVERVIEW

A consequence of taking exogenous androgens in normal males with adequate plasma testosterone levels is the reduction of endogenous testosterone levels. Additionally, exogenous testosterone causes the suppression of gonadotropin-releasing hormone and follicle-stimulating hormone.

1.3.1.2.1. Androstenedione (Andro-Max, Androstat 100, 50 and 100 mg). Androstenedione is an endogenous steroid precursor that is acted upon by the enzyme 17β-hydroxysteroid dehydrogenase to produce testosterone. Synthesis of androstenedione is significantly increased in both men and women following intense anaerobic exercise such as running sprints. Today, androstenedione, is widely marketed as an over-the-counter dietary supplement intended to bolster endogenous levels in the hopes of building skeletal muscle mass. Another factor that has increased interest in androstenedione has been with the baseball slugger from the St. Louis Cardinals, Mark McGwire, when he admitted using it in 1998. Whether androstenedione causes greater increases in muscle mass, especially when used concomitantly with exercise, remains unclear. However, basic and clinical research is required to better understand the dynamics of the hormone/anabolism relationship and to better establish the efficacy (if any) of anabolic supplements. In a clinical trials conducted by King et al. *(23)* and Broeder et al. *(24)*, they tested androstenedione and androstenediol for their physiological and hormonal effects. In these studies, male subjects (ages 19–29 yr and 35–65 yr, respectively) were given 200 or 300 mg/d of androstenedione or androstenediol over an 8- or 12-wk period. They found that androstenedione cause a transient increase in plasma testosterone levels (16% increase during the first month and then levels returned to baseline), but did not result in any increase in muscle mass or strength. It was concluded that the manufacturer-recommended dosages do not produce any appreciable gains in muscle strength. Additionally, the consequences from using androstenedione and/or androstenediol supplements at the prescribed amounts were significant increases in plasma dehydroepiandrosterone sulfate levels, increases in the amount of estrogen-related compounds, decreases in testosterone synthesis through down-regulation, and adverse changes in blood lipid profiles (changes in cholesterol: increased low-density lipoprotein [LDL] and decreased high-density lipoprotein [HDL]). Additionally, it was noted that there was an increased risk of coronary heart disease. It should be noted that since androstenediol and androstenedione are hormones, the IOC, National Collegiate (NCAA), National Football League (NFL), and the U.S. Olympic Committee (USOC) *(6,25)* ban their use from athletic competition.

1.3.1.2.1.1. Indications and Dosages. Although the use of androstenedione as an ergogenic agent for the treatment of andropause has not been approved for use by the Food and Drug Administration (FDA), it may prove useful in the future for treating such conditions. (Andropause is associated with decreases in serum testosterone levels that results in cognitive impairment, lack of energy, loss of bone and muscle mass, increased frailty, loss of balance, sexual dysfunction, and a decrease in the individual's overall general well-being.) Androstenedione is administered orally usually with meals *(26,25)*.

The suggested doses for androstenedione as a nutritional ergogenic supplement in athletes are 50 to 100 mg/d orally. However, clinical studies in adult male volunteers (ages 19–65) suggest that the manufacturer-recommended doses fail to achieve any appreciable gains in muscle strength or endurance (during resistive exercises).

The suggested dosage of androstenedione in males for the treatment of documented andropause is 300 mg/d orally for a period of 7 d. It has been shown that treatment with androstenedione results in increased testosterone levels during the first 4 wk of treatment, then subsequently drops to baseline levels with prolonged treatment (>4 wk). However, no results from clinical studies support the use of androstenedione in the treatment of andropause.

1.3.1.2.2. Danazol (Danocrine®, Danazol (USP), Danocrine capsules (CAP 50, 100, 200 mg). Danazol, a synthetic steroid derived from ethisterone (ethinyl testoster-

14. Anabolic Doping Agents

one), possess weak androgenic effects and is antiestrogenic. Danazol acts indirectly on the pituitary to lower estrogen production through reducing the output of both luteinizing and follicle-stimulating hormones. Danazol also binds to tissue sex hormone receptors, thereby rendering its antiestrogenic, anabolic, and weak androgenic activities. The IOC, NCAA, and the USOC *(6,25)* ban the use of danazol from athletic competition.

1.3.1.2.2.1. Pharmacokinetics. Danazol is administered orally with meals, but plasma levels do not increase proportionally with an increase in dosage. Peak danazol concentrations usually occur in approximately 2 h, but significant treatment time is required for the onset of the therapeutic effects. Daily doses over a period of 6–8 wk are required for treating anovulation or amenorrhea and treatment of 1–3 mo for the pain to subside in fibrocystic breast disease. Danazol is extensively metabolized in the liver to its primary metabolite 2-hydroxymethyl ethisterone, and both are excreted in the urine. The elimination half-life for danazol is 4–5 h *(25)*.

1.3.1.2.2.2. Indications and Dosages. Danazol is indicated for the treatment of angioedema, endometriosis, and fibrocystic breast disease. Although not an approved use by the FDA, danazol can also be used to treat idiopathic thrombocytopenic purpura. However, danazol's mechanism of action for treating idiopathic thrombocytopenic purpura is unclear. Investigations conducted by Ahn *(27)*, Fujisawa et al. *(28)*, and Otawa et al. *(29)* suggest that danazol acts on cell membranes, potentially making them less sensitive to osmotic lysis or by modifying the patient's immune response. Other uses for danazol include treating postcoital contraception and premenstrual syndrome (PMS) *(25)*.

For the prophylactic treatment of hereditary angioedema in adults, danazol is given orally in an initial dose of 200 mg/d. Depending on the patient's response, subsequent doses may be reduced in half at intervals of 1–3 mo, or increased by 200 mg/d if the patient suffers an attack of angioedema during treatment. However, if danazol is used to treat traumatic angioedema, attempts should be made periodically to reduce or discontinue treatment *(25)*.

For treating mild cases of endometriosis in adults, danazol is given orally during menstruation in two divided doses of 200–400 mg/d. In moderate to severe cases of endometriosis, danazol is initially given orally during menstruation in two divided doses of 800 mg/d. Depending on the patient's response, subsequent doses may be reduced gradually. However, daily doses should be given over a period of 3–6 mo, with treatment not extending beyond 9 mo.

For the treatment of fibrocystic breast disease in adults, danazol is given orally during menstruation in two divided doses of 100–400 mg/d. Depending on the patient's response, dosages are adjusted accordingly. It should be noted that therapy should be continued uninterrupted over a period of 6 mo, independent of whether the symptoms are relieved or eliminated. The continuation of treatment over this time is important in order to ensure the elimination of nodularity.

The FDA does not approve the use of danazol in adults for the treatment of chronic idiopathic thrombocytopenic purpura, PMS maladies, and emergency postcoital contraception. However, for the treatment of chronic idiopathic thrombocytopenic purpura, a dosage of 200 mg orally three times/day over a period of 6 mo has been recommended. For the treatment of maladies (e.g., mastalgia, bloating and weight gain [greater than a 1.4 kg increase in weight], anxiety, and depression) associated with PMS, the recommended dosage in adults is 50–100 mg orally two times/d. To achieve the best results, the dose should be titrated. For emergency postcoital contraception, doses of 800–1200 mg orally every 12 h for two doses and a dose of 800 mg orally every 12 h for three doses have been suggested. However, further studies are required because of contradictory data.

1.3.1.2.3. Dihydrotestosterone (DHT) (Andractim™). DHT is classified as a schedule III controlled substance, banned by the NCAA, IOC, and USOC *(6,25)*. DHT is the active metabolite of testosterone believed to be the primary anabolic agent in target tissues (e.g., skeletal muscle and the prostate).

1.3.1.2.3.1. Pharmacokinetics. Results from phase III testing of transdermal DHT patches in hypogonadal men (ages 21–65 yr) indicate treatment for 24 h produces peak concentrations after 13 h (reaching a plateau between 12 and 18 h). On the other hand, peak testosterone levels were achieved in 8 h *(30)*. Serum DHT levels increased from hypogonadal to normal physiological concentrations within 24 h of treatment. Following removal of the patches, plasma DHT levels dropped back down to its baseline hypogonadal range. The half-life for DHT was reported to be approximately 2.83 and 0.97 h, whereas that for testosterone was 1.29 and 0.71 h. Using a sequential crossover design for transdermal DHT, there was negligible variation in uptake from the different application sites (abdomen, back, chest, shin, thigh, or upper arm). However, this was not true for testosterone.

1.3.1.2.3.2. Indications and Dosages. In individuals who have AIDS, DHT is being studied for reversing AIDS-related wasting of muscle mass. Previous attempts to use testosterone to treat AIDS-related wasting was unsuccessful because it is thought that AIDS patients lack 5α-reductase, the enzyme responsible for converting testosterone into DHT in target tissues *(25)*. Furthermore, DHT may be the hormone responsible for stimulating an increase in appetite and is currently in phase III clinical trials as a topical agent for treatment of low circulating testosterone levels (andropause) in men and AIDS-related wasting syndrome *(17,26,31)*. Another benefit gained from the use of topical DHT is that this route of administration avoids the pain associated with im testosterone injection *(18)*.

The suggested dosage to be used by AIDS patients to attenuate the AIDS-related wasting syndrome or hypogonadal men is unclear at this time. However, topical doses of 16, 32, and 64 mg/d have been studied in phase III trials *(25,26,31)*.

1.3.1.2.4. Fluoxymesterone (Fluoxymesterone [Tab 10 mg], Halotestin® [Tab 2, 5, 10 mg], Android-F®, Hysterone®, Ora-Testryl® [10 mg]). Fluoxymesterone is an orally administered androgen and is classified as a Schedule III controlled substance, banned by the NCAA, IOC, and USOC *(6,25)*. Fluoxymesterone promotes normal growth, the development of male sex organs, and the development of secondary sex characteristics. It has twice the anabolic potency as testosterone and has an androgenic to anabolic potency ratio of 1:2. Furthermore, since fluoxymesterone inhibits the formation of estrogen, it could potentially serve as a potent doping agent *(25)*.

1.3.1.2.4.1. Pharmacokinetics. In a clinical study conducted with fluoxymesterone, 10-mg tablets were administered to six male subjects either orally or buccally. Peak serum fluoxymesterone levels of 40–150 ng/mL were achieved in 1–2 h, with a half-life of approximately 2 h *(32,33)*.

14. Anabolic Doping Agents

1.3.1.2.4.2. Indications and Dosages. Fluoxymesterone is indicated for the treatment of inoperable breast carcinoma and hypogonadism in men. The recommended dosage in adults for treating hypogonadism via androgen replacement therapy is 5 mg orally one to four times/daily for a total of 5–20 mg/d. For the treatment of inoperable breast cancer in adults, the recommended dosage is 10–40 mg/d orally. The doses should be divided. Fluoxymesterone can also be used to prevent postpartum breast engorgement. Although this usage is not approved by the FDA, it is suggested that 2.5 mg of fluoxymesterone should be administered orally to adults after delivery, then 5–10 mg orally per day in divided doses for a period of 4–5 d. Fluoxymesterone comes in tablet form in doses of 2, 5, and 10 mg *(25)*.

1.3.1.2.5. Methyltestosterone ([Tablets 10, 25 mg] Android-10®, Testred®, Virilon® [Inj soln 200 mg/mL], and Methitest™). Methyltestosterone is an orally administered androgen and is classified as a Schedule III controlled substance, banned by the NCAA, IOC, and USOC *(6,25)*. Methyltestosterone is a synthetic analog of testosterone, designed to be administered orally without loss of bioactivity, and was first approved for use by the FDA as a topical ointment in 1939 and as an oral androgenic agent in 1940. When compared to testosterone, methylation at the 17 carbon position reduces the rate at which methyltestosterone is metabolized in the liver. Androgens are important for stimulating RNA polymerase and subsequent protein production important in the development of male sex traits. During puberty, androgens promote the growth and development of skeletal muscle, and the redistribution of body fat *(25)*.

1.3.1.2.5.1. Pharmacokinetics. Methyltestosterone is administered either orally or buccally. When methyltestosterone is administrated orally, it undergoes the first-pass effect in the liver where it is metabolized at a rate approximately 50% greater than buccally. Peak serum methyltestosterone levels are achieved after about 2 h, with a half-life of approximately 2.5–3.5 h. The glucuronide and sulfate conjugates are eliminated primarily by renal excretion, with a small degree of the drug unchanged.

1.3.1.2.5.2. Indications and Dosages. Methyltestosterone is indicated for the management of congenital or acquired hypogonadism and can be used for the treatment of delayed puberty and erectile dysfunction. Methyltestosterone is also useful for the treatment of breast carcinoma in postmenopausal women because of its antiestrogenic effects.

Methyltestosterone comes in either capsule or tablet form. The oral dosage required for androgen replacement therapy as well as treatment for erectile dysfunction (impotence) or hypogonadism in adult males is 10–50 mg/d. When taken buccally (i.e., dissolved in buccal cavity), the dose is 5–25 mg/d. In treating delayed puberty in adolescent males, the recommended dosage is 5–25 mg/d orally or 2.5–12.5 mg/d buccally. Treatment occurs over a period of 4–6 mo. In treating breast cancer in adult women, the recommended dosage is 50 mg/d up to four times per week orally or 25 mg/d up to four times per week buccally. Once the desired response is observed, usually within 2–4 wk, the dosage can be reduced to 25 mg twice daily. It should be noted that high doses of methyltestosterone over a long period could result in nonreversible masculine changes in women.

1.3.1.2.6. Nandrolone (Androlone-D 100®, Deca-Durabolin®, Neo-Durabolic®, Anabolin™ LA, Andryl™, Durabolin®, Hybolin™, Nandrocot™, Deca-durabolin Injection [Inj Sol 100 mg/2 mL]; Nandrolone Decanoate Injection [Inj Sol 50 and

100 mg/mL]). Nandrolone is an orally administered androgen and is classified as a Schedule III controlled substance, which is banned by the NCAA, IOC, and USOC *(6, 25)*. Nandrolone is a synthetic androgen used in the treatment of osteoporosis and the anemia associated with chronic renal failure. Nandrolone increases hemoglobin and the mass of red blood cells. However, with the advent of recombinant human erythropoietin, the use of nandrolone in treating the aforementioned anemia is declining. Additionally, since nandrolone produces an anabolic effect, it is used as a doping agent to build muscle mass, increase bone density, and stimulate appetite. Furthermore, nandrolone might also enhance erythropoietic stimulating factor to increase the production of erythrocyte production. Other effects associated with nandrolone include increased levels of LDL and decreased levels of HDL *(25)*.

1.3.1.2.6.1. Pharmacokinetics. Intramuscular administration of nandrolone is slowly released at a relatively constant rate over a period of 4 d. Peak concentrations occur in approximately 3–6 d for a dose of 100 mg im. Plasma esterases hydrolyze nandrolone decanoate to its highly lipid soluble free form, nandrolone. Nandrolone is metabolized in the liver and has a half-life of 6–8 d. The clearance rate of nandrolone is 1.6 L/h/kg body wt.

1.3.1.2.6.2. Indications and Dosages. Nandrolone is indicated for the treatment of the anemia arising from chronic renal failure. Nandrolone can also be used to treat wasting conditions as well as to counter the effects of osteoporosis, but the FDA does not approve these usages. For treating anemia, nandrolone should be taken at intervals of 3–4 wk for up to 12 wk. If a second treatment cycle is required, a 4-wk interval between cycles should be employed. Additionally, because of its erythropoietic effects, adequate iron is required for maximal drug response. For treating the anemia associated with chronic renal failure, adult and adolescent (age 14 yr or more) males and females are administered intramuscularly 50–200 mg and 50–100 mg, respectively, at intervals of 1–4 wk. In children (2–13 yr), the recommended dosage of nandrolone is 25–50 mg im *(25)*.

Nandrolone may be used intramuscularly (50 mg im every 3–4 wk) for the treatment of osteoporosis in postmenopausal women, where it acts to inhibit bone resorption and increases bone density. It should be noted that the FDA does not approve this usage.

1.3.1.2.7. Oxandrolone (Oxandrin®; comes in 2.5-mg tablets). It should be noted that oxandrolone is a Schedule C-III controlled substance and is subsequently banned from athletic competition by the IOC, NCAA, NFL, and USOC *(6,25)*. Oxandrolone is a potent synthetic analogue of testosterone that has approximately eight times the anabolic activity of its parent compound. The ratio of anabolic to androgenic activity (testosterone:oxandrolone) is approximately 1:3 to 1:13, making oxandrolone the most potent of the androgens (Table 2). The deletion of the angular methyl group at the C-19 position results in the molecules greater androgenic potency. Oxandrolone in combination with adequate calories has been used to promote weight gains in individuals with chronic wasting diseases such as Duchenne muscular dystrophy, chronic obstructive pulmonary disease (COPD), and AIDS *(25,34–36)*. Androgens have also proven useful in maintaining muscle mass and body wt in trauma cases or in cases where patients suffered severe burns *(25)*.

At normal prescribed doses, oxandrolone is not ergogenic. It is unclear due to conflicting evidence whether anabolic steroids significantly increase athletic performance

14. Anabolic Doping Agents

when used in high doses. Oxandrolone has been shown to promote increases in lean body mass (increased muscle mass and strength) that is lost with the stoppage of treatment. Oxandrolone is not aromatized to estrogen, thus works directly as an androgen. Furthermore, oxandrolone decrease protein catabolism possibly by competitively inhibiting glucocorticoid receptors or interfering with the glucocorticoid responsive element.

1.3.1.2.7.1. Pharmacokinetics. Oxandrolone is administered orally and is rapidly absorbed. Oxandrolone is highly bound (94–97%) to plasma proteins and has a bioavailability of approximately 97%. Hepatic metabolism of oxandrolone is markedly slower than that of testosterone or other androgens due to the modification of ring A (lack of a 4-ene function) and 17a-alkylation. The elimination half-life for oxandrolone is approximately 9.4 h and peak plasma concentrations are higher than methyltestosterone. Oxandrolone is excreted primarily in the urine as the unchanged parent drug (approximately 28%) and unconjugated product *(25)*.

1.3.1.2.7.2. Indications and Dosages. It is important to note that when treating wasting conditions with oxandrolone (or any other androgen), proper nutrition is essential. Oxandrolone is indicated for the treatment of wasting syndromes associated with chronic diseases and lack of nutrition. Oxandrolone has also been suggested for use in the treatment of AIDS-related wasting syndrome, Duchenne muscular dystrophy, growth failure, and Turner's syndrome. However, the FDA *(25,37)* has not approved these uses. Oxandrolone is indicated for treating wasting conditions (cachexia, resulting from chronic disease and/or infection, severe trauma, prolonged glucocorticoid treatment, or extensive surgery), thereby promoting weight gain and increased protein synthesis. Furthermore, treatment would be indicated with in those individuals who fail to maintain normal body wt. The usual recommended oral dosage in adults is 2.5 mg, taken two to four times daily (5–10 mg/d) over a period of 2–4 wk. Depending on how the patient responds, the treatment may be repeated as needed. If necessary, the dosage may be increased up to 20 mg/d. In children, the recommended oral dose is 0.1 mg/kg (0.045 mg/pound) body wt/d over a period of 2–4 wk. However, the dosage should not exceed the adult dosage.

To treat the wasting syndrome associated with AIDS and the accompanying muscle weakness (not FDA-approved usage), an oral dosage of 5–15 mg/d over 16 wk has been investigated in adults *(38)*. Dosages of 15 mg/d enhanced weight gain whereas the 5 mg/d treatment group and placebo controls experienced either weight maintenance or loss in body wt, respectively. In these subjects, there was not any measurable improvement in muscle strength.

In other clinical studies conducted in children and adolescences suffering from chronic diseases and/or failure of growth (e.g., Duchenne muscular dystrophy, HIV infection, Turner's syndrome in females, and delayed pubertal development in males), oxandrolone was used orally at doses of 0.1 mg/kg/d (0.05 mg/kg/d for Turner's syndrome) over a period of 12 wk *(25,37,39)*. Results indicated that treatment with oxandrolone was successful in countering the weight loss and decreases in muscle mass associated with HIV. With stoppage of treatment, body wt was maintained but there was a decrease in muscle mass.

Treatment with oxandrolone (0.1 mg/kg/d, males) significantly improved muscle strength in children with Duchenne muscular dystrophy, and significantly improved the velocity of growth in boys with delayed pubertal development. Likewise, oxandrolone (0.05 mg/kg/d) significantly increased the rate of growth and final height in girls with Turner's syndrome. Additionally, the concomitant treatment with oxandrolone and growth hormone resulted in a greater final height than with oxandrolone alone.

1.3.1.2.8. Oxymetholone (Anadrol®, Anapolon®; comes in 50-mg tablets). Oxymetholone is an orally administered androgen and is classified as a Schedule III controlled substance, banned by the NCAA, IOC, and USOC *(6,25)*. Oxymetholone, like nandrolone, acts to enhance the production and excretion of erythropoietin, thereby increasing the red blood cell count. In contrast to nandrolone, oxymetholone produces a greater degree of hepatotoxicity.

1.3.1.2.8.1. Indications and Dosages. Oxymetholone is used for the treatment of anemias resulting from aplastic anemia (acquired or congenital), decreased production of red blood cells, bone marrow failure, myelofibrosis, and hypoplastic anemias arising from myelotoxic drugs. Additionally, oxymetholone has been used to treat wasting conditions associated with chronic diseases. In 1997, Anadrol-50 was discontinued. Oxymetholone is not meant to replace other therapeutic approaches to counter anemias such as iron, folic acid, vitamin B_{12} and/or pyridoxine replacement therapy, and blood transfusions.

In adults and children, the recommended oral dosage is 1–5 mg/kg body wt/d. Normally, a dose of 1–2 mg/kg/d is effective but higher doses may be required. As with all androgens, therapy should be tailored to the individuals needs and overall response. Treatment should be given over a period of 3–6 mo with careful monitoring of hepatic functions. Following remission in patients with congenital aplastic anemia, a continued maintenance dose is usually sufficient to maintain normal red blood cell counts.

1.3.1.2.9. Stanozolol (Winstrol®, Winstrol® V [2-mg tablets]). Stanozolol is an orally administered androgen and is classified as a schedule III controlled substance, banned by the NCAA, IOC, and USOC *(6,25)*. It has been used in the treatment of hereditary angioedema, and has been used as an anabolic agent to promote increases in muscle mass, enhance performance, and reverse catabolism. The FDA approved Stanozolol for use in 1962 with 4.5 times greater anabolic potency than testosterone. Additionally, the anabolic activity for stanozolol is three to sixfold greater than its androgenic effects. Stanozolol, as with the other anabolic agents, requires sufficient caloric and protein intake in order to maintain a positive nitrogen balance.

1.3.1.2.9.1. Indications and Dosages. Stanozolol is indicated for use in the treatment of hereditary angioedema. The recommended oral dosage in adults is initially 2 mg taken three times/day. The dosage should be decreased when the frequency of attacks has lessened. A maintenance dose of 2 mg/d or every other day should be taken orally at intervals of 1–3 mo.

1.3.1.2.10. Testosterone (Andro®, AndroGel®, depoAndro®, Depo®-Testosterone, Androderm®, Testoderm®, Testoderm TTS®, Testopel®, Andro Cyp™, Andro-L.A.®, Delatest®, Depandrate™, Depandro®, Duratest™, Durathate™, Histerone™, Meditest™, Testa Span™, Testamone™, Testerone™, Testolin™, Testro™, Testro™ AQ, Testro™ LA.; Testosterone [PELLET 75 mg, INJ SUSP 50 mg/cc]; Testerone suspension [INJ SUSP 50 mg/mL]; Testosterone propionate injection [INJ SOL 100 mg]; Depo testosterone injection [INJ SOL 200 mg/mL]; Testoderm system

14. Anabolic Doping Agents

transdermal [FILM ER 4 mg/d]; Androderm [FILM ER 2.5 mg/d]). Testosterone is the principal endogenous androgen and is classified as a Schedule III controlled substance, banned by the NCAA, IOC, and USOC *(6,25)*. It was first approved for use in 1939 by the FDA and can be administered parenterally by two dosage forms (regular and delayed-release), by transdermal application, or through the implantation of sterile pellets (released over a period of 3–6 mo). Testosterone is metabolized in the liver at a relatively fast rate, thus prompting the search for androgens with prolonged action, as with the analog methyltestosterone. Androgens are important for stimulating RNA polymerase and subsequent protein production important in the development of male sex traits. During puberty, androgens promote the growth and development of skeletal muscle, and the redistribution of body fat *(25)*.

1.3.1.2.10.1. Pharmacokinetics. Oral administration of testosterone would result in the drug being absorbed from the gastrointestinal (GI) tract and being extensively metabolized in the liver (first-pass effect). Since the bioavailability of testosterone is low when taken orally, analogs of testosterone (e.g., methyltestosterone) have been synthesized to act as a prodrug (prohormone) when taken orally, releasing testosterone as the active metabolite when metabolized in the liver. However, the usual routes of administration for testosterone include intramuscularly (im), absorption by transdermal patches, absorption by topical gel application, and pellet implant *(17,25)*.

1.3.1.2.10.1.1. Intramuscular Route (im). When testosterone undecanoate is taken orally for replacement therapy in hypogonadal men, multiple doses are required on a daily basis to achieve the desired affect. Additionally, the resulting serum testosterone levels can vary by a wide margin potentially due to variations in absorption from the GI tract and the rapid metabolism of testosterone in the liver. However, the administration of testosterone esters (e.g., testosterone undecanoate) via an im route offers a more sustained duration of action lasting from 2 to 4 wk, owing to its slow absorption from the injection site. Testosterone esters are less polar than testosterone and are absorbed at a slower rate.

In pharmacokinetic studies conducted in orchidectomized cynomolgus monkeys (*Macaca fascicularis*), Partsch et al. *(40)* showed that a single im injection (10 mg/kg) of testosterone undecanoate produced first-day mean serum levels of 58 nmol/L and levels of 40–68 nmol/L for a period of 45 d. Testosterone levels remained normal over another 56 d. However, im injections of testosterone enanthate (10 mg/kg) produced higher initial plasma testosterone levels (100–177 nmol/L) than the undecanoate out to Day 5, then significantly decreased to low normal levels after 31 d. Clinical studies with testosterone undecanoate in Klinefelter's syndrome patients were conducted by Zhang et al. *(18)*. In these studies, they showed plasma testosterone levels increase from 10 nmol/L (hypogonadal levels) to 47.8 and 54.2 nmol/L following im injection of 500 mg or 1000 mg testosterone undecanoate, respectively.

1.3.1.2.10.1.2. Subcutaneous Implantable Pellets. Subcutaneous testosterone pellets have duration of action that ranges from 3 to 4 mo to approximately 6 mo.

1.3.1.2.10.1.3. Topical Absorption (25).

- Gels. Dosing once a day (24-h dosing interval) with a topical testosterone skin gel or ointment, 10% of the applied dosage is systemically absorbed. This information suggests that the skin acts as a reservoir for sustained-release of testosterone. Differences in skin color may affect the amount of drug absorbed into the skin reservoir. It is important to note that with higher melanin concentrations in dark skin, higher drug concentrations will be observed than in skin of a lighter color.

- Transdermal Patches. Skin patches can be applied to areas of the scrotum, arm, back, or upper buttocks. The scrotum provides an area that is fivefold more permeable than other areas. From scrotal patches, serum testosterone concentrations peak after 2–4 h and plateau following 3–4 wk.

1.3.1.2.10.1.4. Indications and Dosages. Testosterone is indicated for the treatment of breast cancer, delayed puberty, erectile dysfunction, and hypogonadism. Although not approved for use by the FDA, testosterone has also been suggested for the treatment of AIDS-associated wasting syndrome, anemia, and microphallus.

1.3.1.2.10.1.5. Androgen Replacement Therapy for the Treatment of Erectile Dysfunction (Impotence). In adult males, the recommended dosage of testosterone suspension or testosterone propionate is 10–25 mg (im) two to three times/week, whereas 50–400 mg (im) once every 2–4 wk is recommended for testosterone cypionate or enanthate.

1.3.1.2.10.1.6. Androgen Replacement Therapy for Hypogonadism (Primary and Hypogonadotropic Types). In adult males, the recommended dosage of testosterone suspension or testosterone propionate is 10–25 mg (im) two to three times/week, whereas 50–400 mg (im) once every 2–4 wk is recommended for testosterone cypionate or enanthate. In children, to initiate pubertal growth 40–50 mg/m^2 of is administered im. Treatment is continued until the growth rate drops to prepubertal levels. The recommended treatment for the terminal growth phase is 100 mg/m^2 im until growth stops. Continuing treatment (100 mg/m^2 im) at a dosage rate of two per month will maintain virilization.

1.3.2. Biosynthesis of Endogenous Androgens

The principal site for the synthesis of endogenous androgens (e.g., DHEA or testosterone) in men is in the Leydig cells of the testes where approximately 95% of all the androgens are produced. In particular, androgens are synthesized in the mitochondria of Leydig cells. In addition to the testes, androgens are also synthesized in the cortex of adrenal glands. The primary androgen synthesized in the adrenals is androstenedione, a precursor to testosterone and dihydrotestosterone. In males, the adrenal cortex accounts for only about 5% of the total hormone produced in the body. In contrast, the adrenal cortex in females accounts for the majority of androgens (e.g., DHEA) produced, whereas theca follicular cells of the ovaries are secondary for androgen production. The mean production rates of testosterone and DHT in normal healthy males are 0.07 and 0.03 mg/d, respectively, whereas in females the corresponding rates of production are 0.03 and 0.006 mg/d *(8,41,42)*.

The synthesis of testosterone (Fig. 6) in the testis is initiated by the conversion of plasma cholesterol and acetate *(8,41,42)*. The resulting cholesterol esters are acted on by the enzyme 20,22-desmolase in the rate-limiting step to form the intermediate pregnenolone. This rate-limiting step in the synthesis of testosterone is most likely subject to regulation by gonadotropins. In turn, pregnenolone undergoes conversion to progesterone by 3β-OH-steroid dehydrogenase (3β-HSD). Pregnenolone and progesterone are both acted on by the enzyme 17-hydroxylase forming 17-OH-pregnenolone and 17-OH-progesterone, respectively. Similarly, the enzyme 17,20-desmolase is responsible

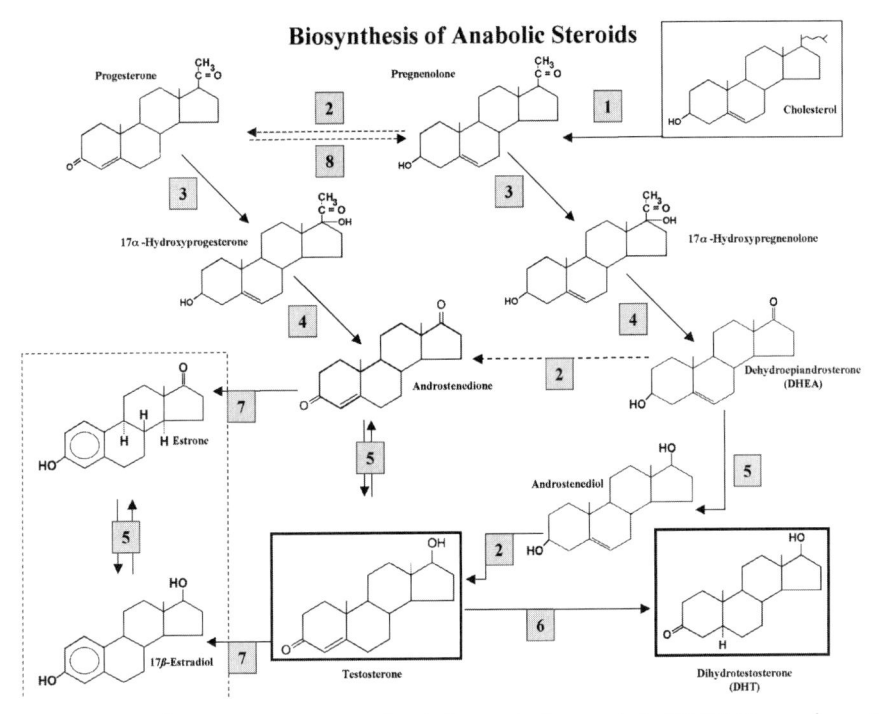

Fig. 6. Enzymes used in testosterone synthesis from cholesterol. **1.** 20,22 Desmolase; **2.** 3β-OH-Steroid Dehydrogenase (3-β-HSD); **3.** 17α-Hydroxylase; **4.** 17,20 Desmolase; **5.** 17β-OH-Steroid Dehydrogenase (17-β-HSD); **6.** 5α-Reductase; **7.** Aromatase; **8.** 5β-Reductase.

for catalyzing the conversion of 17-OH-pregnenolone and 17-OH-progesterone to DHEA and androstenedione, respectively. DHEA and androstenedione both undergo 17β-dehydroxylation by 17β-OH-steroid dehydrogenase to form androstenediol and testosterone. Androstenediol is further acted upon by the enzyme 3β-OH-HSD to yield testosterone *(8,41,42)*.

1.3.3. Mechanism of Action

All of the androgens produce their effect through binding to high-affinity steroid receptors free in the cytoplasm (Fig. 7). Once bound, the hormone-receptor complex translocates into the nucleus and binds to DNA. Other possible interactions may include the passing of the steroid molecule into the nucleus and binding with a nuclear receptor, or possibly dissociating from the steroid receptor and directly interacting with DNA. However, it has been shown that the rate-limiting step in binding steroid hormones to the receptor is not either the cytoplasmic concentration of the steroid or steroid-receptor complex, but the number of cytoplasmic receptors. In the nucleus, anabolic steroids enhance gene transcription resulting in the production of specific mRNA. The mRNA passes out into the cytoplasm, binds to the rough endoplasmic reticulum, and induces protein synthesis. In addition to an anabolic/androgenic action on tissue, catabolic activity is inhibited. Whether inhibition of catabolic activity occurs in the nucleus, through inhibiting the transcription of catabolic enzymes or in the cytoplasm is unclear *(8,41,42)*.

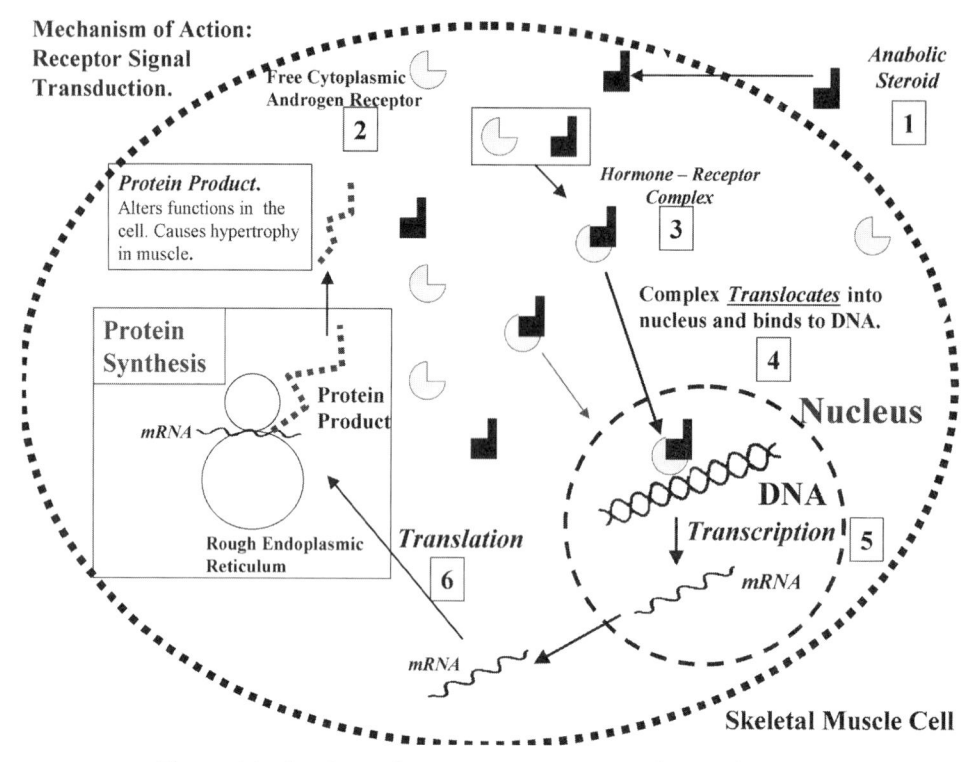

Fig. 7. Mechanism of action: receptor signal transduction.

When androgen receptors are present in a tissue, the tissue is said to be androgen sensitive. Receptor levels in skeletal muscle have been reported to range between 0.5 and 3.0×10^{-12} moles per mg protein, whereas in the prostate receptor levels may be 25-fold greater. Nearly all of the testosterone content in tissues such as the prostate, seminal vesicles, and pubic skin is metabolized to DHT, the active form of testosterone that binds to the nuclear androgen receptors. However, in other tissues (e.g., kidneys, testis, and skeletal muscle) that contain little 5α-reductase, testosterone binds directly to the receptor. DHT is 2.5 to 10 times more potent than testosterone in bioassays (such as capon's comb) and binds to the receptor with a two- to threefold higher affinity (K_d = 0.25–0.5 nM DHT and K_2 = 0.4–1.0 nM testosterone). In skeletal muscle, DHT activity is attenuated by the enzyme 3α-hydroxysteroid oxidoreductase, which converts DHT to the less active androgen 5α-androstane-3, 17β diol. Thus, bioconversion of DHT and other androgens limits their effectiveness in skeletal muscle. A final point to consider for androgen activity is the feedback control mechanism utilizing the testosterone metabolite estradiol (Fig. 8). Estradiol acts to enhance catabolic activity in tissue, thereby attenuating the effects of high levels of testosterone or its analogs *(8,41,42)*.

1.3.4. Transport and Metabolism

1.3.4.1. Transport

Endogenous hormones that are released into the bloodstream subsequently act on remote target tissues responsible for muscle growth and secondary sex characteristics.

14. Anabolic Doping Agents

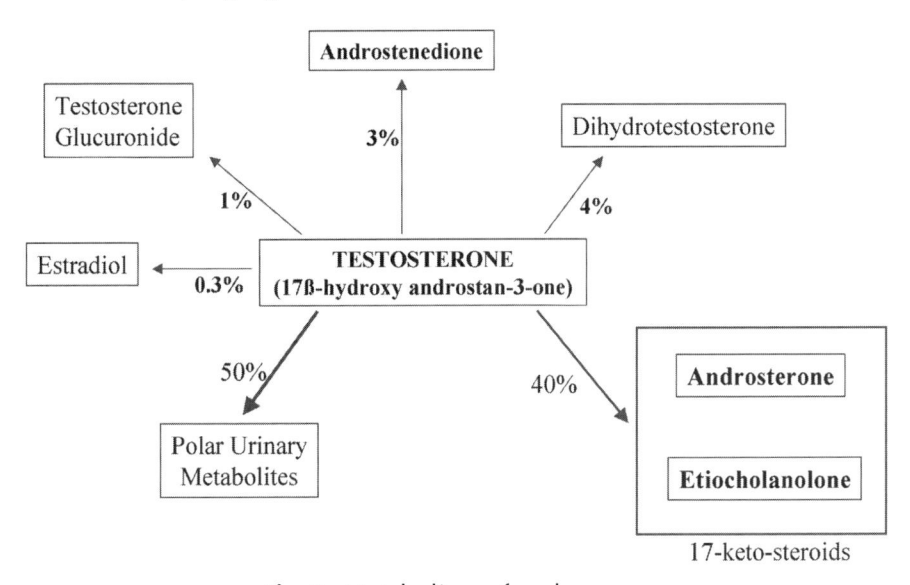

Fig. 8. Metabolism of androgens.

Once entering the plasma, testosterone becomes bound to carrier proteins and is transported to the liver where the complex undergoes catabolism. Of these carrier proteins, testosterone binds with to the sex hormone-binding globulin (SHBG), also known as the testosterone-estradiol binding globulin (TeBG) *(8,42)*. In plasma, approximately 2–3% of testosterone and DHT circulates as unbound (e.g., free), bound to SHBG (~60%), or bound to albumin (~37%). In women, estradiol is also carried by SHBG, whereas in men it is carried by albumin since testosterone and DHT saturate all of the available sites on SHBG. The primary route for testosterone to enter cells is via simple diffusion. However, it is unclear whether testosterone that is bound to SHBG is able to enter cells. It is important to note that changes in the circulating pool of SHBG will have an effect on the proportion of free testosterone in the plasma available to enter target cells. Because testosterone has such a short biological half-life, alkylation (for oral usage) or esterification (for injectable steroids) of the molecule is required in order to prolong its half-life and by slowing down its rate of metabolized *(8,42,43)*.

1.3.4.2. Metabolism (Table 5: Metabolites; Fig. 8)

The primary site for the metabolism of testosterone and other androgens is in the liver. In both testosterone and androstenedione, the double bond located between C4 and C5 are reduced, yielding two stereoisomers with a chiral center at C5. The isomers of androstenedione are etiocholanolone (5β-isomer) and androsterone (5α-isomer). Other isomers that are formed from the hydrogenation of the C-3 keto group include the 3α-hydroxysteroids (androsterone and etiocholanolone) and the 3β-hydroxysteroid (epiandrosterone). Of these 17-ketosteroids, the 3α-hydroxysteroids are found in the highest concentration in the urine. Another metabolite of testosterone, epitestosterone is the 17α-hydroxy androstan-3-one enantiomer of testosterone. In normal adult men, it has been reported that approximately 5–25 mg of 17 keto-steroids are excreted in the urine over a 24-h period *(8,16,42)*.

Table 5
Major Metabolites of Selected Androgens[a]

Androstenedione	Danazol	Dihydrotestosterone	Fluoxymesterone	Methyltestosterone
Testosterone	δ-1-2-hydroxymethyl-ethisterone	Androstanediol	6-hydroxyfluoxy-mesterone	6β-Hydroxy-methyl-testosterone
Estrone	2-hydroxymethyl-ethisterone		6,16-dihydroxyluoxy-mesterone	

Nandrolone	Oxandrolone[c]	Oxymetholone	Stanozolol	Testosterone
19-norandrosterone		17β-hydroxy-17α-methyl-5″-androstan-3-one (mestanolone) 17β-hydroxy-17″-methyl-	16β-hydroxystanozolol	dihydrotestosterone
19-noretiocholanolone		2,3,-seco-5″-androstane-2,3-dioic acid 3″,17β-dihydroxy-17″-methyl-5″,-androstane-2β-carboxylic acid		estradiol androsterone etiocholanolone

[a]Glucuronidated at positions 3 and 17.
[b]Equine. Note: No first-pass effect and cannot be converted to estrogen.
[c]Note: No first-pass effect and cannot be converted to estrogen.

Table 6
Percent Usage of Anabolic Steroids Among Middle and High School Students

	Grades		
Year	8th Grade % Use	10th Grade % Use	12th Grade % Use
1991	1.90	1.80	2.10
1999	2.70	2.70	2.90
2000	3.00	3.50	2.50
Years	8th Grade % Change	10th Grade % Change	12th Grade % Change
(1991–1999)	0.80	0.90	0.80
(1999–2000)	0.30	0.80	−0.40
(1991–2000)	1.10	1.70	0.40

Data from (5).

In addition to the aforementioned metabolites of testosterone, testosterone is also metabolized into a series of hydroxylated (positions 3, 15, and 16) polar compounds that are conjugated to sulfuric and glucuronic acids and excreted in the urine and bile. In addition to the metabolites, approximately 250 mg/day is excreted into the urine unchanged.

Alkylation at position 17 on the D ring for orally active androgens provide a measure of protection against the first-pass clearance in the liver. These drugs include oxandrolone, oxymetholone, methandrostenolone, and stanozolol for the orally active drugs and testosterone enanthate and nandrolone decanoate for the parenterally administered nonmethylated androgens containing a 17-β ester period (8,16,42).

1.4. Toxicology: Adverse Reactions and Contraindications

Use of anabolic steroids, as well as other anabolic agents, is occurring at an increased rate in other segments of the population. The "Monitoring the Future" study conducted by the National Institute on Drug Abuse (NIDA) is an annual survey of drug abuse among American adolescents. Results from this study showed a 6% decrease amongst 12th grade students in associating the magnitude of health risk with the use of anabolic steroids. Over a period of 8 yr (from 1991 to 1999), significant increases in anabolic steroid usage were observed among adolescences (Table 6). More alarmingly, between the years 1998 and 1999, a greater increase in steroid abuse was noted among middle school-aged students. Other reports from Merck indicated that in the United States, the rate of anabolic steroid use in male high school students ranged from 6 to 11%. Surprisingly, this relatively high percentage of users included a number of nonathletes. Additionally, it was reported that steroid usage among female high school students was approximately 2.5%. Furthermore, nonsteroidal anabolic agents such as β_2-adrenergic agonists, growth factors, and growth hormone, are now being used in combination with anabolic steroids in order to gain a more desirable anabolic effect (5).

Results from these studies indicate a rising belief that the gains associated with taking steroids far outweigh any potential risks. A national survey revealed that the most common reasons given for using steroids were to improve athletic performance and/or improve their appearance, and no doubt their self-esteem. This willingness among adolescences to use anabolic steroids reflects a failure of society to recognize the severity of problem amongst the young and/or a lack of programs that sufficiently address the dangers associated with steroid abuse *(14,44)*.

Since 1969, based on seized Stasi (East Germany's State Security Service) records, an extensive doping program (State Plan 14.25) was in existence in the DDR, primarily with the intent of humiliating West Germany at the 1972 Munich Olympics. This East German program may have involved as many as 10,000 athletes, of which many received doping agents without their knowledge. Furthermore, it appears that the practice of state-sponsored doping programs was prevalent through out the Eastern Block countries such as Czechoslovakia, Bulgaria, and the USSR, as well as China. However, Germany is the only country to launch judicial investigations into past doping offenses with the intent of prosecution. Following the fall of the Berlin Wall and the reunification of Germany, the true extent of nationally sponsored anabolic doping programs became evident *(45,46)*.

Today, these former athletes are presenting a host of problems attributed to the use of multiple doping agents (e.g., turinabol, HGH, etc.) that range from liver damage and ovarian inflamation to infertility, tumors, and a continual deterioration of their health. From the use of massive doses of anabolic/androgenic steroids in young female athletes, they have been reported to experience an inhibition of gonadotropin secretion, growth of facial hair, muscle mass, and other virilization traits. It is important to note that virilization occurring in such young women tends to be irreversible (e.g., deepening of voice and clitoral enlargement), even after discontinuation of androgens. Additionally, the impact of massive androgen doses has been reported to cause changes in sexual preference in some women.

In studies conducted in women, it was noted that 100 mg of either DHEA or androstenedione caused plasma testosterone levels to increase by at least six times that of normal human females. This treatment-induced increase in plasma testosterone levels had a duration of 2 h, with peak levels lasting for only a few minutes. In another study conducted with men, it was found that plasma testosterone levels rose by 211 and 237% when treated with either 50 or 100 mg of androstenedione, respectively *(23,24,47,48)*. Androstenedione is classified and sold as a dietary supplement. Because dietary supplements are sold containing androgens, one must be alert to the possibility accidental exposure or alterations to endogenous androgen levels *(49,50)*.

1.4.1. Contraindications

In general, these drugs are Schedule C-III controlled substances and are all banned by the NCAA, USOC, and IOC *(6,25)*. They are sold (with the exception of androstenedione) as prescription only and are categorized as pregnancy category X (should never be used in pregnancy). The drugs listed should not be used in children.

1.4.1.1. ANDROSTENEDIONE

Androstenedione is contraindicated in children, cholestasis, females, hepatic disease, and hepatitis. It should never be used during pregnancy or in cases of prostate cancer.

14. Anabolic Doping Agents

1.4.1.2. DANAZOL

Danazol is contraindicated for the elderly, and in cases of migraine or prostatic hypertrophy. It should never be used in cases of breast cancer, breast-feeding, cardiac disease, elderly, hepatic disease, migraine, porphyria, pregnancy, prostatic hypertrophy, renal disease, seizure disorder, and vaginal bleeding.

1.4.1.3. DIHYDROTESTOSTERONE

Unclear at this time.

1.4.1.4. FLUOXYMESTERONE

Fluoxymesterone is contraindicated in cases of cardiac, hepatic, and renal diseases, men with breast or prostate carcinomas, pregnancy, prostatic hypertrophy, porphyria, and tartrazine dye hypersensitivity.

1.4.1.5. METHYLTESTOSTERONE AND TESTOSTERONE

Testosterone is contraindicated in cases of accidental exposure in women to patients using testosterone gels or creams. Both are contraindicated in women who are breast-feeding or pregnant, children, hypercalcemia, diabetes mellitus, coronary artery disease, diabetes mellitus, females, heart failure, myocardial infarction, and prostatic hypertrophy. It should never be used in cases of breast or prostrate cancer, intravenous administration, cardiac, hepatic and renal diseases, soya lecithin hypersensitivity, and tartrazine dye hypersensitivity.

1.4.1.6. NANDROLONE

Nandrolone decanoate is contraindicated in breast-feeding, children, coronary artery disease, diabetes mellitus, heart failure, hypercalcemia, myocardial infarction, and prostatic hypertrophy. It should never be used in cases of benzyl alcohol hypersensitivity, breast cancer, cardiac and hepatic diseases, females, intravenous administration, pregnancy, and prostate cancer.

1.4.1.7. OXANDROLONE

Contraindicated in cases of arteriosclerosis, breast cancer, breast-feeding, cardiovascular diseases (cardiac disease, coronary artery disease, heart failure, myocardial infarction, peripheral edema), children, cholestasis, diabetes mellitus, females, hepatic and renal diseases, hypercalcemia, hypercholesterolemia, jaundice, peripheral edema, polycythemia, pregnancy, prostate cancer, and prostatic hypertrophy.

1.4.1.8. OXYMETHOLONE

Oxymetholone is contraindicated in cases of breast carcinoma, diabetes, kidney disease (nephrosis, nephrotic phase of nephritis), pregnancy, prostate carcinoma, and seizure disorders. Oxymetholone (Anadrol-50) was discontinued in 1997.

1.4.1.9. STANOZOLOL

Stanozolol is a Schedule C-III controlled substance and is contraindicated in cases of breast carcinoma, diabetes, kidney disease (nephrosis, nephrotic phase of nephritis), pregnancy, prostate carcinoma, and seizure disorders.

1.4.2. General Adverse Effects (25)

Some of the most common side effects include hirsutism, male pattern baldness, acne, increased serum cholesterol, and decreased HDL. Testosterone enanthate, for example, also affects body fluids and electrolytes by causing retention of water, sodium, chloride, potassium, calcium, and inorganic phosphates. The hematological effects of testosterone enanthate include suppression of clotting factors II, V, VII, and X, producing bleeding in patients on anticoagulant therapy, and polycythemia. Other adverse effects include nausea, cholestatic jaundice, alterations in liver function tests, headaches, anxiety, depression, altered libido, and generalized paresthesia. Infrequently, testosterone enanthate can cause hepatocellular neoplasms, hepatis, inflammation, and anaphylactic reactions. High doses of anabolic steroids have been implicated in causing cancer and behavior changes including steroid "roid" rage *(51)*.

1.4.2.1. ENDOCRINE AND UROGENITAL (25)

1.4.2.1.1. Males. In men, the most common side effects associated with androgen usage include gynecomania (an excessive desire for women), and excessive frequency and duration of penile erections. Oligospermia may occur at high dosages.

1.4.2.1.2. Females. In women, the most common side effects associated with androgen therapy are amenorrhea and other menstrual irregularities, inhibition of gonadotropin secretion, and virilization, including deepening of the voice and clitoral enlargement. The observed changes in voice and clitoral enlargement are usually irreversible even after discontinuation of androgens. In pregnant women, treatment with androgens causes virilization of the external genitalia in female fetuses.

1.4.3. Specific Adverse Effects of Selected Androgens

1.4.3.1. ANDROSTENEDIONE

Androstenedione can cause feminization (indirect effect through its metabolites estradione and 17β-estradiol), priapism, secondary malignancy, and virilization (direct anabolic action of androstenedione).

1.4.3.2. DANAZOL

Acne, alopecia, amenorrhea, bleeding, cholestasis, diaphoresis, edema, elevated hepatic enzymes, erythema multiforme, flushing, Guillain-Barre syndrome, headache, hirsutism, hoarseness or deepening of voice, hypercholesterolemia, jaundice, maculopapular rash, nausea/vomiting, peliosis hepatis, pharyngitis, photosensitivity, pruritus, pseudotumor cerebri, seborrhea, Stevens-Johnson syndrome, stroke, teratogenesis, thromboembolism, thrombosis, urticaria, visual impairment, and weight gain.

1.4.3.3. DIHYDROTESTOSTERONE (DHT)

DHT causes male pattern baldness; other adverse effects are unclear at this time.

1.4.3.4. FLUOXYMESTERONE

Amenorrhea, anxiety, change in libido, cholestatic jaundice, clitoral enlargement, depression, edema, elevated hepatic enzymes, excessive frequency and duration of erections, gynecomastia, headache, hirsutism, hoarseness or deepening of voice, hypercalcemia, male pattern baldness, nausea/vomiting, oligospermia, peliosis hepatis, suppression of clotting factors, and virilization.

14. Anabolic Doping Agents

1.4.3.5. METHYLTESTOSTERONE

Acne, alopecia, amenorrhea, anxiety, depression, elevated hepatic enzymes, epididymitis, epiphyseal closure, erythrocytosis, feminization, gynecomastia, hepatitis, hypercalcemia, hypercholesterolemia, jaundice, libido increase/decrease, nausea and vomiting, oligomenorrhea, peliosis hepatis, peripheral edema, priapism, prostatic hypertrophy, secondary malignancy, virilization, and weight gain.

1.4.3.6. NANDROLONE

Nandrolone can cause: acne, acneiform rash, alopecia, amenorrhea, clitoral enlargement, decreased ejaculate volume, depression, diarrhea, edema, elevated hepatic enzymes, epididymitis, epiphyseal closure, excitability, feminization, fluid retention, gynecomastia, hepatic failure, hepatic necrosis, hepatitis, hepatoma, hirsutism, hoarseness or deepening of voice, hypercalcemia, hypercholesterolemia, impotence, injection site reaction, insomnia, jaundice, libido increase/decrease, mastalgia, menstrual irregularity, nausea and vomiting, oligomenorrhea, oligospermia, peliosis hepatis, penile enlargement, peripheral edema, priapism, prolonged bleeding time, prostatic hypertrophy, secondary malignancy, sodium retention, teratogenesis, testicular atrophy, virilization, and weight gain.

1.4.3.7. OXANDROLONE

Oxandrolone can cause: acne, amenorrhea, cholestasis, clitoral enlargement, clotting factor deficiency, coagulopathy, depression, edema, elevated hepatic enzymes, epididymitis, excitability, feminization, fluid retention, gynecomastia, hepatic necrosis and failure, hepatitis, hepatoma, hirsutism, hoarseness or deepening of voice, hypercalcemia, hypercholesterolemia, hyperkalemia, hypernatremia, hyperphosphatemia, impotence, insomnia, jaundice, libido increase/decrease, menstrual irregularity, oligomenorrhea, oligospermia, peliosis hepatis, penile enlargement, peripheral edema, polycythemia, priapism, prolonged bleeding time, prostatic hypertrophy, secondary malignancy, teratogenesis, testicular atrophy, virilization, and weight gain.

1.4.3.8. OXYMETHOLONE

Oxymetholone can cause: acne, blood lipid changes, cholestatic jaundice, clitoral enlargement, diarrhea, edema, excitation, glucose intolerance, gynecomastia, hirsutism, hoarseness or deepening of voice, inhibition of testicular function, insomnia, liver cell tumors, nausea and vomiting, oligospermia, peliosis hepatis, testicular atrophy, and virilization.

1.4.3.9. STANOZOLOL

Stanozolol can cause: acne, blood lipid changes, cholestatic jaundice, clitoral enlargement, diarrhea, edema, excitation, glucose intolerance, gynecomastia, hirsutism, hoarseness or deepening of voice, inhibition of testicular function, insomnia, liver cell tumors, nausea and vomiting, oligospermia, peliosis hepatis, testicular atrophy, and virilization.

1.4.3.10. TESTOSTERONE

Testosterone can cause: acne, alopecia, amenorrhea, anxiety, depression, elevated hepatic enzymes, epididymitis, epiphyseal closure, erythema, erythrocytosis, feminization, gynecomastia, headache, hepatitis, hypercalcemia, hypercholesterolemia, injection site reaction, insomnia, jaundice, libido increase/ decrease, mastalgia, nausea and vomiting, oligomenorrhea, peliosis hepatis, peripheral edema, priapism, prostatic hypertrophy, pruritus, secondary malignancy, skin discoloration, skin irritation, virilization, and weight gain.

1.5. Mechanisms of Interactions (25)

1.5.1. The Following Classes of Drugs May Interact with Androgens When Administering Concurrently

It should be noted that chronic usage of androgens has been shown to lead to dependency and the abuse of other drugs such as alcohol, cocaine, amphetamines, and opioids. Furthermore, studies have shown that androgens are frequently used in varying combinations along with other anabolic agents such as clenbuterol, growth hormone, and nutritional supplements.

1.5.1.1. ANTICOAGULANTS, NONSTEROIDAL ANTIINFLAMMATORY DRUGS, AND SALICYLATES

Androgens such as danazol, fluoxymesterone, methyltestosterone, methandrostenolone, nandrolone, and testosterone have been reported to interact with anticoagulants, nonsteroidal antiinflammatory drugs (NSAIDs), and salicylates by potentiating their anticoagulant effects. With anticoagulants such as warfarin, concomitant usage of androgens can cause an increase in plasma warfarin levels. The specific mechanism by which this takes place is unknown, but it appears not to be related to displacement from plasma proteins. Patients receiving oral anticoagulant, NSAIDs, or salicylate therapy require close monitoring especially when androgens are started or stopped.

1.5.1.2. ANTIDIABETIC DRUGS AND INSULIN

Androgens have been shown to decrease blood glucose levels in diabetics, thereby lowering insulin requirements.

1.5.1.3. ADRENOCORTICOTROPIC HORMONE (ACTH), CORTICOSTEROIDS, HIGH-SODIUM FOODS, AND SODIUM-CONTAINING DRUGS

The interaction of androgens with drugs that promote sodium retention or foods that have high sodium content should be avoided because of risk of edema. Furthermore, individuals with hepatic or cardiac disease should avoid these combinations due to risk of hepatotoxicity, stroke (as a result of hypertension), or heart attack.

1.5.1.4. ALCOHOL (ETHANOL)

Although alcohol does not have any ergogenic effects, it can reduce the anxiety level or tremors prior to competition. Furthermore, it has been shown that ethanol metabolism may interfere with steroid metabolism by interacting with steroid oxidoreductions. In addition to interfering with steroid metabolism, alcohol may potentiate other effects related with androgen abuse. In clinical studies conducted to determine whether personality psychopathology is common among anabolic steroid users, illicit androgen users were compared with age-matched alcoholics and two control groups. Results from these studies showed that androgen users had increased risk for personality psychopathology when compared with community controls. Furthermore, illicit androgen users also demonstrated significant antisocial traits in a manner similar to the alcoholic group *(25,52)*.

14. Anabolic Doping Agents

Pregnant female athletes who are taking androgens and alcohol risk fetal alcohol syndrome (FAS). The testosterone metabolite estradiol has been shown to synergistically interact with ethanol causing renal damage such as hydronephrosis in the developing fetus of humans and animal models. Additionally, renal damage may persist due to suppression of testosterone-stimulated renal growth and development in the fetus.

1.5.1.5. AMPHETAMINES (AMPHETAMINE AND METHAMPHETAMINE)

Abuse of amphetamines and androgens has been well documented with regard to increasing aggressive and antisocial behavior. In addition, a consistent clinical feature associated with methamphetamine-induced organic mental disorders included an organic delusional syndrome with paranoid ideation and hallucinations. Furthermore, with methamphetamine abuse a high propensity for violence is very common. Similarly, violent and aggressive tendencies have been commonly observed in androgen abusers. However, information on the combined effect of androgens and amphetamines on aggressive behavior is lacking and further research is required *(3)*.

The potential consequences arising from the combined use of amphetamines and androgens was addressed initially in the introduction. During the Second World War, all the armies used amphetamines routinely to help increase the soldiers' endurance and alertness, thereby giving them an edge in combat. Additionally, when amphetamines were presumably used in combined with other behavior modifying drugs such as alcohol and/or androgens, the likelihood of a psychotic episode and violence could be greatly enhanced (in either severity or frequency). This would be especially true if these drugs are taken chronically and at high doses.

In related studies focused in investigating androgen effects on brain reward in male rats, results suggested that although androgens do not appear to change the rewarding properties of brain stimulation, they might impact the sensitivity of the brain reward systems. This observation was achieved by implanting electrodes in the lateral hypothalamus using the rate-frequency curve shift paradigm of brain stimulation reward. It was found that androgen (singly or as part of a "cocktail") affects the brain reward system in male rats; it was observed that over a period of 2 wk that methandrostenolone had no effect on either the reward or performance of intracranial self-stimulation. However, when a "cocktail" consisting of testosterone cypionate, nandrolone decanoate, and boldenone undecylenate was given over a period of 15 wk, the bar press rate (to stimulate the electrode) increased slightly but significantly. Treatment with amphetamine prior to and after the 15-wk androgen protocol significantly increased the rate-frequency curve shift. From these results, the investigators were able to conclude that androgens may enhance the sensitivity of the brain to amphetamine-induced brain reward properties *(51)*.

Other areas of research have indicated that amphetamines inhibit spontaneous and HCG-stimulated testosterone secretion in the testes by in part increasing cAMP production and decreasing Ca^{2+} channel activity.

1.5.1.6. ANTIVIRAL NONNUCLEOSIDE REVERSE TRANSCRIPTASE INHIBITOR DRUGS USED IN TREATING AIDS

AIDS patients who are taking the antiviral nonnucleoside reverse transcriptase inhibitors (NNRTIs) agents such as deavirdine, efavirenz, and nevirapine may interact with some anabolic steroid treatments. Results from a study conducted by the Liverpool

HIV Pharmacology Group from the University of Liverpool in conduction with Bristol-Myers Squibb Pharma indicated that no clinically significant interaction occurred with nandrolone, whereas it was unclear whether any potential interactions with oxandrolone would take place. On the other hand, treatment with the androgens stanazolol and testosterone may require close monitoring regarding alterations in drug dosage or the timing of administration (25).

1.5.1.7. ANTIVIRAL PROTEASE INHIBITORS

AIDS patients who are taking the antiviral protease inhibitors such as amprenavir, indinavir, lopinavir, nelfinavir, ritonavir, and saquinavir may interact with some anabolic steroid treatments. Results from a study conducted by the Liverpool HIV Pharmacology Group from the University of Liverpool in conduction with Bristol-Myers Squibb Pharma indicated that no clinically significant interaction occurred with nandrolone, whereas it was unclear whether any potential interactions with oxandrolone would take place. On the other hand, treatment with the androgens stanazolol and testosterone may require close monitoring regarding alterations in drug dosage or the timing of administration.

1.5.1.8. ADRENOCEPTOR AGONISTS

The synergistic effects of clenbuterol and anabolic steroids appear to cause in myocardial infarctions, potentially resulting from coronary spasms. In laboratory animals, there is little information on the anabolic interactions taking between the β-2-adrenergic agonists clenbuterol and salbutamol and the androgens. Clenbuterol had no effect on blood testosterone levels. However, treatment with clonidine (α-2 adrenoceptor agonist) and dobutamine (β-1-adrenoceptor agonist with some β-2 activity, $\beta_1 >>> \beta_2$) caused increases in blood testosterone levels (54,84).

Other studies conducted in intact and castrated male and female Sprague-Dawley rats showed clenbuterol's anabolic effects were highest in males and least in females. In general the efficacy of clenbuterol's anabolic activity was (from highest to lowest): intact males > castrated males > castrated females > intact females. These data suggest an anabolic interaction (potentiation or synergism) may occur between clenbuterol and endogenous androgens or that estrogens may interfere with clenbuterol's anabolic effects (54). However, the exact nature of this interaction remains unclear and further research is needed.

1.5.1.9. CANNABINOIDS

No known anabolic effects or interaction with androgens.

1.5.1.10. CARBAMAZEPINE

Danazol can inhibit carbamazepine metabolism and cause an elevation of plasma carbamazepine levels to potentially toxic concentrations.

1.5.1.11. CLONIDINE

In animals, the effects of clonidine on α-2 adrenergic-induced changes in blood pressure, catecholamine, and growth hormone release were modified by testosterone. In man, however, testosterone is unable to modulate clonidine's effects. However, testosterone was able to restore basal noradrenergic activity in hypogonadal men.

14. Anabolic Doping Agents

1.5.1.12. COCAINE

In selected populations, cocaine and androgens are among the most commonly abused substances. In laboratory studies conducted with rats, cocaine and/or androgens (nandrolone decanoate) treatment when given alone or in combination produced increased aggression. It was found that low-dose (2 mg) androgens taken over a relatively longer period (4 wk) produced even greater aggression than the high intermittent-dosed group (20 mg twice weekly). When animals were given combined optimal doses of cocaine and nandrolone, aggression scores showed that a greater percentage of animals exhibited aggression than did animals receiving a single drug, whereas the level of aggression did not change. Thus, the investigators concluded that the drugs did indeed interact to produce unique effects in development of aggression. Furthermore, cocaine studies conducted in humans (acute) and laboratory animals (chronic) showed that aggression levels were enhanced. It should be noted, however, that further investigations are needed to fully elucidate the complex interactions of cocaine and androgens on aggressive behavior. Additionally, combining androgens and cocaine with ethyl alcohol may contribute to the observed increase in aggression *(75)*.

1.5.1.13. GROWTH HORMONE

Contrary to other reports, the presence of testosterone had no effect on the plasma concentration of growth hormone or its secretion.

1.5.1.14. IMIPRAMINE

The coadministration of the tricyclic antidepressant imipramine with methyltestosterone could result in a dramatic paranoid response in four out of five patients.

1.5.1.15. OPIOIDS

Narcotic analgesics are not ergogenic but can serve to allow athletes with severe injuries to compete. However, the nature of any interactions with androgens is unclear. The nonscheduled opioid agonist/antagonist nalbuphine hydrochloride has been associated with usage dependence among androgen users. From the findings of Wines et al. *(56)*, nalbuphine may represent a new drug of abuse among athletes.

It has been suggested that prolonged use of high-dose androgens may induce a dependency that may involve endogenous opioid systems. A study conducted in rhesus monkeys showed that although the monkeys showed signs of opioid withdrawal when given naloxone (to counter morphine treatments), naloxone was not able to induce any signs of withdrawal symptoms during testosterone treatment. Thus, it does not seem likely that high-dose androgen treatment enhances endogenous opioid activity in rhesus monkeys in a manner resulting in opioid dependence or tolerance.

1.5.1.16. OXYPHENBUTAZONE

The coadministration of oxyphenbutazone, an antirheumatic analgesic rarely used today, along with androgens results in elevated serum oxyphenbutazone levels. Oxyphenbutazone has antiinflammatory, antipyretic, analgesic, and uricosuric actions that can provide symptomatic relief from pain. In general, oxyphenbutazone and its parent molecule phenbutazone have been withdrawn from North America and most European markets because of its toxicity.

1.5.2. Summary of Drug Interactions

1.5.2.1. TESTOSTERONE MIGHT INTERACT WITH CORTICOSTEROIDS, INSULIN, AND OTHER AGENTS (25)

1.5.2.1.1. Concomitant use of testosterone with these compounds may enhance the formation of edema: ACTH, betamethasone (acetate and sodium phosphate), cortisone acetate, dexamethasone (and dexamethasone acetate and sodium phosphate), fludrocortisone acetate, hydrocortisone (and hydrocortisone acetate, sodium phosphate, and sodium succinate), methylprednisolone (acetate and sodium succinate), prednisolone (acetate, sodium phosphate, and tebutate), prednisone, triamcinolone (and triamcinolone acetonide, diacetate, and hexacetonide).

1.5.2.1.2. In diabetic patients the use of testosterone (or other androgens) may result in the lowering of blood glucose levels and subsequently insulin requirements. Thus, the concomitant use of androgens with insulin formulations could result in excessive lowering of blood glucose levels: insulin, human: (zinc suspension, NPH, regular, regular and nph mixture), insulin: (NPH, regular, zinc crystals, zinc suspension), insulin aspart (human regular), insulin glargine, insulin lispro (human), insulin lispro protamine (human).

1.5.2.1.3. Concomitant use of testosterone with oxyphenbutazone may result in elevated serum levels of oxyphenbutazone.

1.5.2.1.4. Concomitant use of testosterone cypionate (injectable) with propranolol hydrochloride may result in an increased clearance of propranolol.

1.5.2.2. SYNTHETIC ANDROGENS (E.G., DANAZOL, FLUOXYMESTERONE, METHYLTESTOSTERONE, NANDROLONE, OXYMETHOLONE, OXANDROLONE, STANOZOLOL) MIGHT INTERACT WITH CORTICOSTEROIDS, ORAL ANTICOAGULANTS, ORAL HYPOGLYCEMIC AGENTS, AND OTHER AGENTS)

1.5.2.2.1. Concomitant use of androgens (e.g., danazol, fluoxymesterone, methyltestosterone, nandrolone, oxymetholone, oxandrolone, stanozolol) with corticosteroids may enhance the formation of edema: ACTH, betamethasone (acetate and sodium phosphate), cortisone acetate, dexamethasone (and dexamethasone acetate and sodium phosphate), fludrocortisone acetate, hydrocortisone (and hydrocortisone acetate, sodium phosphate, and sodium succinate), methylprednisolone (acetate and sodium succinate), prednisolone (acetate, sodium phosphate, and tebutate), prednisone, triamcinolone (and triamcinolone acetonide, diacetate, and hexacetonide) *(25)*.

1.5.2.2.2. Concomitant use of androgens (e.g., danazol, fluoxymesterone, methyltestosterone, nandrolone, oxymetholone, oxandrolone, stanozolol) with oral hypoglycemic agents may result in the inhibition of the metabolism their metabolism (oral hypoglycemic agents): acarbose, chlorpropamide, glimepiride, glipizide, glyburide, metformin hydrochloride, miglitol, pioglitazone hydrochloride, repaglinide, rosiglitazone maleate, tolazamide, tolbutamide, and troglitazone *(25)*.

1.5.2.2.3. Concomitant use of androgens (e.g., danazol, fluoxymesterone, methyltestosterone, nandrolone, oxymetholone, oxandrolone, stanozolol) with oral anticoagulants may result in an increased sensitivity to the anticoagulants, thus requiring a decrease in order to maintain desired prothrombin time: dicumarol, warfarin sodium.

1.5.2.2.4. Concomitant use of androgens (e.g., danazol, fluoxymesterone, methyltestosterone, nandrolone, oxymetholone, oxandrolone, stanozolol) with oxyphenbutazone may result in elevated serum levels of oxyphenbutazone.

2. β-ADRENOCEPTOR AGONISTS

In the 1992 Barcelona Olympics, several athletes from the United States, Germany, China, and Great Britain were asked to leave due to use of banned drugs. Surprisingly, not one of the athletes excused from the games used anabolic steroids, but they were found to have used stimulants such as strychnine or the anabolic agent clenbuterol *(14)*.

Anabolic agents can be used either to enhance athletic performance or to attenuate skeletal muscle atrophy. Muscle atrophy is caused by unloading (unweighting) that can result from prolonged bed rest, joint immobilization, or exposure to the environment of space (microgravity). Under these conditions, mitigation of muscle atrophy and the promotion of muscle growth have been approached pharmacologically by administering anabolic agents such as anabolic steroids, growth hormone, IGFs, and β-adrenergic (adrenoceptor) agonists. Of these anabolic agents, β-adrenoceptor agonists are among the least understood. In general, the tissue-specific distribution of β-adrenergic receptors can be summarized as follows: (a) $β_1$ in the heart; (b) $β_2$ in lung, vascular tissue, and skeletal muscle; and (c) $β_3$ in brown adipose tissue of rats *(10,15,25,58,59,61)*.

Among $β_2$-adrenoceptor agonists used as anabolic agents in humans or livestock, clenbuterol is by far the most popular. Clenbuterol is a relatively selective $β_2$-adrenergic agonist demonstrated to have anabolic effects on skeletal muscle. Developed primarily for the treatment of asthma, clenbuterol has also been used to enhance performance by athletes and body builders and to increase lean body mass in animals raised for food. Controlled clinical studies involving β-agonist-induced muscle effects in adult humans have been rare and results have been ambiguous. In one study, effects on muscle size were not detected although strength recovery after orthopedic surgery was improved. Clenbuterol has been shown to enhance growth and reduces atrophy in unloaded and denervated hind-limb muscles of young rats whose muscles are still growing. In the former studies, and in sexually mature female rats, there is evidence for a drug-induced shift from slow-twitch (type I) toward fast-twitch (type II) fiber types in the slow-fiber-rich soleus muscle. Normal, pregnant rats fed a diet containing clenbuterol show increases in the wet weight of all hind-limb muscles tested except the soleus. Until the current study, there have been no reports of clenbuterol's effects on the hind-limb muscles of fully mature male rats. Additionally, the confounding effects of growth in these mature animals are naturally reduced in comparison to younger animals. Furthermore, studies conducted with mature rats are more likely to reflect the responses of adults under-going disuse atrophy resulting from bed rest, injury, surgery, or microgravity *(10,58,59,61)*.

2.1. Chemistry

The parent molecule to sympathomimetic drugs is phenylethylamine that is composed of a phenyl ring with an ethylamine side chain *(see Fig. 9)*. Variations in the molecular structure of these agents are made to alter the drug's metabolism in order to prolong the drug's activity, to enhance the drug's affinity to α- and β-adrenoceptors as well as the its pharmacokinetic activity. Modifications to the phenylethylamine parent molecule include substitutions on: (a) the phenyl ring, (b) the terminal amino group, and (c) the α- and β-carbons on the ethylamine side chain *(13,15)*.

Substitutions made at positions 3 and 4 on the phenyl ring of phenylethylamine with -OH groups yield the endogenous catecholamines dopamine, norepinephrine, and epinephrine. The least modified molecule, dopamine, is the catecholamine version of phenylethylamine and has greater affinity for the D_1 and D_2 dopamine receptors (D_1 = D_2) than for adrenoceptors (D >> β >> α). Subsequent modifications at other positions can alter the specificity of the molecule for a particular receptor type. These modifications would include the following.

2.1.1. Structure of β₂-Adrenoceptor Agonists (13,15)

2.1.1.1. PHENYL RING SUBSTITUTIONS

Substitutions on the phenyl ring can significantly alter the potency and half-life of a drug. For example, epinephrine and phenylephrine differ only by a hydroxyl group at position 4 of the phenyl ring. Loss of the hydroxyl at position 4 for phenylephrine significantly altered the molecules adrenoceptor affinity: increasing for α ($α_1$ > $α_2$) and near complete loss for β (α >>>> β) except when concentrations are very high.

Additional to altering the molecules potency at either α- or β-adrenoceptors, catecholamines are subject to metabolism by catechol-O-methyltransferase (COMT; *see* section on metabolism). Along with the loss of both hydroxyl groups at positions 3 and 4, the molecule's half-life is increased as well as its distribution into the CNS or other tissues and organ systems.

2.1.1.2. α-CARBON SUBSTITUTIONS

Substitutions on the α carbon of the ethylamine side chain will interfere with metabolism through blocking oxidation of the site by monoamine oxidase (MAO). Blocking metabolism at the α-carbon position tends to increase the molecule's half-life, as is the case with ephedrine and amphetamine.

2.1.1.3. β-CARBON SUBSTITUTIONS

Most of the β-adrenoceptor agonists have hydroxyl groups substituted at the β-carbon position on the ethylamine side chain. It is believed that the presence of the hydroxyl group might be important with respect to storage of the molecule in neural vesicles.

2.1.1.4. AMINO GROUP SUBSTITUTIONS

Substitutions on the amino group with alkyl chains have a tendency to enhance β-adrenoceptor activity and selectivity. The presence of a methyl on amino group of nor-epinephrine yields the hormone epinephrine. Epinephrine has greater affinity for β₂-adrenoceptors than norepinephrine. Increasing the size of the substituent on the amino group increases the molecule's selectivity toward β₂-adrenoceptors, while decreasing selectivity for α-adrenergic receptors. Thus, the presence of an isopropyl (isoproterenol) or isobutyl (albuterol, clenbuterol) on the amino terminus increases β-adrenoceptor selectivity.

2.1.2. Stereochemistry

It should be noted that of the drugs regularly prescribed by physicians, greater than half possess at least one chiral center. In contrast, approximately 99% of the naturally occurring chiral pharmaceutical compounds have a single pharmacologically active enantiomer. Enantiomers can vary greatly in their pharmacological effects upon target tissue(s) as a result of differences in their pharmacodynamic and/or pharmacokinetic parameters because of variations in their binding to receptors or metabolizing enzymes *(10)*.

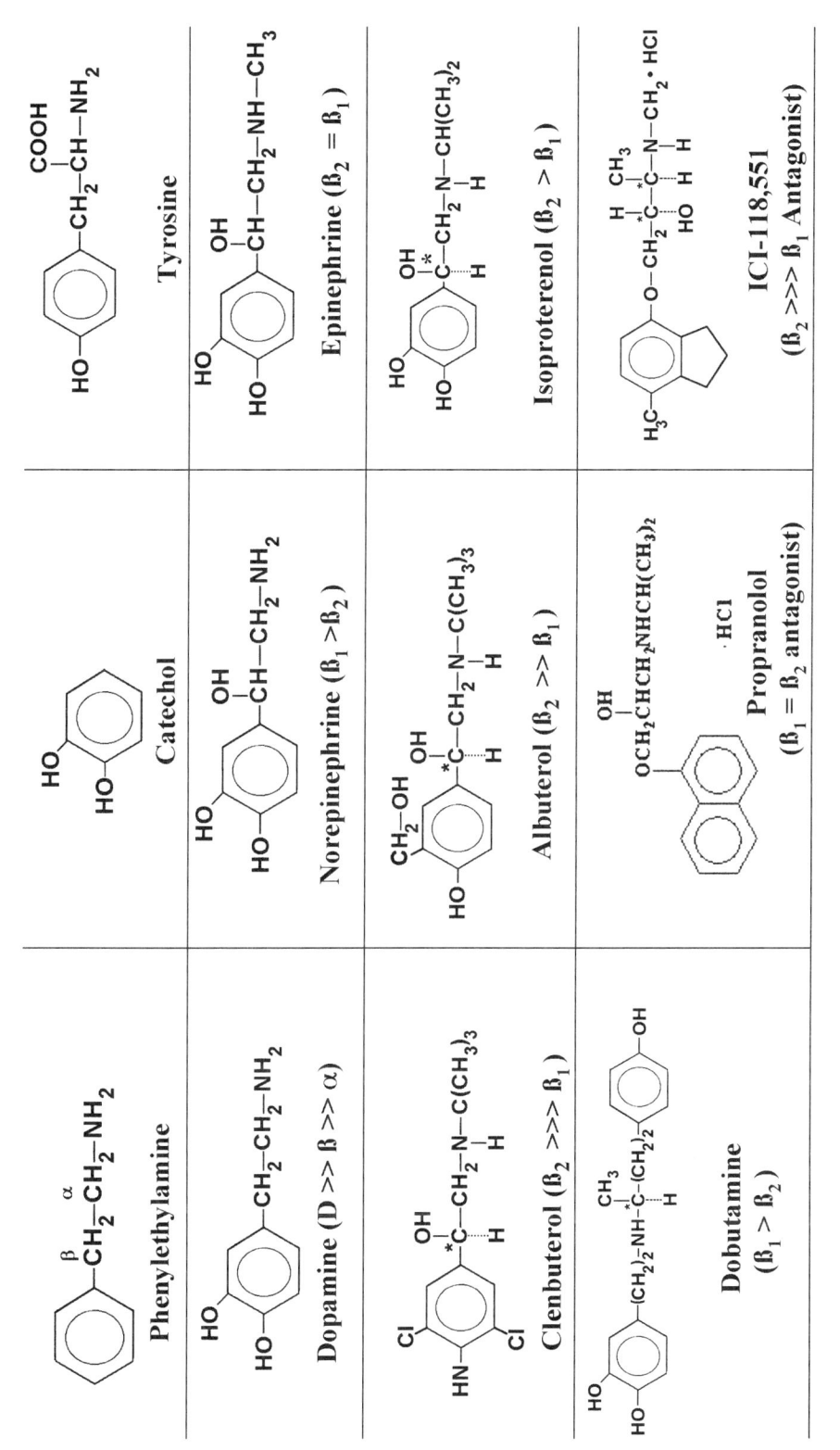

Fig. 9. Common structures for β_2-androceptor agonists and antagonist. Data from (12).

Determining the identity of the active enantiomer (eutomer) in racemic drugs is important because of the potential for avoiding undesirable side effects associated with the less active enantiomer (distomer). As is the case with most β_2-adrenoceptor agonists such as clenbuterol and salbutamol, they are commercially available as a racemic mixture (1:1 ratio) of the two enantiomers, (−)-R and (+)-S. Whether one or both of the enantiomers contribute to a drug's principal action or to its toxic side effect(s) must be determined on a drug-by-drug basis *(10)*.

Furthermore, the less active enantiomer (distomer) may interfere with the activity of the more biologically active species (eutomer) through competitive inhibition. Thus, the distomer may potentially bind to sites other than its primary receptor, thereby potentially causing adverse effects or alter the distribution and/or the activity of the eutomer, resulting in decreased or increased effect or toxicity. Thus, this type of structure can potentially give rise to numerous asymmetrical sites, e.g., chiral centers, yielding molecules with the same chemical formula but different three-dimensional structures *(9,10)* (*see* Tables 7A and B for Physical Properties).

2.2. Basic Physical Properties

Table 7A
Basic Physical Properties of β-Agonists and Other Selected Drugs

Drug	Chemical Formula	Chemical Name	Synonym/Salt Name
Albuterol	C13H21NO3	α1-[[(1,1-dimethylethyl)amino]methyl]4-hydroxy-1,3-benzenedimethanol	Salbutamol
Albuterol Sulfate	C26H44N2O10S	—	Aerolin, Proventil
Cimaterol	C12H17N3O	2-amino-5-[1-hydroxy-2-[(methylethyl)amino]ethyl]benzonitrile	—
Clenbuterol	C12H18C12N2O	4-amino-3,5-dichloro-alpha-[[(1,1-di-methylethyl)amino]methyl]benzene methanol	NAB 365
Clenbuterol HCl	C12H19C13N2O	—	NAB 365 Cl, Spiropent, Ventipulmin
Cocaine	C17H12NO4	[1R-(exo,exo)]-3-(Benzoyloxy)8-methyl-8-azabicyclo[3.2.1]oxtane-2-carboxylic acid methyl ester	free base
Cocaine HCl	C17H22C1NO4	—	HCl
Isoproterenol	C11H17NO3	4-[1-Hydroxy-2-[(1-methylethyl)-amino]ethyl]-1,2-benzenediol	Isoprenaline
Isoproterenol HCl (racemic)	C11H18C1NO3	—	Aerotrol, Euspiran
Isoproterenol sulfate dihydrate (racemic)	C22H36N2O10S	—	Aludrin, Isomist, Propal
The (1) enantiomer (free base)	—	—	—
The (1) enantiomer (HCl)	—	—	—
The (1) enantiomer of isoproterenol (d-) bitartrate dihydrate	—	—	Isolevin

14. Anabolic Doping Agents

Table 7A (continued)

Drug	Chemical Formula	Chemical Name	Synonym/Salt Name
Mabuterol	C13H18C1F3N2O	4-amino-3-chloro-α-[[(1,1-di-methylethyl)amino]methyl]-5-trifluoromethyl)benzenemethanol	—
Mabuterol Hydrochloride (racemic)	C13H19C12F3N2O	—	—
Individual (d) and (1) enantiomers of Mabuterol Hydrochloride	—	—	—
Phenylpropanolamine (PPA)	C9H14C1NO	α-(1-aminoethyl)benzen-methanol-HCl	—
Propranolol	C16H21NO2	1-[(1-Methylethyl)amino]-3-(1-naphthalenyloxy)-2-propanol	—
Propranolol HCl	C16H22C1NO2	—	—
Strychnine	C21H22N2O2	strychnidin-10-one	—
Terbutaline	C12H19NO3	5-[2-[1,1-Dimethylethyl)amino]-1-hydroxyethyl]-1,3-benzenediol	Brethaire, Brethine, Bricanyl, Butaliret, Monovent, Terbasmin, Terbul
Terbutaline-sulfate	(C12H19NO3)2-H2SO4	—	—

Data from (12).

Table 7B
Basic Physical Properties of β-Agonists and Other Selected Drugs

Drug	MNV g/mol	Melting Point °C	Melting Point Solvent/Other	Solubility/Notes
Albuterol	239.31	151 and 157–158	Crystal powder	Salbutamol is soluble in most organic solvents. Salbutamol is also marketed as the pure R enantiomer and is called valbuterol.
Albuterol Sulfate				The sulfate salt is soluble in aqueous solutions.
Cimaterol	219.29	159–161	—	—
Clenbuterol	277.18	177–179	—	Clenbuterol (free base) is soluble in methanol. Soluble in alcohol.
Clenbuterol HCl	313.64	174–176	Colorless microcrystalline powder	The salt is very soluble in water, alcohol, methanol, slightly soluble in chloroform; insoluble in benzene; LD50 in mice, rats, guinea pigs 175, 315, and 67.1 mg/kg orally; 27.6, 35.3, and 12.6 mg/kgIV.
Cocaine	303.35	98	monoclinic tablets from alcohol	One gram dissolves in 600 mL water and 270 mL water at 80°C. Soluble in 6.5 mL alcohol, 0.7 mL chloroform, 3.5 mL ether, 12 mL oil turpentine, 12 mL olive oil, 30–50 mL liquid petrolatum. Also soluble in acetone, ethyl acetate, carbon disulfide. LD50 iv inrts: 17.5 mg/kg
Cocaine HCl	339.82	195	Crystals, granules, or powder	Numbs tongue on application, slightly bitter tasting. One gram dissolves in 0.4 mL water or 3.2 mL cold water. Dissolves in 2 mL hot alcohol, 12.5 mL chloroform. Cocaine HCl also soluble in glycerol, and acetone. Insoluble in ether or oils.

(continued)

Table 7B (*continued*)

Drug	MNV g/mol	Melting Point °C	Melting Point Solvent/Other	Solubility/Notes
Isoproterenol	211.24	155	Crystal powder	—
Isoproterenol HCl (racemic)	247.72	170–171	—	1 g dissolves in 3 mL water or in 50 mL of 95% ethanol. Less soluble in absolute ethanol, practically insoluble in chloroform, ether, and benzene. In a 1% aqueous solution, isoproterenol has a pH of about 5 and will turn a brownish-pink color upon exposure to air or in an alkaline solution.
Isoproterenol sulfate dihydrate (racemic)	520.59	128	—	One gram dissolves in approximately 4 mL of water and is only slightly soluble in alcohol. Practically insoluble in chloroform, ether, and benzene.
The (1) enantiomer (free base)	—	164–165	—	—
The (1) enantiomer (HCl)	—	164–165	—	—
The (1) enantiomer of isoproterenol (d-) bitartrate dihydrate	—	80–83	—	—
Mabuterol	310.75	—	—	Related to Clenbuterol
Mabuterol Hydrochloride (racemic)	345.21	205–206	—	Fairly soluble in water. Related to Clenbuterol. LD50 in male and female mice and rats is 220.8, 119.9, 319.3, and 305.6 mg/kg orally; 41.5, 51.1, 26.4, and 28.1 mg/kg IV.
Individual (d) and (1) enantiomers of Mabuterol Hydrochloride	—	194	—	—
Phenylpropanol-amine (PPA)	187.67	101–102/ 190–194	free base/ HCl salt	PPA is soluble in water and alcohol, and practically insoluble in ether, chloroform, and benzene. The LD50 (rat) for PPA is 1490 mg/kg.
Propranolol	259.34	96	Crystals	Crystals from HCl salt are soluble in water. Practically insoluble in ether, benzene, ethyl acetate. The LD50 in mice; 565 mg/kg orally, 22 mg/kg IV, and 107 mg/kg ip.
Propranolol HCl		163–164	Crystals	—
Strychnine	334.42	275–285	Crystals	The pKa at 25°C is 8.26, and 1 g is soluble in 182 mL ethanol, 6.5 mL chloroform, 150 mL benzene, 250 mL methanol, 83 mL pyridine, and slightly soluble in water. The LD50 in rats: 0.96 mg/kg by slow iv infusion.
Terbutaline	225.29	119–122	Absolute ether	—
Terbutaline-sulfate	323.37	246–248	—	The pKa1 is 8.8, pKa2 is 10.1, and the pKa3 is 11.2. The solubility at 25°C is greater than 20 mg/mL in water, 0.1 NHCl and NaOH. In ethanol the solubility is 1.2 mg/mL and in methanol 2.7 mg/mL.

Data from *(12)*.

2.3. Pharmacology and Kinetics

2.3.1. Drug Usage: Sympathomimetic Preparations and Routes of Administration

Sympathomimetic agents such as albuterol (salbutamol) or clenbuterol are important pharmaceutical agents for the treatment of asthma. In general, these agents cause the relaxation of bronchial smooth muscle and inhibit the release of bronchial constricting substances released from mast cells. The prototypic endogenous sympathomimetic agent epinephrine is a rapidly acting bronchodilator that has been used to treat asthma and anaphylactic shock. Epinephrine can be given as a subcutaneous injection (0.4 mL of a 1:1000 solution) or inhaled as a microaerosol delivered from a pressurized canister (320 µg per puff). Additionally, epinephrine is contained within some local anesthetic preparations as a vasoconstrictor (1:50,000, 1:100,000, or 1:200,000 dilutions), constricting cutaneous vessels and prolonging the local anesthetic action.

2.3.1.1. ALBUTEROL (ACCUNEB™, PROVENTIL®, PROVENTIL® HFA, VENTOLIN®, VENTOLIN® HFA, VENTOLIN® ROTAHALER®, VENTOLIN® SYRUP, VOLMAX®, PROVENTIL®, REPETABS®, RESPIROL RX™, SALBUTAMOL™, VENTOLIN® NEBULES®, VENTOLIN® ROTACAPS®, VENTOLIN® HFA, XOPENEX)

Albuterol and levalbuterol [the (–)-R enantiomer of albuterol and more potent than the racemic mixture] are β_2-selective adrenoceptor agonists ($\beta_2 \gg \beta_1 \ggggg \alpha$) used in the treatment of acute bronchospasm, asthma, and act as a prophylaxis for bronchospasms. In the treatment of asthma or other chronic obstructive airway disease, albuterol acts as a bronchodilator to alleviate the restriction in the airway. Albuterol has a more prolonged bronchodilatory effect than either isoproterenol or metaproterenol, but less of cardiostimulatory effect than terbutaline. Albuterol comes as tablets (4 or 8 mg; *see* Note A), inhalation aerosols (6.8- or 17-g canisters containing 80 or 200 metered inhalations, respectively; *see* Note B), inhalation solution (0.5% solution in 20 mL amber bottle). (**Note A**: Albuterol 4- or 8-mg tablets: comes as timed release (2 or 4 mg in the coating for immediate release, 2 or 4 mg in the core for delayed release) as 4.8 or 9.6 mg of albuterol sulfate. **Note B**: Albuterol 6.8- or 17-g canisters deliver 100 mg of albuterol at the valve and 80 mg at the mouthpiece) *(25,62)*.

Albuterol can be given orally (solution, tablet, or capsule form) or via an oral-inhalation route (metered-dose inhaler). There are numerous treatment regimens that include orally (immediate-release tablets or solution and extended-release tablets), oral inhalation (using Rotahaler inhalation device with inhalation capsules), and oral inhalation using an albuterol nebulizer solution.

2.3.1.1.1. Oral Treatment (Immediate-Release Tablets or Oral Solution). The normal adult dose is 2–4 mg every 6–8 h. The maximum dose in adults and adolescents should not exceed 32 mg/d. In children 6–12 yr and the elderly, 2 mg of albuterol should be taken every 6-8 h with maximum doses of 24 and 32 mg/d, respectively. In children under 6 yr, they should receive an initial dose of 0.1 mg/kg orally every 8 h, not to exceed 8 mg/d. This dose can be increased to 0.2 mg/kg every 8 h if the desired effect is not achieved, but should not exceed 12 mg/d.

2.3.1.1.2. Oral Treatment (Extended-Release Tablets). It should be noted that treatment with 4 mg of the extended-release tablets every 12 h is equivalent to 2 mg of the immediate-release tablets every 6 h. The normal adult dose of the extended-release tablets is 4–8 mg every 12 h. The maximum dose in adults and adolescents should not exceed 16 mg/12 h. In children under 6 yr, they should receive an initial dose of 0.3–0.6 mg/kg orally per day, not to exceed a maximum of 8 mg/d.

2.3.1.1.3. Oral-Inhalation Treatment

1. Metered-Dose Inhaler. Treatment with inhalation doses in adults and children (4 yr and above) should be 90–180 mg (one to two puffs) every 4–6 h as needed.
2. Capsule and Rotahaler Inhaler. Treatment with capsule inhalation doses in adults and children (4 yr and above) should be 200 mg (per capsule) every 4–6 h.
3. Albuterol Nebulizer Solution. Treatment with the nebulizer solution in adults and adolescents should be 2.5 mg every 6–8 h as needed. Treatment should be delivered over a period of 5–15 min. For severe episodes, acute treatment should be 2.5–5 mg initially every 20 min for three doses, followed by doses of 2.5–10 mg every 1–4 h as needed (or 10–15 mg/h by continuous nebulization). In children, treatment should be 1.25–2.5 mg every 4–6 h as needed. As with adults, treatment should be delivered over a period of 5–15 min. Treatment of severe episodes in children should be 0.15 mg/kg (2.5 mg minimum and 5 mg maximum) for three doses every 20 min, followed by 0.15–0.3 mg/kg (10 mg maximum) every 1–4 h as needed *(25,62)*.

2.3.1.1.4. Prophylaxis Treatment in the Prevention of Exercise-Induced Bronchospasms. The use of albuterol to prevent the onset of exercise-induced bronchospasms is not recommended. Longer acting agents such as formoterol, levalbuterol, the (–)-R enantiomer of albuterol, are better suited for this task *(25,57)*.

2.3.1.1.5. Levalbuterol (the (–)-R Enantiomer of Albuterol) Oral-Inhalation Treatment (Nebulizer Solution). The initial treatment with the nebulizer solution in adults, adolescents, and children (12 yr or older) should be 0.63 mg every 6–8 h. Treatment should be given three times per day. For severe asthmatic episodes, treatment should be 1.25 mg three times per day. Higher doses should be monitored for adverse effects. In children 6–11 yr, the initial dose is 0.31 mg every 6–8 h, three times per day. Routine dosing should not exceed 0.63 mg given three times per day *(25)*.

2.3.1.2. AMPHETAMINES (AMPHETAMINE, DEXTROAMPHETAMINE, AND METHAMPHETAMINE)

As a group, the amphetamines are considered CNS stimulants and their effects are mediated centrally and peripherally through the action of norepinephrine. Amphetamines are used to treat attention-deficit hyperactivity disorder (ADHD), as an appetite suppressant for the treatment of obesity, and to treat narcolepsy. However, amphetamines should be used with caution since there is a great potential for abuse and addiction *(25)*.

Methamphetamine is used for the treatment of ADHD in children under 6 yr: 5 mg orally once or twice daily, then increase incrementally by 5 mg/wk. The usual effective dose is 20–25 mg orally daily. For adjunctive treatment of obesity in adults, treat with 5 mg orally 30 min prior to each meal, or treat with 10–15 mg orally with the long-acting form every morning. Treatment should be continued for only a few weeks. Methamphetamine (Desoxyn) comes in tablet form at doses of 5, 10, and 15 mg.

Amphetamine is used for the treatment of narcolepsy in children 3–6 yr by giving 2.5 mg orally once or twice daily then increase incrementally by 2.5 mg/d/wk until the

14. Anabolic Doping Agents

desired response is obtained. In children over 6 yr, 5 mg of amphetamine is given orally once or twice daily, then increase incrementally by 5 mg/wk until the desired response is obtained. For treating narcolepsy in adults, amphetamine is given orally at a dose of 5–20 mg once to three times a day. In children who are being treated for ADHD, amphetamine is given in a fashion somewhat similar to the treatment of narcolepsy. In children 6–12 yr, 2.5 mg amphetamine is given orally twice daily with incremental increases of 5 mg/d/wk until the desired response is obtained. In children 12 yr or older, 5 mg of amphetamine is given orally twice daily. Incremental increases in dose (10 mg/d/wk) are given until the desired response is obtained. Amphetamine comes in tablet form as amphetamine sulfate in doses of 5 or 10 mg.

2.3.1.3. CLENBUTEROL

Clenbuterol is an orally active, sympathomimetic agent (not approved for use in United States) that has specificity for β_2-adrenoceptors ($\beta_2 >>> \beta_1 >>>>> \alpha$), including those in bronchiolar smooth muscle *(60,64)*. Owing to its bronchodilator properties, it is used therapeutically to relieve respiratory disorders in humans (10–20 µg/d taken twice daily) and animals (equine as bronchodilator: 0.8 µg/kg body wt given twice daily for up to 10 d). Clenbuterol can be administered orally or parenterally in horses, but im or iv routes can also be used. Clenbuterol also has been used in veterinary medicine and in human clinical trials as a tocolytic agent *(60,65,66)*. In animals, the recommended treatment with clenbuterol, as a tocolytic agent, is equivalent to 0.8 mg/kg body wt by a single parenteral injection in horses and 0.8 mg/kg body wt orally in cattle *(60)*.

When administered in relatively high therapeutic doses, clenbuterol improves nitrogen retention and thus increases muscle growth. Because clenbuterol also markedly reduces body fat, it has been used illegally by ranchers as a repartitioning agent in beef production, and by athletes, especially body builders, to increase lean body mass *(10,58,61,67–69)*. Experimentally, clenbuterol inhibits skeletal muscle atrophy secondary to disuse, injury, and denervation. Clinical studies in adult humans have shown clenbuterol to be effective in enhancing strength recovery after orthopedic surgery, without altering muscle size *(69)*. In rats, clenbuterol increased the rate of protein synthesis in skeletal muscle *(70–72)*. Thus, clenbuterol therapy could be useful in ameliorating microgravity-induced muscle atrophy in astronauts *(10,58,61,73,74)*.

2.3.1.4. COCAINE

Cocaine is a naturally occurring alkaloid used on mucosal tissue (oral, laryngeal, and nasal cavities) as a topical or local anesthetic. It is also used in the eye as an ophthalmic anesthetic *(13,15,25)*. Cocaine acts by decreasing neural permeability to sodium, thereby decreasing the rate of membrane depolarization and nerve conduction. Centrally, cocaine acts similarly to its peripheral effects, but also inhibits the reuptake of norepinephrine, dopamine, and serotonin, making it an indirect agonist. Adverse effects associated with the use of cocaine (e.g., significant local vasoconstriction, euphoria, abuse, dependence, and the potential for violence) prevent its more widespread clinical use *(75)*. Cocaine is a Schedule C-II controlled substance and is banned by the IOC *(6,25)*.

2.3.1.4.1. Topical Anesthetic Treatment. In adults and children (6 yr or older), a 1–10% cocaine solution is applied to the tissue via sprays, cotton applicators, packs, or instillation. In general, cocaine should be used in the lowest effective dose. However, 4% solutions of cocaine are used most frequently. It should be noted that more concentrated solutions (>4%) of cocaine can result in systemic toxicity. Furthermore, in elderly or debilitated patients, cocaine doses should be reduced. As a topical, cocaine should not be applied to the eye or administered parenterally *(6,25)*.

2.3.1.5. Dobutamine

Dobutamine is a relatively selective β_1-adrenoceptor agonist ($\beta_1 \gg \beta_2 \ggg \alpha$), used for the short-term inotropic treatment of congestive heart failure (low output states), cardiogenic shock, and post cardiac surgery. Dobutamine possesses inotropic, chronotropic, and vasodilatory activity. Dobutamine is administered by iv infusion for a period not to exceed 48 h *(25)*.

2.3.1.5.1. Intravenous Dosage. The initial continuous iv infusion with dobutamine (0.5–1 mg/kg/min) in adults, children, infants, and neonates is subsequently titrated every few minutes to a range of 2–20 mg/kg/min (usual maximum). Adjustments to the dosage are made based on the hemodynamic response. Tachycardia or ventricular ectopy may occur when infusion rates exceed 20 mg/kg/min. However, infusion rates up to 40 mg/kg/min may be required in adults, adolescents, and children on rare instances. In the elderly, variable dose responses to dobutamine may occur; thus the dose should be titrated based on hemodynamic responses *(25)*.

As an anabolic agent, dobutamine has been tested in laboratory animals, but its anabolic responses in muscle and bone were mixed *(76,77)*. Additionally, dobutamine has been investigated as one possible agent in offsetting the onset of microgravity-induced skeletal muscle atrophy *(78)*. However, its effects on skeletal muscle and bone appear to be greater under sedentary conditions than in exercised or trained animals.

2.3.1.6. Isoproterenol (Isuprel®, Medihaler-Iso™)

Isoproterenol is the prototypic synthetic β-adrenoceptor agonist ($\beta_1 = \beta_2 \ggggg \alpha$) approved by the FDA in 1947. It is structurally similar to epinephrine, with inotropic and bronchodilator properties. Isoproterenol is indicated for use in cases of acute bronchospasm, asthma, AV (arterovenous) block, bradycardia, cardiopulmonary resuscitation, Stokes-Adams attack, and torsades de pointes. Isoproterenol can also be used to treat status asthmaticus, although it is not approved for this use by the FDA. In general, isoproterenol relaxes the smooth muscle in the lungs and helps to improve breathing by dilating airways. Isoproterenol is administered by inhalation, parenterally, iv injection or infusion, or sublingually *(13,15,25,63)*.

2.3.1.6.1. Oral-Inhalation Treatment

1. Metered Aerosol. The oral-inhalation dose for the treatment of acute and mild bronchospasms in adults and children with asthma is 120–262 µg isoproterenol HCl (one to two inhalations) four to six times/day at 3- to 4-h intervals. Treatment with isoproterenol sulfate in adults and children is 80–160 mg (one to two inhalations) four to six times/day at 3- to 4-h intervals. The maximum dose for each is 12 inhalations/24 h. It should be noted that the National Asthma Education and Prevention Program Expert Panel recommends against the use of isoproterenol because it could potentially produce excessive cardiac stimulation.
2. Nebulizer. In adults and children the recommended treatment under normal circumstances with isoproterenol is 6–12 inhalations of a 0.25% solution every 15 min up to

three times. The maximum dosage is eight treatments over a period of 24 h. However, the recommended treatment for acute asthma is 5–15 deep inhalations of a 0.5% solution. If necessary, treatment is repeated after 5–10 min. The maximum dosage is five treatments over a period of 24 h. The oral-inhalation dose (via metered dose) for the treatment of acute bronchospasms in adults with COPD is 120–262 mg isoproterenol HCl (one to two inhalations) four to six times/day at 3- to 4-h intervals. The maximum dosage is 12 inhalations/24 h. Treatment in adults and children using a nebulizer is 5–15 deep inhalations of a 0.5% isoproterenol HCl solution. Treatment is repeated if necessary up to every 3–4 h *(25)*.

2.3.1.6.2. Sublingual Treatment. In adults, isoproterenol HCl is given in doses of 10–15 mg, three to four times/day. In children, the isoproterenol HCl is given in doses of 5–10 mg, three times/day. The maximum dosage per day is 60 mg/d in adults and 30 mg/d in children.

2.3.1.6.3. Intravenous Infusion. In adults, isoproterenol is given at a dose of 0.01–0.02 mg (0.5–1.0 mL of a 1:50,000 dilution) iv. Treatment is repeated if necessary. It should be noted that with iv infusion, the individual's cardiac functions should be monitored closely. Treatment should be avoided in individuals receiving general anesthesia with cyclopropane or halogenated hydrocarbon anesthetics.

2.3.1.6.4. Intramuscular (im) and Subcutaneous (sc) Treatment. The treatment of ventricular arrhythmias secondary to AV block in adults is initially 0.2 mg isoproterenol HCl im, followed by 0.02–1 mg as needed. In adults, sc treatment is 0.2 mg initially, followed by treatments of 0.15–0.2 mg as needed. Alternatively, treatment can be given initially by iv bolus of 0.02–0.06 mg, followed by intermittent iv injections of 0.01–0.2 mg *(25)*.

2.3.1.6.5. Phenylpropanolamine (PPA; Acutrim®, Dexatrim®, Phenoxine®, Phenyldrine®, Propagest®, Rhindecon®). This drug has been discontinued in the United States. *Note*: Elderly patients appear to be more likely to have adverse reactions to sympathetic amines.

PPA is a nonprescription sympathomimetic agent used as a nasal decongestant to improve breathing by promoting the drainage of sinus passages, and as an appetite suppressant for the short-term (6–12 wk) treatment of exogenous obesity. PPA has also been used to treat urinary incontinence (non-FDA-approved use). PPA has been included in cold/cough preparations and formulations for appetite suppression *(13,15,25)*.

PPA acts as a CNS stimulant by acting directly on both α- and β-adrenoceptors ($\alpha > \beta$), as well as indirectly through the release of norepinephrine from its storage sites in the nerve terminal. PPA causes vasoconstriction, and subsequently shrinking swollen nasal mucous membranes. PPA also has an indirect effect on β-adrenoceptors in the heart, producing tachycardia and increased blood pressure *(13,15,25)*.

1. Oral dosage using immediate-release tablets or capsules. For adults and adolescents, the dosage was 20–25 mg orally every 4 h, up to 150 mg/d. In children (6–11 yr) the dosage was 10–12.5 mg orally every 4 h with a maximum of 75 mg/d. In younger children (2–5 yr), the dosage for PPA was 6.25 mg orally every 4 h (37.5 mg/d maximum).
2. Oral dosage using extended-release capsules. In adults using the extended-release capsules, the dosage was 75 mg orally every 12 h *(25)*.

PPA was previously indicated as a short-term (6–12 wk) appetite suppressant for treating exogenous obesity concomitantly with a weight loss program. The oral dosage (immediate-release tablets or capsules) in adults used to suppress appetites was 25 mg orally three times daily (up to 75 mg/d). PPA was administered 30 min before meals with one to two full glasses of water. Lower doses of 12.5 mg three times daily may be used in individuals sensitive to sympathomimetics or other stimulants.

2.3.1.7. Propranolol (Betachron®, Inderal®, Inderal® IV, Inderal® LA, Pronol™)

Propranolol is a nonselective β-adrenoceptor antagonist (β-blocker, $\beta_1 = \beta_2 \ggg \alpha$) that reduces chronotropic, inotropic, and vasodilatory responses in a dose-dependent manner. However, the correlation that exists between therapeutic effects, the concentration of propranolol in the plasma, and dose are unclear. Propranolol has a half-life of approximately 4 h. In general, propranolol produces an antihypertensive effect possibly by decreasing cardiac output, inhibiting the release of renin by the kidneys, and reducing sympathetic outflow. An additional effect associated with propranolol is its ability to reduce oxygen requirements of the heart through blocking the effects of β-agonists, as well as possessing antiarrhythmic activity *(13,15,25,63,79)*.

Oral administration of propranolol should be given in divided doses before meals and at bedtime. The dose of the oral concentrate solution should be diluted in water (or juice, etc.) prior to administration. Intravenous administration requires no dilution, but visual inspection of parenteral products should be made for particulate matter and/or discoloration prior to administration. Electrocardiogram (EKG) and central venous pressure during iv administration should not exceed 1 mg/min. In children, propranolol should be infused slowly over a period of 10 min. Propranolol is available as follows: Inderal injection solution (1 mg/mL), Inderal long-acting capsules (60, 80, 120, 160 mg), and Inderal tablets (10, 20, 40, 60, 80 mg). Propranolol, as a doping agent, would most likely have a negative effect on skeletal muscle hypertrophy. However, marksmen or other athletes who require a steady hand *(25,63)* favor it.

β_2-Adrenoceptor antagonists such as propranolol (or the more β_2-specific antagonist ICI-118,551) may provide antioxidant protection to the heart through blocking β_2-adrenoceptor agonist-induced oxidative damage (through increased force of contractions) in individuals with congestive heart failure. Additionally, propranolol has been found to provide a measure of protection in ethanol-induced cardiomyopathy, lowering circulating levels of troponin-T-associated ethanol abuse. Thus, treatment with propranolol prevents the ethanol-induced release of troponin-T (through ethanol-induced oxidative damage). Propranolol antagonized the anabolic effects of albuterol and clenbuterol when given at levels of 10 mg/kg body wt twice daily in rats.

2.3.1.8. Terbutaline (Brethine®, Brethine® SC, Brethaire®, Bricanyl®)

Terbutaline is a β_2-selective adrenoceptor agonists ($\beta_2 \gg \beta_1 \ggggg \alpha$) used in the treatment of acute bronchospasm, asthma, COPD, and as a tocolytic agent (note: this is a non-FDA-approved indication). The stimulation of β_2-adrenoceptors produces relaxation of bronchial smooth muscle and subsequently increased bronchial airflow. Terbutaline has a more prolonged bronchodilatory effect than either isoproterenol or metaproterenol, but not as long as that of albuterol. Terbutaline has a greater cardiostimulatory effect than albuterol *(25)*.

Treatment with terbutaline or other β_2-adrenoceptor agonists produces receptor down-regulation and tolerance to treatment. Furthermore, the continuous use of β_2-

14. Anabolic Doping Agents

adrenoceptor agonists for a period of about 1 yr can accelerate a decline in pulmonary function in asthmatics *(55)*. Additionally, terbutaline produces cardiostimulation, but to a lesser degree than isoproterenol *(25)*.

2.3.1.8.1. Oral Treatment

1. Adults and adolescents (>15 yr). Treatment with 5 mg terbutaline orally three times/ daily every 6 h (15 mg/d maximum dose). Dosage may be reduced to 2.5 mg orally three times daily if adverse effects occur (7.5 mg/d maximum dose).
2. Children (6–12 yr). Treatment with 0.05 mg terbutaline orally every 8 h. Subsequently, the dosage is slowly increased to 0.15 mg/kg orally every 8 h (5 mg/d maximum). Alternatively, the manufacturer recommends the oral dose to be 2.5 mg three times/d (5 mg/d maximum).

2.3.1.8.2. Subcutaneous Treatment

1. Adults and adolescents. Initial treatment is 0.25 mg sc, repeated in 15–30 min if needed (maximum dose is 0.5 mg in 4 h).
2. Children (6–12 yr). Initially, treat sc with 0.006–0.01 mg/kg terbutaline (maximum dosage is 0.25 mg). Subsequently, repeat in 15–30 min if needed (4-h delay prior to subsequent treatments).

2.3.2. Biosynthesis of Endogenous β_2-Adrenoceptor Agonists

The rate-limiting enzyme in catecholamine synthesis is tyrosine hydroxylase, a cytosolic enzyme, which catalyzes the formation of L-dopa (3,4-dihydroxy-L-phenylalanine) from the substrates tyrosine and oxygen. Biopterin is the cofactor for tyrosine hydroxyl-ase and may serve as a regulator controlling the velocity of the reaction. Another function of tyrosine hydroxylase is in production of additional tyrosine through the hydroxylation of phenylalanine *(80)*. However, phenylalanine hydroxylase is the enzyme primary enzyme responsible for the hydroxylation of phenylalanine *(81)*. L-dopa is converted into dopamine through the action of the enzyme dopa decarboxylase, a pyridoxine-dependent enzyme, which removes the carboxyl group from dopa. Dopa decarboxylase, also referred to as aromatic amino acid decarboxylase, can also act on 5-hydroxytryptophan to form serotonin. Dopa decarboxylase is found in both catecholaminergic and serotonergic neurons and nonneuronal tissues (e.g., kidney) throughout the body. Dopamine is then acted on by the enzyme dopamine β-hydroxylase that hydroxylates the β-carbon on the ethylamine side chain forming norepinephrine. Both dopamine β-hydroxylase and tyrosine hydroxylase are mixed function hydroxylase that use molecular oxygen. However, unlike tyrosine hydroxylase that uses pyridoxine-PO$_4$, dopamine β-hydroxylase uses ascorbate and Cu^{2+} as cofactors. Also, the highest concentration of dopamine β-hydroxylase is found in vesicles that store catecholamines. Further conversion of norepinephrine to epinephrine takes place in a few neurons of the brain stem that utilize epinephrine as a neural transmitter and in adrenal medullary cells that secrete epinephrine as the primary neurohormone. The soluble enzyme phenylethanolamine N-methyltransferase (PNMT) is the final step in the synthesis of epinephrine where it transferes a methyl group from S-adenosylmethionine to the terminal amine group of norepinephrine. PNMT is regulated by corticosteroids *(41,82)*.

2.3.3. Mechanism of Action (Fig. 10)

Epinephrine acts on both β_1- and β_2-adrenoceptors, stimulating adenylyl cyclase through activating G stimulatory (G$_S$) protein subunit coupling to the receptor, and

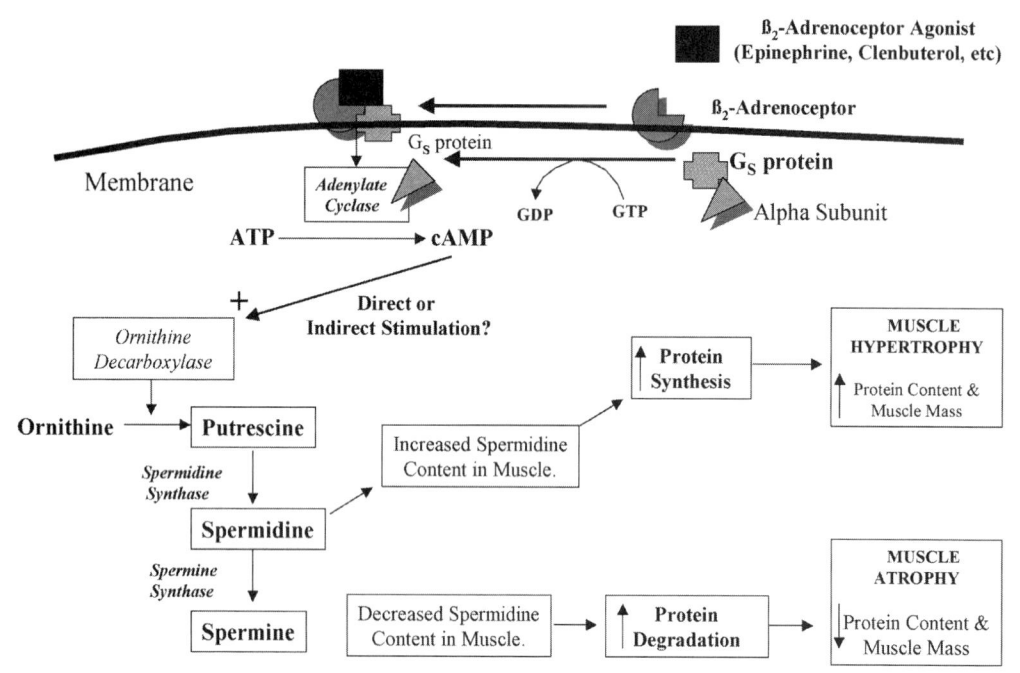

Fig. 10. One possible pathway for β₂-adrenoceptor signal transduction involved with skeletal muscle hypertrophy and atrophy. Note: Spermine may also help resist muscle atrophy by providing a measure of antioxidant protection as it to increases with β₂-adrenoceptor stimulation.

subsequently increasing tissue cAMP levels *(41,82,83)*. In turn, cAMP acts as a second messenger to a number of metabolic pathways. One of the most important pathways is the activation of cAMP dependent protein kinase, which upon activation phosphorylates a number of key proteins. The enzyme ornithine decarboxylase (ODC), which is activated by cAMP, is the rate-limiting enzyme in the synthetic pathway of polyamines *(85–87)*. ODC has been identified as a potentially important link in the β-adrenoceptor signal transduction pathway for inducing cardiac and skeletal muscle hypertrophy *(59, 73,88)*. Other potential means by which β₂-adrenoceptor agonists produce their anabolic effects are unclear. This class of anabolic agents may be acting directly through the stimulation of protein synthesis or through inhibiting the action of proteolytic enzymes. One other effect that has been associated with the use of β₂-adrenoceptor agonists is that they (in particular clenbuterol) are repartitioning agents, by causing an increase in protein production and reducing fat accumulation. The mechanism of action for these effects is again unclear.

It should be noted that β₂-adrenoceptor agonists appear to be more effective in attenuating disuse-induced skeletal muscle atrophy in predominately fast-twitch (Type II) muscles (e.g., extensor digitorum longus [EDL], plantaris, pectineus) than in predominantly slow-twitch (Type I) muscles (e.g., adductor longus [ADL] or soleus). Effects on mixed-fiber-type muscles such as the gastrocnemius are intermediate. In exercised rat models, treatment with β₂-adrenoceptor agonists produces increased muscle mass in all muscles, but their greatest effects were on predominately fast-twitch muscles *(58,59,61)*.

14. Anabolic Doping Agents 545

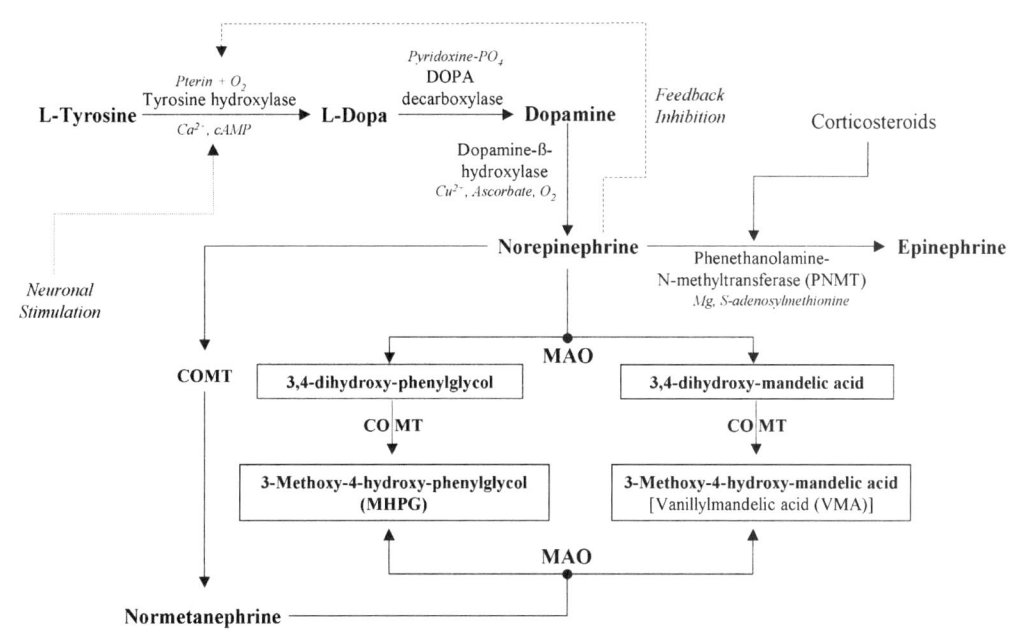

Fig. 11. The biosynthesis of catecholamines in nerve terminals of catecholaminergic neurons. Tyrosine hydroxylase is the rate limiting in the synthesis of catecholamines and is subject to fed-back inhibitory controls by norepinephrine. Corticosteroids induce the synthesis of PNMT in the presence of Mg and S-adenosylmethionine. The metabolism of catecholamines is primarily carried out by the enzymes monoamine oxidase (MAO) and catechol-O-methyltransferase (COMT). MAO-A is responsible for metabolizing primarily deaminates norepinephrine and serotonin, whereas MAO-B is more nonspecific for phenylethylamines. COMT is found on the outer plasma membranes in virtually all cells throughout the body. COMT methylates any catechol group it interacts with.

2.3.4. Metabolism (Fig. 11)

The enzymes MAO and COMT primarily accomplish the metabolism of catecholamines to their inactive forms. These enzymes are distributed extensively throughout the body with MAO located in the outer membrane of mitochondria and COMT on the outer plasma membranes of nearly all cells. In particular, MAO oxidatively deaminates catecholamines to their respective aldehydes, which are acted on in turn by aldehyde dehydrogenases that convert the aldehydes to their analogous acids. MAO acts on free catecholamines within the nerve terminal and not on those stored within vesicles. However, marked increases in deaminated metabolites can be caused by drugs that interfere with catecholamine storage (e.g., reserpine) or by indirect-acting sympathomimetics (e.g., amphetamines). Additionally, MAO is found in the gut and liver to metabolize ingested indirect sympathomimetics (e.g., tyramine and phenylethylamine) found in foods. Inpatients treated with MAO inhibitors can potentially be at risk of suffering severe hypertensive crisis when eating foods rich in tyramine. Additionally, as was stated previously in the section under chemistry, a substitution with a methyl group on the α-carbon would block deamination by MAO, as is the case with amphetamine. The enzyme COMT is responsible for acting on extra-neuronal catecholamines by transferring a methyl group from a cosubstrate, S-adeno-sylmethionine, to the hydroxyl group located at position 3 on the phenyl ring *(41,82)*.

2.4. Toxicology: Contraindications and Adverse Reactions

2.4.1. Contraindications

Sympathomimetic drugs are sold as prescription only and/or are considered as drugs of abuse, as in the case of the amphetamines and cocaine. In general, these drugs are categorized as: pregnancy category C, Schedule C-II controlled substances (amphetamines, cocaine). The NCAA, USOC, and IOC *(6,25)* ban them. Clenbuterol, cimaterol, fenoterol, mabuterol, and procaterol are not approved for human use in the United States. Clenbuterol is prohibited for use in food animals (bovine, swine, etc). However, of all these β_2-adrenoceptor agonists, clenbuterol is the agent most likely to be encountered.

2.4.1.1. ALBUTEROL

Albuterol is contraindicated in cases of: women who are breast-feeding, cardiac arrhythmias, cardiac disease, children, coronary artery disease, diabetes mellitus, elderly, hypertension, hyperthyroidism, pheochromocytoma as a result of hypersensitivity to sympathomimetics, pregnancy, seizure disorders (history of seizures), and tachycardia.

2.4.1.2. AMPHETAMINES (AMPHETAMINE AND METHAMPHETAMINE)

Amphetamine/methamphetamine are contraindicated in cases of advanced arteriosclerosis, agitated states, during or within 14 d of MAO inhibitors, glaucoma, history of drug abuse, hyperthyroidism, moderate to severe hypertension, and symptomatic cardiovascular disease.

2.4.1.3. CLENBUTEROL (EQUINE)

In the United States, clenbuterol is not approved for human use. In horses, it is contraindicated for use in pregnant mares that are near to term, horses suspected of having cardiovascular impairment due to the likelihood of tachycardia, and antagonizes the effects of oxytocin and prostaglandin $F_{2-\alpha}$.

2.4.1.4. COCAINE

Cocaine is a Schedule C-II controlled substance and its use is by prescription only. Cocaine is contraindicated in cases of women who are breast-feeding, cardiac arrhythmias, cardiac disease, cerebrovascular disease, children, coronary artery disease, elderly, hepatic disease, hypertension, infection, pseudocholinesterase deficiency, pregnancy, seizure disorders (history of seizures), thyrotoxicosis, and Tourette's syndrome. Cocaine should not be used in children under 6 yr in age.

2.4.1.5. DOBUTAMINE

Dobutamine is contraindicated in cases of when individuals are experiencing angina, atrial fibrillation, acute myocardial infarction, cardiac arrhythmias, cardiac or coronary disease, children, elderly, hypovolemia, idiopathic hypertrophic subaortic stenosis, neonates, pregnancy, and sulfite hypersensitivity.

14. Anabolic Doping Agents

2.4.1.6. ISOPROTERENOL

Isoproterenol is contraindicated in cases when angina, asthma, atrial fibrillation, atrial flutter, breast-feeding, cardiac arrhythmias, cardiac disease, children, coronary artery disease, corticosteroid therapy, diabetes mellitus, digitalis toxicity, elderly, hypertension, hyperthyroidism, hypoxemia, metabolic acidosis, pheochromocytoma, pregnancy, respiratory acidosis, sulfite hypersensitivity, tachycardia, thyroid disease, ventricular fibrillation, and ventricular tachycardia.

2.4.1.7. PHENYLPROPANOLAMINE

The use of PPA has been discontinued in the United States and is banned by the IOC. PPA is contraindicated in cases of acute myocardial infarction, angina, women who are breast-feeding, cardiac arrhythmias and disease, cardiomyopathy, children, closed-angle glaucoma, coronary artery disease, diabetes mellitus, elderly, females, glaucoma, heart failure, hypertension, hyperthyroidism, infants, myocardial infarction and heart failure, pregnancy, prostatic hypertrophy, renal impairment and failure, substance abuse, tachycardia, and urinary retention.

2.4.1.8. PROPRANOLOL (INDERAL®)

The NCAA, USOC, and the IOC *(6,25)* have banned the use of β_2-adrenoceptor blockers. Propranolol is contraindicated in cases of bronchial asthma, cardiogenic shock, congestive heart failure (except when failure is secondary to tachyarrhythmia treatable with propranolol), and sinus bradycardia. It has been reported that in some patients lacking a history of heart failure, the continued use of β-adrenoceptor antagonists can potentially result in cardiac failure. Furthermore, in cases of congestive heart failure, use of β-adrenoceptor antagonists may be contraindicated because sympathetic stimulation may be essential for supporting circulatory function.

2.4.1.9. TERBUTALINE

Terbutaline is contraindicated in cases where women are breast-feeding, cardiac arrhythmias, cardiac and coronary artery diseases, children, diabetes mellitus, elderly, hypertension, hyperthyroidism, pheochromocytoma, pregnancy, seizure disorder, seizures, and tachycardia.

2.4.2. General Adverse Reactions

Adverse effects associated with use of β_2-adrenergic agonists such as albuterol, clenbuterol, and isoproterenol can lead to severe CNS disturbances that include dizziness, headaches, insomnia, nervousness, syncope, tremor, and weakness. Additionally, they can also affect the cardiovascular system by causing angina, bradycardia, excitability, hyperkinesis, hypertension, hypotension, muscle cramps, palpitations, sinus tachycardia, and ventricular arrhythmias. As a group, β_2-adrenergic agonists can also cause dry mouth, alteration of taste, as well as GI symptoms that include nausea, vomiting, and heartburn. Furthermore, this class of drugs can also have adverse effects on the respiratory system that includes coughing, dyspnea, pulmonary edema, and bronchospasms. Bronchospasms arise from the action of the "inactive" (+)-S enantiomer. Other general adverse effects include dermatitis, diaphoresis, flushing, pallor, rash, pruritus, and urticaria *(25,60)*.

2.4.3. Specific Adverse Effects of Selected β_2-Adrenoceptor Agonists

2.4.3.1. ALBUTEROL (SALBUTAMOL™)

Albuterol's adverse reactions are dose dependent and occur more commonly with oral (tablets or syrup) rather than aerosol or inhalation administration. When albuterol is taken *orally*, the most common adverse effects are tremor (10–20%) and anxiety (9–20%). Other adverse effects include those listed in section under general adverse reactions. These reactions can include: angina, angioedema, anxiety, arrhythmia exacerbation, bronchospasm, cough, diaphoresis, diarrhea, dizziness, drowsiness, dyspepsia, epistaxis, excitability, fever, flushing, headache, hoarseness, hostility, hyperglycemia, hyperkinesis, hypertension, hypokalemia, insomnia, irritability, maculopapular rash, muscle cramps, nausea/vomiting, nightmares, palpitations, peripheral vasodilation, pharyngitis, rash (unspecified), restlessness, rhinitis, sinus tachycardia, throat irritation, tremor, urinary retention, and urticaria *(25,63)*.

When albuterol is administered through *inhalation aerosols*, the most common adverse effects include palpitations, sinus tachycardia, anxiety, tremor, and increased blood pressure that occasionally result in hypertension. Other adverse effects that can be associated with inhalation aerosols include nausea/vomiting, throat irritation, dyspepsia, insomnia, headache, epistaxis, cough, dizziness, nightmares, and hostility. Infrequently cases of urticaria, angioedema, maculopapular rash, bronchospasm, hoarseness, and oropharyngeal edema might also be observed with inhalation aerosols. However, the adverse effects associated with the use of the pure (–)-R enantiomer, levalbuterol (0.63- or 1.25-mg doses), are nervousness, tremor, and rhinitis. In children (6–11 yr old), the adverse effects associated with levalbuterol include accidental injury, asthma (bronchospasm), diarrhea, fever, headache, pharyngitis, rash, and rhinitis. It should be noted that many of the adverse effects associated with the use of albuterol could be attributed to the (+)-S enantiomer *(62)*.

2.4.3.2. AMPHETAMINES (AMPHETAMINE, DEXTROAMPHETAMINE, AND METHAMPHETAMINE)

Although amphetamines are not anabolic agents, they are frequently used as dietary aids or as performance enhancers (increased alertness, etc.). Adverse reactions to amphetamines can include: anorexia, constipation, diarrhea, dizziness, dyskinesia, dysphoria, euphoria, hypertension, impotence, insomnia, over stimulation, palpitations, restlessness, sinus tachycardia, weight loss, and xerostomia *(25)*.

2.4.3.3. CLENBUTEROL

When taken in normal dosages (human), clenbuterol is well tolerated. Clenbuterol is used in humans for treating chronic obstructive airway disease at doses of 10–20 µg twice daily. In a study conducted with healthy human subjects, no adverse cardiovascular effects were observed and respiratory functions improved.

Clenbuterol is also used to treat horses (tocolysis and respiratory ailments) and cattle (tocolytic agent). Use of clenbuterol can potentially result in CNS disturbances that include headache, insomnia, nervousness, palpitations, restlessness, syncope, distal tremor, and weakness. When taken in high doses or on a chronic basis, adverse effects can include hypoglycemia, hypokalemia, hypomagnesemia, hypophosphatemia, and leucocytosis, palpitations, tachypnea-dyspnea, sinus tachycardia, ventricular arrhythmias,

14. Anabolic Doping Agents

and hypertrophy *(53,60)*. Additionally, clenbuterol was found to block epinephrine-induced inhibition of insulin-stimulated glucose uptake in rat skeletal muscles. When given in very high doses (carcinogenic study, 25 mg/kg/body wt) to Sprague Dawley rats, no carcinogenicity was found. However, cardiac hypertrophy was observed in a dose-dependent manner.

Acute toxicity has been observed in subjects who ate livers (clenbuterol accumulates in liver) from cattle treated with clenbuterol. Clinical symptoms were distal tremors, headache, moderate hyperglycemia, hypokalemia, leucocytosis, palpitations, and tachypnea-dyspnea. Following 3–5 d the symptoms disappeared.

2.4.3.4. COCAINE

Although cocaine is not an anabolic agent, it is frequently used as a recreational drug in combination with androgens and potentially β_2-adrenoceptor agonists. Cocaine is a Schedule C-II controlled substance that is addictive. In general, cocaine toxicity can occur in three stages: early stimulation, advanced stimulation, and depression. Higher doses normally lead to progression to more advances stages of toxicity. Cocaine used in doses of 20 mg can lead to adverse reactions, whereas doses of 1.2 g are known to be fatal *(25)*.

Adverse reactions to cocaine use can include: abdominal pain, agitation, agnosia, anxiety, apnea, bowel ischemia, cardiac arrest, Cheyne-Stokes respiration, confusion, delirium, diaphoresis, dizziness, emotional lability, exophthalmos, fecal incontinence, hallucinations (can be auditory, gustatory, olfactory, or visual), headache, hyperreflexia, hypertension, hyperthermia, hyporeflexia, intracranial bleeding, irritability, muscle paralysis, mydriasis, myoglobinuria, nasal congestion, nausea/vomiting, premature labor, psychosis, pulmonary edema, renal tubular obstruction, restlessness, rhabdomyolysis, rhinitis, seizures, septal perforation, serotonin syndrome, sinusitis, spontaneous abortion, tachypnea, tremor, urinary, and incontinence.

As a consequence of cocaine use, serious adverse cardiac effects can occur that include: (a) *early-stage effects*, which can include hypertension, premature ventricular contractions (PVCs), generalized vasoconstriction, ventricular tachycardia, and sinus bradycardia when used in low doses; (b) *advanced-stage adverse effects*, which include cardiac arrhythmias (e.g., ventricular tachycardia and ventricular fibrillation), myocardial ischemia and/or infarction, and ultimately congestive heart failure; and (c) *late-stage depressive cardiovascular effects*, which include cardiac arrest and circulatory collapse. Concomitant use of cocaine with other CNS stimulants can result in an inordinate degree of anxiety, irritability, seizures, and/or cardiac arrhythmias.

2.4.3.5. DOBUTAMINE

Adverse effects attributed to the use of dobutamine (β_1 and β_2-adrenergic agonist, where $\beta_1 \gg \beta_2$) are similar to the other sympathomimetic drugs. These effects are usually transient and unless they become intolerable, medical treatment is not required. Adverse effects normally associated with the use of β-adrenoceptor agonists include: angina, dyspnea, fatigue, headache, hypertension, hypokalemia, hypotension, injection site reaction (local phlebitis), nausea/vomiting, palpitations, paresthesias, phlebitis, PVCs, and sinus tachycardia. Except for a possible persistent tachycardia, these adverse effects are normally short-lived. In addition, terbutaline can cause metabolic disturbances that include hyperglycemia and hypokalemia, especially at high doses. Infrequently, the use of terbutaline has been reported to cause seizures. However, seizures cease upon the withdrawal of treatment. Infrequently, dobutamine might cause electrolyte disturbances that could result in serious adverse cardiac effects *(25)*.

2.4.3.6. ISOPROTERENOL

Isoproterenol's adverse reactions are dose dependent. Adverse effects associated with the CNS include anxiety, diaphoresis, dizziness, headache, insomnia, lightheadedness, mild tremor, restlessness, and weakness. Normally these reactions are transient and do not require medical attention, unless they become prolonged. Chronic use of isoproterenol over long periods can result in tolerance to the drug effect. It is recommended that if this occurs alternative therapy should be initiated. Additionally, hypersensitivity responses have been reported in individuals with sulfite allergies when they use isoproterenol formulations containing sulfite *(25,63)*.

Adverse effects associated with the cardiovascular system include cardiac arrhythmias, heart failure, myocardial infarction, sinus tachycardia, and ventricular arrhythmias (ventricular tachycardia). Also, proarrhythmias can result from drugs that sensitize the myocardium to arrhythmias (e.g., other sympathomimetics or antiarrhythmic agents) or due to a precondition that results from electrolyte imbalances (e.g., hypomagnesemia, hypokalemia, or hyperkalemia). In children receiving intravenous infusions (rates of 0.05–2.7 mg/kg/min) of isoproterenol to treat refractory asthma, clinical deterioration, myocardial infarction (necrosis), congestive heart failure, and death has been reported. Furthermore, factors such as acidosis, hypoxemia, and the coadministration of corticosteroids or methylxanthines (e.g., theophylline, aminophylline, or theobro-mine) appear to increase the risks of cardiac toxicity.

Other adverse effects associated with oral inhalation of isoproterenol may include bronchial irritation, edema, cough, and oropharyngeal dryness. Isoproterenol when taken either orally or by inhalation can also cause GI disturbances such as nausea and vomiting. On occasion isoproterenol can cause a reddish discoloration of the saliva when taken either sublingually or by inhalation. The red color does not indicate any harmful effect of the medication or loss of potency, but is the result of oxidation.

2.4.3.7. PHENYLPROPANOLAMINE (PPA)

The use of PPA has been discontinued in the United States. Adverse effects associated with the use of PPA can include: angina, exacerbated arrhythmia, diaphoresis, dysuria, hypertension, interstitial nephritis, intracranial bleeding, mydriasis, myocardial infarction, nausea and vomiting, palpitations, premature atrial contractions (PACs), PVCs, unspecified renal failure, restlessness, rhabdomyolysis, sinus tachycardia, stroke, tachypnea, and xerostomia. In addition, since PPA is a sympathomimetic, it can produce CNS stimulatory effects that can include anorexia, anxiety, dizziness, hallucinations, headache, insomnia, irritability, psychosis, restlessness, and seizures. These effects are commonly associated with excessive use, overdosage, and substance abuse. Furthermore, the elderly appear to have an increased sensitivity to the CNS stimulatory effects of PPA compared with younger individuals *(25,63)*.

PPA has often been used as a dietary aid and the potential for misuse is very high. When PPA is used in higher than recommended doses (overdose) or in combination

14. Anabolic Doping Agents

with monoamine oxidase inhibitors (MAOIs) or caffeine, hypertension or a hypertensive crisis may result. Signs of hypertension could include severe headache, intracranial bleeding, and stroke (nonfatal and fatal). In particular, intracerebral and/or subarachnoid hemorrhage has been well documented with the use of PPA and PPA products (formulations for cough-cold combinations and appetite suppressants). In the Yale Hemorrhagic Stroke Project *(25)*, the FDA was unable to predict who (based on age, race, sex, etc.) was at risk of stroke. However, it was noted that females were significantly at risk.

2.4.3.8. Propranolol

In general, the adverse effects associated with the use of propranolol are transient and mild, and usually are the result of the drug's therapeutic effects. Bradycardia and hypotension are mild adverse cardiovascular effects associated with propranolol that can be treated with iv atropine if necessary. Adverse cardiovascular effects of a more serious nature effects can include AV block and heart failure. Propranolol can have adverse effects on the GI system by causing diarrhea, nausea, and vomiting. Other adverse reactions can include alopecia, bronchospasm, diabetes mellitus, exfoliative dermatitis, fatigue, hallucinations, hyperglycemia, hypertriglyceridemia, hypoglycemia by interfering with glycogenolysis, hypotension, impotence, libido decrease, musculoskeletal pain, myalgia, nightmares, pruritus, skin hyperpigmentation, and xerosis *(25,63)*.

Propranolol has been shown to mask the signs of hypoglycemia (e.g., tachycardia, palpitations, and tremors) and can result in a prolonging (or enhancing) of hypoglycemia through interfering with glycogenolysis.

2.4.3.9. Terbutaline

Adverse effects attributed to the use of terbutaline are similar to the other sympathomimetic drugs. These effects are usually transient and unless they become intolerable, medical treatment is not required. Adverse effects normally associated with the use of β-adrenoceptor agonists include: angina, anxiety, arrhythmia, diaphoresis, dizziness, drowsiness, dyspnea, headache, hypokalemia, lethargy, muscle cramps, nausea/vomiting, palpitations, PVCs, restlessness, seizures, sinus tachycardia, tremor, and xerostomia. Except for a possible persistent tachycardia, these adverse effects are normally short-lived. In addition, terbutaline can cause metabolic disturbances that include hyperglycemia and hypokalemia, especially at high doses. Infrequently, the use of terbutaline has been reported to cause seizures. Once terbutaline has been withdrawn, seizures stop *(25)*.

2.5. Mechanisms of Interactions

2.5.1. The Following Classes of Drugs May Interact with $β_2$-Adrenoceptor Agonists and Other Sympathomimetics When Administered Concurrently

It has been discussed that $β_2$-adrenoceptor agonists are commonly used in very high concentrations in combination with androgen cocktails. Furthermore, to render greater anabolic effects β-adrenoceptor agonists may be used in conjunction with HGH, as well as IGF-1 as well as nutritional supplements *(25,63)*.

Although the amphetamines and cocaine are sympathomimetic agents, they are not β_2-adrenoceptor agonists. Additionally, they have been used as performance enhancers and are Schedule C-II controlled substances that have been banned by both the IOC and USOC.

2.5.1.1. ANDROGENS

The synergistic effects of clenbuterol and anabolic steroids appear to cause myocardial infarctions, potentially resulting from coronary spasms. In laboratory animals, there is little information on the anabolic interactions taking between the β-2-adrenergic agonists clenbuterol and salbutamol and the androgens. Clenbuterol had no effect on blood testosterone levels. However, treatment with dobutamine (β_1-adrenoceptor agonist) caused increases in blood testosterone levels.

2.5.1.2. AMPHETAMINES

Concomitant use of amphetamines with other sympathomimetics (e.g., β_2-adrenoceptor agonists, cocaine, ephedrine, norepinephrine, pseudoephedrine) can cause excessive cardiovascular or CNS stimulation. Furthermore, the use of amphetamines in the presence of other sympathomimetics and cardiac glycosides (e.g., digoxin) can result in increased blood pressure, cardiac arrhythmias, and heart rate.

The use of amphetamines with β-adrenoceptor antagonists such as propranolol or ophthalmic β-adrenoceptor antagonist solutions can produce unopposed α-adrenergic activity. Through increased α-adrenergic activity, an increase in blood pressure, bradycardia, or heart block could occur. Other substances that can interact with amphetamines include:

Guanethidine: Causes a decrease in guanethidine's antihypertensive effects.
MAOIs: Can cause an increase in the pressor response of amphetamines through causing the release of norepinephrine.
Tricyclic antidepressants: Concomitant use of tricyclics with amphetamines can decrease the effects of amphetamines.
Urinary acidifiers: Concomitant use of urinary acidifiers with amphetamines decreases the half-life of amphetamines, thereby shortening the clinical effects.
Urinary alkalinizers: Concomitant use of urinary alkalinizers with amphetamines increases the half-life of amphetamines, thereby prolonging the clinical effects.

2.5.1.3. AMPHOTERICIN B

The interaction of Amphotericin B with β_2-adrenoceptor agonists such as isoproterenol can increase the risk of developing arrhythmias by causing hypokalemia and hypomagnesemia.

2.5.1.4. ANTIHYPERTENSIVE AGENTS

There is a potential for decreasing the effectiveness of antihypertensive therapy with concomitant use of β_2-adrenoceptor agonists.

2.5.1.5. CARDIAC GLYCOSIDES

The risk of developing cardiac arrhythmias is significantly increased with the concomitant use of β_2-adrenoceptor agonists and cardiac glycosides.

14. Anabolic Doping Agents

2.5.1.6. COCAINE

Briefly, the concomitant use of cocaine with other sympathomimetics (e.g., β_2-adrenoceptor agonists, cocaine, ephedrine, norepinephrine, pseudoephedrine) can cause excessive cardiovascular or CNS stimulation. Furthermore, the use of cocaine in the presence of other sympathomimetics and cardiac glycosides (e.g., digoxin) can result in increased blood pressure, cardiac arrhythmias, and heart rate. The use of cocaine concomitantly with tricyclic antidepressants, cardiac glycosides, or levodopa can increase the risk of developing cardiac arrhythmias. The simultaneous use of cocaine with cholinesterase inhibitors can reduce cocaine's metabolism and increase the risk of cocaine toxicity. Because cocaine stimulates a generalized adrenergic response, it can interact with many drugs in a fashion similar to that of β_2-adrenoceptor agonists (e.g., nitrates, MAOIs, halogenated anesthetics).

2.5.1.7. CORTICOSTEROIDS

The interaction of corticosteroids with β_2-adrenoceptor agonists such as isoproterenol can increase the risk of developing arrhythmias by causing hypokalemia.

2.5.1.8. ENTACAPONE

The combined use of drugs metabolized by COMT such as isoproterenol and entacapone could result in an increase in heart rates, possibility for arrhythmias, and inordinate changes in blood pressure.

2.5.1.9. ERGOT ALKALOIDS

The interaction of ergot alkaloids with β_2-adrenoceptor agonists such as isoproterenol can cause peripheral vasoconstriction and increased cardiac output that leads to an increase in blood pressure.

2.5.1.10. GENERAL ANESTHETICS

The concomitant use of general anesthetics (hydrocarbon derivatives such as cyclopropane, isoflurane, halothane) with β_1- and β_2-adrenoceptor agonists significantly increases the potential for the development of lethal cardiac arrhythmias. This is true for most β-adrenoceptor agonists including albuterol, dobutamine, terbutaline, and especially isoproterenol.

2.5.1.11. GINGER, ZINGIBER OFFICINALE

Results from in vitro investigations suggest that there is a possible interaction that may occur between ginger, *Zingiber officinale*, and β_2-adrenoceptor agonists. This interaction might result in an additive positive inotropic effect. However, there are no clinical data available to substantiate this observation.

2.5.1.12. GUANETHIDINE

The concomitant use of guanethidine and dobutamine could result in a potentiation of dobutamine's pressor, thereby resulting in hypertension and arrhythmias.

2.5.1.13. INSULIN

The interaction of insulin and glucose with β_2-adrenoceptor agonists such as isoproterenol can increase the risk of developing arrhythmias by causing hypokalemia.

2.5.1.14. Levodopa

Isoproterenol can increase the risk of proarrhythmia if administered with levodopa.

2.5.1.15. Loop Diuretics

The interaction of loop diuretics with β_2-adrenoceptor agonists such as isoproterenol can increase the risk of developing arrhythmias by causing hypomagnesemia.

2.5.1.16. MAOIs

The concomitant use of β_2-adrenoceptor agonists with MAOIs or drugs that possess MAOI activity (e.g., furazolidone, linezolid, and procarbazine) can result in severe cardiovascular effects that can result in severe hypotension (albuterol) or a prolonging and intensification of the cardiac stimulatory and vasopressor effects associated with isoproterenol (isoprenaline). Terbutaline's effects on the vascular system have also been reported to increase in the presence of MAOIs. Other MAOIs such as phenelzine and tranylcypromine possess amphetamine-like activity that results in the release of norepinephrine. The combination of these MAOIs with isoproterenol can exacerbate isoproterenol's β-adrenergic effects and subsequently lead to severe cardio- and cerebrovascular responses. It is recommended that a 14-d washout period be allowed between the use of these types of drugs.

2.5.1.17. Nitrates

Treatment with β_2-adrenoceptor agonists can compromise the antianginal effects of nitrates on the myocardium. Increased oxygen demands can be placed on the myocardium with β_2-adrenoceptor agonists such as albuterol, clenbuterol, isoproterenol, and terbutaline. Using β_2-adrenoceptor agonists in patients requiring antianginal therapy can counteract the therapeutic activity of nitrates.

2.5.1.18. Penicillins

The interaction of some penicillins (e.g., as piperacillin or mezlocillin when administered in high doses) with β_2-adrenoceptor agonists such as isoproterenol can increase the risk of developing arrhythmias by causing hypokalemia.

2.5.1.19. Sympathomimetics

In general, the use of β_2-adrenoceptor agonists along with other sympathomimetics or CNS stimulants can result in the release in endogenous catecholamines and produce additive effects that can result in CNS or cardiovascular toxicity. The use of β-adrenoceptor agonists with cocaine can intensify cocaine's effects.

2.5.1.20. Theophylline, Aminophylline

Although clinically methylxanthines and β_2-adrenoceptor agonists are routinely used together, it should be noted that there is an increase risk of additive CNS stimulation, with sensations of tremor or nervousness. Additionally, the interaction of β_2-adrenoceptor agonists with methylxanthine derivatives such as caffeine, theophylline, aminophylline, or theobromine, could potentially lead to an increase in adverse reactions including myocardial infarction, congestive heart failure, and death.

2.5.1.21. Thiazide Diuretics

The interaction of some thiazide diuretics with β_2-adrenoceptor agonists such as isoproterenol can increase the risk of developing arrhythmias by causing hypokalemia.

14. Anabolic Doping Agents

Table 8
Trade Names for Cyclofenil

Trade Name	Dose Available	Manufacturer	Country
Fertodur (OTC)	200 mg tab.	Schering	D, CH, I
Fertodur	200 mg tab.	Schering	PT, GR, TK, M
Neoclym	200 mg tab.	Poli	I
Ondogyne (OTC)	400 mg tab.	Roussel	F
Rehibin	100 mg tab.	Serono	GB
Sexovid	100 mg tab.	Teikiku Zoki	J
Sexovid (OTC)	100 mg tab.	Leo	ES

OTC = over the counter.

2.5.1.22. THYROID HORMONES

The concomitant use of β_2-adrenoceptor agonists with thyroid hormones can result in an intensification of either drug effects on the cardiovascular system. The combined use of these drugs could result in a further risk of coronary insufficiency in patients suffering from coronary artery disease.

2.5.1.23. TRICYCLIC ANTIDEPRESSANTS AND MAPROTILINE

Since maprotiline, a tetracyclic antidepressant, inhibits the reuptake of norepinephrine at the neuronal membrane. The result of this interaction would be an exacerbation of β- and α-adrenoceptor agonist activities that could lead to peripheral vasoconstriction and a subsequent increase in blood pressure, arrhythmias, and hyperpyrexia.

3. CYCLOFENIL

Cyclofenil, though not an anabolic/androgenic steroid, acts as an antiestrogen and increases testosterone production. It is a weak/mild estrogen receptor antagonist (84,89).

3.1. Pharmacology and Kinetics

3.1.1. Drug Usage: Preparations and Routes of Administration

When the athlete is trying to obtain a harder appearance, cylcofenil is used either during steroid treatment, after the treatment, or before competitions with doping tests. The dosage used lies between 400 and 600 mg/d, and below this, the results are poor. It takes a period of 1 wk to begin to see effects. Athletes report strength gains, an increase in energy, and faster regeneration.Cyclofenil is not readily available, but can be found in other countries under the trade names listed in Table 8.

3.1.2. Mechanism of Action

Cyclofenil weakly interacts with estrogen receptors, thus antagonizing estrogen's ability to bind to the receptor.

3.2. Toxicology: Contraindications and Adverse Reactions

3.2.1. Contraindications

It is ineffective among women.

3.2.2. Adverse Reactions

The following adverse reactions have been reported during use: light acne, hot flashes. When cyclophenil is discontinued, some athletes report a depressed mood and a slight decrease in physical strength. In addition, those who take cyclofenil as an antiestrogen during steroid treatment could experience a rebound effect when the compound is discontinued.

3.3. Mechanisms of Interactions

Cyclofenil is used in combination with steroid treatment to obtain a harder appearance. This combination maintains a low estrogen level with lower water retention and less gynecomastia.

4. HUMAN GROWTH HORMONE

Human growth hormones (HGH) include the following: somatotropin; Genotropin®, Humatrope®, Norditropin®, Nutropin®, Saizen®, Serostim®, Tev-Tropin™, Biotropin®, Nutropin Depot™, Nutropin® AQ. HGH is secreted by the pituitary gland and is a heterogeneous mixture of peptides. It stimulates normal skeletal, connective tissue, muscle, and organ growth in children and adolescents *(25)*.

HGH has been purified and is produced by recombinant DNA technology. It is produced from either a mammalian cell line (mouse C127) or *Escherichia coli*. Its amino acid sequence and structure are identical to the dominant form of human pituitary growth hormone. Prior to the mid-1980s, growth hormone was obtained from human cadavers. Today, several somatotropin products are available in either normal or long-acting extended-release forms.

4.1. Pharmacology and Kinetics

4.1.1. Drug Usage: Preparations and Routes of Administration

In both children and adults, somatotropin or its analogs are administered as injectables to treat various growth failures due to growth hormone deficiency, chronic renal disease, Prader-Willi syndrome or Turner's syndrome, and cachexia or AIDS wasting.

Several somatotropin products are available (listed above) that are normal or long-acting extended-release forms (i.e., Nutropin Depot™). These extended-release forms involve insertion of micronized particles of somatotropin into microspheres.

Somatotropin is administered by either intramuscular or subcutaneous injection. In normal males, the mean half-life of intravenous somatotropin is 0.6 h, whereas via subcutaneous or intramuscular routes, the half-life is 1.75 and 3.4 h, respectively. Slower absorption of the drug after subcutaneous or intramuscular administration is responsible for the longer half-lives. Approximately 20% of circulating somatotropin is bound to growth hormone-binding protein. Bioavailability after subcutaneous administration ranges between 70 and 90%. Little excretion of the compound occurs via urine *(25)*.

The depot form of the drug has a bioavailability that ranges for 30–55% depending on the dosing regimen. Once released from the microspheres, the kinetics are the same as somatotropin formulated for daily administration. Serum growth hormone levels above 1 mg/L persist for 11–14 d following single doses of 0.75–1.5 mg/kg *(25)*.

14. Anabolic Doping Agents

The pharmacokinetics is similar in children and adults and not affected by gender. In individuals with renal or hepatic insufficiency, there is a decreased clearance of the drug.

For treatment of growth failure or growth hormone deficiency, children would typically receive 0.16–0.24 mg/kg/wk subcutaneously divided into seven equal daily injections. For adults, the dosage would be a maximum of 0.006 mg/kg/d subcutaneously. For depot forms, the dosage for children typically would be 1.5 mg/kg subcutaneously on the same day each month or 0.75 mg/kg twice each month on the same two days (i.e., Days 1 and 15). For patients over 45 kg, twice-per-month dosing is recommended. Dosage and administration would be adjusted for individual patients.

For treatment of AIDS wasting, daily bedtime subcutaneous injections of Serostim for adults are given as follows: 6 mg for individuals greater than 55 kg body wt, 5 mg for 45–55 kg, 4 mg for 35–45 kg, and 0.1 mg/kg for less than 35 kg.

In body building, "HGH enhancers" are used to raise HGH levels. These over-the-counter supplements can contain cow's colostrum (rich in growth factors, i.e., growth hormone and IGF-1, immune factors, etc.) or an herbal extract of Tribulus terrestris (which stimulates production of luteinizing hormone [LH], testosterone, follicle-stimulating hormone [FSH], and estradiol) *(25)*.

In addition, under conditions such as acromegaly where HGH levels are elevated, somatostatin analogs (inhibitors of growth hormone release) such as octreotide (i.e., Sandostatin or Sandostatin Lar Depot) are used.

4.1.2. Biosynthesis of Endogenous Human Growth Hormone

HGH is secreted from the pituitary gland and is a heterogeneous mixture of peptides. The principal form is a 191 amino acid polypeptide with a molecular mass of 22 kDa. Growth hormone secretion is pulsatile and occurs in discrete bursts. This release is enhanced by growth hormone-releasing hormone and reduced by somatostatin, both of which bind to receptors. In addition, stimulators of growth hormone release include dopamine, serotonin, α-adrenergic agonists, whereas inhibitory factors include β-adrenergic agonists, IGF-1 and growth hormone.

4.1.3. Mechanism of Action

Pituitary growth hormone directly stimulates the production of somatomedins or IGFs in the liver and other tissues. It increases triglyceride hydrolysis in adipose tissue and hepatic glucose output. These direct actions are potentiated by glucocorticoids and oppose the actions of insulin on fat and carbohydrate metabolism. The anabolic and growth-promoting effects of growth hormone are mediated through IGFs *(90)*. These include increases in the production of skeletal growth (growth and metabolism of the epiphyseal plates), the number and size of skeletal muscle cells, and the red cell mass *(25,37,90)*. In addition, the metabolism of proteins, carbohydrates and lipids, mineral retention, and the synthesis of chondroitin sulfate and collagen in connective tissue are stimulated. These indirect effects are insulin-like and opposed by glucocorticoids. Overall, they stimulate normal skeletal, connective tissue, muscle, and organ growth in children and adolescents.

4.1.4. Metabolism

Growth hormone is catabolized in the liver and kidneys.

4.2. Toxicology: Contraindications and Adverse Reactions (25)

4.2.1. Contraindications

Somatotropin is contraindicated in patients who are pregnant or breast-feeding. In elderly or neonatal patients, somatotrophin treatment is not recommended.

Somatotrophin is not recommended for patients undergoing chemotherapy, radiation therapy, or surgery, or if they have experienced trauma.

It should not be used in patients with the following conditions: benzyl alcohol hypersensitivity, cresol hypersensitivity, diabetes mellitus, epiphyseal closure, glycerin hypersensitivity, hypothyroidism, increased intracranial pressure, neoplastic disease, otitis media, acute respiratory failure, and scoliosis.

4.2.2. Adverse Reactions

The following adverse reactions have been reported: antibody formation, arthralgia, bleeding, carpal tunnel syndrome, fluid retention, glycosuria, gynecomastia, headache, hgematuria, hyperglycemia, hypothyroidism, increased intracranial pressure, injection site reaction, myalgia, nausea/vomiting, pancreatitis, paresthesias, peripheral edema, unspecified rash, secondary malignancy, seizures, skin hyperpigmentation, and weakness.

4.3. Mechanisms of Interactions

The following classes of drug may interact with HGH (somatotropin) when administered concurrently.

4.3.1. Corticosteroids (i.e., Cyclosporin)

Corticosteroids can inhibit the growth-promoting effects of somatotropin, thus the corticosteroid dosage should be carefully adjusted.

4.3.2. Sex Steroids (i.e., Testosterone, Estrogen)

4.3.3. Cytochrome P450 Pathway

Somatotropin stimulates the activity of cytochrome-mediated metabolism of antipyrine and other drugs.

5. GONADOTROPHIN-RELEASING HORMONE

5.1. Pharmacology and Kinetics

5.1.1. Drug Usage: Preparations and Routes of Administration

There are several forms of synthetic gonadotrophin-releasing factors: sermorelin (Geref, a synthetic, parenteral growth hormone-releasing hormone) and gonadorelin (Factrel, a synthetic luteinizing hormone-releasing hormone) given by injection and implantable form leuprolide acetate, a synthetic leuteinizing hormone-releasing hormone (Viadur) *(25)*.

14. Anabolic Doping Agents

Factrel is used to diagnose gonadotropin deficiency. It is given to adults and children over 12 yr of age at a dose of 100 mg either subcutaneously or intravenously. In younger children, the dose is 100 mg intravenously.

Geref is used to treat growth hormone deficiency as well as diagnose growth hormone secretion by the pituitary gland. To treat growth hormone deficiency in children, a subcutaneous dose of 0.03 mg/kg (30 µg/kg) is given once daily at bedtime. Once the epiphyses are fused, discontinue treatment. For diagnosing growth hormone deficiency, adults are given 1 mg/kg in a single intravenous dose following an overnight fast.

Viadur is a 12-mo implant (120 mg/d) that continuously delivers leuprolide acetate for the treatment of prostate cancer. After an initial stimulation, gonadotrophin secretion is inhibited, leading to decreased levels of LH and FSH. In males, testosterone is reduced to castrate levels. These decreases occur after 2–4 wk of administration.

Nafarelin is a synthetic analog of endogenous gonadotropin-releasing hormone (GnRH) with 200 times the potency. It is used to treat precocious puberty of central origin and endometriosis (25). In addition, nafarelin is used to treat women with uterine leiomyoma or hirsutism and to shrink prostatic tissue in men with benign prostatic hyperplasia (BPH). It is also used in in vitro fertilization. Nafarelin is administered intranasally (25) and acts by stimulating the release of LH and FSH from the anterior pituitary. However, over time this action is attenuated.

Treatment with nafarelin results in decreases in serum estradiol levels in women and spermatogenesis in men. The recommended doses of nafarelin are 400 µg/d for treating symptoms associated with endometriosis. Nafarelin has an overall efficacy equivalent to that of other GnRH agonists (91).

5.1.2. Mechanism of Action

The synthetic hormone stimulates release of the gonadotrophins at the level of the pituitary gland.

5.2. Toxicology: Contraindications and Adverse Reactions

5.2.1. Contraindications

Use of gonadotrophin-releasing factors is not recommended in pregnant and nursing mothers. Nafarelin is contraindicated in pregnant or lactating females, undiagnosed abnormal vaginal bleeding, or in individuals that are hypersensitive to GnRH or GnRH-agonists.

5.2.2. Adverse Reactions

For gonadotrophin-releasing factors, the following adverse reactions have been reported: abdominal discomfort, flushing, headache, lightheadedness, nausea/vomiting, and swelling and pain at the injection site. For nafarelin, the adverse reactions are more extensive than that observed in the gonadotrophin-releasing factors. These include: anxiety, breast pain and edema, dizziness, depression, decreases in bone density, hot flashes, headaches, impotence, nasal irritation, vaginal dryness, nervousness, changes in mood or libido, insomnia, vaginal bleeding (including vaginal irritation, odor, pruritus, infection, or pain), hypertrophy of female genitalia, vaginitis, dysmenorrhea, pyrexia, weight gain, fatigue, and acute generalized hypersensitivity reaction.

5.3. Mechanisms of Interactions

No significant drug interactions have been noted with nafarelin *(25)*. However, the following drugs may interact with the releasing hormones when administered concurrently:

5.3.1. Androgens, Estrogens, Glucocorticoids, and Progestins

They affect secretion of gonadotrophins.

5.3.2. Digoxin and Oral Contraceptives

Gonadotrophin concentrations are suppressed.

5.3.3. Levodopa and Spironolactone

Gonadotrophin concentrations can be transiently elevated.

5.3.4. Phenothiazines and Dopamine Antagonists

Increased prolactin levels can blunt the response to gonadotrophins.

6. INSULIN-LIKE GROWTH FACTOR-1 (IGF-1)

IGF-1, also known as somatomedin-C, functions as the principal mediator of the action of HGH. IGF-1 has a single chain, 70 amino acid polypeptide that has a 50% homology with insulin. IGFs mediate the anabolic and growth-promoting effects of growth hormone, including increases in the production of skeletal growth (growth and metabolism of the epiphyseal plates), the number and size of skeletal muscle cells, and the red cell mass. It is believed that reestablishment of lost neuromuscular contacts, due to nerve degeneration, are facilitated by IGF-1 *(25,90)*.

6.1. Pharmacology and Kinetics

6.1.1. Drug Usage: Preparations and Routes of Administration

There is a recombinant form of human IGF-1, mecasermin (Myotrophin, Cephalon/Chiron), which is under review for FDA approval for use to slow the progression of muscle paralysis associated with amyotrophic lateral sclerosis. In addition, there is a new clinical trial scheduled to start winter 2002. In the phase III trial, a single daily dose of mecasermin 0.05 and 0.1 mg/kg given subcutaneously was suggested.

Since IGF increases lean body mass, reduces fat, and builds bone, muscle, and nerves, it is popular with bodybuilders. It is a major ingredient in many HGH enhancers. In addition, recombinant IGF-1 is also sold as an oral spray (i.e., IGF-1, Peachtree Health Products, FL) and in tablet form (i.e., Homeopathic IGF-1; *92*). The spray is applied under the tongue three times per day, at least 30 min before or after meals. The tablet is taken once per day, at least 30–90 min after eating.

6.1.2. Biosynthesis of IGF-1

There are two IGFs, IGF-1 and IGF-2. They are polypeptides with molecular masses of 7500 Da and are homologous to proinsulin. IGF-2 has more insulin-like activity than IGF-1, whereas IGF-1 is more growth hormone-dependent and is more potent as a growth factor.

Many tissues (including the CNS and muscle) synthesize IGF-1, but the liver is the major source of circulating IGF-1. The extra hepatic synthesis and secretion of IGFs is growth hormone dependent, but these IGFs are believed to act locally as paracrine modulators. Thyroid hormone and insulin also regulate IGF synthesis. Circulating IGFs are bound to a family of binding proteins that act as transport proteins and also modulate the actions of IGFs on target tissues.

6.1.3. Mechanism of Action

IGF-1 acts through an IGF-1 receptor, which is structurally related to the insulin receptor. It has intrinsic tyrosine kinase activity, which mediates the hormonal signal. IGF-1 receptors are found in a variety of tissues including the CNS, peripheral nerves, and muscle.

6.2. Toxicology: Contraindications and Adverse Reactions

6.2.1. Contraindications

No contraindications are reported.

6.2.2. Adverse Reactions

The following adverse reactions have been reported: injection site reaction, diaphoresis, knee pain, and changes in hair growth or texture were seen in phase III.

6.3. Mechanisms of Interactions

Bodybuilders recommend concurrent administration of IGF-1 with multiminerals to obtain better results.

7. CLOMIPHENE (CLOMID®, SEROPHENE®)

Clomiphene citrate (2-[p- (2-chloro-1, 2-diphenylvinyl) phenoxy] triethylamine citrate) is an orally administered, nonsteroidal, ovulatory stimulant with a molecular weight of 598.09 g/mol. Clomiphene is recommended for the induction of pregnancy in patients with polycystic ovary syndrome, amenorrhea-galactorrhea syndrome, psychogenic amenorrhea, post-oral-contraceptive amenorrhea, and certain cases of secondary amenorrhea of undetermined etiology.

7.1. Pharmacology and Kinetics

7.1.1. Drug Usage: Preparations and Routes of Administration

Clomiphene is available in 50-mg tablets. Treatment should begin with a dose of 50-mg daily for 5 d. If ovulation does not appear to occur after the first course of therapy, the dose should be increased to 100 mg once per day for 5 d. This course may be started as early as 30 d after the previous one after precautions are taken to exclude the presence of pregnancy. The maximum daily dose is 100 mg. If ovulation does not occur, further treatment is not recommended. Coitus should be timed to coincide with the expected time of ovulation. In patients, unusual sensitivity to pituitary gonadotropin, such as those with polycystic ovary syndrome, the 50-mg dose is particularly recommended.

7.1.2. Mechanism of Action

Clomiphene interacts with estrogen-receptor-containing tissues, including the hypothalamus, pituitary, ovary, endometrium, vagina, and cervix. It may also compete with estrogen for estrogen-receptor-binding sites and may delay replenishment of intracellular estrogen receptors. It blocks the normal negative feedback of circulating estradiol preventing the estrogen-mediated decrease in output of GnRH. Clomiphene treatment results in an increased release of pituitary gonadotrophins, initiating steroidogenesis and folliculogenesis. These cause growth of the ovarian follicle and raise circulating estradiol levels. Clomiphene may allow several oocytes to reach maturity. After ovulation, plasma progesterone and estradiol rise and fall as during the normal ovulatory cycle and prepare the endometrium for implantation.

It has been suggested that both clomiphene's estrogenic and antiestrogenic properties participate in initiation of ovulation, but the estrogenic effects of clomiphene are secondary to the primary effects on hypothalamic-pituitary-ovarian function. Clomiphene has no apparent androgenic, anti-androgenic, or progestational effects, nor does it affect pituitary-thyroid or pituitary-adrenal function. After clomiphene therapy discontinuation, there is usually no continued pharmacological effect on subsequent menstrual cycles. However, in some females, spontaneous ovulation has continued. It should be noted that since clomiphene is a hormone-like substance, the IOC, NCAA, and the USOC *(6,25)* ban its use from athletic competition. Because of its antiestrogenic properties, clomiphene could potentially be used to enhance the effectiveness of androgens by blocking their secondary estrogenic effects.

7.1.3. Metabolism

Orally administered clomiphene is readily absorbed and primarily excreted via feces (42%) and a smaller portion via urine (8%). The half-life of clomiphene is 5 d, however, it has been reported in the feces 6 wk after administration.

It should be noted that clomiphene is a combination of racemic isomers, enclomiphene and zuclomiphene, whose pharmacokinetic and pharmacodynamic parameters have not been elucidated. Zuclomiphene is thought to be the more estrogenic isomer. Clomiphene appears to undergo hepatic metabolism. Both unchanged drug and its metabolites are excreted in the feces via the bile. There may be stereo-specific entero-hepatic recycling or sequestering. The zuclomiphene isomer appears to accumulate over several cycles of treatment; however, the combined maximum plasma levels of enclomiphene and zuclomiphene do not appear to exceed 100 mmol/L.

7.2. Toxicology: Contraindications and Adverse Reactions (25)

7.2.1. Contraindications

Clomiphene is not recommended in patients without an intact hypothalamic-pituitary tract and ovarian response (i.e., untreated adrenal insufficiency, pituitary insufficiency or primary pituitary failure, pituitary adenomas or other pituitary tumor, primary ovarian failure, or untreated thyroid disease), since these patients will not respond to treatment.

14. Anabolic Doping Agents

In females with diabetes mellitus, hirsutism (or hyperandrogenism), hyperinsulinemia, obesity, or lowered endogenous estrogen levels, there may be reduced response to clomiphene.

Clomiphene is contraindicated in patients with abnormal or dysfunctional uterine bleeding of undetermined origin, ovarian cancer or endometrial cancer, endometriosis, ovarian enlargements, or preexisting ovarian cysts not due to polycystic ovarian syndrome.

Clomiphene should not be used in women after conception has occurred.

Clomiphene is not recommended in patients with hepatic disease or dysfunction, since the reduced clearance of the drug will result in higher plasma concentrations and increased risk of certain side effects. Liver function should be evaluated in all patients prior to the start of treatment.

Patients should be advised to avoid drinking alcoholic beverages or tobacco smoking during treatment, as both will decrease its effectiveness.

In patients with active thrombophlebitis or other active thromboembolic disease, clomiphene should be used very cautiously.

Additional contraindications are abdominal pain, breast cancer, breast-feeding, major depression or psychosis, driving or operating machinery, testicular failure, visual disturbance, and vomiting.

7.2.2. Adverse Reactions

The following adverse reactions have been reported: abdominal pain, alopecia, anxiety, appetite stimulation, ascites, blurred vision, cervical mucus thickening, diarrhea, diplopia, dizziness, dyspnea, elevated hepatic enzymes, erythema multiforme, fatigue, headache, hepatitis, hot flashes, hypotension, increased urinary frequency, insomnia, mastalgia, menstrual irregularity, mittelschmerz, nausea and vomiting, oliguria, ovarian enlargement, ovarian hyperstimulation syndrome (OHSS), pelvic pain, photophobia, pleural effusion, pruritus, psychosis, pulmonary edema, pulmonary embolism, restlessness, scotomata, secondary malignancy, teratogenesis, thromboembolism, thrombosis, urticaria, visual impairment, and weight gain.

7.3. Mechanisms of Interactions (25)

The following drugs and classes of drug may interact with clomiphene when administered concurrently:

7.3.1. Black Cohosh (Cimicifuga racemosa)

This drug may suppress production of LH and thus antagonize clomiphene treatment.

7.3.2. Androgens

Hyperandrogenism and infertility have been associated with increased levels of the hormone prasterone, and DHEA. Thus, they may antagonize clomiphene treatment.

7.3.3. Soy Isoflavones

There may be competition at the estrogen receptor, thus reducing effectiveness of the treatment.

8. TAMOXIFEN (NOLVADEX®)

Tamoxifen is a nonsteroidal antiestrogen agent in a class of drugs called selective estrogen receptor modulators. Tamoxifen's structure is based on the same nucleus as diethylstilbestrol, but its additional side chain (trans isomer) imparts antiestrogenic activity. Tamoxifen is chemically related to another antiestrogen, clomiphene.

Tamoxifen is a primary therapy for metastatic breast cancer in both men and postmenopausal women. In premenopausal women with metastatic breast cancer, it is an alternative to ovarian ablation. Tamoxifen is more effective for patients with estrogen receptor positive disease. It is also indicated as adjuvant therapy in postmenopausal women with node-positive and node-negative breast cancer following total mastectomy or segmental mastectomy, axillary dissection, and breast irradiation. Other potential benefits of tamoxifen include lowered serum cholesterol concentrations, reduced incidence of myocardial infarctions, and increased bone mineral density (25).

8.1. Pharmacology and Kinetics

8.1.1. Drug Usage: Preparations and Routes of Administration

Tamoxifen is available as tamoxifen citrate (NOLVADEX®, AstraZeneca) in 10-mg and 20-mg tablets. In patients who have breast cancer, the recommended daily dose is 20–40 mg/d is recommended; when greater than 20 mg/d the dose is divided into two (morning and evening). Similarly, in patients with ductal carcinoma *in situ* or for the reduction in the incidence of breast cancer in high-risk women, the recommended daily dose is 20 mg/d given over a period of 5 yr (25).

Dosage adjustment in patients with renal dysfunction is unnecessary, but patients with biliary stasis may need a lower dose.

Orally administered tamoxifen is rapidly absorbed with a peak plasma concentration after 4–5 h. Bioavailability is comparable between the 10-mg tablet twice daily and a single 20-mg daily dose. Its main cytochrome P450 metabolite, Bdesmethyl tamoxifen, is biologically similar to tamoxifen. After repeated doses, tamoxifen accumulates and reaches steady state in the plasma in 4 wk; whereas Bdesmethyl tamoxifen reaches steady state in 8 wk. Tamoxifen has an initial half-life of 7–14 h and an extended secondary phase of 4–7 d; whereas the metabolite has one of approximately 14 d. It should be noted that tamoxifen is banned from use (males) in athletic competition by the IOC, USOC, and the NCAA (6,25).

8.1.2. Mechanism of Action

Tamoxifen is a competitive inhibitor of estradiol binding at the estrogen receptor. It induces a change in the three-dimensional shape of the receptor and inhibits its binding to the estrogen-responsive element on DNA. Tamoxifen has mixed estrogen antagonist and agonist properties. In bone, it stimulates estrogen receptors and may prevent postmenaopausal osteoporosis; whereas in breast tissue, it has antiestrogenic effects. Additionally, cell cycling is slowed by tamoxifen's activity in the nucleus. Tamoxifen's interaction with nuclear chromatin blocks or alters the expression of estrogen dependent genes (RNA transcription) and results in reduced DNA polymerase activity, impaired thymidine utilization, blockade of estradiol uptake, and decreased estrogen response.

Tamoxifen decreases IGF-1, which stimulates cancer cell growth and development, and stimulates the secretion of transforming growth factor beta associated with inhibiting the activity of breast cancer cells.

8.1.3. Metabolism

Tamoxifen distributes widely throughout the body and is extensively metabolized in the liver by the cytochrome P450 system. In plasma, N-desmethyl tamoxifen is the main metabolite and is biologically similar to tamoxifen. Tamoxifen undergoes some enterohepatic circulation. Though excretion of both the unchanged drug and its metabolites is primarily in the feces, conjugated parent compound and metabolites make up more than 70% of the total excreted (25).

8.2. Toxicology: Contraindications and Adverse Reactions

8.2.1. Contraindications

Tamoxifen is contraindicated in patients who are pregnant or breast-feeding. In children, the safety and effectiveness has not been determined.

8.2.1.1. ANTICOAGULANTS

Tamoxifen treatment is contraindicated in patients requiring anticoagulation therapy and those with a history of thromboembolic disease.

8.2.1.2. ENDOMETRIAL CANCER

It should not be used in patients with endometrial cancer or endometrial changes including hyperplasia and polyps.

8.2.1.3. INTRAMUSCULAR INJECTIONS

Intramuscular injections should not be given during tamoxifen treatment to avoid bleeding, bruising, or hematomas.

8.2.1.4. CAUTIONS

It should be used with caution in patients with the following conditions: preexisting bone marrow suppression (i.e., neutropenia, leukopenia, or thrombocytopenia), abnormal gynecological symptoms (i.e., menstrual irregularities, abnormal vaginal bleeding, changes in vaginal discharge, pelvic pain or pressure), visual disturbance (i.e., cataracts), lipoprotein abnormalities (i.e., hypercholesterolemia, hyperlipoproteinemia), or hypercalcemia.

8.2.2. Adverse Reactions

Adverse reactions to tamoxifen treatment are usually mild and transient.

1. Menopausal symptoms (i.e., hot flashes, night sweats, nausea/vomiting), amenorrhea, dysmenorrhea, menstrual irregularity, vaginal bleeding, vaginal discharge, and vaginal irritation (dryness) have been reported, but do not require discontinuance of treatment.
2. Endometrial and uterine changes (i.e., endometrial hyperplasia, polyps, endometriosis, uterine fibroids, and ovarian cysts) may occur during treatment. Increased incidence of uterine and endometrial cancer may also occur.

3. Early Pregnancy. In women exposed to tamoxifen during early pregnancy, teratogenesis, abnormal reproductive anatomy, fetal death, spontaneous abortions, vaginal bleeding, and DES-like syndrome have been reported.
4. Though *bone marrow suppression* is rare, anemia, leukopenia, neutropenia, and thrombocytopenia have been reported.
5. *Thromboembolism* (i.e., pulmonary embolism, deep vein thrombosis, and stroke) has been reported as significantly increased with tamoxifen treatment.
6. *Ocular effects* (i.e., cataracts, corneal deposits, corneal opacification, optic neuritis, retinopathy, and visual impairment) have been reported.
7. During initial tamoxifen treatment for metastatic breast cancer, bone pain, tumor pain, and/or hypercalcemia can occur. Secondary malignancies have been reported.
8. Elevated hepatic enzymes and hyperbilirubinemia may occur and could indicate severe hepatoxicity. Rare effects, but possibly fatal, are cholestasis, hepatitis, hepatic necrosis, and fatty changes in the liver. Also rare are hyperlipidemia and pancreatitis.
9. Occasionally, males treated for breast cancer report a decrease in libido and impotence.
10. Additional adverse reactions include: alopecia, anaphylactoid reactions (i.e., angioedema, erythemia multiforme, Stevens-Johnson syndrome and pemphigus-like, bullous rash), cough, depression, edema, fatigue, rash (unspecified), and weight loss.

8.3. Mechanisms of Interactions

The following drugs and classes of drug may interact with tamoxifen when administered concurrently.

8.3.1. Anticoagulants

There is increased incidence of abnormal bleeding.

8.3.2. Antineoplastic Agents and Other Chemotherapy Agents (i.e., cyclophosphamide, ifosfamide, and the nonsynthetic chemotherapy agents anthracyclines, docetaxel, etoposide, VP-16, paclitaxel, vinca alkaloids)

There is increased risk of a thromboembolic event. Tamoxifen inhibits cytochrome P450 mixed-function oxidases and blocks the multidrug resistance glycoprotein that is part of the mechanism of resistance to naturally occurring (nonsynthetic) chemotherapy agents *(25)*. To establish whether this desirable effect is clinically significant, trials have been conducted in tumor-bearing dogs that suggest the use of tamoxifen and similar agents may be effective in countering multidrug resistance to chemotheraputic agents *(93,94)*. However, tamoxifen may interfere with the activation of other chemotherapeutic agents such as cyclophosphamide and ifosfamide through the inhibition of the mixed-function oxidases.

8.3.3. Metabolism Inhibitors

Antiretroviral protease inhibitors, cyclosporine, delavirdine, efavirenez, erythromycin, imatinib, nifedipine, STI-571, and diltiazem. These inhibit metabolism of tamoxifen by inhibiting the cytochrome P450 3A4 isozyme.

8.3.4. Metabolism Inducers

Carbamazepine, barbiturates, bexarotene, bosentan, ethosuximide, fosphenytoin, nevirapine, phenytoin and troglitazone: These induced the metabolism of tamoxifen by stimulating the cytochrome P450 3A4 isozyme.

8.3.5. Benzodiazepines

These induce or compete with tamoxifen metabolism.

8.3.6. Estrogens and Oral Contraceptives

These are pharmacological opposites of tamoxifen.

8.3.7. Bromocriptine

This will increase serum concentrations of tamxofen and Bdesmethyl tamoxifen.

8.3.8. Rifabutin, Rifampin, and Rifapentine

Reduce the half-life and maximum concentration of tamoxifen in the body. This could reduce tamoxifen's effectiveness.

8.3.9. Soy Isoflavones

Compete with tamoxifen at the estrogen receptor.

8.3.10. Melatonin

Enhances tamoxifen's effects.

8.3.11. Phytoestrogen Compounds (i.e., Black Cohosh [Cimicifuga racemosa])

These may potentiate or interfere with tamoxifen's actions at the estrogen receptor.

9. AROMATASE INHIBITORS

Inhibitors of the aromatase enzyme system block the conversion of androgens to estrogens. The growth of many breast cancers is estrogen receptor mediated and, thus, can be stimulated by estrogen. In postmenopausal women, the principal source of circulating estrogen (primarily estradiol) is conversion of adrenally generated androstenedione to estrone by aromatase in peripheral tissues, such as adipose tissue, with further conversion of estrone to estradiol. By blocking estrogen production, estrogen-sensitive tumors can be reduced in size and their progression delayed in some women. This class of drugs are permitted by the NCAA, but banned by the IOC and USOC *(6,25)*. Furthermore, use of aromatase inhibitors in men is forbidden because it would potentially present an unfair advantage by reducing levels of estrogen and subsequently prolonging testosterone bioavailability. One example of the aromatase inhibitor activity in boys is the delaying of epiphyseal fusion, thereby promoting an increase in height. However, more studies are required to fully establish the indirect anabolic nature of aromatase inhibitors as a group. Nevertheless, although there is not a large pool of information concerning the use of aromatase inhibitors as doping agents, the potential for their abuse as part of a current or future anabolic cocktail is great *(25,95)*.

9.1. Pharmacology and Kinetics

9.1.1. Drug Usage: Preparations and Routes of Administration

This class of drugs is steroidal and nonsteroidal inhibitors of the aromatase enzyme system. Drugs of this class are used as the first-line treatment of locally advanced metastatic breast cancer (hormone receptor positive or hormone receptor unknown) in postmenopausal women. Aromatase inhibitors are also used for treatment of advanced breast cancer in postmenopausal women with disease progression following antiestrogen treatment.

9.1.1.1. ANASTROZOLE

Anastrozole (Arimidex®, AstraZeneca) is orally administered in 1-mg tablet form. Absorption is not affected by food. For first-line therapy, it is taken once per day. Treatment continues until tumor progression is evident. For second-line therapy, Arimidex is administered as a single 1-mg tablet once per day. For patients with mild/moderate hepatic impairment, no dose change is recommended, however, patients should be monitored for side effects. Arimidex has not been studied in patients with severe hepatic impairment. No dose changes are necessary either for patients with renal impairment or in elderly patients *(25)*. Anastrozole, the parent drug, is the primary inhibitor of aromatase activity. The major circulating metabolite, triazole, has no pharmacological activity. From an oral dose, anastrozole is well absorbed into the systemic circulation and is primarily excreted in the feces (85%) after hepatic metabolism and to a lesser extent in the urine (11%). The terminal elimination half-life is approximately 50 h in postmenopausal women. When taken for 7 d once per day, plasma concentrations approach steady-state levels, which are three to fourfold higher than levels observed after a single dose of Arimidex. Plasma proteins bind 40% of the circulating anastrozole. When given at a dose of 1 mg or greater daily, estradiol was suppressed to the lower limit of detection (3.7 pg/L). Within 24 h, estradiol was reduced 70% whereas after 14 d, an 80% reduction was attained.

Anastrozole was not found to affect levels of cortisol, aldosterone, or thyroid-stimulating hormone (TSH). It does not possess direct progestogenic, androgenic, or estrogenic activity, but does affect circulating levels of progesterone, androgens, and estrogens.

9.1.1.2. LETROZOLE

Letrozole (Femara®, Novartis) is available in a one 2.5-mg tablet administered orally. For adults and elderly patients, the 2.5-mg tablet is given once per day. Treatment should continue until tumor progression is evident. No adjustment in dosage is required for patients with renal impairment, if their creatinine clearance is greater than or equal to 10 mL/min. In patients with mild to moderate hepatic impairment, no dosage change is necessary; however, in patients with severe hepatic impairment, caution should be used in dosing *(25)*.

Letrozole is rapidly and completely absorbed from the GI tract and unaffected by food. It is metabolized slowly to an inactive metabolite, a glucuronide conjugate, which is excreted renally. The terminal elimination half-life is 2 d. After daily dosing at 2.5 mg, the steady-state plasma level is reached in 2–6 wk and is 1.5–2 times higher than a single-dose administration. Letrozole is weakly protein bound.

In postmenopausal women with advanced breast cancer, daily doses of 0.5–5 mg resulted in estrogen suppression below the limits of detection. There is no impairment of adrenal steroidogenesis, androgens, or TSH.

14. Anabolic Doping Agents

9.1.1.3. EXEMESTANE

Exemestane (Aromasin®, Pharmacia and Upjohn Co.) is available in 25-mg tablets. It is used in the treatment of advanced breast cancer in postmenopausal women whose disease has progressed following tamoxifen therapy. For adults and the elderly, one 25-mg tablet is taken by mouth once a day after meals. This dosage is the maximum daily dose; higher doses are tolerated, but do not increase estrogen suppression. Treatment is continued until tumor progression is evident. No safe and effective use has been established for children and adolescents. In patients with hepatic impairment or renal impairment, the dosage does not need to be changed.

Exemestane is rapidly absorbed with a T_{max} of 1.2 h and a bioavailability of 42%. It is extensively distributed into tissues. Exemestane is bound to plasma proteins (90%). Maximal aromatase suppression occurs at doses of 10–25 mg. Maximum suppression of circulating estrogens occurs 2–3 d after the start of treatment (25 mg/d by mouth) and persists for 4–5 d *(25)*.

Exemestane has no effect on synthesis of steroids, androgens, LH, and FSH.

9.1.1.4. AMINOGLUTETHIMIDE

Aminoglutethimide (Cytadren®, Novartis) is an oral adrenal steroid inhibitor. It is used for the suppression of adrenal function in Cushing's syndrome. Although not FDA labeled, it has been used in the treatment of breast carcinoma and prostate carcinoma. Aminoglutethimide is available as a 250-mg tablet. For treatment of Cushing's syndrome, adults receive an initial dose of 250 mg by mouth twice to three times a day for approximately 2 wk. The maintenance dose is 250 mg by mouth every 6 h; if necessary this dose can be increased to a maximum of 2 g/d. In children, safety and efficacy has not been established. For treatment of breast or prostatic cancer, adults receive an initial dose of 250 mg by mouth two to three times a day for 2 wk in combination with 40 mg/d of hydrocortisone (10 mg in the morning and at 5 PM, 20 mg at bedtime). The maintenance dose is 250 mg by mouth every 6 h in combination with hydrocortisone (40 mg as described above) *(25)*.

9.1.1.5. VOROZOLE

Vorozole (Rivizor®, Johnson & Johnson; Janssen Pharmaceutica) is classified as an aromatase inhibitor. It was studied as an agent for managing advanced breast cancer in postmenopausal women with disease progression following antiestrogen therapy. However, the data from phase III clinical testing did not show a significant benefit, so it was withdrawn from consideration. No dosage information is available. Vorozole is roughly 1000-fold more potent than aminoglutethimide as an aromatase inhibitor.

9.1.2. Mechanism of Action

These aromatase inhibitors act by suppressing production of estrogen in the adrenal, peripheral tissues and in the cancer tissue itself. Anastrozole and letrozole are potent and selective nonsteroidal inhibitors of aromatase. They act by competitively binding to the heme of the cytochrome P450 subunit of the enzyme. Exemestane is an irreversible, steroidal aromatase inhibitor. Since it is structurally related to androstenedione, it functions as false substrate for aromatase. It is converted into an intermediate that binds irreversibly to the active site of aromatase causing its inactivation, also known as "suicide inhibition" (25).

Aminoglutethimide inhibits the enzymatic conversion of cholesterol to pregnenolone, thereby reducing the synthesis of glucocorticoids, mineralocorticoids, estrogens, and androgens. There is a compensatory increase in secretion of ACTH by the pituitary, requiring glucocorticoid administration to maintain the effects of aminoglutethimide. Aminoglutethimide also inhibits estrogen production from androgens in peripheral tissues by blocking the aromatase enzyme.

9.1.3. Metabolism (95,96)

9.1.3.1. ANASTROZOLE

Anastrozole is extensively metabolized in the liver and excreted as metabolites. The known metabolites are triazole, a glucuronide conjugate of hydroxy-anastrozole, and a glucuronide of anastrozole itself. The major route of elimination is via the feces, whereas renal elimination represents a minor fraction.

9.1.3.2. LETROZOLE

Letrozole is metabolized to a pharmacologically inactive carbinol metabolite that is excreted renally as a glucuronide conjugate in the urine.

9.1.3.3. EXEMESTANE

Exemestane is extensively metabolized via oxidation of the methylene group and reduction of the 17-keto group with subsequent formation of many secondary metabolites. The principle isozyme is cytochrome P450 (CYP) 3A4. The metabolites are inactive or inhibit aromatase to a lesser degree than the parent drug. The 17-dihydro-metabolite may have androgenic activity.

9.1.3.4. AMINOGLUTETHIMIDE (AG)

In a study conducted by Alshowaier et al. (97), they determined the pharmacokinetics of both enantiomers (R-AG and S-AG, dose 500 mg racemic AG, serial plasma and urine samples collected over 48 h) and their acetyl metabolites (R-AcAG and S-AcAG) in breast cancer patients. Half-lives were similar for both enantiomers, but plasma concentrations (analysis by HPLC/UV detection) of the R-enantiomer was 1.5 times higher than the S-AG, and the pharmacokinetic profile for both AG enantiomers followed a one-compartment open model. Of the 500 mg dose, 41% was excreted in the urine as the parent compound (15% R-AG and 26% S-AG) and 5.1% as the acetylated metabolites (2.9% R-AcAG and 2.2% S-AcAG). They also found that the renal clearance of the S-AG was 2.3-fold greater than the R-enantiomer (97). However, the R-AG enantiomer was found to be significantly more potent than S-AG. The investigators concluded that the primary factor contributing to the potency of racemic AG was primarily due to the R-enantiomer rather than its pharmacokinetic differences.

9.1.3.5. VOROZOLE

Vorozole, a triazol derivative, is a new third-generation aromatase inhibitor. In animal studies conducted by Lidstrom et al. in rhesus monkeys showed that the biodistribution of radiolabeled vorozole ([N-methyl-11C] Vorozole) was high in the liver and reached a constant level (20%) of the injected dose after 10 min. Additionally, labeled vorozole showed high specific binding to aromatase-rich tissue, whereas binding to other tissues was lower and less specific. The dissociation constant (Kd) for vorozole was 17 n*M* (95).

In studies conducted by Gross (98) using an in vitro model for cytochrome P450 aromatase. It was shown that the IC50 against aromatase was 0.44 n*M* (cultured rat ovarian granulose cells) and 1.38 n*M* (human placental aromatase). Vorozole was shown to be selective for aromatase and did not effect other cytochrome P450-dependent reactions. Furthermore, vorozole did not exhibit any agonistic or antagonistic activity toward steroid (estrogen, progestin, androgen, or glucocorticoid) receptors.

Treatment with vorozole produced a dose-dependent decrease in aromatase activity and circulating levels of estrogens. Furthermore, tissue levels of estrone and estradiol decreased by 64 and 80%, respectively. Clearance values of vorozole were constant in all age groups up to 50 yr. In age groups greater than 50 yr, clearance rates decreased at a rate of 0.047 L/h/yr. Following a single dose, clearance values were lower in breast cancer patients (4.8 L/h) than in healthy male and female volunteers (8.6 L/h). Additionally, drug clearance was independent of demographic variables related to body size (total body wt, body surface area, lean body mass), whereas the apparent distributional flow (Q) and central volumes of distribution (Vc) were proportional to the total body wt (0.17 L/h/kg and 0.43 L/kg, respectively). The peripheral volume of distribution (Vp) was found also found to be proportional to total body weight and was higher in women than in men (0.64 and 0.40 L/kg, respectively). They found that neither race nor duration of therapy (0.5–28 mo) was a factor with respect to drug effect. They concluded that although there was a relatively high degree of residual interpatient variability in vorozole clearance, it was unlikely that age was of any clinical significance (98).

9.2. Toxicology: Contraindications and Adverse Reactions (25)

9.2.1. Contraindications

9.2.1.1. ANASTROZOLE

Anastrozole is to be used with caution in patients with hepatic cirrhosis or mild to moderate hepatic impairment. It has not been tested in patients with severe hepatic impairment. Anastrozole is contraindicated in premenopausal females and in patients who are pregnant or breast-feeding. It causes pregnancy loss and fetal harm, but is not tetratogenic. Also, it may be excreted into the breast milk.

9.2.1.2. LETROZOLE

Letrozole is contraindicated in patients hypersensitivity to letrozole or its excipients. Letrozole may cause fetal harm when administered to pregnant women. It is embryotoxic and fetotoxic and may be teratogenic. Letrozole should not be administered to women who are breast-feeding as it may be excreted into breast milk.

9.2.1.3. EXEMESTANE

Exemestane should not be given to premenopausal females and in patients who are pregnant or breast-feeding. In animal studies, it causes fetal abnormalities and death in fetuses and was detected in the breast milk. The safety and efficacy of exemestane in children have not been established.

9.2.1.4. AMINOGLUTETHIMIDE

In patients under stress (i.e., surgery, trauma, or acute illness), be aware of the possibility of cortical hypofunction.

9.2.1.5. VOROZOLE

Contraindications are unclear.

9.2.2. Adverse Reactions (25)

The following adverse reactions have been reported:

9.2.2.1. ANASTROZOLE

The major adverse effects were hot flashes, GI disturbance (i.e., diarrhea, abdominal pain, constipation, nausea/vomiting, and dry mouth), vaginal bleeding, thromboembolism, and nervous effects (i.e., anxiety, confusion, depression, dizziness, headache, hypertonia, insomnia and paresthesias). Less frequent effects are asthenia, back pain, bone pain, pelvic pain, arthralgia, dyspnea, hypertension, increased cough, pharyngitis, rash (unspecified), vasodilation, and edema.

9.2.2.2. LETROZOLE

The most frequent adverse reactions are bone pain, back pain, hot flashes, nausea, arthralgia, and dyspnea. Other less frequent effects were peripheral thromboembolic events (i.e., venous thrombosis, thromboplebitis, portal vein thrombosis, and pulmonary embolism), cardiovascular events (i.e., angina, myocardial infarction, myocardial ischemia, and coronary heart disease), and cerebrovascular events (i.e., transient ischemic attacks, thrombotic or hemorrhagic strokes).

9.2.2.3. EXEMESTANE

The most common adverse effects include hot flashes, fatigue, pain (unspecified), depression, insomnia, anxiety, dyspnea, dizziness, headache, and weight gain. Common GI effects include nausea/vomiting, abdominal pain, anorexia, constipation, and diarrhea. Less frequent adverse effects include arthralgia, alopecia, confusion, dyspepsia, respiratory infections, and urinary tract infections.

9.2.2.4. AMINOGLUTETHIMIDE

Adverse reactions include drowsiness, morbilliform skin rash, nausea/vomiting, anorexia, adrenal insufficiency, hypothyroidism, masculinization, hirsutism, headache, dizziness, hypotension, pruritus, myalgia, and fever.

9.2.2.5. VOROZOLE

Adverse reactions are unclear.

9.3. Mechanisms of Interactions

The following classes of drug may interact with aromatase inhibitors when administered concurrently (25):

9.3.1. Estrogen-Containing Products (Including Oral Contraceptives, Androstenedione, Prasterone, Dehydroepiandrosterone)

These products will interfere with the pharmacological actions of aromatase inhibitors.

9.3.2. Inducers of Cytochrome P450 3A4

There will be a decrease in plasma levels of exemestane.

9.3.3. Dexamethasone

Aminoglutethimide accelerates its metabolism.

9.3.4. Warfarin

Aminoglutethimide diminishes its effects.

9.3.5. Ethanol

It can potentiate the effects of aminoglutethimide.

9.3.6. Oral Anticoagulants, Theophylline, Digitoxin, Medroxyprogesterone

Decreased pharmacologic effects due to increased hepatic microsomal enzymes by aminoglutethimide.

10. ERYTHROPOIETIN

Erythropoietin, produced in the kidney, stimulates red blood cell production by the bone marrow. Its synthesis is stimulated by tissue hypoxia. Recombinant forms of erythropoietin, epoetin alfa and darbepoetin alpha, have been developed, with FDA approval, for treatment of anemia in zidovudine-treated HIV patients, chronic renal failure patients, and patients receiving cancer chemotherapy. Also, it is FDA approved to reduce the need for allogeneic blood transfusions in surgery patients. Epoetin alfa is banned by the NCAA, IOC, and USOC *(6,25)*.

10.1. Pharmacology and Kinetics

10.1.1. Drug Usage: Preparations and Routes of Administration

10.1.1.1. EPOETIN ALFA (EPOGEN®, PROCRIT®; PROCRIT, ORTHO BIOTECH)

Epoetin alfa is a recombinant form of the renal hormone erythropoietin, produced by Chinese hamster ovarian cells with the erythropoietin gene inserted. Native erythropoietin is a glycosylated protein with a mol wt of about 36,000 Dalton. The recombinant form is biologically and immunologically indistinguishable from the native form with a mol wt of 30,400 Dalton. Epoetin alfa is available as an injectable in solutions of 2000, 3000, 4000, 10,000, 20,000, and 40,000 U/mL. For the treatment of anemia in patients with chronic renal failure (both those on dialysis and those dialysis-free): In adults and adolescents over 16 yr of age, the initial dose is 50 to 100 U/kg given either intravenously (iv) or subcutaneously (sc) three times per week. After 2 wk of therapy, the hematocrit should rise more than 4 points. If the hematocrit does not increase by 5–6 points after 8 wk, then the dose needs to be increased. Clinically significant changes in hematocrit may take 2–6 wk to occur. Dosage changes should not be made more frequently than once per month. The dosage must be individualized to maintain the hematocrit within the suggested target range (30–36%). If after a dosage adjustment the hematocrit does not improve, iron stores must be reevaluated. The median maintenance dose is 75 U/kg iv/sc three times per week (range: 12.5–525 U/kg). In adult chronic renal failure patients not on dialysis, divided doses of 75–150 U/kg/wk are given by iv/sc *(25,63)*.

In adolescents younger than 16 yr old, children and infants with more than 1 mo on dialysis, the initial dosage is 50 U/kg given iv/sc three times per week. For pediatric hemodialysis patients, the median maintenance dose was 167 U/kg/wk (range: 49–447 U/kg/wk). For peritoneal dialysis patients, the median maintenance dose was 76 U/kg/wk (range: 24–323 U/kg/wk).

In adolescents younger than 16 yr old, children and infants with more than 1 mo not on dialysis, the initial dosage is 50–250 U/kg iv/sc three times per week. The maintenance dosage must be individualized to keep the hematocrit within the suggested target range (30–36%).

For the treatment of zidovudine-induced anemia in HIV-infected patients (with erythropoietin levels less than 500 mU/mL who receive zidovudine at a dose of less than or equal to 4200 mg/wk): For adults, an initial dose of 100 U/kg iv/sc is given three times per week. Hematocrit should be monitored weekly during the first 8 wk. The dose may be increased by 50–100 U/kg, up to a maximum of 300 U/kg, if the response is poor after 8 wk. Every 4–8 wk, the hematocrit should be evaluated and the dose adjusted accordingly. If a patient at the maximum dose does not respond, then higher doses will probably not be effective. Once the desired hematocrit (30–36%) is obtained, the dose should be adjusted to maintain this level.

For adolescents, children, and infants 8 mo old or older (not FDA approved), a dose of 50–400 U/kg iv/sc two to three times per week should be given *(25,63)*.

For the treatment of anemia in patients with nonmyeloid malignancies (where the anemia is due to at least 2 mo of concomitantly administered chemotherapy [erythropoietin levels above 200 mU/mL]): In adults, an initial dose of 150 U/kg subcutaneously three times per week. The dosage may be increased to 300 U/kg three times per week if the response is poor. If they still respond poorly at this maximum dose, it is unlikely that they will respond to higher doses. The dose should be adjusted to maintain a hematocrit of 30–36%. For adolescents, children, and infants older than 6 mo (not FDA approved), dosages of 25–300 U/kg iv/sc three to seven times per week can be given.

To reduce the need for allogenic blood transfusions in anemic patients (hemoglobin levels between 10 and 13 g/dL) scheduled to undergo elective, noncardiac, nonvascular surgery: Ten days before surgery, on the day of surgery, and for 4 d after surgery, adults are given a dosage of 300 IU/kg/d subcutaneously. An alternative to this regimen is 600 IU/kg subcutaneously once weekly, 21, 14, and 7 d before surgery plus one dose on the day of surgery. During this therapy, all patients should receive adequate iron supplementation. Please note that this therapy is for patients at high risk for perioperative transfusions where significant blood loss is anticipated, and not for anemic patients who are willing to donate their blood.

For the treatment of anemia of prematurity (not FDA approved) combined with iron supplementation: In premature neonates, a dosage of 25–100 U/kg subcutaneously three times per week is given. Alternative regimens include 100 U/kg sc five times per week or 200 U/kg sc every other day for 10 d.

For the treatment of anemia associated with myelodysplastic syndrome (MDS) (not FDA approved): In adults, a dosage of 150–300 mL/kg subcutaneously three times per week is given.

14. Anabolic Doping Agents

For the treatment of orthostatic hypotension (not FDA approved) associated with primary autonomic failure: For adults, a dosage of 25–50 U/kg subcutaneously three times per week was given. For all of the above treatments, patients with either hepatic or renal impairments did not appear to require an adjustment of the dosages.

Epoetin alfa is administered by intravenous or subcutaneous injection. Peak plasma concentrations occur between 5 and 24 h after subcutaneous injection, this route gives a more sustained response. The circulating half-life is 4–13 h with detectable levels maintained for at least 24 h. The intravenous route results in a rapid rise in plasma concentration. At 50–300 mL/kg, given three times per week, there is a dose-dependent response; above 300 mL/kg, there is no significant increase in response. The pharmacokinetics profile of epoetin alfa in children and adolescents appears to be similar to that of adults.

10.1.1.2. DARBEPOETIN ALFA

Darbepoetin alfa is a second-generation recombinant form of the renal hormone erythropoietin, produced by Chinese hamster ovarian cells with the erythropoietin gene inserted. The recombinant form is biologically and immunologically indistinguishable from the native form with a molecular weight of 30,400 Dalton.

Darbepoetin alfa is available as an injectable in solutions of 25, 40, 60, and 200 µg/mL *(25,63)*.

For the treatment of anemia in patients with chronic renal failure (both on dialysis and dialysis-free) who are not currently receiving epoetin alfa: In adults, an initial dose of 0.45 :g/kg iv/sc once per week. The dose must be adjusted to obtain and maintain the desired effect. In hemodialysis patients, the median maintenance dose is 0.41 mg/kg sc/iv once weekly (range: 0.26–0.65 mg/kg once weekly).

For anemia in patients with chronic renal failure (both on dialysis and dialysis-free) who are receiving epoetin alfa at doses of <2500, 5000–10,000, and 34,000–89,999 U/wk, equivalent doses of darbepoetin would be 6.25, 25, and 100 µg/wk.

For anemia in patients with nonmyeloid malignancies (not FDA approved): In a study of adult anemia patients not receiving chemotherapy, patients responded to doses of 1, 2.25, and 4.5 mg/kg iv/sc once per week for 12 wk. In a second study, patients received chemotherapy 0.5, 1.5, or 2.25 mg/kg iv/sc once per week.

For all of the above treatments, patients with either hepatic or renal impairments did not appear to require an adjustment of the dosages. Darbepoetin alfa can be administered either intravenously or subcutaneously. With the subcutaneous route, the response is more sustained and the peak plasma concentrations occur between 24 and 72 h after administration. The iv route produces a more rapid peak plasma concentration. At doses up to 0.45 mg/kg once per week, there is a dose-dependent response. The pharmacokinetic profile of darbepoetin alfa in children and adolescents has not been assessed.

10.1.2. Mechanism of Action

Erythropoietin, a glycoprotein, stimulates the division and differentiation of committed erythroid progenitor cells in the bone marrow to produce red blood cells. Epoetin alfa has the same biological activity as native compound. In adults, the majority of erythropoietin is produced in the kidney and the rest by the liver. During fetal development, the liver is the primary source of erythropoietin, and at birth production is transferred to the kidney. The cells that produced erythropoietin are interstitial cells of the inner cortex that are close to the proximal tubules. As the hematocrit decreases, reducing tissue oxygenation, more cells are recruited to produce erythropoietin. This production can increase by 100- to 1000-fold. In patients with chronic renal failure, this production is impaired leading to anemia.

10.1.3. Metabolism

The metabolism and elimination of erythropoietin and the two recombinant compounds (epoetin alfa and darbepoetin alfa) are not completely known. The glycosylation of erythropoietin prevents it from being cleared rapidly from the blood. Nonglycosylated compound has a half-life in vivo of a few minutes. It is not removed by hemodialysis. About 10% of the dose appears to be excreted in the urine *(25,63)*.

10.2. Toxicology: Contraindications and Adverse Reactions (25,63)

10.2.1. Contraindications

Contraindications for epoetin alfa and darbepoetin alfa are identical.

10.2.1.1. UNCONTROLLED HYPERTENSION OR ALLERGIC CONDITIONS

These therapies should not be used in patients with uncontrolled hypertension, or who are allergic to hamster protein, albumin, or benzyl alcohol. There is an increased risk of thrombotic events (including myocardial infarction, seizures, stroke, or death).

10.2.1.2. HEMODIALYSIS

In hemodialysis patients, there may be a need for anticoagulation therapy during treatment.

10.2.1.3. PORPHYRIA

This therapy is contraindicated in patients with porphyria. Patients may develop functional or absolute iron deficiency. It is not indicated in patients with iron-deficiency anemia or anemias due to acute or chronic blood loss. Emphasis on dietary and dialysis requirements is important. Some patients have been reported to develop hyperkalemia.

10.2.1.4. BREAST-FEEDING

These therapies are contraindicated for pregnant patients or those who are breast-feeding.

10.2.1.5. CONTRAINDICATED DRUG COMBINATIONS

Combinations of drugs (i.e., androgens, darbepoetin alfa, epoetin alfa) that stimulate erythropoiesis with epoetin alfa should be avoided.

10.2.1.6. INTERFERENCE

Interference by the following conditions has been reported: acute or chronic infection or inflammation, aluminum overload, cystic fibrosis, erythrocyte enzyme deficiency, folate deficiency, hematological disease (e.g., thalassemia, refractory anemia, or other myelodysplastic disorder), hyperparathyroidism, hypersplenism, occult blood loss, osteitis fibrosa cystica, or vitamin B_{12} deficiency.

10.2.2. Adverse Reactions

The following adverse reactions have been reported for both compounds: arthralgia, asthenia, bronchospasm, chest pain (unspecified), cough, diarrhea, dizziness, edema, encephalopathy, erythema, fatigue, fever, headache, hypertension, infection, injection site reaction, myalgia, myocardial infarction, nausea/vomiting, paresthesias, phlebitis, pruritus, rash (unspecified), seizures, thromboembolism, thrombosis, urticaria, and weakness.

10.3. Mechanisms of Interactions

The following classes of drug may interact with erythropoietin analogs when administered concurrently:

10.3.1. Androgens

Since androgens stimulate erythropoiesis, concurrent administration can increase the patient's response to these therapies; reducing dosage is required. This combination of drugs should be avoided if possible.

10.3.2. Darbepoetin Alfa, Epoetin Alfa

The combination of the two erythropoiesis stimulators should be avoided.

10.3.3. Desmopressin

Reduced bleeding time from desmopressin usage results in patients with end-stage renal disease.

10.3.4. Probenicid, Amphotericin B

Inhibit secretion of endogenous erythropoietin.

10.3.5. Iron Supplements

Iron stores in the body must be replete. Inadequate stores will reduce the response to these therapies.

11. DETECTION AND LABORATORY TEST INTERFERENCES

This is a brief overview of analytical approaches to detecting anabolic/androgenic steroids in various biological samples *(8)*.

11.1. Biosamples

The presence of androgens can be detected in samples such as whole blood, plasma, and urine. Other matrices (tissues) for analysis of anabolic steroids can include bone, hair, liver, cardiac and skeletal muscles, saliva, and sweat of humans or laboratory animals (rats, mice, etc.).

11.1.1. Urine

Urine provides an ideal matrix for the qualitative and quantitative determination of androgens by providing large volumes and relatively high concentrations of the parent compound and metabolites for analysis. Additionally, early researchers used human male urine to isolate and purify androgen crystals. From these crystals, they were able to eventually identify and characterize individual hormones and their metabolites, as well as establish their androgenic and anabolic properties. Historically, the identity of testosterone, the prototypical anabolic steroid, was first established from crystals isolated from volumes (~15 L) of human male urine. Testosterone was the most potent endogenous anabolic and androgenic steroid known at that time. Subsequent work showed that DHT, the active form of testosterone in tissue, was actually more potent than testosterone though having the same affinity for the androgen receptor (8).

On a functional level, urinary androgens reflect an incomplete but relevant indication of endocrine secretory activity. However, care must be taken when attempting to interpret urine androgen values since multiple sources for androgenic properties or androgenic/anabolic effects on excretion are involved. Additionally, caution must be used with respect to interpreting the qualitative and quantitative results for urinary androgen metabolites because: (a) active parent molecules are metabolized through multiple pathways, (b) drugs can alter androgen metabolism, and (c) foods and food supplements can alter androgen metabolism. Other problems associated with urinary androgen assays include the time it takes for collecting 24-h urine samples.

The ratio of concentrations for testosterone glucuronide to epitestosterone glucuronide (T/E ratio) in urine is the most frequently used method for establishing testosterone abuse in athletes (100). Results showing T/E ratios >6 have been considered proof of past abuse of testosterone. However, questions have been raised regarding the validity of using T/E ratios alone as a marker of testosterone abuse in urine-doping analysis since naturally occurring ratios >6 have been reported. Additionally, one must consider the question whether great athletes have higher than average testosterone levels, thereby giving rise to these higher T/E ratios. Thus, in light of these problems, the possibility of reporting false positives becomes of great concern. To address the problem, alternative methods for determining testosterone abuse have been addressed including urinary testosterone/luteinizing hormone ratio, hair analysis, HPLC/MS, and GC/combustion-isotope-ratio mass spectrometry.

In studies conducted by Kjeld et al. (101,102), they showed that urinary unconjugated testosterone, DHT, estradiol, and progesterone levels changed under various storage conditions (temperature, presence of enzyme inhibitors, bacteriostatic agents, and various salts). Unconjugated testosterone levels did not change when samples were stored at temperatures of –20°C. When samples were stored at 4°C, they remained stable for up to 5 d. However, when samples were stored at 18°C, testosterone levels were found to increase by an average of 100% over 2–3 d, whereas DHT levels increased by approximately 200%. When the samples were stored at 37°C, the rate of increase for testosterone was two to three times faster than when stored at 18°C. In addition, the rate of increase of unconjugated androgens can be altered by the addition of enzyme inhibitors, bacteriostatic agents, and various salts. Changes in sample pH were found to impact levels of unconjugated androgens. At pH 8.6 there was no significant effect, but at pH 2, levels of free androgens were found to increase by approximately fourfold over a period of 10 min. Similar results were observed for estradiol and progesterone. Thus, storing urine samples at –20°C will help preserve their profile with respect to free to glucuronidated doping agents as well as the quality of the parent drug. This is true for the androgens, estrogens, as well as other drugs (β-adrenoceptor agonists/antagonists, cocaine, amphetamines, etc.). *However, when analyzing urine samples for the presence of doping agents,*

14. Anabolic Doping Agents

the total drug concentration is of primary interest. Nevertheless, proper storage will help ensure high-quality samples that may be used multiple testing if the occasion arises. Furthermore, it a sample is frequently used, smaller aliquots should taken and stored to prevent freeze-thaw damage. Samples should never be refrozen following thawing. Thus, when in doubt about the stability of the compound to be analyzed, the specimen should be frozen at –20°C or less. In addition, if the specimen is a protein or peptide hormone, the specimen should be frozen and stored at –70°C or less. It is important to note that the specimens should be stored at a constant temperature; therefore, self-defrosting freezers should be avoided if possible. This is especially true for protein hormones and growth factors *(8)*.

Independent of the type of analysis, another problem frequently encountered with urine samples is bacterial contamination. Bacterial growth in urine can be prevented by the addition of a general bacterial static agent such as 1% boric acid, chloroform, or toluene.

11.1.2. Whole Blood, Plasma, and Saliva

The collection of urine over a 24-h period can be inconvenient for the individual and often problems with renal function may contribute to erroneous results. In contrast, the collection of plasma, its transport, and analysis are much more convenient for all concerned *(8)*.

In general, it is accepted that analysis of biological samples constitutes an ideal and objective means for establishing the use of doping agents (or other drugs). Analyses are usually preformed on urine samples by immunoassay screens, followed by GC/MS conformation of positive specimens. However, with the advent of more sensitive techniques (e.g., ELISA), analysis of plasma for specific drugs is replacing many of the urine assays. Additionally, plasma (or serum) is ideal for pharmacokinetic studies where repeated sampling is required over a short period of time. An example of sampling times for bioavailability would be: 15 min before bolus IV dose of drug (time 0), followed by postdosage times of 5, 10, 15, 30 min, 1, 2, 3, out to 72 h or greater. However, it should be noted that plasma sampling is representative of only that time in which it was drawn due to the rapid fluctuations that occur in hormone levels or changes in the bioavailability of doping agents following irregular dosing with various anabolic cocktails.

The use of other biological specimens such as saliva and hair (*see* Subheading 11.6.1.3) for the analysis of anabolic steroids and other drugs of abuse has been meet with varying degrees of success. Rantonen et al. *(103)* have shown that a good correlation exists between plasma and saliva cortisol ($r = 0.47$, $p < 0.001$) and HGH ($r = 0.59$, $p < 0.001$) levels in pediatric cases. However, they found that HGH levels in the saliva were approximately 1000-fold less than that observed in the plasma.

Studies conducted by Vapaatalo et al. *(104)* found that when using TLC (thin-layer chromatography) for screening saliva in test subjects for the drugs amphepramone, amphetamine, ephedrine, and prolintane, they were only able to detect ephedrine on a consistent basis. In contrast, urine analysis showed that all drugs and/or their metabolites were present in the urine. Thus, they concluded that screening the saliva for doping agents was inferior to urine. However, in years since Vapaatalo's study, technological advances in instruments and analytical techniques allowed for screening the saliva for drugs of abuse, therapeutic drugs, and nonpeptide hormones. Hofman *(105)* showed that there was generally a good correlation existing between plasma and saliva drug levels. However, because of diurnal and monthly variations in steroid hormone levels, multiple samples should be collected (morning and evening) to give meaningful results. In these situations, the collection of saliva is considerably more convenient than with plasma.

Saliva can be collected by having the individual spit into a tube or absorption onto a cotton ball. It should be noted, however, that the collection of saliva on cotton balls has been shown to cause significant increases in the levels of DHEA, testosterone, and progesterone. In addition, since most of the analytes are stable at ambient temperatures, samples can be shipped without refrigeration. However, since these specimens are not sterile and are subject to degradation over time by bacteria, samples can be sterile filtered to exclude most of the bacterial contamination.

It has been shown that salivary levels of steroid hormones and other compounds that are protein bound in the serum reflect the unbound and active concentration of those hormones/drugs. Furthermore, Hofman concluded that the use of saliva is an excellent source for the detection and monitoring of hormone and drug levels that offers several advantages (e.g., less expensive and noninvasive) over that of serum testing.

11.1.3. Hair

As of yet, hair analysis is not fully recognized by international sporting committees as an acceptable means to confirm doping abuse. However, analysis of human or animal hair has been shown by several investigators as being a readily available sample source that complements the analysis of more traditional sample types (e.g., urine, serum). The testing of hair samples for the presence of anabolic substances was shown to be comparable to results from urine samples. Additionally, hair analysis might be useful for retesting samples for verification abuse or to distinguish between exogenous abuses from other forms of unintentional exposure to banned substances. Unintentional exposure to banned substances, as a result of taking legal food supplements (contain banned substances not stated on the label), would be suspected when urine samples were positive and hair samples were negative. In contrast, chronic abuse would be suspected when both urine and hair samples are positive.

Urine drug testing has been used to monitor compliance with the banned substance rules introduced in the mid-1970s by sports authorities. Urine is tested prior to competition, but prolonged periods (latency period) before analysis can defeat these tests. Hair analysis, on the other hand, provides a less time-sensitive complement to the more traditional urine analysis. In studies conducted by Gaillard et al. *(106)*, they developed methods for analyzing hair samples for amphetamines, anabolic steroids, and their esters and corticosteroids.

Hair samples of 50 and 100 mg, respectively, were used to analyze for amphetamines and anabolic steroids (as well as anabolic steroid esters). The procedure for analysis of amphetamines involved an initial digestion with 1 N NaOH, extracted by ethyl acetate, derivatized by TFA, and subsequently analyzed by GC equipped with positive chemical-ionization mass spectrometry. Analysis of anabolic steroids and their esters was somewhat similar to that of the amphetamines. A modification of the amphetamine procedure was used to analyze for anabolic steroids and their esters.

14. Anabolic Doping Agents

For the analysis of anabolic steroids and their esters, samples digested 1 N NaOH and highly purified using solid phase extraction on aminopropyl and silica cartridges. Prior to injection, samples were derivatized with N-methyl-N-trimethylsilyltrifluoroacetamide (MSTFA). Analysis was performed on a gas chromatograph coupled to a triple quadrupole mass spectrometer.

Results from these tests showed that amphetamines were detected more frequently in the hair (10 out of 19 analyses) than in the urine (6 out of 30 analyses). Furthermore, the anabolic steroids nandrolone and testosterone undecanoate were each found once in hair (2 out of 25 analyses) whereas none were found in urine (0 out of 30 analyses).

In studies conducted by Dumestre-Toulet et al. *(107)*, they obtained urine and hair samples from several internationally renowned bodybuilders (who were allegedly trafficking doping agents in France). Samples were analyzed by GC/MS (gas chromatography-mass spectrometry) for anabolic compounds that included steroids and metabolites, β_2-adenergic agonists (salbutamol [albuterol], clenbuterol), ephedrine, and other doping agents. They detected various doping agents in the urine that included several androgens and sympathomimetics. The androgens found were norandrosterone (seven subjects, 4.7–100.7 ng/mL), norethiocholanolone (six subjects, 0.9–161.8 ng/mL), stanozolol (four subjects, 1–25.8 ng/mL), methenolone (four subjects, 2.5–29.7 ng/mL), testosterone (seven subjects, 3–59.6 ng/mL), epitestosterone (seven subjects, 1–20.4 ng/mL). The testosterone/epitestosterone ratio was found to be greater than 6 (four subjects, 18.5–59.6). The sympathomimetics found were ephedrine (two subjects, 29 and 36 ng/mL) and clenbuterol (three subjects, 0.2–0.3 ng/mL).

However, analysis of hair samples showed a similar but somewhat different pattern of doping agents that included the androgens nandrolone (three subjects, 1–7.5 pg/mg), stanozolol (four subjects, 2–84 pg/mg), methenolone (two subjects, 17 and 34 ng/mL), testosterone enanthate (five subjects, 0.6–18.8 ng/mg), and testosterone cypionate (two subjects, 3.3–4.8 ng/mg). In addition to the androgens, they also found ephedrine (two subjects, 0.67 and 10.70 ng/mg), salbutamol (three subjects, 15–31 pg/mg), and clenbuterol (six subjects, 15–122 pg/mg) in the hair samples. Thus, from these results the investigators concluded that by analyzing both urine and hair samples they were able to confirm the usage and repetitive exposure to doping substances. Furthermore, by analyzing hair samples concomitant with urinalysis, they were able to reveal substances that were not detected by urine screens alone. The period of detection for different doping agents varies depending on the sample used and drug being analyzed (Table 9).

11.2. Analytical Approaches

In a study conducted by Kintz et al. *(108)*, they analyzed urine and hair from two male bodybuilders by GC/MS (electron impact) for steroids abuse. The samples were positive for nandrolone, stanozolol, and testosterone, and their respective metabolites, thereby suggesting that hair analysis was a useful supplementary test for urine drug testing in athletes by the IOC. Steroid concentrations in the hair were nandrolone (196 and 260 pg/mg hair), stanozolol (135 and 156 pg/mg hair), and testosterone (46 and 71 pg/mg hair). For purposes of analysis, the hair samples were decontaminated using methylene chloride and approximately 100 mg was hydrolyzed by 1 N sodium hydroxide (15 min at 95°C) in the presence of deuterated internal standards. The drugs were extracted by ethyl acetate and subsequently silylinated.

Table 9
Period of Detection for Selected Doping Agents

Agent	Sample Type	Routine Testing Period of Detection	Zero-Tolerance Detection Period
Amphetamines	Urine	3 days	5 days
Amphetamines	Hair	N/A	90 days[a]
Androgens-Oral	Urine	N/A	21 days[a]
Androgens-Injection	Urine	N/A	9 months
Cocaine/Crack	Urine	3 days	5 days
Cocaine/Crack	Hair	Up to days post use	90 days[a]

[a]Time factor depending on hair length.
Data from Aegis Sciences Corporation, http://a1.solidweb.com/ps/AegisLab...e/frm+About_Site_Page.

11.2.1. Clenbuterol Analyses

Analysis of tissue and mean 24-h plasma concentrations of clenbuterol were determined by enzyme immunoassay (EIA) and confirmed by GC/MS. Comparative analytical studies of both methods were conducted previously and the LODs, limits of quantitation (LOQs), and other parameters for both methods have been published. Both quantitation methods were equivalent and the standard deviations of clenbuterol concentrations for standards and samples were less than 5%. Accordingly, *rac*-clenbuterol concentrations were determined by EIA *(110)*.

11.2.2. Enzyme Immunoassay

Analysis by EIA requires only 20 µL of plasma or tissue homogenate volume and has sensitivity to 10 pg/mL clenbuterol. Briefly, wells of a 96-well microtiter tray are incubated with the antibody provided with the kit (1:11 dilution) for 30 min and washed thrice with distilled water. The wells are subsequently dried and either 20 µL of standards (0, 10, 25, 50, 100, 300, 900, 2700, and 8100 pg/mL clenbuterol) or samples are added in triplicate. To the samples and standards, 100 µL of conjugate (1:11 dilution) is added and then incubated for 15 min at room temperature. The contents are subsequently discarded, and wells are washed thrice with distilled water (250 µL), followed by the addition of 100 µL substrate/chromogen mix. Trays are incubated at room temperature in the dark for another 15 min, and the reactions terminated by the addition of 100 µL stopping reagent (sulfuric acid solution provided with the kit). Absorbances are read within 1 h at 450 nm on a microtiter plate reader.

11.2.3. Extraction and Derivatization of Clenbuterol for GC/MS Assay

The extraction of clenbuterol from tissue homogenates or plasma is described previously by Abukhalaf et al. *(110)*. Briefly, 1.0 mL of clenbuterol standards (5, 50, 100, and 200 ng/mL) or samples were loaded into tubes and 25 µL of 2 µg/mL brombuterol (internal standard) was added to a final concentration of 50 ng/mL. Subsequently, 4 mL of 100 mM potassium phosphate buffer (pH 6.0) was added and the buffered extracts were loaded onto pre-equilibrated solid phase silica extraction columns. The columns were then sequentially rinsed with potassium phosphate buffer (pH 6.0), 0.1 N glacial acetic acid, and methanol, respectively. Columns were aspirated for at least 5 min to ensure that the column bed was completely dry and all column washes were discarded. Clenbuterol and brombuterol were eluted from the column with methylene chloride-isopropyl alcohol-ammonium hydroxide (78:20:2 v/v/v). The addition of fresh elution solvent (methylene chloride) to the residue ensured complete removal of water when evaporated to dryness. To the dried clenbuterol samples and standards, 50 μL of freshly prepared trimethylboroxine derivatizing solution (8 μmol trimethylboroxine/mL in dry ethyl acetate) was added, and then incubated for 20 min at 60°C.

Tubes containing derivatized clenbuterol and brombuterol were allowed to cool to room temperature, and transferred to auto-sample vials (2 μL injection volume). Analysis was performed on a HP 5890 gas chromatograph equipped with a 5972 mass selective detector (MSD). The analytes were resolved with an HP 1 MS capillary column crosslinked with 1% phenylmethylsilicone (15 m × 0.25 mm with 0.25 μm film thickness). Inlet pressure programming mode was used to enhance sensitivity. The electron multiplier was operated at 200 V above the tune value. The carrier gas used was ultra-high-purity helium (99.99%) and splitless injection was used. The splitless valve remained closed for 1 min and the initial inlet pressure was 25 psi. The column head pressure was held for 0.5 min, then decreased to 16 psi at a rate of 25 psi/min, and finally maintained at this pressure for the duration of the analysis. This resulted in a flow rate of 1.1 mL/min during the run. The injector temperature was 280°C. The initial oven temperature was 150°C and was held for 1 min; the temperature was programmed to increase at 15°C/min to 215°C, and then increased to 300°C at 35°C/min, and held there for 2 min. The total run time was 9.76 min. The transfer line temperature was held at 280°C. Selected ion monitoring was used to enhance the assay sensitivity. Under these conditions, brombuterol and clenbuterol yielded abundant diagnostic ions with high m/z values.

Hammond et al. *(111)* determined normal circulating levels of several endogenous steroids in venous blood from human male subjects. Hormone levels were determined by employing specific radioimmunoassays following fractionation of the steroids on microcolumns (hydroxyalkoxypropyl Sephadex) microcolumns (Table 10).

11.3. Involuntary Doping and False Positives

Currently, the IOC does not support the use of hair analysis in screening doping cases in athletes. The use of such a technique to augment urine analysis could prove to be important especially in discriminating cases of involuntary doping from those of chronic usage. For example, in cases where hair results are negative for doping agents but urine tests are positive, acute exposure (substance introduced involuntarily through food or beverage) rather than chronic is suggested. Additionally, in cases where urine samples are positive for doping agents, analysis of plasma/saliva and hair samples could be used to confirm the presence of doping agents, thereby helping to avoid reporting false positives.

Many athletes use legal, nonprescription nutritional supplements in order to help them in their training programs. However, in the studies conducted by Geyer et al. *(49)*, they showed that some dietary supplements containing Chrysin, Tribulus Terrestris, and Guarana contained several banned substances not stated on the product label. The

Table 10
Blood Steroid Levels in Male Subjects

Steroid	Peripheral Venous Levels Mean ng/mL	Peripheral Venous Levels Range ng/mL	Spermatic Venous Levels Mean ng/mL	Spermatic Venous Levels Range ng/mL
Testosterone	3.84	0.63–10.64	255.10	2.85–619.10
Dihydrotestosterone	0.19	0.07–0.28	3.74	0.04–9.71
Androsterone	0.27	0.12–0.47	0.97	0.20–2.15
Androstenedione	1.01	0.26–2.65	11.87	0.97–30.18
17β-Hydroxyprogesterone	1.04	0.48–2.20	37.33	1.68–141.00
Progesterone	0.31	0.02–0.57	10.17	1.51–33.24
Pregnenolone	1.34	0.29–2.39	10.97	0.83–30.10

Data from (110).

Chrysin-containing product contained the androgens norandrostenedione and norandrostenediol, whereas a Tribulus–Terrestris containing product contained the androgens androstenedione, androstenediol, androstenediol, norandrostenedione, and norandrostenediol. Further investigation showed that some Guarana-containing products contained the androgens androstenedione, androstenediol, testosterone, and norandrostenedione. Furthermore, the total amount of androgens varied significantly from capsule to capsule, with concentrations ranging from 0.3–5000 mg per capsule. Subsequently, when these dietary supplements were administered to healthy volunteers, all urine samples were found to be positive for norandrosterone, a metabolite of the androgen nandrolone. Geyer et al. (49) further reported that 3–4 h postdose norandrosterone levels ranged between 4 and 623 ng/mL. Additionally, they reported that a female volunteer increased her testosterone/epitestosterone ratio from 0.6 to 4.2.

Green et al. (50) showed that 11 of 12 over-the-counter dietary supplements did not conform to labeling requirements established in 1994 by the Dietary Supplement Health and Education Act. The supplements tested were androstenedione, androstenediol, and 19nor congeners (nor4 and 5androstene3, 17dione and 19nor4 and 5androstene3β, 17βdiol). One of the brands tested contained 10 mg of the controlled androgen testosterone, whereas another brand was 77% higher than the amount stated on the label. Furthermore, of 12 brands tested, 11 contained amounts less than the stated amounts. Thus, results from these two tests showed that the labeling on dietary supplements could not be trusted with respect to the content and/or purity. Furthermore, athletes, sports-governing bodies, and the medical community need to know this information because of the potential consequences (health risks, positive urine tests, etc.) that may be encountered. Lists of banned substances can be found on the World Anti-Doping Agency website (www.wada-ama.org).

11.4. Functional Testing

In addition, functional testing of androgenic or anabolic properties, as well as anti-androgenic activity, can be studied in target tissues (e.g., skeletal muscle, gonadal tissue, tumors, etc.) through whole-animal models *(8)*. Some examples of suitable animal models for studying anabolic and/or androgenic effects are the capon's comb and castrated rats. Additionally, organ cultures and cell culture systems have been employed in numerous experiments and tests as an aid in characterizing the effects of anabolic/androgenic agents. These approaches are especially helpful when trying to establish or confirm anabolic/androgenic activity to an unknown substance that has been characterized by GC/MS and subsequently isolated and purified by HPLC (high-performance liquid chromatography) *(110)*.

An example of an organ culture system is with the fine structure of the rabbit epididymis. In the absence of androgenic/anabolic steroid hormones, the cells show signs of cellular regression (e.g., cell shrinkage, increase number of autophagic vacuoles, loss of smooth endoplasmic reticulum, and loss of stereocilia border), whereas in the presence of the appropriate hormones, the cells retain a more normal appearance. The quality (i.e., potency) of the individual androgens can be determined in this type of culture system by the degree of protection given against cellular regression. For example, the potency of support in maintaining the cells in the epididymis were: 5α-dihydrotestosterone (DHT) ≥ 3α-androstanediol > testosterone > 3β-androstanediol.

Cell culture models for establishing androgenic or anabolic effects can include cultured skeletal muscle cells. Changes in cellular proteins such as the creatine kinase mm isozyme (CK_{mm}) and structural proteins (myosin heavy chain Types I and II) reflect the degree of anabolism or catabolism occurring. With the use of imaging systems in conjunction with inverted phase contrast microscopy and powerful imaging software, changes in cell size (e.g., hypertrophy or atrophy) can be determined. Systems such as this can also prove useful in toxicology testing where cell vitality can be addressed with such techniques as analysis for apoptosis, trypan blue dye exclusion, changes in the rate of cell proliferation, as well as changes in total cellular protein content. Another advantage of in vitro testing (organ or cell culture) could be in determining the effects of direct drug interactions on target tissues. However, when doing these kinds of tests, it is extremely important to employ proper positive and negative controls. The negative control is that which contains just the bare minimum to just keep the cells alive (e.g., defined, serum-free medium). On the other hand, positive controls are a modification of the negative controls in which necessary growth supplements such as hormones and growth factors are added to support proper growth. Fetal bovine serum can also be added to support growth, but this may mask the true nature of the substances that are being studied since the serum may contain anabolic hormones that support growth. However, the serum may be used as long as a modified negative control also contains serum. An example of dissection medium used for the isolation of follicular cells from ovaries would be Dulbecco's minimal essential medium (DMEM) supplemented with 25 mmol HEPES/L, 100 IU penicillin/mL, 0.1 ng streptomycin/mL, 50 mg gentamicin/mL, and 10 mg amphoteric in B/mL medium. An example of a medium for supporting growth would be DMEM/Ham's F12 medium buffered with 15 mmol HEPES/L and $NaHCO_3$. The medium is further supplemented with 3 mmol (l)-glutamine/L, 100 IU penicillin/mL, 0.1 ng streptomycin/mL, 2.5 mg transferrin/mL, 4 ng sodium selenite/mL, and 0.1% (w/v) bovine serum albumin (BSA fraction V). Cell viability can be established by using trypan blue exclusion *(112)*.

11.5. Laboratory Test Interferences

11.5.1. Anabolic/Androgenic Steroids

Treatment with anabolic/androgenic steroids may alter clinical laboratory test results.

11.5.1.1. THYROID FUNCTION TESTS

Androgens have been found to interfere with thyroid function tests by causing decreases in thyroxine-binding globulin. This interaction results in decreases in serum T-4 levels and increases in resin uptake of T-3 and T-4. When measuring free thyroid hormone levels, no changes were observed and no clinical evidence of thyroid dysfunction was observed.

11.5.1.2. LYSOPHOSPHATIDYLCHOLINE INTERFERENCE IN HORMONE IMMUNOASSAYS

Lysophosphatidylcholine (LPC) has been shown by Lepage et al. (1993) to interfere with the formation of antigen-antibody complex in steroid hormone (aldosterone, cortisol, and progesterone) immunoassays, causing plasma levels to be approximately 30% higher than what is actually present. Potentially, this could be true for the androgens as well. It was also shown that the addition of albumin to the samples reduced LPC interference to 7%, whereas the addition of cholesterol reduced it by 50%. Conclusions from these tests suggested that the ratio existing between serum albumin and LPC should be taken into account.

11.5.1.3. HYDROXYCORTICOSTEROIDS

Danazol has been reported by Konishi et al. *(113)* to interfere with the Porter-Silber method for determining total urinary 17-hydroxycorticosteroids.

11.5.2. β-Adrenoceptor Agonists and Antagonists

Treatment with sympathomimetic agents (β-adrenoceptor agonists or antagonists, amphetamines, cocaine) may alter clinical laboratory test results.

11.5.2.1. AMPHETAMINES

In general, amphetamines can cause a circadian-like increase in plasma levels of corticosteroids, with levels being highest in the evening. Additionally, amphetamines can potentially interfere the analysis of steroids in the urine.

11.5.2.2. PROPRANOLOL

Propranolol can cause elevated blood urea levels in patients with severe heart disease, elevated serum transaminase, alkaline phosphatase, or lactate dehydrogenase.

ACKNOWLEDGMENTS

This work was supported, in part, by NASA Grant NCC9-112 and NIH Grants RCRII 2P20, RR11104-08, and 5P20RR11104-7.

14. Anabolic Doping Agents

REFERENCES

1. Hallakarva Gunnora "Berserkergang." Stefan's Florilegium Berserkergang-art. http://www.florilegium.org.
2. Lombardo JA. Anabolic-androgenic steroids. In: Lin GC and Erinoff L, eds. Anabolic steroid abuse. NIDA Research Monograph 102:60–73 (1990).
3. Times Record News; Wichita Falls, Texas; June 18, 2001. Speed's long history: amphetamine drugs have caused trouble for decades. Jeff Hall, Times Record News www.trnonline.com/archives/2001archives/06182001/local_news/25530.shtml. Jeff Hall may be contacted at (940)-763-7596 or by e-mail at hallj@wtr.com.
4. Goodman LS and Gilman A. Goodman and Gilman's The pharmacological basis of therapeuics, 1st ed. New York:McGraw-Hill, 1941:1207–1226.
5. NIDA report, www.nida.nih.gov/ResearchReports/Steroids/anabolic steroids.htm
6. World Anti-Doping Agency (WADA), www.wada.org
7. Kochakian CD. History of anabolic-androgenic steroids. In: Lin GC and Erinoff L, eds. Anabolic steroid abuse. NIDA Research Monograph 102:29–59 (1990).
8. Burtis CA and Ashwood ER. Tietz's textbook of clinical chemistry, 2nd ed. Philadelphia: Saunders, 1994:1783–1795, 1843–1856.
9. Morrison RT and Boyd RN. Organic chemistry, 3rd ed. Boston: Allyn & Bacon, 1974: 115–142, 225–247, 515.
10. von Deutsch DA, Abukhalaf IK, Aboul-Enein HY, Wineski LE, Oster RA, Paulsen DF, and Potter DE. β-Agonist-induced alterations in organ weights and protein content: comparison of racemic clenbuterol and its enantiomers. Chirality 12:137–148 (2000).
11. Mukherjee A, Kirkovsky L, Yao XT, Yates RC, Miller DD, and Dalton JT. Enantioselective binding of Casodex to the androgen receptor. Xenobiotica 26:117–122 (1996).
12. Budavari S, O'Neil MJ, Smith A, Heckelman PE, and Kinneary JF. The Merck index, An encyclopedia of chemicals, drugs, and biologicals, 12th ed. Whitehouse Station, NY: Merck Research Laboratories Division of Merck & Co., Inc., 1996.
13. Katzung BG. Basic & clinical pharmacology, 8th ed. New York: McGraw-Hill, 2001:20–137, 138–154, 625–643, 679–710.
14. Time Report, Dope into Gold, Jan. 19, 1998, vol. 151, No. 3.
15. Hardman JG and Limbird LE. Goodman and Gilman's The pharmacological basis of therapeuics, 10th ed. New York: McGraw-Hill, 2001:199–248, 282–284, 1441–1458.
16. Meikle AW, Arver S, Dobs AS, Sanders SW, Rajaram L, and Mazer NA. Pharmacokinetics and metabolism of a permeation-enhanced testosterone transdermal system in hypogonadal men: influence of application site—a clinical research center study. J Clin Endocrinol Metab 81:1832–1840 (1996).
17. Wang C, Berman N, Longstreth JA, Chuapoco B, Hull L, Steiner B, et al. Pharmacokinetics of transdermal testosterone gel in hypogonadal men: application of gel at one site versus four sites: a General Clinical Research Center Study. J Clin Endocrinol Metab 85:964–969 (2000).
18. Zhang GY, Gu YQ, Wang XH, Cui YG, and Bremner WJ. A pharmacokinetic study of injectable testosterone undecanoate in hypogonadal men. J Androl 19:761–768 (1998).
19. Segura J, Ventura R, and Jurado C. Derivatization procedures for gas chromatographic-mass spectrometric determination of xenobiotics in biological samples, with special attention to drugs of abuse and doping agents. matogr. B Biomed Sci Appl 713:61–90 (1998).
20. Simionescu L, Neacsu E, Zimel A, and Caragheorgheopol A. The development of a radioimmunoassay system for testosterone (T) and dihydrotestosterone (DHT). Part 2. The preparation of antisera to T. Endocrinologie 28:107–125 (1990).

21. Peng SH, Segura J, Farre M, Gonzalez JC, and de la Torre X. Plasma and urinary markers of oral testosterone undecanoate misuse. Steroids 67:39–50 (2002).
22. SmartBodyz Nutrition; http://www.smartbodyz.com; Fort Worth, Texas 76102; Toll Free: 187; SmartBodyz (1-877-627-8263); Telephone: 817-335-1982; E-mail: webmaster@smartbodyz.com
23. King DS, Sharp RL, Vukovich MD, Brown GA, Reifenrath TA, Uhl NL, and Parsons KA. Effect of oral androstenedione on serum testosterone and adaptations to resistance training in young men. JAMA 281:2020–2028 (1999).
24. Broeder CE, Quindry J, Brittingham K, Panton L, Thomson J, Appakondu S, et al. Physiological and hormonal influences of androstenedione supplementation in men 35 to 65 years old participating in a high-intensity resistance training program. Arch Intern Med 160:3093–3104 (2000).
25. Gold Standard Clinical Pharmacology 2000. http://cpip.gsm.com/
26. Wang C and Swerdloff RS. Should the nonaromatizable androgen dihydrotestosterone be considered as an alternative to testosterone in the treatment of the andropause? J Clin Endocrinol Metab 87:1462–1466 (2002). Review.
27. Ahn YS. Efficacy of danazol in hematologic disorders. Acta Haematol 84:122–129 (2000).
28. Fujisawa K, Tani P, Piro L, and McMillan R. The effect of therapy on platelet-associated autoantibody in chronic immune thrombocytopenic purpura. Blood 81:2872–2877 (1993).
29. Otawa M, Kuriyama Y, Iwase O, Kawanishi Y, Miyazawa K, Aizawa S, et al. [Possible role of immunocompetent cells on periodic exacerbation of idiopathic thrombocytopenic purpura]. Rinsho Ketsueki 38:331–335 (1997).
30. Rittmaster RS, Thompson DL, Listwak S, and Loriaux DL. Androstanediol glucuronide isomers in normal men and women and in men infused with labeled dihydrotestosterone. J Clin Endocrinol Metab 66:212–216 (1988).
31. Wang C, Iranmanesh A, Berman N, McDonald V, Steiner B, Ziel F, et al. Comparative pharmacokinetics of three doses of percutaneous dihydrotestosterone gel in healthy elderly men—a clinical research center study. J Clin Endocrinol Metab 83:2749–2757 (1998).
32. Kammerer RC, Merdink JL, Jagels M, Catlin DH, and Hui KK. Testing for fluoxymesterone (Halotestin) administration to man: identification of urinary metabolites by gas chromatography-mass spectrometry. J Steroid Biochem 36:659–666 (1990).
33. Capponi VJ, Cox SR, Harrington EL, Wright CE, Antal EJ, and Albert KS. Liquid chromatographic assay for fluoxymesterone in human serum with application to a preliminary bioavailability study. J Pharm Sci 74:308–311 (1985).
34. Fenichel G, Pestronk A, Florence J, Robison V, and Hemelt V. A beneficial effect of oxandrolone in the treatment of Duchenne muscular dystrophy: a pilot study. Neurology 48:1225–1226 (1997).
35. Fenichel GM, Griggs RC, Kissel J, Kramer TI, Mendell JR, Moxley RT, et al. A randomized efficacy and safety trial of oxandrolone in the treatment of Duchenne dystrophy. Neurology 56:1075–1107 (2001).
36. Fox-Wheeler S, Heller L, Salata CM, Kaufman F, Loro ML, Gilsanz V, et al. Evaluation of the effects of oxandrolone on malnourished HIV-positive pediatric patients. Pediatrics 104:e73 (1999).
37. Nilsson KO, Albertsson-Wikland K, Alm J, Aronson S, Gustafsson J, Hagenas L, et al. Improved final height in girls with Turner's syndrome treated with growth hormone and oxandrolone. J Clin Endocrinol Metab 81:635–640 (1996).
38. Berger JR, Pall L, Hall CD, Simpson DM, Berry PS, and Dudley R. Oxandrolone in AIDS-wasting myopathy. AIDS 10:657–662 (1996).

14. Anabolic Doping Agents

39. Guarneri MP, Abusrewil SA, Bernasconi S, Bona G, Cavallo L, Cicognani A, et al. Turner's syndrome. J Pediatr Endocrinol Metab 14:959–965 (2001).
40. Partsch CJ, Weinbauer GF, Fang R, and Nieschlag E. Injectable testosterone undecanoate has more favourable pharmacokinetics and pharmacodynamics than testosterone enanthate. Eur J Endocrinol 132:514–519 (1995).
41. Malan PG and Gould RP. Essentials of endocrinology. O'Riordan JLH, ed. Oxford, England: Blackwell Scientific, 1982:95–98.
42. Winters SJ. Androgens: endocrine physiology and pharmacology. In: Lin GC and Erinoff L, eds. Anabolic steroid abuse. NIDA Research Monograph 102:113–130 (1990).
43. Dunn JF, Nisula BC, and Rodbard D. Transport of steroid hormones: binding of 21 endogenous steroids to both testosterone-binding globulin and corticosteroid-binding globulin in human plasma. J Clin Endocrinol Metab 53:58–68 (1981).
44. Berendonk B. Doping Dokumente: Von der Forschung zum Betrug. Berlin: Springer-Verlag, 1991:91–171.
45. East Germany Doping Scandal, wysiwyg://8/http://abcnews.go.com /...01013_egerman athletes_feature.html.
46. ABCNEWS.com:20/20: East Germany Doping Scandal, wysiwyg://8/ http://abcnews.go.com /...01013_egermanathletes_feature.html.
47. Palusinski R and Barud W. Effects of androstenedione in young men (Letter to the Editor). JAMA 283:741 (2000).
48. Leder BZ, Longcope C, Catlin DH, Ahrens B, Schoenfeld DA, and Finkelstein JS. Oral androstenedione administration and serum testosterone concentrations in young men. JAMA 283:779–782 (2000).
49. Geyer H, Mareck-Engelke U, Reinhart U, Thevis M, and Schänzer W. Positive doping cases with norandrosterone after application of contaminated nutritional supplements [Positive Dopingfälle mit Norandrosteron durch verunreinigte Nahrungsergänzungsmittel]. Deutsche zeitschrift für sportmedizin 51:378–382 (2000).
50. Green GA, Catlin DH, and Starcevic B. Analysis of over-the-counter dietary supplements. Clin J Sport Med 11:254–259 (2001).
51. Tarter RE, Ammerman RT, and Ott Peggy J. Handbook of Substance Abuse: Neurobehavioral Pharmacology. Plenum Press, New York and London, 1998, Chapters 31–34.
52. Preedy VR, Patel VB, Reilly ME, Richardson PJ, Falkous G, and Mantle D. Oxidants, antioxidants and alcohol: implications for skeletal and cardiac muscle. Front Biosci 4:e58–e66 (1999).
53. Hoffman RJ, Hoffman RS, Freyberg CL, Poppenga RH, and Nelson LS. Clenbuterol ingestion causing prolonged tachycardia, hypokalemia, and hypophosphatemia with confirmation by quantitative levels. J Toxicol Clin Toxicol 39:339–344 (2001).
54. DeRamundo BM and Volpe A. Effect of steroid hormones and antihormones on hypothalamic beta-endorphin concentrations in intact and castrated female rats. J Endocrinol Invest 13:91–96 (1990).
55. Convertino VA, Polet JL, Engelke KA, Hoffler GW, Lane LD, and Blomqvist CG. Increased beta-adrenergic responsiveness induced by 14 days exposure to simulated microgravity. J Gravit Physiol 2:P66–P67 (1995).
56. Wines JD Jr, Gruber AJ, Pope HG Jr, and Lukas SE. Nalbuphine hydrochloride dependence in anabolic steroid users. Am J Addict 8:161–164 (1999).
57. von Berg A and Berdel D. [A new beta-2 sympathomimetic drug with longer effectiveness. Comparison with current beta-2 sympathomimetic drugs in therapy of bronchial asthma in childhood]. Monatsschr Kinderheilkd 141:53–58 (1993).

58. von Deutsch DA, Abukhalaf IK, Wineski LE, Aboul-Enein HY, Potter DE, and Paulsen DF. Distribution and muscle-sparing effects of clenbuterol in hindlimb suspended rats. Pharmacol 65:38–48 (2002).
59. von Deutsch DA, Abukhalaf IK, Wineski LE, Silvestrov NA, Bayorh M, and Potter DE. Changes in muscle proteins and spermidine content in response to unloading and clenbuterol treatment. C J Physiol Pharmacol 81:28–39 (2003).
60. Eudra, (European Agency for the Evaluation of Medical Products: Veterinary Medicines and Information Technology Unit); EMEA/MRL/723/99-FINAL Feb 2000. Westferry Circus, 7 Canary Wharf, E14 4HB LONDON, (Tel: +44 207 418-8569 Fax: +44 207 418-8416)/ E-mail: mail@emea.eudra.org; http://www.eudra.org/emea.html.
61. Wineski LE, von Deutsch DA, Abukhalaf IK, Pitts SA, Potter DE, and Paulsen DF. Muscle-specific effects of hindlimb suspension and clenbuterol in mature, male rats. Cells Tissues Organs 171:188–198 (2002).
62. Schmekel B, Rydberg I, Norlander B, Sjoswand KN, Ahlner J, and Andersson RG. Stereoselective pharmacokinetics of S-salbutamol after administration of the racemate in healthy volunteers. Eur Respir J 13:1230–1235 (1999).
63. Tryniszewski C. Nurse's drug looseleaf. Blue Bell, PA: Blanchard & Loeb, 2001.
64. Morales-Olivas FJ, Brugger AJ, Bedate H, Garcia-Diez JM, Morcillo E, and Esplugues J. [Clenbuterol: a new partial antagonist of the beta adrenergic receptors (author's transl)]. Arch Farmacol Toxicol 6:131–138 (1980).
65. Perez R, Garcia M, Arias P, Gallardo M, Valenzuela S, and Rudolph MI. Inhibition of xylazine induced uterine contractility by clenbuterol and nifedipine. Res Vet Sci 63:73–76 (1997).
66. Stegmann GF and Bester L. Some cardiopulmonary effects of midazolam premedication in clenbuterol-treated bitches during surgical endoscopic examination of the uterus and ovariohysterectomy. J S Afr Vet Assoc 72:33–76 (2001).
67. Maltin CA, Delday MI, Hay SM, Innes GM, and Williams PE. Effects of bovine pituitary growth hormone alone or in combination with the beta-agonist clenbuterol on muscle growth and composition in veal calves. Br J Nutr 63:535–545 (1990).
68. Smith DJ. The pharmacokinetics, metabolism, and tissue residues of beta-adrenergic agonists in livestock. J Anim Sci 76:173–194 (1998).
69. Maltin CA, Delday MI, Watson JS, Heys SD, Nevison IM, Ritchie IK, and Gibson PH. Clenbuterol, a β-adrenoreceptor agonist, increases relative muscle strength in orthopedic patients. Clin Sci 84:651–654 (1993).
70. Bates PC and Pell JM. Action and interaction of growth hormone and the beta-agonist, clenbuterol, on growth, body composition and protein turnover in dwarf mice. Br J Nutr 65:115–129 (1991).
71. Reeds PJ, Hay SM, Dorwood PM, and Palmer RM. Stimulation of muscle growth by clenbuterol: lack of effect on muscle protein biosynthesis. Br J Nutr 56:249–258 (1986).
72. Reichel K, Rehfeldt C, Weikard R, Schadereit R, and Krawielitzki K. [Effect of a beta-agonist and a beta-agonist/beta-antagonist combination on muscle growth, body composition and protein metabolism in rats]. Arch Tierernahr 45:211–225 (1993).
73. Abukhalaf IK, von Deutsch DA, Wineski LE, Silvestrov NA, Abera SA, Sahlu SW, and Potter DE. Effect of hindlimb suspension and clenbuterol treatment on polyamine levels in skeletal muscle. Pharmacol 65:145–154 (2002).
74. Apseloff G, Girten B, Walker M, Shepard DR, Krecic ME, Stern LS, and Gerber N. Aminohydroxybutane bisphosphonate and clenbuterol prevent bone changes and retard muscle atrophy respectively in tail-suspended rats. J Pharmacol Exp Therap 264:1071–1078 (1993).
75. Spealman RD. Noradrenergic involvement in the discriminative stimulus effects of cocaine in squirrel monkeys. J Pharmacol Exp Ther 275:53–62 (1995).

14. Anabolic Doping Agents

76. Girten B, Oloff C, Plato P, Eveland E, Merola AJ, and Kazarian L. Skeletal muscle antioxidant enzyme levels in rats after simulated weightlessness, exercise and dobutamine. Physiologist 32(Suppl 1):S59–S60 (1989).
77. Bloomfield SA, Girten BE, and Weisbrode SE. Effects of vigorous exercise training and beta-agonist administration on bone response to hindlimb suspension. J Appl Physiol 83:172–178 (1997).
78. Desplanches D, Favier R, Sempore B, and Hoppeler H. Whole body and muscle respiratory capacity with dobutamine and hindlimb suspension. J Appl Physiol 71:2419–2424 (1991).
79. Takeo S, Elmoselhi AB, Goel R, Sentex E, Wang J, and Dhalla NS. Attenuation of changes in sarcoplasmic reticular gene expression in cardiac hypertrophy by propranolol and verapamil. Mol Cell Biochem 213:111–118 (2000).
80. Katz I, Lloyd T, and Kaufman S. Studies on phenylalanine and tyrosine hydroxylation by rat brain tyrosine hydroxylase. Biochim Biophys Acta 445:567–578 (1976).
81. Fitzpatrick PF. The aromatic amino acid hydroxylases. Adv Enzymol Relat Areas Mol Biol 74:235–294 (2000).
82. Siegel GJ, Albers RW, Alganoff BW, and Katzman R. Basic neurochemistry, 3rd ed. Boston: Little, Brown, 1981:205–218.
83. Hardin AO and Lima JJ. Beta 2-Adrenoceptor agonist-induced down-regulation after short-term exposure. J Recept Signal Transduct Res 19:835–852 (1999).
84. Cepero M, Cubria JC, Reguera R, Balana-Fouce R, Ordonez C, and Ordonez D. Plasma and muscle polyamine levels in aerobically exercised rats treated with salbutamol. Pharm Pharmacol 50:1059–1064 (1998).
85. Genazzani AR, Petraglia F, Mercuri N, Brilli G, Genazzani AD, Bergamaschi M, et al. Effect of steroid hormones and antihormones on hypothalamic beta-endorphin concentrations in intact and castrated female rats. J Endocrinol Invest 13:91–96 (1990).
86. Cepero M, Perez-Pertejo Y, Cubria JC, Reguera R, Balana-Fouce R, Ordonez C, et al. Muscle and serum changes with salbutamol administration in aerobically exercised rats. Comp Biochem Physiol C Toxicol Pharmacol 126:45–51 (2000).
87. Cubria JC, Ordonez C, Reguera RM, Tekwani BL, Balana-Fouce R, and Ordonez D. Early alterations of polyamine metabolism induced after acute administration of clenbuterol in mouse heart. Life Sci 64:1739–1752 (1999).
88. Turchanowa L, Rogozkin VA, Milovic V, Feldkoren BI, Caspary WF, and Stein J. Influence of physical exercise on polyamine synthesis in the rat skeletal muscle. Eur J Clin Invest 30:72–78 (2000).
89. www.cyberflex.co.uk/steroidcyclofenil.htm
90. Lewis MI, LoRusso TJ, and Fournier M. Anabolic influences of insulin-like growth factor I and/or growth hormone on the diaphragm of young rats. J Appl Physiol 82:1972–1978 (1997).
91. Wong JM, Forrest KA, Snabes SZ, Zhao SZ, Gersh GE, and Kennedy SH. Efficacy of nafarelin in assisted reproductive technology: a meta-analysis. Hum Reprod Update 7:92–101 (2001).
92. www.achilleshealthmart.com
93. Ishii I and Kitada M. [Multidrug-resistance by induction of inactivation for anticancer drugs]. Nippon Rinsho 55:1044–1049 (1997).
94. Waddle JR, Fine RL, Case BC, Trogdon ML, Tyczkowska K, Frazier D, and Page RL. Phase I and pharmacokinetic analysis of high-dose tamoxifen and chemotherapy in normal and tumor-bearing dogs. Cancer Chemother Pharmacol 44:74–80 (1999).
95. Lidstrom P, Bonasera TA, Kirilovas D, Lindblom B, Lu L, Bergstrom E, et al. Synthesis, in vivo rhesus monkey biodistribution and in vitro evaluation of a 11C-labelled potent aromatase inhibitor: [N-methyl-11C]vorozole. Nucl Med Biol 25:497–501 (1998).

96. Piotrovsky VK, Huang ML, Van Peer A, and Langenaecken C. Effects of demographic variables on vorozole pharmacokinetics in healthy volunteers and in breast cancer patients. Cancer Chemother Pharmacol 42:221–228 (1998).
97. Alshowaier IA, el-Yazigi A, Ezzat A, Abd el-Warith A, and Nicholls PJ. Pharmacokinetics of S- and R-enantiomers of aminoglutethimide following oral administration of racemic drug in breast cancer patients. J Clin Pharmacol 39:1136–1142 (1999).
98. Goss PE. Pre-clinical and clinical review of vorozole, a new third generation aromatase inhibitor. Breast Cancer Res Treat 49(Suppl 1):S59–S65; discussion S73–S77 (1998).
99. Wiseman LR and Spencer CM. Vorozole. Drugs Aging 11:245–250; discussion 251–252 (1997).
100. van de Kerkhof DH, de Boer D, Thijssen JH, and Maes RA. Evaluation of testosterone/epitestosterone ratio influential factors as determined in doping analysis. J Anal Toxicol 24:102–115 (2000).
101. Kjeld JM, Puah CM, and Joplin GF. Rise of unconjugated sex hormones in human urine on storage. Clin Chim Acta 80:285–291 (1977).
102. Kjeld JM, Puah CM, and Joplin GF. Labile testosterone conjugate in human urine: further evidence. Clin Chim Acta 93:227–233 (1979).
103. Rantonen PJ, Penttila I, Meurman JH, Savolainen K, Narvanen S, Helenius T. Growth hormone and cortisol in serum and saliva. Acta Odontol Scand 58:299–303 (2000),
104. Vapaatalo H, Karkainen S, and Senius KE. Comparison of saliva and urine samples in thin-layer chromatographic detection of central nervous stimulants. Int J Clin Pharmacol Res 4:5–8 (1984).
105. Hofman LF. Human saliva as a diagnostic specimen. J Nutr 131:1621S–1625S (2001).
106. Gaillard Y, Vayssette F, and Pepin G. Compared interest between hair analysis and urinalysis in doping controls. Results for amphetamines, corticosteroids and anabolic steroids in racing cyclists. Forensic Sci Int 107:361–379 (2000).
107. Dumestre-Toulet V, Cirimele V, Ludes B, Gromb S, and Kintz P. Hair analysis of seven bodybuilders for anabolic steroids, ephedrine, and clenbuterol. J Forensic Sci 47:211–214 (2002).
108. Kintz P, Cirimele V, Sachs H, Jeanneau T, and Ludes B. Testing for anabolic steroids in hair from two bodybuilders. Forensic Sci Int 101:209–216 (1999).
109. Kintz P, Cirimele V, Dumestre-Toulet V, Villain M, and Ludes B. Doping control for methenolone using hair analysis by gas chromatography-tandem mass spectrometry. J Chromatogr B Analyt Technol Biomed Life Sci 766:161–167 (2002).
110. Abukhalaf IK, von Deutsch DA, Parks BA, Wineski LE, Paulsen DF, Abul-Enein HY, and Potter DE. Comparative analytical quantitation of clenbuterol in biological matrices using GC-MS and EIA. Biomed Chromatogr 14:99–105 (2000).
111. Hammond GL, Ruokonen A, Kontturi M, Koskela E, and Vihko R. The simultaneous radioimmunoassay of seven steroids in human spermatic and peripheral venous blood. J Clin Endocrinol Metab 45:16–24 (1977).
112. Harper JM, Mackinson I, and Buttery PJ. The effects of beta agonists on muscle cells in culture. Domest Anim Endocrinol 7:477–484 (1990).
113. Konishi H, Minouchi T, and Yamaji A. Interference by danazol with the Porter-Silber method for determination of urinary 17-hydroxycorticosteroids. Ann Clin Biochem 38:277–279 (2001).

Additional Reading

Akahane K, Furukawa Y, Ogiwara Y, Haniuda M, and Chiba S. Beta-adrenoceptor blocking effects of a selective beta 2-agonist, mabuterol, on the isolated, blood-perfused right atrium of the dog. Br J Pharmacol 97:709–716 (1989).

Amemiya K, Kudoh M, Suzuki H, Saga K, and Hosaka K. Toxicology of mabuterol. Arzneimittelforschung 34:1680–1684 (1984).

Amemiya K, Asano T, Arika T, Nakamura M, and Kudoh M. Special toxicology-physical dependence potential, antigenicity and mutagenicity of mabuterol. Arzneimittelforschung 34: 1685–1686 (1984).

Baronti A, Lelli M, Manini G, and Verdiani P. Procaterol metered aerosol in patients with chronic obstructive pulmonary disease. Int J Clin Pharmacol Res 7:363–368 (1987).

Baselt RC and Cravey RH. Disposition of toxic drugs and chemical in man, 4th ed. Foster City, CA: Chemical Toxicology Institute 1995:1, 7, 16, 44, 76, 108, 186, 222, 293, 405, 407, 448, 476, 478, 686, 693, 703, 720.

Beastall GH, Ratcliffe WA, Thomson M, and Semple CG. Trilostane interference with steroid assays. Lancet 1:727–728 (1981).

Bowers LD. Analytical advances in detection of performance-enhancing compounds. Clin Chem 43:1299–1304 (1997).

Brambilla G, Cenci T, Franconi F, Galarini R, Macri A, Rondoni F, et al. Clinical and pharmacological profile in a clenbuterol epidemic poisoning of contaminated beef meat in Italy. Toxicol Lett 114:47–53 (2000).

Brasch J and Flader S. Human androgenic steroids affect growth of dermatophytes in vitro. Mycoses 39:387–392 (1996).

Brown J, Clasper C, Smith T, and Lomax MA. Effects of a beta 2-adrenergic agonist, cimaterol and corticosterone on growth and carcass composition of male rats. Comp Biochem Physiol 102:217–220 (1992).

Byrem TM, Beermann DH, and Robinson TF. The beta-agonist cimaterol directly enhances chronic protein accretion in skeletal muscle. J Anim Sci 76:988–998 (1998).

Byrem TM, Robinson TF, Boisclair YR, Bell AW, Schwark WS, and Beermann DH. Analysis and pharmacokinetics of cimaterol in growing Holstein steers. J Anim Sci 70:3812–3819 (1992).

Cardoso LA and Stock MJ. Effect of clenbuterol on growth and body composition during food restriction in rats. J Anim Sci 74:2245–2252 (1996).

Chance WT, Zhang X, Zuo L, and Balasubramaniam A. Reduction of gut hypoplasia and cachexia in tumor-bearing rats maintained on total parenteral nutrition and treated with peptide YY and clenbuterol. Nutrition 14:502–507 (1998).

Chikhou F, Moloney AP, Austin FH, Roche JF, and Enright WJ. Effects of cimaterol administration on plasma concentrations of various hormones and metabolites in Friesian steers. Domest Anim Endocrinol 8:471–480 (1991).

Dawson R. Editorial, BMC News, 2000.

Eisen EJ, Croom WJ Jr, and Helton SW. Differential response to the beta-adrenergic agonist cimaterol in mice selected for rapid gain and unselected controls. Anim Sci 66:361–371 1988.

Fischer W, Lasek R, and Muller M. Anticonvulsant effects of propranolol and their pharmacological modulation. Pol J Pharmacol Pharm 37:883–896 (1985).

Galan Martin AM, Marino JI, Garcia de Tiedra MP, Marabe JJ, Caballero Loscos MJ, and Marino MM. Determination of nandrolone and metabolites in urine samples from sedentary persons and sportsmen. J Chromatogr B Biomed Sci Appl 761:229–236 (2001).

Germouty J, Aubert J, Clavier J, Paramelle B, and Voisin C. [Long-term tolerability of formoterol in chronic obstructive bronchopathies]. Allerg Immunol (Paris) 24:342–347 (1992).

Gleixner A, Sauerwein H, and Meyer HH. Probenecid, sulfinpyrazone and pyrazinamide do not inhibit urinary excretion of the beta 2-adrenoceptor agonist clenbuterol in cattle. Food Addit Contam 13:603–608 (1996).

Gleixner A. Probenecid markedly reduces urinary excretion of ethinylestradiol and trimethoprim slightly reduces urinary excretion of clenbuterol. Food Addit Contam 15:415–420 (1998).

Grassi V, Daniotti S, Schiassi M, Dottorini M, and Tantucci C. Oral beta 2-selective adrenergic bronchodilators. Int J Clin Pharmacol Res 6:93–103 (1986).

Gregorevic P, Williams DA, and Lynch GS. Effects of leukemia inhibitory factor on rat skeletal muscles are modulated by clenbuterol. Muscle Nerve 25:194–201 (2002).

Groot MJ, Schilt R, Ossenkoppele JS, Berende PL, and Haasnoot W. Combinations of growth promoters in veal calves: consequences for screening and confirmation methods. Zentralbl Veterinarmed A 45:425–440 (1998).

Guentert TW, Buskin JN, and Galeazzi RL. Single dose pharmacokinetics of mabuterol in man. Arzneimittelforschung 34:1691–1696 (1984).

Hamada K, Kihana T, Kataoka M, Yoshioka S, Nishio S, Matsuura S, and Ito M. Urinary disturbance after therapy for cervical cancer: urodynamic evaluation and beta2-agonist medication. Int Urogynecol J Pelvic Floor Dysfunct 10:365–370 (1999).

Harri M. Beta blockade and physical training in rats. Ann Clin Res 14(Suppl 34):168–172 (1982).

Hernandez-Carrasquilla M. External contamination of bovine hair with beta2-agonist compounds: evaluation of decontamination strategies. J Chromatogr B Biomed Sci Appl 767: 235–243 (2002).

Horiba M, Murai T, Nomura K, Yuge T, Sanai K, and Osada E. Pharmacokinetic studies of mabuterol, a new selective beta 2-stimulant. II: urinary metabolites of mabuterol in rats and their pharmacological effects. Arzneimittelforschung 34:1668–1679 (1984).

Huang H, Gazzola C, Pegg GG, and Sillence MN. Differential effects of dexamethasone and clenbuterol on rat growth and on beta2-adrenoceptors in lung and skeletal muscle. J Anim Sci 78:604–608 (2000).

Hunt DG, Ding Z, and Ivy JL. Clenbuterol prevents epinephrine from antagonizing insulin-stimulated muscle glucose uptake. J Appl Physiol 92:1285–1292 (2002).

Ishizaki O, Daidohji S, Kimura K, Shibuya K, Horiguchi T, and Sekiwa M. Reproduction studies with mabuterol in rats. Arzneimittelforschung 34:1687–1690 (1984).

Kawakami Y. First clinical studies on mabuterol. A summarizing report. Arzneimittelforschung 34:1699–1700 (1984).

Kazlauskas R and Trout G. Drugs in sports: analytical trends. Ther Drug Monit 22:103–109 (2000).

Kim J, Shigetomi S, Tanaka K, Yamada ZO, Hashimoto S, and Fukuchi S. [The role of beta 2-adrenoceptor on the pathogenesis of insulin resistance in essential hypertension]. Nippon Naibunpi Gakkai Zasshi 70:521–528 (1994).

Lacey RJ, Cable HC, James RF, London NJ, Scarpello JH, and Morgan NG. Concentration-dependent effects of adrenaline on the profile of insulin secretion from isolated human islets of Langerhans. J Endocrinol 138:555–563 (1993).

Lavoie JL, Calderone A, and Beliveau L. A farnesyltransferase inhibitor attenuated beta-adrenergic receptor down regulation in rat skeletal muscle. Am J Physiol Regul Integr Comp Physiol 282:R317–R322 (2002).

Le Bizec B, Bryand F, Gaudin I, Monteau F, Poulain F, and Andre F. Endogenous nandrolone metabolites in human urine: preliminary results to discriminate between endogenous and exogenous origin. Steroids 67:105–110 (2002).

Lepage N, Roberts KD, and Langlais J. Interference of lysophosphatidylcholine in hormone radioimmunoassays. Clin Chem 39:865–869 (1993).

Longcope C. Adrenal and gonadal androgen secretion in normal females. Clin Endocrinol Metab 15:213–228 (1986).

Matsumoto K, Ojima K, Ohta H, and Watanabe H. Beta 2- but not beta 1-adrenoceptors are involved in desipramine enhancement of aggressive behavior in long-term isolated mice. Pharmacol Biochem Behav 49:13–18 (1994).

14. Anabolic Doping Agents

McEvoy JD, McCaughey WJ, Cooper J, Kennedy DG, and McCartan BM. Nortestosterone is not a naturally occurring compound in male cattle. Vet Q 21:8–15 (1999).

Merck Manual. www.merck.com/pubs/mmanual/section22/ chapter305/305a.htm

Miyata T, Kai H, Furusawa K, Nakamura H, Saito M, Okano Y, and Takahama K. Secretomotor and mucolytic effects of mabuterol, a novel bronchodilator. Arch Int Pharmacodyn Ther 288:147–160 (1987).

Mueller RK, Grosse J, Lang R, and Thieme D. Chromatographic techniques—the basis of doping control. J Chromatogr B Biomed Appl 674:1–11 (1995).

Murakami K, Nakagawa T, Yamashiro G, Araki K, and Akasofu K. Adrenal steroids in serum during danazol therapy, taking into account cross-reactions between danazol metabolites and serum androgens. Endocr J 40:659–664 (1993).

Murtha PE, Zhu W, Zhang J, Zhang S, and Young CY. Effects of Ca++ mobilization on expression of androgen-regulated genes: interference with androgen receptor-mediated transactivation by AP-I proteins. Prostate 33:264–270 (1997).

Nakamura M, Yamaya M, Fukushima T, Sekizawa K, Sasaki H, and Takishima T. Effect of mabuterol on tracheal mucociliary clearance of magnetized iron particles in anesthetized dogs. Respiration 58:33–36 (1991).

Nielen MW, Vissers JP, Fuchs RE, van Velde JW, and Lommen A. Screening for anabolic steroids and related compounds in illegal cocktails by liquid chromatography/time-of-flight mass spectrometry and liquid chromatography/quadrupole time-of-flight tandem mass spectrometry with accurate mass measurement. Rapid Commun Mass Spectrom 15:1577–1585 (2001).

O'Connor RM, Butler WR, Finnerty KD, Hogue DE, and Beermann DH. Acute and chronic hormone and metabolite changes in lambs fed the beta-agonist, cimaterol. Domest Anim Endocrinol 8:537–548 (1991).

Puls I, Beck M, Giess R, Magnus T, Ochs G, and Toyka KV. [Clenbuterol in amyotrophic lateral sclerosis. No indication for a positive effect]. Nervenarzt 70:1112–1115 (1999).

Ramos F, Castilho MC, and Silveira MI. Occurrence of beta 2-adrenergic agonist residues in urine of animal meat producers in Portugal. J AOAC Int 81:544–548 (1998).

Sainz RD and Wolff JE. Effects of the beta-agonist, cimaterol, on growth, body composition and energy expenditure in rats. Br J Nutr 60:85–90 (1988).

Saugy M, Cardis C, Robinson N, and Schweizer C. Test methods: anabolics. Baillieres Best Pract Res Clin Endocrinol Metab 14:111–133 (2000).

Schmidt EW, Ulmer WT, and Rominger KL. Pharmacokinetics and pharmacodynamics of beta 2-agonists (in the light of fenoterol). Respiration 62:190–200 (1995).

Shinohara Y and Baba S. Stable isotope methodology in the pharmacokinetic studies of androgenic steroids in humans. Steroids 55:170–176 (1990).

Simon M and Babich-Armstrong M. 17-Hydroxycorticosteroids in urine. Clin Chim Acta 103: 101–108 (1980).

Stallion A, Zhang FS, Chance WT, Foley-Nelson T, and Fischer JE. Reversal of cancer cachexia in rats by cimaterol and supplemental nutrition. Surgery 110:678–684 (1991).

Taguchi S, Yoshida S, Tanaka Y, and Hori S. [Simple and rapid analysis of trenbolone and zeranol residues in cattle muscle and liver by stack-cartridge solid-phase extraction and HPLC using on-line clean-up with EC and UV detection]. Shokuhin Eiseigaku Zasshi 42: 226–230 (2001).

Thomas DP, McCormick KM, and Jenkins RR. Effects of beta-adrenergic blockade on training-induced structural adaptations in rat left ventricle. Eur J Appl Physiol Occup Physiol 57:671–676 (1988).

Touchstone JC. Steroids. In: Zweig G and Sherma J, eds. Handbook of chromatography. Boca Raton, FL: CRC Press, 1986:3–25, 41–64.

Walker HC and Romsos DR. Effects of cimaterol, a beta-adrenergic agonist, on energy metabolism in ob/ob mice. Am J Physiol 255:R952–R960 (1988).

Wu AH. Mechanism of interferences for gas chromatography/mass spectrometry analysis of urine for drugs of abuse. Ann Clin Lab Sci 25:319–329 (1995).

Yen JT, Mersmann HJ, Nienaber JA, Hill DA, and Pond WG. Responses to cimaterol in genetically obese and lean pigs. J Anim Sci 68:2698–2706 (1990).

Yoon JM and Lee KH. Gas chromatographic and mass spectrometric analysis of conjugated steroids in urine. J Biosci 26:627–634 (2001).

Yoshimura T, Kurita C, Nagao T, Usami E, Nakao T, Watanabe S, et al. Inhibition of tumor necrosis factor-alpha and interleukin-1-beta production by beta-adrenoceptor agonists from lipopolysaccharide-stimulated human peripheral blood mononuclear cells. Pharmacol 54:144–152 (1997).

Websites

www.musclesurf.com
www.teenbodybuilding.com
www.vermontnutrition.com

PART VI
Legal Aspects

Chapter 15

Drug Interaction Litigation

Stephen A. Brunette, PC

1. OVERVIEW

This chapter provides an overview of theories of liability and defenses that have emerged in drug interaction litigation in recent years, in a "case study" format. It includes exemplary civil cases filed by individuals against physicians (Subheading 2), pharmacists (Subheading 3), and drug manufacturers (Subheading 4), and by a physician against a drug manufacturer (Subheading 5). Exemplary cases of judicial scrutiny of forensic evidence of causation in drug interaction litigation are also reviewed (Subheading 6). Cases that do not involve drug interactions are not within the scope of this chapter.

Drug interaction law varies among jurisdictions, and within jurisdictions over time. Accordingly, the reader is advised to consult local counsel to ascertain the law applicable to a particular case in which the reader may be involved.

2. ACTIONS AGAINST PHYSICIANS

A civil action against a physician based on an injury allegedly caused by an adverse drug interaction must establish that the physician owed a particular duty to the plaintiff, the standard of care that governed fulfillment of that duty, that the physician breached that duty, and that the breach of duty was the cause in fact and proximate cause of the plaintiff's injury.

A physician may be found negligent for prescribing drugs that he knows to have potentially adverse interaction effects, failing to monitor a patient after prescribing such drugs, and failing to warn the patient of the potential adverse interaction effects. In *Whittle v. United States,* 669 F. Supp. 501 (D DC 1987), for example, a patient went to an Army medical center for treatment of headaches and depression. She was seen

From: *Handbook of Drug Interactions: A Clinical and Forensic Guide*
A. Mozayani and L. P. Raymon, eds. © Humana Press Inc., Totowa, NJ

by a psychiatric resident, who diagnosed various psychological disorders and possible migraine headaches. He prescribed Nardil, an antidepressant monoamine oxidase inhibitor (MAOI), and Fiorinal, a barbiturate consisting of butalbital, caffeine, and aspirin. She died of butalbital poisoning after a few months on these prescriptions.

The decedent's husband filed a medical malpractice action. The undisputed evidence established that MAOIs interfere with the ability of the liver to metabolize barbiturates, allowing the barbiturates to remain in the bloodstream at high levels for a longer period of time; that as a result of this "prolongation" effect, taking Nardil in combination with a barbiturate such as Fiorinal increases the possibility that a second, supplemental ingestion of Fiorinal will push the barbiturate level in the blood to toxic levels; and that the MAOI can convert the nontoxic Fiorinal regimen into a potentially toxic one. The evidence also showed that because of the "prolongation" or "potentiation" effect, the pharmacological literature recommends that barbiturates should be administered at a reduced dose when taken concurrently with Nardil.

The defendant physician's records showed that he was aware of the potential adverse interaction effects of Nardil and Fiorinal, but he testified that his intention was to discontinue the Fiorinal when the Nardil reached therapeutic levels. The evidence established that the physician had not informed the patient of potential adverse interaction effects of these drugs, and was negligent in continuing to prescribe large volumes of Fiorinal to the decedent at a time when she was also taking Nardil, and in failing to take any steps to reduce or to monitor the decedent's usage of Fiorinal at a time when she was taking a maximum or near maximum daily dose of Nardil.

A physician may not have a duty to warn of risks of possible drug interactions that are unproven, or where the likelihood of the risk occurring is extremely remote. In *Jones v. United States,* 933 F. Supp. 894 (N.D. Cal. 1996), for example, a husband and wife filed a wrongful birth action against the United States under the Federal Tort Claims Act, seeking costs and damages associated with raising their daughter, alleging that the child was born because U.S. Army doctors negligently failed to warn the mother that Penicillin-VK, prescribed prophylactically prior to oral surgery, could interfere with the effectiveness of her Triphasil-28 birth control pills.

The plaintiffs offered expert testimony of two expert witnesses—a board-certified obstetrician-gynecologist and a pharmacist—to show that penicillin interferes with the effectiveness of the birth control pills. Following a *Daubert* hearing, the court ruled their testimony inadmissible. (*See* Subheading 6, below, for a detailed discussion of this court's *Daubert* analysis.)

Concerning the defendant physicians' duty, the court reasoned that, under California law, a physician has a duty of reasonable disclosure of the available choices with respect to a proposed therapy and of the dangers inherently and potentially involved, but this duty does not require the physician to conduct a "mini course in medical science" or to discuss "the relatively minor risks inherent in common procedures, when it is common knowledge that such risks inherent in the procedure are of very low incidence." The physician must disclose any known risks of death or serious bodily injury, must explain in lay terms the complications that might possibly occur, and must disclose "such additional information as a skilled practitioner of good standing would provide under similar circumstances." Expert testimony as to the standard of care in this case led the court to conclude that, because the existence of the alleged drug interaction is unproven and its likelihood extremely remote, the standard of care in Monterey County in 1992 did not require a warning in the extremely common practice of prescribing antibiotics.

See also Crisostomo v. Stanley, 857 F.2d 1146 (7th Cir. 1988) (action allowed to proceed against physician who prescribed Zyloprim where physician failed to advise patient to discontinue use if adverse reaction occurred; action against manufacturer dismissed where plaintiff failed to establish that manufacturer knew of drug's danger; evidence suggested that Zyloprim may cause skin rash independently or in interaction with ampicillin).

Where there is no specific contraindication for a possible adverse drug interaction on the manufacturer's label, the physician may have a viable defense to an action based on an alleged failure to warn. In *Silves v. King,* 970 P.2d 790 (Wash. App. 1999), an emergency room physician prescribed indomethacin, a nonsteroidal antiinflammatory drug, to a patient for treatment of gouty arthritis in his toe. The physician knew the patient was also taking heparin, an anticoagulant, for blood clotting problems, and that the Physician's Desk Reference (PDR) advises caution when prescribing indomethacin to patients with coagulation defects. The PDR contained no specific contraindication for prescribing both indomethacin and heparin. Approximately 2 wk after taking both drugs, the patient suffered pulmonary hemorrhage and was thereafter unable to return to work. A jury found the physician had not violated the standard of care in prescribing both drugs. The jury did find, however, that the physician had failed to obtain the patient's informed consent, but that her failure to obtain informed consent was not the proximate cause of the patient's injury. The verdict in favor of the physician was affirmed on appeal.

In addition to possible civil litigation for negligence in prescribing drugs with potential adverse interaction effects, a physician's license to practice medicine may be revoked under appropriate circumstances. In *Johnson v. State Medical Board of Ohio,* 1999 Ohio App LEXIS 4487 (Ohio App 1999), a physician admitted that he had, over the years, developed a style of practice that incorporated a "poly-pharmacy" approach to the prescription of medication, in which he would prescribe two narcotic analgesics, generally from different schedules, for patients with complaints of pain who he "was sure" were not drug abusers. He testified that he instructed the patients to use the medications only as needed for comfort and to use the lower scheduled drug when possible. He believed that his patients abided by his instructions, took the medications only as needed, and did not abuse the medications.

The medical board's expert testified that the practice of "poly-pharmacy" is not appropriate; that there is no justification for prescribing narcotic analgesics and benzodiazepines concurrently due to the risk of additive central nervous system depressant effects; that when prescribing two narcotics with the intention that the drugs be used alternatively, a physician should not prescribe a complete renewal of both prescriptions; that there is little therapeutic benefit in prescribing two narcotics over a long period of years; that a physician should prescribe narcotic medications for a diagnosis of chronic pain only after the physician has done everything that can be done in a diagnostic, therapeutic, and curative sense and has documented the results; and that abrupt termination of narcotic and benzodiazepine medications, after having been maintained on those medications for years, is dangerous because the patient may have become either physically and/or psychologically addicted to the medications.

The hearing examiner issued a report containing a detailed patient-by-patient summary of the facts concerning the medical care provided by the physician, and a patient-by-patient summary of the testimony of the physician and the board's expert. The examiner concluded that the physician had demonstrated a "reckless and unjustifiable disregard" of his patients' obvious drug-seeking behavior, alcohol abuse, depression, and suicidal tendencies, and had disregarded the advice and concerns of consultants, specialists, psychiatrists, psychologists, and family members. The examiner also concluded that the physician had prescribed medications that may have caused or exacerbated the symptoms he was treating, and failed to perform diagnostic workups to determine the cause of his patients' problems and/or to seek a cure for them. The examiner rejected the physician's testimony that he had prescribed multiple controlled substances based on his deep concern with his patients' well-being, noting that despite the fact that he had maintained the patients on multiple narcotic analgesics and multiple benzodiazepines for many years, he abruptly discontinued those medications without explanation and without considering that the patients may have become either physically and/or psychologically addicted to the medications. The examiner also noted that when patients complained of symptoms that may have been indicative of serious withdrawal, the physician neither evaluated the patients nor attempted to minimize the effects of withdrawal. The examiner recommended revocation of the physician's license to practice medicine; the board accepted this recommendation and revoked his license; the court of appeals affirmed the revocation. *See also Clausing v. State,* 955 P.2d 394 (Wash. App. 1998) (license revocation affirmed; physician negligently prescribed legend drugs for other than legitimate or therapeutic purposes).

3. ACTIONS AGAINST PHARMACISTS

There are three basic views that govern civil litigation against pharmacists in jurisdictions in the United States. One view is that pharmacists have no duty to warn their customers of potential adverse drug interactions, and are shielded from liability under the "learned intermediary" doctrine (Subheading 3.1). Another view is that pharmacists have duties to their customers to the extent that they voluntarily undertake such duties (Subheading 3.2). The third view is that pharmacists, like physicians, have a duty to exercise ordinary care in accord with the standard of care for their profession, and are subject to civil liability for breaching that duty (Subheading 3.3).

3.1. No Duty to Warn: Learned Intermediary Doctrine

Several jurisdictions hold that a retail pharmacy has no general duty to warn a customer or the customer's physicians of potential adverse prescription drug interactions. The case frequently cited as the leading authority for this view—though not a drug interaction case—is *McKee v. American Home Products Corp.,* 782 P.2d 1045 (Wash. 1989). The court affirmed a summary judgment in favor of a pharmacist, where the plaintiff had not filed an affidavit by a pharmacist who knew standards of practice and care applicable to pharmacists in the state of Washington, to support his claim that a pharmacist had a duty to warn a customer of adverse side effects of long-term administration of Plegine, an appetite suppressant. The court held that because the requisite affidavit had not been filed, there were no issues of material fact concerning the pharmacist's duty to warn, and summary judgment was therefore appropriate.

15. Drug Interaction Litigation

The court went beyond its narrow holding, discussed the law of several jurisdictions concerning the duty of a pharmacist to warn of adverse effects of drugs dispensed by the pharmacist, adopted the learned intermediary doctrine for application to pharmacists, and issued an advisory ruling that a pharmacist has a duty to accurately fill a prescription and to be alert for clear errors or mistakes in a prescription, but has no duty to question the judgment of a physician or to warn customers of hazardous side effects of prescription drugs, either orally or by providing the manufacturer's package insert. The dissent would have remanded for trial, and for jury determination of whether the pharmacist's conduct violated the standard of care for pharmacists, as specified in state statutes, regulations, and an affidavit filed by the plaintiff's nonpharmacist medical expert.

Various jurisprudential rationales for applying the learned intermediary doctrine to pharmacists were summarized recently by the Massachusetts Supreme Court in *Cottam v. CVS Pharmacy,* 764 N.E.2d 814 (Mass. 2002). The court reasoned that the physician has superior knowledge of the patient's medical history and unique condition, and is therefore in a better position than a pharmacist to decide which information is most pertinent to a particular patient; that imposing a duty to warn on pharmacists would place too heavy a burden on them by requiring that they retain and catalog every document received concerning a drug, and assure that each document is distributed with the drug; that requiring the pharmacist to provide warnings may cause "risk-averse" pharmacists to institute a policy of warning a customer of all known risks, even minute or unproven risks, which might overwhelm a patient into deciding not to take a medication prescribed by a physician; that pharmacists do not choose which products to make available to consumers, and patients do not choose which products to buy; and that a pharmacist does not have discretion to alter or refuse to fill a prescription because the risks and benefits of that prescription for that particular patient have already been weighed by the physician.

The doctrine was applied in *Silves v. King,* 970 P.2d 790 (Wash. App. 1999), in which an emergency room physician prescribed indomethacin, a nonsteroidal antiinflammatory drug, to a patient for treatment of gouty arthritis in his toe. The physician knew the patient was also taking heparin, an anticoagulant, for blood-clotting problems, and that the PDR advises caution when prescribing indomethacin to patients with coagulation defects. A pharmacist employed by the hospital dispensed the prescription, and testified that if she had known the patient was also taking heparin she would have called the physician, but would have dispensed the prescription if the physician advised her to do so, because there were no specific contraindications for taking indomethacin with heparin. Approximately 2 wk after taking both drugs, the patient suffered pulmonary hemorrhage and was thereafter unable to return to work. Citing *McKee v. American Home Products Corp.,* 782 P.2d 1045 (Wash. 1989), the court of appeals in *Silves* ruled that the pharmacist had no duty to warn the patient of possible adverse interaction effects of indomethacin and heparin, or to consult with the physician, because there were no specific contraindications for taking both drugs.

In *Johnson v. Walgreen Co.,* 675 So.2d 1036 (Fla. 1st D.C.A. 1996), the decedent suffered from several health problems, had several physicians who prescribed various medications to him, and died of multiple drug toxicity. His widow sued the pharmacy that filled the prescriptions, alleging negligence in failing to warn of adverse drug interactions. The court dismissed the complaint on grounds that the pharmacy's sole duty was to accurately and properly fill all lawful prescriptions, and that it had no duty to warn of potential adverse drug interactions.

The plaintiff in *Johnson* also argued that there was a private right of action against the pharmacist under a state licensing statute that requires pharmacists, in dispensing a prescription, to assess the prescription for potential adverse reactions and interactions with other drugs, and to provide counseling to persons receiving prescriptions if, in the exercise of professional judgment, such counseling is necessary. The court declined to find a private right of action under the statute, but observed that a pharmacist is in a unique position to maintain a comprehensive record of all medications prescribed to a patient, regardless of the number of physicians who may be prescribing medications for the patient, and that recent trends in federal and state regulatory law do require pharmacists to screen for possible drug interactions. The court concluded that it is for legislatures, not courts, to create a private right of action against a pharmacist for negligence in failing to warn of potential adverse drug interactions of which the pharmacist has knowledge. *Johnson, supra.*

See also Morgan v. WalMart Stores, Inc., 30 S.W.2d 455 (Tex. App. 2000) (acknowledging that pharmacist's role has changed from mere dispenser of medications to professional with vital role in patient treatment, that modern pharmacies use computer systems that can analyze drug interactions and contraindications in seconds, and that pharmacists may undertake to warn customers of same, but holding that under the learned intermediary doctrine, pharmacists have no legal duty to warn of potential adverse effects of prescription medications, absent special circumstances not present in case).

If a pharmacy has actual knowledge of a customer's allergies, and that the prescription in question is likely to have adverse effects on the customer, the learned intermediary doctrine may be inapplicable, and the pharmacy may have a duty to warn a customer and his physician of possible adverse effects of the prescription. *See Happel v. WalMart Stores, Inc.,* 766 N.E.2d 1118 (Ill. 2002).

3.2. Voluntary Undertaking

The general rule that a pharmacist owes no duty to warn of possible adverse drug interactions may not apply if the pharmacy voluntarily undertakes to monitor possible drug interactions in filling prescriptions.

The "voluntary undertaking" theory of liability may, for example, impose a duty on the pharmacy to exercise reasonable care in the implementation of a system adopted to monitor drug interactions, and subject the pharmacy to liability for negligence, fraud, and violation of a state consumer protection statute. *See, generally,* Restatement (Second) of Torts, §§323, 324A (1965). In *Baker v. Arbor Drugs, Inc.,* 544 N.W.2d 727 (Mich. App. 1996), the Michigan Court of Appeals reversed a summary judgment entered in favor of a pharmacy, and remanded for trial of the plaintiff's claims that the pharmacy and one of its pharmacists were negligent in the use of a prescription computer system that the pharmacy advertised would detect drug interactions. The patient had been taking Parnate (a monoamine oxidase inhibitor), and was prescribed Ceftin (an antibiotic) and Tavist-D (a decongestant) for treatment of a cold. The pharmacist who filled the prescription testified that the computer system had detected a possible drug interaction, as indicated by the appearance of the letter "I" next to the price on the prescription label for the Tavist-D, but that she had not personally seen the report of the drug interaction because a pharmacy technician overrode the computer system. The pharmacist testified further that she knew that Parnate and Tavist-D should not be taken together, and had she known that the patient was taking Parnate, she would not have filled the prescription for the Tavist-D. The court reasoned that the pharmacy had voluntarily assumed a duty to monitor drug interactions in the prescriptions it filled by implementing the computer system, and advertising to the general public that its computer system would detect harmful drug interactions for its customers. In assuming this duty, the pharmacy is held to a standard of due care in the implementation of the system, and it was for a jury to determine whether the pharmacy breached this duty and was, therefore, negligent under the circumstances. The court also ruled that the case could go to trial on the claims under the Michigan Consumer Protection Act, and for fraud.

See also *Sanderson v. Eckerd Corporation,* 780 So.2d 930 (Fla. App. 2001) (adopted "voluntary undertaking" theory in action against pharmacy alleging negligent use of advertised drug interaction system).

Even under the "voluntary undertaking" theory, however, the extent of the pharmacist's duty will be limited to the extent of the undertaking. In *Frye v. Medicare-Glaser Corporation,* 605 N.E. 2d 557 (Ill. 1992), a decedent's estate alleged that a pharmacy and pharmacist negligently undertook to warn the decedent of the dangers of combining his prescription for Fiorinal with alcohol. The pharmacy's computer system generated suggestions for discretionary warnings that a pharmacist may place on the prescription container, and here suggested three warning labels—one to warn about drowsiness, another to warn about the use of alcohol with the drug, and a third to warn about impairment of the ability to drive. The pharmacist who filled the prescription testified that she knew of possible adverse effects of the interaction of alcohol and Fiorinal, but she did not include a warning about these effects because she thought the label would offend people and cause them to drink, and she had been "chewed out" in the past for placing this label on prescription containers.

The Illinois Pharmacists Association and the National Association of Boards of Pharmacy filed *Amicus Curiae* briefs in the case, urging the Illinois Supreme Court to impose an affirmative duty on pharmacists to counsel consumers on the dangerous effects of prescription drugs, and arguing that the "learned intermediary" doctrine, which generally imposes the duty to warn on physicians, should not prevent the Court from also imposing a duty to warn on pharmacists. The Court declined to address this issue in its ruling, because neither party had argued for the imposition of such a duty. The Court ruled that the pharmacists' duty was limited to the extent of their undertaking, which in this case consisted only of placing a warning that the prescription may cause drowsiness. The Court declined to rule that the pharmacy had undertaken a duty to warn of all possible interaction effects by using a computer system that warned of only some possible interaction effects, but did not warn of other possible interaction effects with, e.g., aspirin, caffeine, or barbiturates, and other central nervous system depressants. The Court reasoned that if it imposed a broad duty to warn under the "voluntary undertaking" theory, pharmacies might choose to provide no warnings rather than risk being found negligent in providing incomplete warnings, and this would not support a public policy of encouraging pharmacies to undertake to provide warnings.

The court reasoned further that consumers should rely principally on the prescribing physician to warn of all possible drug interaction effects, not on their pharmacies. A dissenting opinion in the case would not have restricted the "voluntary undertaking" theory in this manner, and would have allowed the case to go to trial on the issue of negligence.

Defining the scope of the duty assumed by a pharmacy under the "voluntary undertaking" theory is a fact-specific inquiry, based on the totality of the pharmacy's communications with the patient, and the patient's reasonable understanding, based on those communications, of what the pharmacy has undertaken to provide. Providing a label containing a single warning of a single risk may not be reasonably construed as an undertaking to warn of all adverse effects, but where a pharmacy provides a detailed list of warnings, contraindications, or possible adverse interactions—or by way of advertising promises a consumer that it will provide such information—the pharmacy may he found to have a duty to provide a comprehensive list of possible adverse drug interactions. *See Cottam v. CVS Pharmacy,* 764 N.E.2d 814 (Mass. 2002).

Expert testimony may not be necessary to establish the extent of a pharmacy's undertaking, or negligence in failing to warn of possible adverse drug interactions, where the pharmacist's specialized or technical knowledge or performance are not at issue. Where the issues involve only whether a pharmacy made representations that would be deemed an undertaking of a duty to warn, or whether the warning was understandable by a reasonable person, a jury may be allowed to determine these issues without the assistance of expert testimony. *See Cottam v. CVS Pharmacy,* 764 N.E.2d 814 (Mass. 2002).

3.3. Reasonable Care Required

An increasing number of jurisdictions are holding pharmacists to the professional standard of care that applies to any profession. In *Lasley v. Shrake's Country Club Pharmacy, Inc.,* 880 P.2d 1129 (Ariz. 1994), the Arizona Supreme Court reversed a trial court's ruling that a pharmacy has no duty to warn as a matter of law, and ruled that a pharmacy owes its customers a duty of reasonable care to warn of potential adverse drug interactions. The patient had been prescribed Doriden and codeine for approximately 30 yr, received his prescriptions from the defendant pharmacy for approximately 10 yr, and eventually required in-patient hospitalization for Doriden detoxification, and psychiatric treatment for addiction, major clinical depression, and related disorders. He and his family complained that the pharmacy owed a duty of reasonable care in, *inter alia,* advising customers and physicians of potential adverse drug interactions, and relied on an affidavit of an expert and standards of the American Pharmaceutical Association Standards of Practice for the Profession of Pharmacy, to show that the standard of care for pharmacists includes a duty to advise customers of the highly addictive nature of prescribed drugs, and of the hazards of ingesting two or more drugs that adversely interact with one another. The trial court dismissed the complaint, on grounds that a pharmacy has no such duty.

The Arizona Supreme Court reviewed authority from the majority of jurisdictions, which hold that a pharmacy has no duty to warn, under various factual circumstances. The Court rejected this majority view, reasoning that it misconstrues the relationship between "standard of care" and "duty" in tort law, in that it first determines details of the standard of conduct for pharmacies, and then concludes that a duty to warn does not exist. The Court reasoned that the threshold question is, instead, whether a duty exists as a matter of law. If the court finds that a duty exists, the second inquiry is whether a defendant who owed a duty to a plaintiff violated the standard of conduct applicable to the field.

Applied to the facts in the case, the court ruled as a matter of law that a pharmacy owes a duty of reasonable care to its customers, and found that the evidence presented to the trial court—consisting of the affidavit and standards described above—was sufficient to raise a question of fact as to whether the pharmacy violated the standard of care in failing to warn its customer of potential adverse interactions and addiction.

Similarly, in *Dooley v. Revco Discount Drug Centers, Inc.,* 805 S.W.2d 380 (Tenn. App. 1990), a 5-yr-old, who had been taking Theophylline for 2 yr for treatment of asthma, was prescribed erythromycin by the same physician, and the prescription was filled by the same pharmacy. The erythromycin package insert warned of possible theophylline toxicity in patients prescribed erythromycin, and advised that theophylline dosages be reduced if erythromycin is prescribed. The pharmacy did not warn the plaintiffs of this possible interaction, and the pharmacist who filled the prescription testified that he was not aware of it. The patient suffered cerebral seizures as a result of toxic levels of theophylline after the erythromycin was introduced.

The plaintiff introduced an affidavit and testimony of an expert pharmacist, who stated that the standard of care for pharmacists in the locale required them to maintain a patient profile and alert a patient and his physician when a prescription is ordered for a drug that may adversely interact with another prescription of the patient, and that there exists computer technology that allows pharmacists to identify potential adverse drug interactions, and specifically the adverse interaction between theophylline and erythromycin. The court ruled that this evidence raised a question of fact as to whether the pharmacy owed a duty to its customers, including the plaintiff, to discover and warn of potential adverse drug interactions, and ordered the case to go to trial.

In *Horner v. Spolito,* 1 S.W.3rd 519 (Mo. App. 1999), a pharmacist filled two prescriptions for a customer—one for 50 750-mg doses of Placidyl, a strong hypnotic drug, which the prescribing physician instructed to be taken once every 8 h; the other for 50 10-mg doses of diazepam, a central nervous system depressant, which the prescribing physician instructed to be taken once every 8 h. Before filling the prescriptions, the pharmacist consulted Facts and Comparisons, an authoritative pharmacy manual, which indicated that the normal dose for Placidyl was one 500-mg dose or one 750-mg dose before bedtime. The manual also warned that the drug's effects were enhanced when combined with other central nervous system drugs, such as diazepam.

Concerned about the prescribing physician's instructions, the pharmacist called his office and was told the prescription was "okay" because the patient "needed to be sedated throughout the day." The pharmacist filled the prescriptions; the patient was found dead 6 d later; the autopsy revealed that death was caused by multiple medications, especially Placidyl (ethchlorvynol), which was "near the toxic range."

The trial court granted summary judgment in favor of the pharmacist, ruling that he owed no duty to the patient other than to properly fill a legal prescription that had no discrepancies on its face. The Missouri Court of Appeals reversed and remanded for trial, ruling that a pharmacist—like any other professional—has a duty to exercise the care and prudence that a reasonably careful and prudent pharmacist would exercise under the circumstances, and it is up to the jury to determine whether a pharmacist breached that duty in a particular case. That duty may require only that the pharmacist properly fill a legal prescription in some cases, but in others it may require the pharmacist to do more to protect customers from risk that the pharmacist can reasonably foresee. The court relied on state law governing the practice of pharmacy (Mo. Rev. Stat. §338.010.1), and state and federal law and regulations that require a pharmacist to offer to discuss with each customer or his physician the safe and effective use of a prescription drug, based on the pharmacist's education, experience, and review of available information about the drug and the patient. The court noted that the federal Omnibus Budget Reconciliation Act of 1990 required states to establish standards for pharmacists to provide such counseling to customers and prescribing physicians. *See* Kenneth R. Baker, *The OBRA 90 Mandate and Its Developing Impact on the Pharmacist's Standard of Care*, 44 Drake L. Rev. 503 (1996).

See also Happel v. Wal-Mart Stores, Inc., 766 N.E.2d 1118 (Ill. 2002) (pharmacy may have duty to warn of possible adverse reactions where pharmacy has actual knowledge of customer's condition and that prescription is contraindicated).

Compare, Morgan v. WalMart Stores, Inc., 30 S.W.2d 455 (Tex. App. 2000) (acknowledging that pharmacist's role has changed from mere dispenser of medications to professional with vital role in patient treatment, that modern pharmacies use computer systems that can analyze drug interactions and contraindications in seconds, and that pharmacists may undertake to warn customers of same, but holding that under learned intermediary doctrine, pharmacists have no legal duty to warn of potential adverse effects of prescription medications, absent special circumstances not present in case).

A pharmacist may, of course, have a duty to warn of interaction effects if the pharmacist prescribes the remedy. In a case from the archives, *Fuhs v. Barber,* 36 P.2d 962 (Kan. 1934), a physician had prescribed a lead-based ointment for treatment of a skin irritation. When the patient returned to the pharmacist for a refill, the pharmacist recommended a sulphur-based ointment he had invented. The plaintiff's skin turned black from the reaction of the lead and sulphur. The Kansas Supreme Court held the pharmacist had a duty to warn of the possible interaction.

4. ACTIONS AGAINST PHARMACEUTICAL MANUFACTURERS

If a pharmaceutical manufacturer has complied with federal legislative and regulatory requirements for testing and labeling a drug, and if the label provides adequate warnings of all known potential adverse interaction effects, the manufacturer may be shielded from liability under the learned intermediary doctrine (Subheading 4.1). If the manufacturer has been negligent in the testing, manufacturing, or marketing of the drug, the manufacturer may be liable to a consumer for this negligence or strict liability (Subheading 4.2). Where circumstances warrant, a manufacturer may face challenges under various other theories of liability, such as breach of implied warranty, breach of express warranty, fraud, negligent misrepresentation, fraud by concealment, civil conspiracy, and concert in action (Subheading 4.3). Theories of liability are typically incorporated in a single action, and variations in state law may produce different legal tests, and different outcomes under similar circumstances. The following discussion is not intended to explain peculiarities of state law in these areas. Rather, it reports the law as stated in the drug interaction cases within the scope of this chapter. The reader is advised to seek local counsel in the jurisdiction in which an action is filed for a review of the law applicable to the action.

4.1. Learned Intermediary

In *Eck v. Parke, Davis & Co.*, 256 F.3d 1013 (10th Cir. 2001), a patient and his family filed a product liability action against the manufacturers of two prescription drugs —Isocet and Dilantin. The plaintiff's physician had prescribed Isocet to the patient to treat his complaints of tension headaches in 1994 and 1995. In 1997, the patient was referred to an epilepsy specialist who prescribed Dilantin to control the patient's seizures. The first physician was involved in administering and monitoring the levels of Dilantin. While taking the Dilantin, the patient experienced a tension headache and took two Isocet tablets from his earlier prescription, and shortly thereafter was diagnosed with acute liver failure. The epilepsy specialist testified that she was aware of the medical risk of the interaction of Isocet and Dilantin, but still would have prescribed Dilantin because of the greater risk posed by the patient's seizures. The court held that the plaintiffs failed to controvert this testimony, that the defendant manufacturers were shielded from liability under the "learned intermediary doctrine," and that any failure to warn on the part of the defendants was therefore not the proximate cause of Mr. Eck's liver failure.

The plaintiffs had alleged that the defendant manufacturers had failed to label their products with adequate warnings of Dilantin's propensity to interact with acetaminophen, placed defective and unreasonably dangerous products in the marketplace that caused Mr. Eck's liver failure, and were negligent in the designing, testing, warning, and marketing of their products through their failure to provide adequate instructions or warnings, and by misrepresenting the safety of their products when used in conjunction with one another.

Applying Oklahoma law, the court reasoned that, in order to recover in a failure to warn case against a drug manufacturer, a plaintiff must establish both cause-in-fact (that the product in question caused the injury) and proximate cause (that the manufacturer of the product breached a duty to warn of possible detrimental reactions, and this breach was a substantial contributing factor in causing the harm). Under Restatement (Second) Torts § 402A comment K, certain products, including prescription drugs, are "unavoidably unsafe products" that cannot be made completely safe, but serve a public benefit, so drug manufacturers cannot be held strictly liable merely because of the dangerous propensities of their products. Although the manufacturer has a duty to warn ultimate consumers of known dangers of prescription drugs and their interactions, there is an exception to this duty—the "learned intermediary doctrine"—under which the manufacturer is shielded from liability where the product is properly prepared and marketed and proper warning is given to prescribing physicians. The prescribing physician acts as a learned intermediary between the patient and the prescription drug manufacturer by assessing the medical risks in light of the patient's needs.

See also Ashman v. SK&F Lab Co., 72 F. Supp. 1401 (N.D. Ill. 1988) (learned intermediary doctrine shielded manufacturer from liability for injury resulting from physician's failure to warn of possible adverse interaction of Tagamet and Halcion; manufacturer's label included warning of possible adverse interaction); *Cottam v. CVS Pharmacy,* 764 N.E.2d 814 (Mass. 2002) (learned intermediary doctrine is exception to general rule that manufacturer or retailer of unavoidably dangerous product must directly warn all foreseeable consumers of dangers of its product; rationale for doctrine is that physicians have duty to inform themselves about drug and warn patients of dangers they deem necessary and relevant for patients to make informed decision; requiring manufacturer to provide warnings directly to consumer would interfere with doctor–patient relationship); *Singleton v. Airco, Inc.,* 314 S.E. 2d 680 (Ga. App. 1984) (though not invoking learned intermediary doctrine, court ruled that manufacturer has duty to warn only physician, and that warnings of risks of interaction of Anectine (succinylcholine chloride) and Ethrane (enflurane) were adequate; summary judgment in favor of manufacturers affirmed).

The learned intermediary doctrine may not shield a manufacturer from liability where the warning to the medical community was not timely, or was delayed for an unreasonable time after the manufacturer learned of the product defects. In *Linnen v. A. H. Robbins Company, Inc.,* 1999 Mass. Super LEXIS 552 (1999), the court declined to enter summary judgment in favor of the manufacturer of fen-phen (fenfluramine and phentermine) under the learned intermediary doctrine, where the evidence suggested that the manufacturer had actual knowledge of the risk of pulmonary hypertension associated with the drugs for more than 1 yr before it changed its package insert to advise physicians of this risk, and there was, accordingly, a question of fact as to whether the physician would have warned her patient of this risk before prescribing the drug. The patient died of pulmonary hypertension, allegedly as a result of using the drugs.

4.2. Negligence and Strict Liability

In *Bocci v. Key Pharmaceuticals, Inc.,* 974 P.2d 758 (Or. App. 1999), a patient who suffered permanent brain damage due to theophylline toxicity caused by interaction of theophylline (an asthma medication) and ciprofloxican (an antibiotic frequently prescribed to asthmatics for respiratory infections), filed an action against the physician who prescribed theophylline for negligence and failure to diagnose, and against the pharmaceutical company for negligence and strict products liability. The claim against the physician was dismissed; the claim against the pharmaceutical company was resolved at jury trial in favor of the patient. The findings of fact of the case are complex, but necessary for review in order to understand the court's disposition of the case.

The court in *Bocci* found that the drug theophylline is a bronchodilator that has been used to treat asthma for many decades. Theophylline has a narrow therapeutic range: in order to prevent asthma symptoms, the serum levels of the drug in the blood generally must be at least 10 µg/mL, but serum levels above 20 µg/mL can be toxic. Saturation kinetics play a part in the way in which this drug may be metabolized; when the level of the drug in the body increases but the liver's ability to metabolize it does not increase, or when the amount of the drug entering the body stays the same but the liver's ability to metabolize it decreases for some reason, saturation can occur. This causes the serum levels of theophylline in the blood to increase. The ability of a body to metabolize theophylline may be affected by many things, such as smoking or the presence of a virus. Interactions between theophylline and other drugs may cause a

15. Drug Interaction Litigation 611

body to metabolize theophylline at a slower rate, thus increasing the serum levels of theophylline in the blood and leading to theophylline toxicity. Theophylline toxicity can cause nausea, vomiting, headaches, diarrhea, tachycardia, seizures, and death.

Before the 1970s, theophylline therapy was difficult because a great deal of monitoring and adjustment of dosage was necessary to keep stable the amount of the drug in a patient's blood at any given time. In the 1970s, Key introduced a new theophylline product, Theo-Dur, a timed-release capsule that it claimed had zero-order absorption. Zero-order absorption occurs when a drug is constantly absorbed by the system and eliminated at the same rate, thus keeping the serum levels of the drug in the blood stable. Key promoted Theo-Dur as being safer than other theophylline products; because of its zero-rate absorption, Key claimed, the risk of "toxic peaks" could be avoided. Key aggressively promoted Theo-Dur to physicians through sales representatives, journal advertising, and direct-mail campaigns. Promotional materials also urged patients, physicians, and pharmacists not to accept generic or brand-name substitute theophylline products, as switching from Theo-Dur could cause "excessive toxicity." In 1987, the Food and Drug Administration (FDA) informed Key that it must cease claiming that Theo-Dur was superior to other theophylline products because of zero-order absorption, because the claim was not sufficiently supported by clinical data. In 1989, the FDA again found that Key was making false and misleading claims that Theo-Dur was superior to other theophylline products.

In October 1987, Key became aware of several medical journal articles reporting a drug interaction causing theophylline toxicity when both theophylline and ciprofloxacin, a newly available antibiotic often used to treat respiratory tract infections common among asthmatics, were administered. A Key internal memorandum dated October 30, 1987, stated: "Ciprofloxacin produces a 30–113% decrease in theophylline clearance. These effects are significant enough to cause a patient that is stabilized on theophylline to potentially become toxic." In March 1988, Key proposed to the FDA that a warning be added to its Theo-Dur package insert concerning the interaction between theophylline and ciprofloxacin. Key's application for the labeling change, however, was not submitted in proper form, and it was not until March 1989 that the labeling change was approved. The labeling change was not reflected in the 1990 volume of the PDR, although it was included in a May 1990 PDR supplement.

Information such as a warning about theophylline–ciprofloxacin interaction is generally imparted to the medical community by drug manufacturers through "Dear Doctor" and "Dear Pharmacist" letters or statograms, through promotional materials sent to physicians, or through representatives of pharmaceutical companies (detailers) who call on physicians. Federal regulations allow for distribution of such warnings to physicians before revised labeling is approved by the FDA, and also allow a pharmaceutical company to change its labeling without preauthorization from the FDA in order to add warnings, precautions, or information concerning adverse reactions.

Between October 1987, when Key became aware of the theophylline–ciprofloxacin interaction, and Bocci's injury in October 1990, Key took no steps to inform physicians or patients of this potential toxicity problem, although it knew of several cases of serious toxicity and one death caused by the interaction of theophylline and ciprofloxacin. During this period, Key continued to promote Theo-Dur as the only theophylline product that "protects against toxicity."

Bocci began taking Theo-Dur when he was 7 yr old. On October 21, 1990, when Bocci was 20 yr old, he went to a medical clinic for treatment of a skin rash and was treated by Dr. Davis. Bocci indicated to Dr. Davis that he was not taking any medications, although he was taking 900 mg of Theo-Dur a day. Dr. Davis prescribed ciprofloxacin for the skin rash; Bocci took both ciprofloxacin and Theo-Dur from October 21 to October 26, 1990. On October 27, 1990, Bocci went to an urgent care clinic with symptoms including nausea, vomiting, and diarrhea, and was seen by Dr. Edwards. Dr. Edwards discovered that Bocci had been on a stable dose of Theo-Dur for a long time, and, although he considered a diagnosis of theophylline toxicity, he did not diagnose that condition, and did not consult the PDR or the PDR supplement. Dr. Edwards did not think that a patient on a stable dose of Theo-Dur could experience severe theophylline toxicity that could lead to brain damage unless the patient had taken an overdose, because Theo-Dur had been marketed and promoted to him as a "safe" drug. The detailer who had promoted the drug to Dr. Edwards and clinic in 1989 and 1990 testified that he would routinely tell physicians that Theo-Dur had zero-order absorption and that it was safe.

Dr. Edwards testified that he did not make a connection between a patient on a stable dose of a safe drug such as Theo-Dur and a serious toxicity problem. He therefore diagnosed gastroenteritis, treated Bocci with antinausea medication and intravenous fluids, and then sent him home. Several hours later, Bocci had violent seizures and was taken to a hospital emergency room. Anticonvulsant medications were administered but failed to control the seizures, and the physicians attending him had difficulty diagnosing the cause of the seizures. Late that evening, after learning that Bocci had been taking asthma medication, they tested for theophylline toxicity and discovered that Bocci's theophylline level was 63 µg/mL, well into the toxic range. The theophylline was removed from Bocci's blood through dialysis and the seizures ceased, but Bocci suffered permanent brain damage as a result of the seizures.

A number of physicians testified about their knowledge and understanding of Theo-Dur as of October 1990, when Bocci sustained his injury. Those physicians did not know about the theophylline–ciprofloxacin interaction and did not know that patients stabilized on standard doses of Theo-Dur could experience toxicity problems causing severe seizures such as those experienced by Bocci. Those physicians did not know that blood levels of theophylline should be obtained on patients using theophylline products if the patients experienced nausea and vomiting.

On Bocci's claims, the jury returned a verdict finding that Key was 65% at fault and Bocci was 35% at fault. On Dr. Edwards' cross-claims, the jury found that Key was negligent and that Key's negligence caused Edwards' damages and found that Key had made fraudulent misrepresentations to Dr. Edwards that caused him damage. The jury further found that Key caused 100% of Dr. Edwards' damages. The jury also found clear and convincing evidence that Key had acted with wanton disregard for the health and safety of others and had knowingly withheld from or misrepresented to the FDA or prescribing physicians information known to be material and relevant to theophylline toxicity, in violation of applicable FDA regulations. The court entered a judgment in Bocci's favor including compensatory damages of $5,621,648.20 and punitive damages of $35 million, and in Dr. Edwards' favor for compensatory damages of $500,000 and $22.5 million in punitive damages.

Failure to comply with state or federal regulations governing the testing, manufacturing, and marketing of drugs may establish a prima facie case of negligence. *Batteast v. Wyeth Laboratories, Inc.,* 526 N.E.2d 428 (Ill. App. 1988) (the manufacturer was sued for negligence, strict liability, and willful and wanton conduct; physicians were sued for negligence and willful and wanton conduct). In *Batteast,* the defendant began manufacturing aminophylline suppositories in 1945, at which time correspondence from the FDA indicated that the suppositories would not be considered a new drug. The manufacturer received no written or verbal FDA approval following this correspondence, and introduced no other evidence that the drug was ever approved for safety. Prior to 1975, the defendants conducted two animal studies on the suppositories, and one human study of absorption rates of the suppositories with a cocoa butter base vs a hydrogenated base. The defendant ceased manufacturing the aminophylline suppositories in 1982, without ever having received FDA approval for marketing the drug and without ever having established the safety and efficacy of the drug, but continued to distribute aminophylline suppositories manufactured by another pharmaceutical company.

In 1972 and 1973, the FDA published two notices stating that aminophylline suppositories require an approved New Drug Application (NDA), and that it would be unlawful to ship suppositories that were not subject to an NDA. The defendant did not respond to these two notices. In 1974, the FDA published a third notice concerning the manufacturing and distribution of aminophylline suppositories, requiring submission of either an NDA or an ANDA (Abbreviated New Drug Application) by drug manufacturers. The defendant filed its first ANDA with the FDA for approval of its drug in response to this notice. The FDA replied to the application with a notice that biologic availability studies were required before the suppositories could be approved for marketing, and a suggestion that a research protocol be submitted prior to initiation of any studies. The defendant did not submit a protocol in response to this request, received a second request 1 yr later, became aware that its ANDA for the aminophylline suppositories would be rejected, but continued marketing the drug until its ANDA was officially rejected by the FDA in 1983. The court ruled that evidence of this chronology was admissible as proof of negligence under state law, which provided that violation of a statute or ordinance designed to protect human life or property is prima facie evidence of negligence. The court rejected the defendant's argument that the FDA regulations were not intended to protect the infant plaintiff. *Batteast v. Wyeth Laboratories, Inc.,* 526 N.E.2d 428 (Ill. App. 1988).

A drug may be deemed unreasonably dangerous because of the absence of an adequate warning or sufficient information accompanying the product, because the product may be "unavoidably unsafe" without such warning or information. *Batteast v. Wyeth Laboratories, Inc.,* 526 N.E.2d 428 (Ill. App. 1988) [*See* Restatement (Second) of Torts § 402A, comment k (1965)]. The determination as to the adequacy of warnings that are included in a package insert of a drug distributed to the medical profession is a question that is within the province of the trier of fact. In *Batteast,* the court found the evidence sufficient to support the plaintiffs' contention that a manufacturer's aminophylline suppositories were unreasonably dangerous due to the lack of adequate warnings accompanying the product. Numerous communications from the FDA concerning risks of the product, and requests that the manufacturer change its package insert to advise physicians of those risks, established that the manufacturer was aware of certain risks involved in administering aminophylline suppositories to children but failed to warn the medical profession of those risks. Specifically, the court found that the package insert failed to warn physicians of the following risks: (a) severe intoxication and death have followed rectal administration because of hypersensitivity or overdosage; (b) adverse reactions include circulatory failure and respiratory arrest; (c) absorption from rectal administration is unreliable and there is great variation from patient to patient in dosage needed in order to achieve a therapeutic blood level; (d) when prolonged or repeated use is planned, blood levels must be monitored to establish and maintain an individualized dosage; (e) toxic synergism may result when aminophylline is combined with other sympathomimetic bronchodilator drugs; (f) tonic and clonic convulsions are an adverse reaction to the use of aminophylline treatment; (g) indications of aminophylline poisoning are often masked by the patient's other symptoms; (h) no formal recommendation had ever been made concerning the advisability of cutting any dosage of an aminophylline suppository in half; and (i) enemas should be utilized for rectally administered overdosage.

The *Batteast* court reasoned further that full and complete disclosure concerning the potential adverse reactions of a drug is necessary to enable a health care provider to render an informed decision regarding utilization of the drug, and that in this case the lack of knowledge of these warnings seriously impaired the treating physician's ability to properly formulate a risk benefit analysis for the drug aminophylline, to determine whether aminophylline should be utilized, and to institute appropriate measures to ensure that the drug was used effectively and safely. The court concluded that the warnings contained in the package insert distributed with the defendant's aminophylline suppositories were clearly inadequate for the medical profession as a whole, and specifically for the plaintiff's physician.

Even if a drug is found to be unreasonably dangerous, its defective condition must be established to be a proximate cause of the injury before a plaintiff can recover. *Batteast v. Wyeth Laboratories, Inc.,* 526 N.E.2d 428 (Ill. App. 1988). A proximate cause of an injury is any cause that, in natural or probable sequence, produced the injury. It need not be the only cause, nor the last or nearest cause; it is sufficient if it concurs with some other cause acting at the same time, which in combination with it, causes the injury. In *Batteast,* the evidence supported a jury finding that the manufacturer's distribution of an inherently dangerous drug, without obtaining FDA approval and without providing instructions or warnings of possible adverse interaction effects, was the proximate cause of the plaintiff's injury. The treating physician testified that he would not have ordered the defendant's aminophylline suppositories for the infant plaintiff if he had been made aware of the risk of death to children from hypersensitivity to the drug, or if he had known of the potential dangers listed in the "Adverse Reactions" section of FDA guidelines that were not incorporated into the manufacturer's labeling. The physician testified further that when he was treating the infant, he was not aware of the patient-to-patient variation in absorption of aminophylline, and that if the manufacturer had alerted him to this fact, and of the difference in dosages necessary to achieve the therapeutic range, he would have been able to treat the infant with individual dosages monitored by blood studies. Under these circumstances, and the fact that other causes may have contributed to the infant's injury did not absolve the manufacturer of liability for its failure to market the drug in a safe condition through the utilization of adequate warnings, and a jury finding that the failure to provide such warnings was the proximate cause of the infant's injuries was reasonable. *Batteast v. Wyeth Laboratories, Inc.,* 526 N.E.2d 428 (Ill. App. 1988).

A manufacturer will not be liable if the plaintiff fails to establish that the defendant's drug was the proximate cause of the plaintiff's injury. In *Haggerty v. The Upjohn Company,* 950 F. Supp. 1160 (S.D. Fl. 1996), for example, the plaintiff failed to establish causation where the plaintiff's expert failed to rule out other possible causes of the plaintiff's behavior, including, *inter alia,* that the plaintiff's injuries—incurred when the plaintiff jumped from a balcony—may have been caused by the plaintiff's consumption of alcohol and an unknown number of Valium tablets, along with one tablet of Halcion manufactured by the defendant, before he jumped from the balcony. (*See* detailed discussion of the court's *Daubert* analysis in Subheading 6, below).

Causation will not be established of the evidence shows that the patient knew of the risk of adverse drug interaction, but consented to take the drug after having been informed of the risk. *See Eck v. Parke, Davis & Co.*, 256 F.3d 1013 (10th Cir. 2001) (evidence established that defendant's drugs interacted to cause a patient's liver failure, but manufacturer was not liable because evidence also established that patient was aware of risk of drug interaction but decided to take drug despite risk).

Where a person's death may have been caused by taking excessive doses of a combination of prescribed pain medications, the fact that the patient took excessive doses may not bar a plaintiff's recovery where the evidence establishes that it is not unusual for a patient in extreme pain to take more than the prescribed dosage, and that a physician may even have verbally advised the patient to take more then the prescribed dosage if necessary to alleviate the pain. In *Dean v. K-Mart Corp.,* 720 So.2d 349 (La. App. 1998), a patient died from respiratory failure due to the combination of prescribed opiates, benzodiaprezines and propoxyphene, which the patient was taking to alleviate the pain from a work-related injury. The court ruled that even if the patent were taking excessive doses, this would not break the causal chain between his work-related injury and his death from the prescribed medications. One caveat: this was a workers' compensation case, in which a claimant must establish causation but need not establish fault on the part of the defendant in order to receive benefits. It may have limited value as precedent in a tort case in which the plaintiff must establish both negligence and causation by a preponderance of the evidence.

4.3. Multiple Theories of Liability

A cluster of cases have challenged the manufacturer of Parlodel, a drug used to inhibit postpartum lactation, and Methergine, a drug used to reduce the size of the uterus and postpartum hemorrhage, in actions based, *inter alia,* on strict liability in tort, negligence, breach of implied warranty, breach of express warranty, fraud, negligent misrepresentation, fraud by concealment, civil conspiracy, concert in action, loss of consortium, and seek punitive damages based on the defendant's conduct. *See, e.g., Eve v. Sandoz Pharmaceutical Corp.*, 2001 U.S. Dist. LEXIS 4531 (S.D. Ind. 2001); *Globetti v. Sandoz Pharm. Corp.,* 111 F. Supp. 2d 1174, 1176 (N.D. Ala. 2000); *Glastetter v. Novartis Pharm.*, 107 F. Supp. 2d 1015 (E.D. Mo. 2000); *Brumbaugh v. Sandoz Pharm.*

Co., 77 F. Supp. 2d 1153 (D. Mont. 1999); *Hollander v. Sandoz Pharm. Corp.*, 95 F. Supp. 2d 1230, 1238-39 (W.D. Okla. 2000).

In each of these cases, the defendant filed pretrial motions in limine and requested *Daubert* hearings, to challenge the scientific reliability of the plaintiffs' evidence of medical causation. In some of these cases the defendants succeeded in striking the plaintiffs' medical and scientific evidence of causation (e.g., *Glastetter*; *Brumbaugh*; *Hollander*); in others, the trial court ruled the medical and scientific evidence admissible, and allowed the cases to go forward (e.g., *Eve; Globetti*). The evidence offered by both sides was essentially the same in all of the cases, and is summarized in detail in the context of the *Daubert* analyses in Subheading 6, below.

5. CROSS-CLAIMS BY PHYSICIANS OR PHARMACISTS AGAINST PHARMACEUTICAL MANUFACTURERS

In *Bocci v. Key Pharmaceuticals, Inc.*, 974 P.2d 758 (Or. App. 1999), the defendant physician filed a cross-claim against the defendant pharmaceutical manufacturer for negligence and fraud, where the manufacturer's promotions had endorsed its product, Theo-Dur (theophylline), as a safe drug; the promotions had been the subject of an FDA letter of adverse findings that advised the manufacturer to cease promoting the drug as safe, and there was other evidence that the company knew about adverse and fatal interactions between theophylline and ciprofloxacin that were not communicated to the physician. The physician claimed that the manufacturer's promotions were a substantial contributing factor to his failure to diagnose and treat the plaintiff's theophylline toxicity, and were therefore cause in fact and proximate cause of the plaintiff's brain injury that was caused by the misdiagnosis. This cross-claim resulted in a $23 million verdict for compensatory and punitive damages in favor of the physician. The $23 million award to the physician was upheld as not excessive in *Bocci v. Key Pharmaceuticals, Inc.*, 22 P.3d 758 (Or. App. 2001).

6. RELIABILITY OF FORENSIC EVIDENCE OF CAUSATION

The Parlodel/Methergine cases described in Subheading 4, above, provide an excellent example—taken as a whole—of the factors a trial court may consider in ruling on the admissibility of medical and scientific evidence of causation, and of the fact that cases with essentially the same facts may be resolved differently, depending on the manner in which a particular court exercises its discretion in ruling on the admissibility of medical and scientific evidence. The complex undisputed facts, as summarized by the *Eve* court, established as follows.

In the fall of 1989, the plaintiff—a healthy 29-yr-old woman with no obstetrical or other preexisting health problems—delivered a child by caesarean section, and was given a routine 3-d prescription for Methergine to stop postpartum hemorrhage. She had elected not to breast-feed her baby, so was also given a 2-wk prescription for Parlodel (an ergot alkaloid) to prevent lactation. She took the prescriptions simultaneously while in the hospital without incident, and was discharged with instructions to take the remaining Parlodel pills until the prescription was gone. She began experiencing severe headaches the day after discharge, took Tylenol (acetaminophen) without success, then tried Sudafed (pseudoephedrine), also without success.

One day later, "the really big pain came in," it "felt like there was some liquid started to run through the back of my head and it felt like somebody had a brick pounding it inside my head." She was admitted to the emergency room for treatment of the headache, presented as dysthartic, slightly confused, aphasic with right hemiparesis, blood pressure of 166/89, and a computed tomography (CT) scan revealed that she had suffered an intracerebral hemorrhage (ICH), or stroke.

A routine drug screen conducted on admission indicated the presence of pseudoephedrine and acetaminophen (which, in limited circumstances, can be vasoconstrictors and can elevate blood pressure) and caffeine. During her hospitalizations for the stroke and subsequent rehabilitation, several cerebral angiograms, magnetic resonance imaging (MRI), and CT scans revealed no evidence of alternative causes of her ICH— such as aneurysm, alteriol venous malformation (AVM), microemboli, or micotic emboli —so her physicians concluded that the etiology of the stroke was unknown.

The plaintiff's physician testified that both Parlodel and Methergine are considered to be vasoconstrictors, and opined to a reasonable degree of medical probability, based on the vasoconstrictive action of these drugs, that Parlodel and possibly the Methergine were contributing factors to her stroke, and that in a normal delivery, the postpartum period itself would not significantly increase the risk of stroke. Plaintiffs' experts—a physician and a toxicologist—had worked directly with Parlodel safety issues prior to any Parlodel litigation. The physician had served on the FDA when Parlodel was first approved for Parkinson's disease, and the toxicologist had researched the toxicology of Parlodel and published an article on the subject in a peer-reviewed journal. Using differential diagnosis, these experts ruled out, to a reasonable degree of medical certainty, alternative causes of her stroke other than Parlodel.

Concerning the pharmacology and history of Parlodel, it was undisputed that the active ingredient of Parlodel is bromocriptine mesylate ("bromocriptine"), one of several ergot alkaloids; it differs structurally and physically from other ergot alkaloids in that a bromine atom has been added; it prevents lactation from occurring by blocking the secretion of the hormone prolactin, which acts on the breasts to induce the secretion of milk; it is typically prescribed for 14 d for this purpose. It had been sold since 1978; the FDA had approved it in 1980 for use in preventing postpartum lactation in women who could not or elected not to breast-feed; the manufacturer withdrew the Parlodel indication for prevention of physiological lactation in 1994, after receiving notice that the FDA would be filing a notice of opportunity and hearing to withdraw Parlodel for that indication. Parlodel remained FDA approved at the time of trial for the treatment of Parkinson's disease, amenorrhea (absence of menses), galactorrhea (abnormal production of breast milk), and acromegaly (chronic hyperpituitarism).

Concerning the pharmacology and history of Methergine, it was undisputed that the active ingredient of Methergine is methylergonovine maleate, also an ergot alkaloid; it is vasoconstrictor that has been reported in some patients to cause immediate and transient elevations in blood pressure. Methergine had been sold by the defendant and used for routine management after delivery of the placenta, postpartum atony, postpartum hemorrhage, and postpartum subinvolution, since the late 1940s, and remained FDA approved for these purposes at the time of trial. There were no epidemiologic or controlled scientific studies showing an increased risk of stroke among patients of any type who take Methergine, either in conjunction with Parlodel or otherwise.

Concerning the Plaintiffs' claims alleging fraud, misrepresentation, and failures to warn, it was undisputed that the FDA reported problems among women receiving Parlodel in conjunction with other ergot derivatives such as Methergine in 1983, and suggested revisions in both the Adverse Reactions and Warnings sections of the defendant's package insert to include the reports of adverse reactions, as well as a statement regarding use of Parlodel in women who had already received or were receiving other ergot alkaloids. Specifically, an FDA Bulletin on December 1, 1983, discussed the adverse drug reactions (ADRs) reported to it regarding Parlodel taken with other ergots in a publication entitled "ADR Highlights," noting that "in the present bromocriptine labeling it may be difficult for the physician to identify bromocriptine as another ergot alkaloid," and that use of bromocriptine "with other ergot alkaloids as well as its use with vasoconstrictive drugs may represent a hazard to the postpartum women." It was also undisputed that in October 1983, the defendant received a doctoral thesis written by a French physician, Dr. Bousbacher, regarding the side effects of Parlodel in postpartum women. In March 1985, the FDA specifically requested that Parlodel should be "contraindicated" for women diagnosed with "toxemia of pregnancy" and for those who had also received other ergot alkaloids after delivery, including specifically, Methergine and Cafergot, and specifically instructed the defendant to make these revisions within 6 mo or by the next package insert printing, whichever came first.

The defendant refused to contraindicate Parlodel and other ergots in 1985 and for the entire period Parlodel was marketed for prevention of postpartum lactation. Within 1 wk of the FDA request, the defendant's marketing department was asked to quantify the use of Methergine or Ergotrate to determine the effect on sales of the FDA-requested contraindication with Parlodel. "The feeling among Marketing Management was that Methergine or Ergotrate was always used in delivery so that a contraindication would virtually wipe out Parlodel's use" in prevention of postpartum lactation. The defendant expected to generate $35 million in Parlodel sales for this use in 1985, and concluded at an internal meeting in 1985 that the Methergine/Cafergot-Parlodel contraindications request was "prejudicial" to the defendant "by naming two of [defendant's] products." The defendant replied to the FDA with an opposition to any revision of its labeling, but said it was willing to contraindicate use of Parlodel in women with "toxemia of pregnancy."

The FDA sought additional adverse reaction reports follow-up, reiterated its belief that the defendant was withholding information and substituting its interpretation of diagnoses for the treating physicians' diagnoses, approved a change in the Methergine package insert but requested a new revision to include a drug interaction subsection "with information about concurrent administration of other vasoconstrictors," such as Methergine. Some of the defendant's medical personnel urged that the Parlodel/Methergine contraindication be included in the package insert; the defendant's management deemed the labeling changes would be "catastrophic"; the final Methergine package insert never adopted the explicit language warning against the concomitant administration of Parlodel with Methergine.

The plaintiff's physician testified that his understanding regarding the recommendations for the concomitant use of ergot alkaloids was that "for any prolonged period of time, the two used together was not recommended," so he was not aware, in 1989, of any problem in prescribing Methergine for only 2 d along with Parlodel.

In 1987, at the FDA's request, the defendant updated the Parlodel package insert to include a reference to adverse effects such as seizure, stroke, and myocardial infarction (MI), and issued a "Dear Doctor" letter to inform physicians of the labeling changes. The FDA "did not like the appearance of the 'Dear Doctor' letter" and found that it "reflected" a "promotional tone." Further, an FDA physician did not receive a copy of the "Dear Doctor" letter, and "a canvas of ten ACOG [American College of Gynecologist] members attending [an FDA meeting] revealed that only one member recalled receiving the letter." The defendant commissioned a study in 1988 entitled "Physicians Reactions to a New Communication on the Use of Parlodel in Postpartum Lactation," which concluded that "Despite the previous mass mailing of a letter to OB/GYNs that described the remote possibility of serious side effects with patients who take Parlodel for postpartum lactation, this information did not reach a slight majority of the physicians in this study." The plaintiff's treating physician testified that he did not receive one.

The defendant aggressively marketed Parlodel throughout the late 1980s, and in 1987 issued an internal memo to its sales force explaining that although it had "modified the Parlodel package insert," the sales representatives were instructed: "Remember, this issue should not be mentioned unless a discussion is initiated by the physician." One of the defendant's sales representatives testified that he recalled the memo, and that "by August of 1987 we knew that the medication was hurting a lot of people, and we knew the FDA wanted the company to pull the medication and the more pressure the FDA put on the company to pull the medication, the more ardently the company [was] 'wining and dining the sales reps' to encourage us to promote the drug harder because there was a, I would generalize it as, a general fog over the sales reps because we knew what we were doing was wrong, it's as simple as that." One of the defendant's physician "thought leaders" admitted in his deposition that despite his touting the benefit of Parlodel for lactation suppression to other doctors at hospital meetings, he never prescribed Parlodel or any lactation suppressant to any of his obstetrical patients.

In 1988, the FDA Fertility and Maternal Health Drugs Advisory Committee found that "drugs are not to be used routinely to suppress lactation....Drugs should only be available to women with specific conditions, such as women who deliver stillborns."

The defendant commissioned an epidemiology study to examine the relationship between Parlodel and strokes and seizures in postpartum women, the results of which suggested, in 1988, that women taking Parlodel were at an increased risk of having strokes (relative risk 8.44) and late-occurring seizures (finding a "substantial positive association" of 60% increased risk), and that for patients taking Parlodel with ergonovine/Methergine "there is an extremely positive association between bromocriptine and late-occurring seizures among those who received ergonovine," and that these women were at a 49-fold increased risk of having a late-occurring seizure. The author of the study agreed under oath that, based on the study data, Parlodel is a risk factor for postpartum women for late-occurring seizures, alone and in conjunction with ergonovine/Methergine. The previously mentioned study of physicians' reactions to the "Dear Doctor" letter also found that the results of the epidemiological study would be a deciding factor in influencing physicians' future prescribing practices for Parlodel.

The defendant publicly maintained the position that the epidemiological study "reinforces the safety" of Parlodel. The defendant's "Parlodel Business Plan" for 1989 assured that "a comprehensive defense plan has been established hinging on positive results of the [epidemiological] study. Promotional efforts will increase...." In late 1988, the defendant issued a "Parlodel Update" to the "field force personnel," stating that the epidemiological study "did not find an association between the use of Parlodel and reports of seizures—which can occur spontaneously in women who have recently given birth," and that "In our opinion, the data clearly reinforce the safety of Parlodel in treating postpartum lactation."

A January 1989 memo from the president of the defendant's research institute noted that the epidemiological study found a "strong positive association between ergonovine use, Parlodel and seizure."

An epidemiologist of the defendant who attended the data presentation meeting opined that the data "is supportive of an interaction between bromocriptine and ergonovine." The defendant's associate director of medical operations wrote, with respect to the epidemiological study, "There was a subset of the group, however, with a significantly elevated risk for late-occurring postpartum seizure: this group comprised of those who also received ergonovine had a 49-fold greater risk of seizures. With this in mind, I recommend that we amend our package insert so that Parlodel is contraindicated in women who have also received ergonovine." One day after the data presentation meeting, an officer of the defendant requested that the defendant "recut the data on late-onset seizures using 48 and 96 hours as the cut off. This may change all data on ergonovine combination problems." He also urged "in the final report, the information on the risk of drug interaction should not be the major conclusion."

The defendant never placed a contraindication regarding bromocriptine and ergonovines in its package insert, and did not mention the "extremely strong positive association" for late-occurring seizures in women who had received Methergine/ergonovine after delivery in its sales brochure, "A Comforting Thought." The only information provided to prescribing physicians in the sales brochure was that there was no effect, and even a possible protective effect, for seizures from Parlodel use.

In mid-1989, the 12-member Fertility and Maternal Health Drugs Advisory Committee ("FDA Advisory Committee") unanimously reaffirmed its 1988 recommendations, stated that there is no need for prophylactic treatment other than analgesics and breast support for postpartum breast engorgement, that it had not been provided with evidence that bromocriptine was a safe and effective treatment for symptoms of postpartum breast engorgement, and unanimously recommended that neither hormones nor bromocriptine "should be used for this indication because they have not been shown to be equally or more effective than analgesics and breast support, and because they may induce adverse medical effects."

The defendant reacted to these findings and recommendations with an internal memorandum to its sales force that the FDA Advisory Committee recommendation that drugs no longer be used for postpartum lactation prevention "was based on beliefs of the committee members that there is 'no need' for pharmacologic therapy for lactation suppression," that the recommendations were "advisory only," and that Parlodel "can continue to be prescribed with confidence." The defendant's "selling strategy"

15. Drug Interaction Litigation

for the third and fourth quarters of 1989 told sales representatives to continue to sell Parlodel aggressively. A sales representative testified that "we were just advised that Parlodel was obviously receiving a lot of heat in the journals and from the FDA and that we needed to bleed every dollar that we could get out of Parlodel before the FDA just put a stop to it." He testified further that sales representatives were "never instructed to stop pushing Parlodel" because the "reality of the situation is that Parlodel represented millions and billions of dollars over time, and it was, in fact, the company's cash cow...."

In late 1989, the FDA again found that no drugs, including Parlodel should be used for prevention of postpartum lactation, "because they have not been shown to be equally effective than [aspirin and breast binding], and they may induce adverse medical effects." In September 1989—the month before the plaintiff's prescription—the FDA requested that the defendant withdraw Parlodel from the market for this purpose. In October 1989, the defendant refused, and stated that: "Parlodel should not be used routinely but should remain available for specific circumstances under which the physician and patient decide that the drug is indicated...We believe in choice of therapy...must be left to an informed decision made jointly by a patient and her physician."

The plaintiff's physician testified he was never informed that in 1989, the FDA requested that the defendant withdraw Parlodel and that the defendant refused. He testified that he would have liked to have known the FDA's concerns, but no drug representative contacted him.

The 1989 package inserts for Parlodel and Methergine contained FDA-required and FDA-approved language. The package insert in effect for Parlodel at the time of the plaintiff's prescription stated, in pertinent part, as follows:

> WARNINGS . . . .
>
> Fifteen cases of stroke during Parlodel(R) (bromocriptine mesylate) therapy have been reported mostly in postpartum patients whose prenatal and obstetric courses had been uncomplicated. Many of these patients experiencing seizures and/or strokes reported developing a constant and often progressively severe headache hours to days prior to the acute event. Some cases of stroke and seizures during therapy with Parlodel(R) (bromocriptine mesylate) were also preceded by visual disturbances (blurred vision, and transient cortical blindness). Four cases of acute myocaridal infarction have been reported, including 3 cases receiving Parlodel(R) (bromocriptine mesylate) for the prevention of physiological lactation. The relationship of these adverse reactions to Parlodel(R) (bromocriptine) mesylate is not certain.
>
> ADVERSE REACTIONS . . . .
> Physiological Lactation
>
> Serious adverse reactions include 38 cases of seizures (including 4 cases of status epilepticus), 15 cases of stroke, and 3 cases of myocardial infarction among postpartum patients. Seizure cases were not necessarily accompanied by the development of hypertension. An unremitting and often progressively severe headache, sometimes accompanied by visual disturbance, often preceded by hours to days many cases of seizure and/or stroke. Most patients show no evidence of toxemia during the pregnancy.

The package insert in effect for Parlodel at the time of the plaintiff's prescription included the following language providing a warning regarding the administration of Parlodel with other ergot alkaloids such as Methergine:

Although there is no conclusive evidence which demonstrates the interaction between Parlodel (bromocriptine mesylate) and other ergot alkaloids, concomitant use of these medications is not recommended. Particular attention should be paid to patients who have recently received other drugs that can alter blood pressure.

The package insert in effect for Methergine at the time of the plaintiff's prescription included the following language:

Drug Interactions. Caution should be exercised when Methergine (methylergonovine maleate) is used concurrently with other vasoconstrictors or ergot alkaloids.

The 1989 PDR contained the same information about Parlodel as the package insert.

The plaintiff's physician testified that he relied on the PDR or the promotional literature distributed by the drug representative before prescribing a drug, and that he was aware at the time of the prescription in 1989 that "uncontrolled hypertension, toxemia of pregnancy, [and] sensitivity to any ergot alkaloids" were contraindications for prescribing Parlodel.

When the FDA initially approved the defendant's first application to market the drug Parlodel in 1978, the FDA conditioned its approval on the basis that the defendant would conduct a clinical study of the safety and efficacy of Parlodel in humans. The defendant completed the clinical testing for this study in 1981, but, despite FDA requests, had not submitted the report of this study as of 1994 at which time an internal memorandum stated that the study "...is a skeleton in our closet that could cause embarrassment given the current sensitive situation with Parlodel. [The study] is a long term safety and efficacy study run as a condition of approval of the original FDA back in 1978. It still has not been submitted to the FDA." The defendant submitted the data to the FDA in 1996, after the FDA withdrew Parlodel from the market for use in preventing postpartum lactation. The final report of the study did not include the causal assessments based on a number of ADRs, which showed that the defendant had concluded that at least one patient did in fact suffer from Parlodel-related hypertension.

Plaintiffs' expert toxicologist, after reviewing the case reports of the patients in the study, found that: "11/57 [of] patients in the second limb of that study demonstrated increases of their blood pressure...one patient was listed in the [defendant's] internal report as having developed hypertension, with Parlodel listed as the cause. This causation assessment, done by [defendant], was not included in their report of the FDA." Other defects identified in the study and the report by the plaintiff's experts included: the defendant dropped hypertensive patients from the studies, buried blood pressure readings in reams of clinical data, without providing corresponding reference in the summary reports provided to the FDA; 28 cases of hypertension were not presented to the FDA in the respective clinical trial summary reports; in one Parlodel clinical trial, a critically important incident of "extreme, uncontrolled hypertension" suffered by a patient after taking Parlodel was neither reported nor presented to the FDA in summary reports for that study; the defendant concealed from the FDA the existence of animal studies, conducted prior to Parlodel's approval for human use, that revealed Parlodel's vasoconstrictive properties; and the author of one of the animal studies testified before FDA subcommittees in 1988 and 1989, and repeatedly told physicians, that the drug is not a vasoconstrictor, and can only cause vasodilation. A scientist of the

15. Drug Interaction Litigation

defendant, charged with collecting Parlodel data for submission to the FDA, admitted that the defendant knew it was required by law to submit all animal studies to the FDA as part of the drug application process.

Concerning the relevance of the foregoing facts to the defendant's motion in limine, the court found that epidemiology is the study of disease patterns and risks in human populations; in a typical epidemiologic study, an epidemiologist compares the health of people exposed to a substance to that of persons not so exposed to determine whether the exposure to the substance is associated with an increased rate of disease; epidemiologic studies typically provide an estimate of "relative risk," which is the ratio of the incidence of a disease in exposed individuals to the incidence in unexposed individuals; a relative risk of 1.0 means that the incidence in the groups is the same, that is, the exposure has no association with the disease, and if the study is properly performed, a relative risk below 1.0 means that the exposure is associated with the absence of the disease, whereas a relative risk significantly above 1.0 means that exposure is associated with an increased risk of the disease.

The court found that an adverse event report (AER) is a report made to a drug company or the FDA that a particular patient who was taking a particular drug experienced a particular medical problem; and these reports can be made by laypersons as well as doctors, but most are submitted by doctors.

The court found that case reports are "reports in medical journals describing clinical events in one or more individuals. They report unusual or new disease presentations, treatments, manifestations, or suspected associations between two diseases, effects of medication, or external causes" [citing Federal Judicial Center, *Reference Manual on Scientific Evidence*, at 374 (2d ed. 2000)].

The court found that "relative risk" cannot be derived from case reports; that no epidemiologic or controlled scientific studies have been performed showing an increased risk of stroke among patients of any type who take Methergine, either in conjunction with Parlodel or otherwise; and that there are no studies in live, intact animals showing that Methergine causes stroke.

Given this background, the court considered the defendant's motion in limine and request for a *Daubert* hearing on the admissibility of these witnesses' opinions, and exercised its discretion to admit the testimony under the *Daubert* trilogy. See *Daubert v. Merrell Dow Pharm.*, 509 U.S. 579, 125 L. Ed. 2d 469, 113 S. Ct. 2786 (1993); *General Elec. Co. v. Joiner*, 522 U.S. 136, 139 L. Ed. 2d 508, 118 S. Ct. 512 (1997); *Kumho Tire Co., Ltd. v. Carmichael*, 526 U.S. 137, 152, 143 L. Ed. 2d 238, 119 S. Ct. 1167 (1999). The court reviewed other rulings in Parlodel litigation in which the admissibility of the same plaintiffs' experts had been ruled either admissible [*citing*, e.g., *Kittleson v. Sandoz Pharm. Corp.*, No. CIV 98-2277, 2000 WL 562553 (N.D. Minn. Mar. 3, 2000); *Globetti v. Sandoz Pharm. Corp.*, 111 F. Supp. 2d 1174, 1176 (N.D. Ala. 2000)] or inadmissible [*citing*, e.g., *Glastetter v. Novartis Pharm.*, 107 F. Supp. 2d 1015 (E.D. Mo. 2000); *Brumbaugh v. Sandoz Pharm. Co.*, 77 F. Supp. 2d 1153 (D. Mont. 1999); *Hollander v. Sandoz Pharm. Corp.*, 95 F. Supp. 2d 1230, 1238-39 (W.D. Okla. 2000)], and ruled the testimony admissible in this case.

There was no dispute in any of the Parlodel cases that there was no epidemiological evidence to support the witnesses' opinions, that their opinions were based only on case reports, rechallenge reports, animal studies, comparisons of the ergot bromocriptine to other ergots, FDA regulatory actions, and internal documents of the defendant. The court in *Eve* reasoned that epidemiological evidence may be the best scientific evidence that can be presented, but noted that *Daubert* simply requires reliable evidence. The court found that the witnesses relied on the methodology of differential diagnosis, a method widely used by medical clinicians to identify medical conditions so they may be treated, and that the cumulative evidence upon which the witnesses relied satisfied the *Daubert* requirements of scientific reliability. The court specifically relied on the reasoning of *Globetti, supra,* in making its ruling, as follows:

> Plaintiffs argue powerfully that an epidemiological study of the association of Parlodel and AMI [acute myocardial infarction] is not practical because of the relative rarity of AMIs among postpartum women. To gather a population of postpartum women with a sufficient sub-population of those who have suffered an AMI to be statistically significant would require hundreds of thousands, if not millions, of women. The evidence suggests that AMI occurs in postpartum women at the rare rate of 1 to 1.5 per 100,000 live births. Thus, even in a study of one million women, the sub-populations of those suffering an AMI would be only ten to fifteen women, far from enough to allow drawing any statistically significant conclusions. In short, the best scientific evidence is that presented by plaintiff's experts. *Globetti*, 111 F. Supp. 2d at 1179 (footnote omitted)(emphasis added).

> In a footnote, the *Globetti* court further noted, "While not suggested by defendant, the court notes that it would be medically and scientifically unethical to attempt a control-group experiment. To do so would require administering Parlodel to women and exposing them to the possibility of life-threatening events like AMI and stroke. Indeed, to prove the association between Parlodel and AMI or stroke, the scientist would have to expect a certain number of deaths among the test subjects." *Globetti*, 111 F. Supp. 2d at 1179 n.5.

Eve, supra. The reader is referred to cases cited above for judicial reasoning that resulted in exclusion of the evidence that was admitted in the *Eve* case.

Another good example of the application of the *Daubert* trilogy to the medical and scientific evidence in drug interaction litigation is *Jones v. United States,* 933 F. Supp. 894 (N.D. Cal. 1996). Here, a husband and wife filed a wrongful birth action against the United States under the Federal Tort Claims Act, seeking costs and damages associated with raising their daughter, alleging that the child was born because U.S. Army doctors negligently failed to warn the mother that Penicillin-VK, prescribed prophylactically prior to oral surgery, could interfere with the effectiveness of her Triphasil-28 birth control pills. The plaintiffs offered expert testimony of two expert witnesses—a board-certified obstetrician-gynecologist and a pharmacist—to show that penicillin interferes with the effectiveness of the birth control pills.

The court held a *Daubert* hearing to determine whether the expert testimony was sufficiently reliable to be admitted. The court found that neither of the witnesses had conducted independent research in the area of antibiotic/oral contraceptive interaction, that the physician's opinion was based solely on published articles he read during the 7 h in which he did research in preparation for his testimony, and concluded that their opinions were not based on objective, verifiable evidence that was derived from scientifically valid principles. The court found that the evidence showed, at most, that there is anecdotal support for the hypothesis that an unexplained interaction between certain antibiotics and oral contraceptives may reduce the effectiveness of the contraceptives, but did not establish a proven, cause-and-effect relationship that the court considered necessary to satisfy the *Daubert* standard.

15. Drug Interaction Litigation

Specifically, the court found that although the witnesses claimed that their opinions were supported by numerous scientific articles, a careful reading of the articles revealed that many of their authors came to conclusions that differed from the conclusions of the plaintiffs' witnesses; that the witnesses extracted data from articles that found no statistically significant correlation between antibiotic use and increased failure of oral contraceptives, and relied on the data to reach conclusions contrary to conclusions reached by the authors of the articles. The court stated that "This tactic does not qualify as good science." Furthermore, the court found that the only articles that supported the experts' opinions were are not based on controlled, scientific studies, but on anecdotal case reports, reviews of research done by other people, or studies that lacked a control group, and were therefore not based on scientific method.

The plaintiffs also relied on the package labeling of the Triphasil-28 as evidence of causation. The label warned that certain antibiotics may "possibly" have an effect on oral contraceptive effectiveness. The court found this warning to be even less probative of causation than the inconclusive studies upon which plaintiffs' experts relied, and stated that "...a boilerplate warning on a drug package insert may reflect no more than an overly cautious response to possible liability, not scientific proof of causation." The court concluded that the plaintiffs' experts "...did not rely on a single, controlled study that showed a statistically significant correlation between antibiotic use and decreased effectiveness of oral contraceptives. Consequently, the Court finds that Plaintiffs' evidence does not satisfy the first prong of the *Daubert* standard."

The court reasoned further that under California law, a plaintiff must establish both general causation—"that the Defendant's conduct increased the likelihood of injury—and specific causation—"that the defendant's conduct was the probable, not merely a possible, cause of the injury."

To establish general causation, the court stated that the plaintiffs would have to show that there is a scientifically validated interaction between Penicillin-VK and Triphasil-28 birth control pills that made it more likely that the plaintiff would become pregnant while taking both drugs than if she were taking birth control pills alone, and that the evidence did not meet this requirement. The court found to the contrary, based on the testimony of the plaintiffs' experts. They testified that antibiotics kill bacteria in the digestive system, thereby interfering with the mechanism by which oral contraceptives release estrogen into the woman's body, thereby lowering estrogen levels in a manner that reduces the contraceptive effect of the birth control pills and allows the woman to ovulate and become pregnant. The court observed, however, that Triphasil-28 birth control pills have two components, estrogen and progestin, and that each component has independent contraceptive effect. The progestin component is metabolized differently than the estrogen component, and the plaintiffs' experts presented no scientific evidence to show that antibiotics interfere with metabolization of progestin. Even if scientific evidence showed that antibiotics interfered with the estrogen component, the court inferred that the progestin component would still prevent pregnancy.

To establish specific causation, the court stated that the plaintiffs would have to show that the interaction between Penicillin-VK and Triphasil-28 birth control pills was the probable, not merely a possible, cause of plaintiff's pregnancy, which would require them to show that such an interaction occurs at more than double the rate of the known failure rate for oral contraceptives alone. The court found no competent testimony on this issue, and found that none of the articles relied upon by the plaintiffs' experts were controlled, broad-based studies of the existence of an interaction between antibiotics and oral contraceptives, let alone the rate at which such an interaction occurs.

The court concluded that the plaintiff failed to prove by a preponderance of the evidence that she became pregnant during the time that she was taking Penicillin-VK. Expert testimony concerning the length of time between conception and the ability of the pregnancy test to detect a pregnancy, and the date of administration of the antibiotic, supported a contrary conclusion, that she conceived before she began taking the antibiotics. Proximate cause was, accordingly, not established.

Similar scrutiny was applied by the court in rejecting the plaintiff's causation expert in *Haggerty v. The Upjohn Company,* 950 F. Supp. 1160 (S.D. Fl. 1996). The plaintiff injured his neck while working as a drywall installer, underwent surgery for a herniated disc, and was released with a postsurgical prescription for Halcion (triazolam, a benzodiazepine) to help him sleep. He claimed that the warnings that accompanied the Halcion were inadequate and failed to warn him of potential side effects, which allegedly caused him to engage in bizarre behavior, with severe consequences.

Specifically, he claimed that one night, approximately two months after his release from the hospital, he took one Halcion tablet, went to bed at approximately 6:30 PM, and that his next recollection was waking up in a hospital room the following morning with a fractured back. He alleged that ingestion of the Halcion tablet significantly altered his behavior, causing him to become belligerent, aggressive, suffer from hallucinations, and conduct himself in a bizarre and agitated fashion, culminating in his leaping from the balcony on the second story of his apartment complex. Additionally, on that same evening, the plaintiff reportedly assaulted and threatened his live-in girlfriend with a knife, assaulted his 8-yr-old son and a neighbor, and walked around his apartment and building without clothing. He alleged further that as a result of his Halcion-induced conduct on the evening of April 20th, his live-in girlfriend obtained a restraining order to prevent him from returning to his apartment, his two children from a prior marriage who had been residing with him were adjudicated dependent and placed in foster care, and upon his discharge from the hospital he was arrested for aggravated assault, battery, aggravated battery, and indecent exposure, for which he was ultimately imprisoned and lost his parental rights over his two children.

The defendant manufacturer contended that the plaintiff misused Halcion by ingesting numerous tablets of the drug concurrently with large quantities of alcohol and an unknown number of Valium tablets. The defendant also presented evidence of the plaintiff's long history of alcohol and poly-substance abuse, frequent physical attacks on the women with whom he had lived, usually occurring while he was under the influence of alcohol, and testimony of several experts that the defendant suffered from various psychiatric personality disorders.

The defendant filed a motion in limine to exclude the testimony of the plaintiff's causation expert, who possessed a Ph.D. in pharmacology, and a motion for summary judgment on grounds that her opinion was inadmissible, and the plaintiff therefore lacked any evidence that the defendant's drug caused his injuries.

The plaintiff's expert testified at the hearing on the motion in limine that, in her opinion, Halcion caused the psychiatric and behavioral effects experienced by the plaintiff in the evening in question. She testified that her opinion was based on a review of spontaneous reports of adverse medical events involving Halcion collected by the FDA in its Spontaneous Reporting System (SRS), along with anecdotal case reports appearing in the medical literature, references in textbooks to non-Halcion studies of psychomotor agitation in rats and mice, peer reviewed articles summarizing primary clinical findings that she had not personally reviewed, newspaper articles from the lay press, correspondence to the FDA from a public-interest group, a secondary summary prepared by Dr. Anthony Kales that provided a detailed listing of primary citations with abstracts of primary findings, and European postmarketing surveillance reports. She testified further that she had not performed any independent research on the alleged adverse side effects of Halcion.

The plaintiff's expert also testified that she employed an inductive reasoning process to arrive at her conclusions, which she called "differential etiology" or "differential diagnosis," by which she arrived at a conclusion about the cause of the plaintiff's conduct by considering possible causes and attempting to eliminate all other possible causes but the Halcion. The court found it significant, however, that the witness cited no epidemiological studies to support a causal relationship between Halcion and the plaintiff's conduct; that she did not perform a clinical examination of, or even meet, the plaintiff before forming her opinion on causation; that she did not consider any psychiatric or psychological evaluations or diagnoses of the plaintiff before forming her opinion and was unaware of a psychological evaluation that resulted in a diagnosis of borderline personality disorder in the plaintiff; that she had not read two psychological evaluations that indicated that, because of his personality defects, the plaintiff was likely to express his anger in an unpredictable and explosive manner, and was at risk for displaying unprovoked and exaggerated aggressive outbursts. The witness testified further that another possible cause of the plaintiff's conduct, which ought to have been considered in her differential diagnosis, was significant drug interaction or abuse of alcohol, and that all of the plaintiff's behavior on the evening in question could have been the result of alcohol intoxication, which would have worsened any existing psychological or psychiatric disorder he may have. Finally, the witness had not reviewed the rescue report from the evening in question, which indicated the plaintiff drank six or seven beers and had taken an unknown number of Valium tablets on that evening.

Based on the foregoing, the court found that the plaintiff's expert's opinion was not based on scientifically valid principles, was inadmissible, and granted the defendant's motion for summary judgment.

TABLE OF CASES

United States Supreme Court
Daubert v. Merrell Dow Pharm., 509 U.S. 579, 125 L. Ed. 2d 469, 113 S. Ct. 2786 (1993)
General Elec. Co. v. Joiner, 522 U.S. 136, 139 L. Ed. 2d 508, 118 S. Ct. 512 (1997)
Kumho Tire Co., Ltd. v. Carmichael, 526 U.S. 137, 143 L. Ed. 2d 238, 119 S. Ct. 1167 (1999).

Seventh Circuit
Crisostomo v. Stanley, 857 F.2d 1146 (7th Cir. 1988)
Ashman v. SK&F Lab Co., 72 F. Supp. 1401 (N.D. Ill. 1988)
Eve v. Sandoz Pharmaceutical Corp., 2001 U.S. Dist. LEXIS 4531 (S.D. Ind. 2001)

Eighth Circuit
Glastetter v. Novartis Pharm., 107 F. Supp. 2d 1015 (E.D. Mo. 2000)
Kittleson v. Sandoz Pharm. Corp., No. CIV 98-2277, 2000 WL 562553 (N.D. Minn. Mar. 3, 2000)

Ninth Circuit
Brumbaugh v. Sandoz Pharm. Co., 77 F. Supp. 2d 1153 (D. Mont. 1999)
Jones v. United States, 933 F. Supp. 894 (N.D. Cal. 1996)

Tenth Circuit
Eck v. Parke, Davis & Co., 256 F.3d 1013 (10th Cir. 2001).
Hollander v. Sandoz Pharm. Corp., 95 F. Supp. 2d 1230, (W.D. Okla. 2000)

Eleventh Circuit
Globetti v. Sandoz Pharm. Corp., 111 F. Supp. 2d 1174, (N.D. Ala. 2000)
Haggerty v. The Upjohn Company, 950 F. Supp. 1160 (S.D. Fl. 1996)

District of Columbia Circuit
Whittle v. United States, 669 F. Supp. 501 (D DC 1987)

Arizona
Lasley v. Shrake's Country Club Pharmacy, Inc., 880 P.2d 1129 (Ariz. 1994)

Florida
Johnson v. Walgreen Co., 675 So.2d 1036 (Fla. 1st D.C.A. 1996)
Sanderson v. Eckerd Corporation, 780 So.2d 930 (Fla. App. 2001)

Georgia
Singleton v. Airco, Inc., 314 S.E. 2d 680 (Ga. App. 1984)

Illinois
Batteast v. Wyeth Laboratories, Inc., 526 N.E.2d 428 (Ill. App. 1988)
Frye v. Medicare-Glaser Corporation, 605 N.E. 2d 557 (Ill. 1992)
Happel v. Wal-Mart Stores, Inc., 766 N.E.2d 1118 (Ill. 2002).

Kansas
Fuhs v. Barber, 36 P.2d 962 (Kan. 1934)

Louisana
Dean v. K-Mart Corp., 720 So.2d 349 (La. App. 1998)

Massachusetts
Cottam v. CVS Pharmacy, 764 N.E.2d 814 (Mass. 2002)
Linnen v. A. H. Robbins Company, Inc., 1999 Mass. Super LEXIS 552 (1999)

Michigan
Baker v. Arbor Drugs, Inc., 544 N.W.2d 727 (Mich. App. 1996)

Missouri
Horner v. Spolito, 1 S.W.3d 519 (Mo. App. 1999)

Ohio
Johnson v. State Medical Board of Ohio, 1999 Ohio App LEXIS 4487 (Ohio App 1999)

Oregon
Bocci v. Key Pharmaceuticals, Inc., 974 P.2d 758 (Or. App. 1999); *later proceeding*, 22 P.3d 758 (Or. App. 2001)

Tennessee
Dooley v. Revco Discount Drug Centers, Inc., 805 S.W.2d 380 (Tenn. App. 1990)
Texas
Morgan v. WalMart Stores, Inc., 30 S.W.2d 455 (Tex. App. 2000)
Washington
Clausing v. State, 955 P.2d 394 (Wash. App. 1998)
McKee v. American Home Products Corp., 782 P.2d 1045 (Wash. 1989)
Silves v. King, 970 P.2d 790 (Wash. App. 1999)

REFERENCES

Baker KR. The OBRA 90 mandate and its developing impact on the pharmacist's standard of care. 44 Drake L. Rev. 503 (1996).

Reference Manual on Scientific Evidence (Federal Judicial Center, 2000).

Restatement (Second) of Torts, §§323, 324A.

Restatement (Second) of Torts § 402A, comment k.

Attorneys' fees in product liability suits. 53 ALR4th 414.

Cause of action against drug manufacturer for failure to warn of side effects associated with prescription drug. 3 COA 815.

Duty of medical practitioner to warn patient of subsequently discovered danger from treatment previously given. 12 ALR4th 41.

Federal pre-emption of state common law products liability claims pertaining to drugs, medical devices, and other health-related items. 98 ALR Fed 124.

Liability of hospital, or medical practitioner, under doctrine of strict liability in tort, or breach of warranty, for harm caused by drug, medical instruments, or similar device used in treating patient. 54 ALR3d 258.

Liability of manufacturer or seller for injury caused by drug or medicine sold. 79 ALR2d 301.

Liability of manufacturer or seller for injury or death allegedly caused by failure to warn regarding danger in use of vaccine or prescription drug. 94 ALR3d 748.

Liability of United States under federal tort claims act for damages caused by ingestion or administration of drugs, vaccines, and the like, approved as safe for use by government agency. 24 ALR Fed 467.

Physician's liability for injury or death resulting from side effects of drugs intentionally administered to or prescribed for patient. 45 ALR3d 928.

Products liability: admissibility of expert or opinion evidence as to adequacy of warning provided to user of product. 26 ALR4th 377.

Products liability: strict liability in tort where injury results from allergenic (side-effect) reaction to product. 53 ALR3d 298.

Promotional efforts directed towards prescribing physician as affecting prescription drug manufacturer's liability for product-caused injury. 94 ALR3d 1080.

Strict products liability: liability for failure to warn as dependent on defendant's knowledge of danger. 33 ALR4th 368.

Chapter 16

Psychotropic Medications and Crime

The Seasoning of the Prozac Defense

Michael Welner, MD

1. INTRODUCTION

Psychiatrists are asked to assess criminal responsibility for prospective insanity and diminished capacity defenses, and as part of presentencing efforts in capital cases. The examinees may present with a history of having been treated with psychotropics at the time of the offense. A treatment history introduces the need to appraise the influence of the psychotropic medication on the crime through the following questions:

Was the treatment responsible for the crime?
Was the disease being treated responsible for the crime?
Were both the treatment and disease responsible for the crime?
Were neither responsible for the crime?
Were both responsible in some ways, and neither responsible in other respects?

Such is the complexity of human choices and criminal behavior, and the influence of neurophysiology interacting with the environment. Untangling the potential confounding factors is a fascinating challenge.

2. PROZAC

Defense strategies attributing crime to antidepressants, fluoxetine (Prozac) in particular, drew widespread attention in the 1990s *(1)*. Inspired by 1990 case reports published by a respected Harvard psychiatrist suggesting a specific causal link between Prozac and suicidal preoccupation *(2)*, criminal defense attorneys made the leap to attributing homicidal violence to psychotropic medicines. The controversy over a connection

From: *Handbook of Drug Interactions: A Clinical and Forensic Guide*
A. Mozayani and L. P. Raymon, eds. © Humana Press Inc., Totowa, NJ

heightened when plaintiffs brought civil damages suits against Eli Lilly and Company, manufacturer of Prozac, following violent events and suicides.

The most celebrated of these Prozac cases involved no criminal defense at all. Joseph Wesbecker, a depressed employee of Standard Gravure Printing Company in Louisville, Kentucky, walked into company offices in September 1989 armed with an AK-47 and four other weapons. He proceeded to shoot dead eight coworkers and wound 12 others, before killing himself *(3)*.

Mr. Wesbecker had a long and bitter relationship with his employer. He had been speaking of mass homicide as early as one year prior to the attack. Several weeks before the rampage, he began taking Prozac. His medical history took on posthumous relevance when, 5 yr later, 28 plaintiffs filed a $50 million lawsuit against Eli Lilly.

Although the case settled—while a jury deliberated to a verdict exonerating Prozac—the controversial backdoor wrangling did little to quell the overall controversy. Approximately 200 civil suits have followed; other medicines were also charged in civil complaints, including selective serotonin reuptake inhibitors (SSRI) cousins sertraline (Zoloft) *(3)* and paroxetine (Paxil) *(4)*. The pharamaceutical companies scored an impressive streak of victories, and civil lawsuits petered out. Still, enough points of debate within the medical community endured to this day, and questions have not been fully relegated to the past.

The attention drawn to these notorious cases prompted psychiatry to scrutinize the causal relationship of medicine to violent crime. In the early 1990s, reports of higher rates of suicides or attempted suicides promoted uncertainty within the medical community and concern and debate among lawmakers, while Eli Lilly scrambled to protect the reputation of its wildly successful medicine.

The subsequent deliberation included research, and even the convening of a special panel by the Food and Drug Administration (FDA). In 1991, that panel concluded there was no credible link between antidepressants, including Prozac, and violence. The FDA panel added that bad outcomes were more likely a product of poor monitoring of depression by treating professionals *(5)*. The Committee on Safety of Medicines in the United Kingdom issued similar findings. Furthermore, antidepressants, including SSRIs, have a demonstrated efficacy in reducing violence in a number of individuals *(6)*.

Nevertheless, skeptics have been emboldened by reviews of medical examiner files that correlate the finding of suicide in those whose postmortem toxicology demonstrates the presence of tricyclic antidepressants and fluoxetine. More pertinent to criminal questions, those same studies find violent methods to have been far more frequently associated with fluoxetine suicides than suicides in those taking tricyclics *(7)*.

Review of available evidence on this topic has to account for drug company sponsorship behind some of the exonerating studies and reviews *(8)*. That said, the most compelling evidence of SSRI's easing violence as opposed to exacerbating it arises from the study of "anger attacks," episodes of disproportionate anger that occur more frequently in the depressed *(9)*. Anger attacks were more frequently associated with anxiety, hostility, and personality disorders *(10)*. And though fluoxetine had a pronounced effect on reducing the incidence of anger attacks in research, it was associated with producing such attacks in those who did not report them previously in only 4–7% of study subjects *(11)*. This number, by the way, was substantially less than the incidence of new-onset anger attacks, 20% in those treated with placebo *(12)*.

Additional study has demonstrated a beneficial effect of fluoxetine on anger independent of diagnosis (13). In addition, antiaggression effects are most demonstrable at two-to-three months of treatment (14).

Whether because of available research exonerating Prozac and its cousin SSRI medicines from homicidality and suicidality—or the product of tremendous legal resources invested by pharmaceutical companies to confront even criminal cases that blamed their product—criminal court verdicts have consistently rejected Prozac defenses. For this reason, those cases actually resulting in successful criminal defense are especially worth noting.

On September 7, 1999, Douglas D. Lund of Annapolis, Maryland, reportedly attacked his wife, and police charged him with attempted murder. His case was to become, to this day, the most successful use of a medication defense. Mr. Lund had no previous history of violence. He had been diagnosed in the past with attention-deficit hyperactivity disorder, and had recently received a diagnosis of depression; his treatment included the antidepressant sertraline.

At the time of the crime, Mr. Lund was experiencing sleeplessness, and had asked his wife Jo Ann to go for a drive at 3 AM. While driving, and without a word, Mr. Lund unhooked her seat belt, crashed the car into a steel fence post, pushed her out of the car, and began striking her head into the pavement and choking her. Then, he carried her to the nearby grass, as she pleaded with him to spare her life and to put her down. Without explanation, Lund then flagged down a passing motorist, who called 911. Mrs. Lund suffered a broken back, collarbone, and finger.

Based on medical testimony that Mr. Lund's diagnosis was bipolar disorder, manic, a judge found Mr. Lund not guilty by reason of insanity. Mr. Lund was released to the community in February 2001. His wife, an assistant state's attorney who supported him through his prosecution, did nevertheless file for divorce (15).

Some medicines, in precipitating mania, have directly spurred the onset of acute mental illness, which in turn may fuel violent behavior. In such settings, legal insanity might be a viable defense. In Mr. Lund's case, a diagnosis of mania was perfectly plausible given the inherent risk that taking an antidepressant does occasionally flip a person into a manic episode (though bupropion, when causing this effect, apparently manifests with milder severity) (16).

Even for those who do not have so extreme a reaction as mania, or the more muted hypomania, agitation may result from virtually all antidepressants. Such a behavioral change, though not rising to a level of insanity, could sufficiently mitigate criminal responsibility to affect sentencing. Table 1 lists serotonergic antidepressants with their frequency of causing agitation (17).

Sometimes, psychiatrists have observed suicidal risk to actually coincide with clinical improvement. Patients may describe having the energy to finally act upon impulses they already experienced when they were even more depressed and withdrawn (18). This mechanism should be considered, realistically, in assessing violent crime, particularly of a suicidal nature, that occurs during a period where clinical records show symptomatic improvement.

Another behavioral change worth noting is the serotonin syndrome. This phenomenon of serotonin overload causes frank confusion and disorientation (19). The serotonin syndrome may occur even on seemingly low doses of medication (20), reflecting

Table 1
Serotonergic Antidepressants and Frequency of Agitation[a]

Antidepressant	Incidence of Agitation
Celexa	3%
Luvox	2%
Paxil	1.1%
Prozac	>1%*
Zoloft	1%

[a]PDR notes frequency in text, not table, (17).

the metabolic capabilities and relative sensitivities of the individual. It is best considered when a crime reflects very disorganized and disoriented behavior, and the victim is engaged without premeditated plotting. The perpetrator continues confused subsequent to the crime, but that confusion abates as the offending medicine is metabolized out of the system, providing that the offender stops taking it. A hypothetical scenario would follow something like this:

> Sheila M. is living with her boyfriend Mark. Their relationship is warm and supportive. After developing panic attacks, Sheila is placed on an SSRI. One day, Sheila begins to show signs of frank confusion and disorientation. Mark calls Sheila's mother to come over and to stay with them.
>
> As all three are in the kitchen, preparing dinner, Sheila picks up a knife and begins stabbing her mother in the back. Mark restrains her and yells for help. A neighbor calls police. Taken into custody, Sheila babbles about having to cook dinner tonight and wanting to go buy tomatoes for the salad. Over the next 48 h, she becomes completely normal. Doctors interviewing her at the jail learn that she has not been taking her medicine since arrest. She exhibits profound regret over the incident when she realizes that it really happened.

A manic cause would be reflected in less cognitive confusion, and in sustained behavioral and mental disorganization, even after the medicine is used up by her system. The motiveless (rational or irrational) crime carried out with a weapon within her reach and towards a closely located and nonthreatening figure are also key history points.

Serotonin syndrome also strengthens the uncommon approach of proving legal insanity based upon a lack of awareness of "nature and consequences" of actions. Most insanity defense cases revolve around the questioned lack of appreciation of wrong. A higher level of disorganization is needed in order to disable a person from recognizing that she was unable to appreciate the very nature of her actions, nor their consequences.

One case recently trumpeted as a successful Prozac defense was not exactly that. Still, the case of Chris DeAngelo bears close consideration for the issues it raises about interactions, illness, and the role of intoxicants.

Mr. DeAngelo, a married insurance salesman from Derby, Connecticut, had no criminal history and no known financial trouble. Yet, he was ultimately implicated in several bank robberies, and left himself open to being shot by officers who had responded to the incident that resulted in his finally being caught. Subsequently, police learned that Mr. DeAngelo had been treated with Prozac and alprazolam. He raised an insanity defense, and the prosecutor on the case agreed to the plea (21).

Closer scrutiny of Mr. DeAngelo accompanied his subsequent hospitalization, especially as doctors deliberated whether he should be released to the community. Although Mr. DeAngelo had been diagnosed with having had a manic episode induced by the Prozac he had been prescribed, more details continued to emerge about his problematic drinking. Eventually, his inability to maintain sobriety on passes outside the hospital became a pivotal issue interfering with his release. The history now available on Mr. DeAngelo now muddies what really led to his crimes. Was it the Prozac? The illness? The booze? Or the alprazolam? What originally appeared to be a successful Prozac defense may have been a fortuitous outcome abetted by prosecutorial naivete or dishonest forensic investigation, or both. Reminders of the need for inclusive diligence are as important a lesson as to be gained.

3. OTHER PSYCHOTROPICS

Overshadowed by the SSRIs, benzodiazepines—especially alprazolam—are appreciated within the medical literature as responsible for unusual and sometimes quite dramatic changes in behavior (22). Given that these medicines are designed to calm, and even to induce sleep, violent behavior is absolutely idiosyncratic and unintended. Idiosyncratic rage reactions in people taking benzodiazepines are not dose dependent, but rather reflect a person's peculiar sensitivity.

The first report of such a reaction appeared in 1960, concerning chlordiazepoxide (Librium) taken by a man who went on to assault his wife for the first time in their 20 yr marriage (23). Since then, paradoxical rage has been reported with a variety of benzodiazepines (24). Alprazolam has, however uncommon, been more frequently implicated than other medicines of this class, and particularly in those with histories of idiosyncratic reactions to alcohol and other medicines, and with borderline personality disorder (25).

Case reports and literature have identified assaults resulting from alprazolam, but not homicides; this may reflect the divide between the populations that inspire clinical research and those examined within the different priorities of the forensic system. The physician who studies or reports his patient who has subsequently killed displays unprecedented humility.

Bond demonstrated, in a sample of 23 patients treated with alprazolam for panic disorder, an increased likelihood of aggressive response to provocation (26). This finding describes disinhibition, a phenomenon also attributed to alcohol. It is the same disinhibition exploited by rapists who secure their prey by slipping benzodiazepines such as flunitrazepam into vulnerable victims' drinks (27). The same drug has been used by gangs to ease their disinhibition to carry out violent crimes (28). Disinhibited by accident? Disinhibited by design? Was the crime provoked? How provoked? Unprovoked? The complexity of disinhibition mandates caution and scrutiny as to the circumstances preceding the instant crimes.

Not to be overlooked is the increased likelihood of benzodiazepines to cause frank confusion, especially in the elderly (29) and the brain injured (30). Confusion from benzodiazepines results from their action as a general central nervous system depressant, affecting γ-aminobutyric acid (GABA) nerve cell receptors located all over the brain (31). This effect differs from mania or agitation, but may have a significant impact on violence and crime that occurs in institutional settings, or by geriatric defendants.

In the current climate of psychopharmacology, benzodiazepines have fallen out of favor despite their tremendous advantages in the treatment of acute anxiety. The quality of relief provided by benzodiazepines is such that some come to abuse these medicines *(31)*. The abuse can, if unchecked, advance to a physical dependence *(31)*. Even those who responsibly take benzodiazepines may become physically dependent upon them to the end of developing terrible withdrawal reactions if forced to suddenly stop them *(31)* because of travel, surgery, and postoperative hospitalization, or simply running out of pills.

Other medicines have been developed, including the SSRIs, that do not lead to physical tolerance. Still, because of the speed with which benzodiazepines produce relief of anxiety and panic, they retain a secure place in the psychotropic armamentarium. For this reason, their relevance to future questions of medication-induced crime continues, perhaps with the most legitimate defense potential.

Given the unexpectedness of a rage reaction, alprazolam seems ideally suited to the defense of involuntary intoxication. Indeed the precedent setting case of Florida, *State v. Boswell*, involved a defendant who was taking Prozac (fluoxetine) and Xanax (alprazolam) at the time he shot a police officer *(32)*.

The Prozac–Xanax combination seen in the *Boswell* and *DeAngelo* cases similarly raises the question of whether the alprazolam was more responsible for unusual behavior than the fluoxetine. Fluoxetine, a potent inhibitor of CYP 3A4, raises blood levels of circulating alprazolam. An individual who experiences disinhibiting effects from alprazolam, or frank paradoxical rage, may unwittingly be at higher risk from this commonly prescribed medication regimen.

Involuntary intoxication has a long history in courts, often inspiring cynicism. Psychiatric diagnostic classification accounted for alcohol idiosyncratic intoxication *(33)* until *DSM–IV*, when the concept was discarded as controversial *(34)*. Still, there is ample documented understanding that some are exquisitely sensitive to the effects of alcohol, in that they become explosive upon drinking *(35)*.

4. WHAT IS INVOLUNTARY INTOXICATION (LEGALLY)?

Guided by enduring common law, cases from the 19th century (36) invoked the following definition for involuntary intoxication: "That if a person by the unskilfulness of his physician, or by the contrivance of his enemies, eat or drink such a thing as causeth such a temporary or permanent phrenzy…this puts him into the same condition, in reference to crimes, as any other phrenzy, and equally excuseth him" *(37)*.

In practice, defenses of involuntary intoxication have been generally supported in American courts when accident, fraud or contrivance, coercion, or mistake led to the intoxication. However, many cases predated sophistication about the effects of medications, and dealt with a pharmacopaea that included bootlegged moonshine *(38)*. The very notion of drug interactions was as remote as the computer.

Not surprisingly, most court rulings of note on involuntary intoxication have involved cases where the defendant consumed alcohol or illicit drugs. Consistent interpretation of law is found where the defendant willingly consumed the intoxicant *(39)*, and/or was aware of its possible effects *(40)*; or had previous experience and familiarity with a combination of medicine and intoxicant *(41)*. In those instances, courts have ruled the intoxication voluntary.

What about intoxication that transpires when someone slips something into a drink, or laces a marijuana cigarette, for example? Involuntary or voluntary? Courts have ruled that spiking a substance that the defendant knew was intoxicating, and ingested nonetheless, does not allow for a defense of involuntary intoxication, even when he is surprised by the ultimate effects on his behavior or thinking *(42)*. On the other hand, when a more ordinary item, such as coffee, was laced, courts have upheld involuntary intoxication *(43)*.

When the intoxicant's effects are unexpected, and attributed to debilitating illness, courts have likewise ruled intoxication voluntary when the defendant was aware of his disability, but still chose to take in the intoxicant *(44)*.

On the other hand, laws may be more accommodating if a defendant drank alcohol or took an illicit drug with the expectation of relief, especially if he were suffering from illness, and the existing prescribed regimen was ineffective *(45)*.

Courts have also addressed questions of involuntary intoxication where no alcohol or intoxicant was among the agents taken. Depending on the state, rulings have yielded important precedents. Defense claims have been supported when a wrong medicine was administered by an associate *(46)*, and when a person compliant with a regular prescription suffered unexpected effects *(47)*. The latter echoes the aforementioned scenario of idiosyncratic rage fueled by alprazolam or another benzodiazepine.

Nevertheless, courts in some states have ruled against the defense in cases where the defendant knew the effects of a medicine at higher doses than prescribed *(48)*; knew he had an inherited predisposition to a sensitive reaction to a medicine *(49)*; had been erratically compliant with the prescribed medicine *(50)*; or, in cases where the defendant had engaged in activities incompatible with the known side effects of the medicine *(51)*.

The latter case is especially important to those charged with driving while intoxicated who invoke medication defenses, given that standard practice of informed consent is for physicians to advise their patients taking psychotropics of the potential effects on their ability to operate a motor vehicle or heavy machinery *(52)*. In actuality, most psychotropics, properly dosed, should not so interfere. Drug companies emphasize such warnings in their product literature to limit their own prospective liability and to pacify the demanding FDA, which controls access to the American marketplace.

However, many medicines, including SSRIs, may cause alcohol to accumulate in the system *(53)*. Those who drink even amounts they feel are not intoxicating later discover—after they are pulled over and given Breathalyzer tests—that their alcohol blood levels were higher than they had anticipated.

Even as we understand more about drug interactions and metabolism, the cases from earlier years underscore what we even see today: the most common legitimate connection between psychotropic drugs and crime arises when the medicines interact with illicit drugs and alcohol to produce unexpected effects *(54)*. Because this scenario does not necessarily mitigate responsibility, especially if the defendant knowingly consumed a potential intoxicant, a full inventory of the contributing conditions and agents consumed is pivotal.

Other than the distinction between known intoxicants and medicines, the most important aspect of the law in this area concerns what criteria relating to the defendant's thinking are needed to establish involuntary intoxication. In some states, even if eligible otherwise, the defendant must prove that the intoxication rendered him unable to appreciate right from wrong, or the criteria for that state's insanity defense *(55)*. Other states do not impose such a burden on the defendant once the court is satisfied that intoxication was involuntary *(56)*.

Other classes and types of psychotropic medicines, including antipsychotics and mood stabilizers, are far less likely to influence behavior to disinhibition or paradoxical rage, or to impact criminal and moral responsibility for even white-collar crimes. Irritability may be attributed to antipsychotics if akathisia is present *(57)*, but the legal significance of such an effect is pertinent only to mitigation—if at all clinically significant. The leap from irritability to impact on choices and appreciation of wrong strains credulity. However, attorneys should note that the atypical antipsychotic risperidone has been reported to rarely cause mania *(58)*.

Of the mood stabilizers, only carbamazepine has been associated in case reports with paradoxical rage *(59)*. This may be more likely, if still very uncommon, in children and adolescents. Carbamazepine is also an antiseizure medicine; it is therefore important to establish the reason the defendant was taking the medicine in the first place. The possibility of an idiosyncratic reaction cannot supercede the more likely scenario of undertreatment for the emotional or behavioral condition prompting the prescription of the drug in the first place.

Antipsychotics are essentially calming medicines that are administered to organize thoughts and to promote an attachment to reality *(60)*. Mood-stabilizing medicines have powerful beneficial effects on impulse control *(61)*. Some medicines are even likely responsible for preventing violence. Clozapine *(62)* and lithium, in particular, have antiaggressive effects *(63)* as well as antisuicidal effects *(64)*.

Accutane, an antiacne medicine *(65)*, has followed a similar, if less notorious track as the SSRIs. Case reports in the literature have identified individuals who developed depression while taking this medicine *(66)*. The drug has been proposed as a criminal defense *(67)*, with violence attributed to it. Recent research specifically focusing on the question of an accutane–suicide–violence link has failed to establish a connection *(68)*. Nevertheless, one high-profile civil lawsuit in Florida will revisit this question in the months ahead.

The case concerns a teenager who flew a private plane into a Tampa skyscraper, killing himself. He expressed, in a suicide note found on his person, his identification with Osama bin-Laden and the September 11 attacks on America. However, the teen pilot was not an Arab, not a Muslim, and had no apparent affiliation to Arab anti-American groups known to be operating in Florida. The teenager's family has subsequently sued the drug company that manufactures Accutane *(69)*, charging that his actions occurred as a result of the effects of the drug.

Given the unexpected nature of many adolescent crimes, and the prevalence of acne and teenagers' search for relief, the Accutane–crime link figures to draw more attention in future legal proceedings.

Another drug attracting attention for a potential link to violence is mefloquine. This widely prescribed antimalarial has been associated, in medical literature, with two syndromes pertinent to criminal and civil cases. Though rare *(70)*, some patients may experience an acute disorientation and confusion *(71)*. This has been linked, to date, to an anticholinergic syndrome *(72)*. More pertinent to criminal cases, a second constellation of side effects involves hallucinations, acute psychosis, and/or aggression *(73)*. Key in assessing such questions is timing; side effects characteristically emerge during or shortly after receiving prophylaxis while traveling, or actual treatment *(74,75)*.

One recent criminal appellate ruling found the causal relevance of Lariam to be inconsequential to a fraud defendant's capacity to deceive *(76)*. However, mefloquine is being studied closely in the aftermath of three domestic homicide cases involving soldiers at the Ft. Bragg military base who had previously received mefloquine treatment *(77)*.

5. THE DISEASE IS BIGGER THAN THE TREATMENT

Far more likely an issue, for an individual prescribed medicines, is the influence of the condition itself—or an untreated co-occurring condition—on criminal responsibility. Undertreatment is already acknowledged as a problem in researched studies of clinical populations *(78)*. That some of those who are undertreated eventually break the law should not be surprising, especially in considering how densely populated the corrections system is with folks who have significant psychiatric histories *(79)*.

Therefore, medicines that accelerate the metabolism of the psychotropic may be pertinent to a criminal defense, especially if behavioral changes coincided with the time course of the regimen. If the patient followed a doctor's instructions, then the unexpected ineffectiveness of the medicine may be even further supportive to the defense *(80)*.

When patients drink alcohol or take illicit drugs, along with the antipsychotic, attorneys should question whether the criminal behavior originated from the drugs themselves, or the interaction between the drugs and the antipsychotics. The literature supporting a link between alcohol and illicit drugs and crime is so clear *(81)* as to relegate the more indirect possibility of a drug's impact on metabolism of a psychotropic.

A defendant compliant with medicines and still undertreated warrants greater appreciation for his limited contribution to the deterioration of his condition than someone who chooses noncompliance. Therefore, attorneys should probe the defendant's insight into the implications of his noncompliance and awareness of potential drug interactions.

Notwithstanding the legal mandate of informed consent, psychiatry in practice rarely addresses the potentials for criminality that might arise, hypothetically, should patients abuse drugs while taking medicines, or skip doses of their prescribed regimen. "You have to take this every day," and "you're not supposed to drink when you are on this, it will make you sick," may not be enough of an explanation why.

The recent trial in Houston, Texas, of Andrea Yates demonstrated the relationship between undertreatment and crime. Would Mrs. Yates have stopped taking her medicines if she fully appreciated that she might have become homicidal to her five children? Likely not. Tragically, such crimes are so unfathomable—especially in foresight—that we need to be cautious of our expectations about the breadth of informed consent one can expect.

Ultimately, issues of responsibility for sentencing are left to the trier of fact, and the point of what a patient should have known about medication compliance and illness relapse is ultimately best resolved by the evidence at hand.

6. GUIDELINES FOR ASSESSMENT

Given the many possibilities that must be sorted out in a criminal responsibility evaluation, a few general principles are helpful to guide every evaluation.

Past patterns of violence reflect future patterns of violence. Violence and criminality resemble other important positive and negative behaviors in that they are an expression unique to an individual. Those with a past history of violence express their destructiveness under circumstances that reflected their neurochemistry, their interpersonal tendencies, their illness, medicines they took, individual sensitivities, and many other things. Although the aforementioned factors may not have been at all a part of the instant offense, ill-advised choices often reenact the same dynamics.

This principle is why no history of previous violence may be a particularly compelling argument in support of a disturbance in brain chemistry, possibly caused by medication. An unnatural defendant—which has nothing to do with race, socioeconomics, or education—is an unnatural defendant for a reason.

Full medical history. Attention to an examinee's medical history elicits physiological vulnerabilities and drug allergies, as well as factors that might suggest his vulnerability to a paradoxical or unexpected reaction to a medicine. Imaging studies to consider frontal or amygdala pathology may demonstrate gross structural brain impairment that would make a person more vulnerable to the effects of certain psychotropics, or to environmental provocation.

Other conditions associated with brain damage but that might not show findings on a CT (computed tomography), EEG (electroencephalogram), MRI (magnetic resonance imaging), or PET (positron emission tomography) scan, are AIDS and neurological diseases. Examining medical problems and a comprehensive review of body systems helps the examiner to learn of any conditions that the defendant was self-medicating, or how he or she has been buffeted by unremitting pain and chronic illness—both associated with suicidality.

Probe particular patterns of behavior when taking medicines, and which patterns are intended. Determine changes of dose, starting, stopping, and pattern of noncompliance as well. The timing of dose is important. In addition, explore behaviors and patterns off the psychotropics.

History of drug use needs to be gathered in this context, including observations about whether drugs taken had different effects on the defendant than usual and whether these changes coincided with medication changes or dosing. Though it is important to assess intoxication, withdrawal can contribute to criminal choices, irritability, and poor impulse control. Illicit drug craving is commonly responsible, for example, for robbery and violent crime.

Metabolic potential worsens as a person advances into old age *(82)* and in patients with liver disease *(83)*. These populations are at higher risk for drug interactions, or problems arising from accumulated medicines. Even with no previous history of violent behavior, the changes to their physiology may render them vulnerable to untoward effects of medicines prescribed at even modest doses.

Females show faster metabolic activity of isoenzyme CYP3A4, particularly in the premenopausal period *(84)*. Therefore, consideration of criminal responsibility and drug interaction questions in such a defendant would be more a question of inadequate treat-

16. Psychotropic Medications and Crime

ment of illness than intoxication. The following is a list of the 3A4 medications: alprazolam, diazepam, midazolam, triazolam, diltiazem, felodipine, nicardipine, nifedipine, nitrendipine, verapamil, cyclophosphamide, tamoxifen, paclitaxel, vinblastine, estradiol, cortisol, testosterone, amiodarone, lidocaine, carbamazepine, cisapride, cyclosporine, erythromycin, macrolide antibiotics, terfenadine, astemizole, nefazodone, quinidine, methadone, ritonavir, indinavir, saquinavir, colchicine, progesterone, alfentanil, sertraline, metoprolol, timolol, mexilitene, propafenone, codeine, dextromethorphan, sildenafil, haloperidol, and buspirone.

Full event history. To the extent possible, a moment-by-moment reconstruction of the period leading up to the crime, the period involving the crime, and the period immediately after is essential. The painstaking investigation thus gathers information about what was ingested, why it was ingested, and what emotions were present and when and how they changed.

The role of the victim in contributing to the crime warrants a toxicology profile of the victim as well, along with a corresponding history of ingestion history.

Because the significance of so many intoxicants and offending medicines relates to impulsive actions, the examiner should carefully discern the time lag from triggering events (if there were any) to criminal acts.

Consideration of motive is also a must. The less likely a motive can account for the crime, the more likely the crime was caused by a physiological phenomenon, including medicines. And, the more likely the involuntariness of an intoxication, if medicines were that physiological pilot light. Level of regret may herald a lack of motive. Motiveless crimes are characteristically associated with profound remorse *(85)*.

Collaterals. A defendant will understandably try to present his or her case in as self-serving a manner as possible. That being the case, the examiner who relies up the defendant as the sole informant does truth a disservice. Identifying and getting access to witnesses, historians, and others with clear and detailed information can confirm the validity of the history. Because so many variables can affect the overall conclusions of the examiner, confirming the truth is essential.

The crime scene can reveal many details about the level of disorganization of the offender. Likewise, an examination of the offender's home, or pictures from where he or she used drugs, may confirm use when blood levels cannot be determined.

Testing. Drug and medication tests should be performed upon arrest, when apprehending a defendant shortly after the crime has been committed. Of course, civil liberty issues would be confronted, and costs would be problematic. But we can certainly do a better job than at present; only in select fortunate cases of some defendants who are taken to the emergency room are any toxicology tests done. Of that small percentage, the toxicology battery is quite often incomplete.

The mystery of forensic assessments of drug interactions typically deepens because blood analyses are often not done during the period that would yield reliable and useful results. Consequently, toxicologists are often called upon to extrapolate blood levels based on time of ingestion, other medicines and drugs taken, time of eating, and other factors that might accelerate or decelerate breakdown of the medication.

Even when the consulting toxicologist is fortunate enough to gather sufficient information to arrive at a numerical figure for a blood level, that number cannot be considered in a vacuum. Likewise, in a clinical setting, there are those who, at very low levels of a medicine, show pronounced physical and mental effects. Alternatively, there are those for whom drugs well above a normal blood level hardly affect them at all. And postmortem levels of certain drugs frequently differ from expected antemortem levels (86).

Blood levels are therefore one piece of evidence in an overall clinical assessment. Uncommonly, numerical values of the blood levels of a prescribed medicine will yield absolute answers in the investigation of questioned death and criminal and civil responsibility.

Supplementing laboratory study with a complete background investigation about an individual, lethal ideation, and possible motives, will attach contextual relevance to the numbers available or arrived at. So, too, will additional testing, such as hair analysis, which provides a contextual appreciation of the test results of a snapshot in time compared to what the defendant had been taking in recent months.

Testing the defendant's capacity to metabolize drugs through the CYP isoenzyme 2D6 can assist investigations of drug interactions and criminal responsibility (87).Of course, this is pertinent only if the drugs in question are actually metabolized on the 2D6 isoenzyme. The following list serves as a useful guide, to date, of those 2D6 medicines with the potential for problematic behavioral effects: alprenolol, amitriptyline, chlorpheniramine, clomipramine, codeine, desipramine, dextromethorphan, encainide, fluoxetine, haloperidol, imipramine, indoramin, metoprolol, nortriptyline, ondansetron, oxycodone, paroxetine, propranolol, and propafenone.

Poor female 2D6 metabolizers may be further hampered by lower activity during the luteal phase of the menstrual cycle (88). The association of this metabolic change with more dramatic behavioral changes of late-luteal-phase dysphoria, or with postpartum events, has yet to be demonstrated.

Psychotropic drugs are metabolized through the isoenzymes CYP 1A2, 2D6, 2C19, and 3A4. Many of these drugs are metabolized through more than one system; therefore, changes in the activation or inhibition of one isoenzyme will not necessarily dramatically alter blood concentrations. Future research will undoubtedly trace more definitive cause–effect relationships between specific isoenzyme activity, specific medicines, interactions, and the influence on a crime. At this stage, the presumption of such a link in a given case is just that, without more than the established theoretical pathways. We have not yet identified all of the pathways for all of the drugs.

Further discoveries will also yield important insights on the metabolism distinctions within ethnic groups and subpopulations, just as study of the genetic code has yielded unique sequences. Part of the problem is the paucity of available psychotropic and psychopharmacology research data from a sizeable sample of non-Caucasian, female subjects. We are still some years from the practical application of these ideas to yield conclusions of medical certainty on a given case.

REFERENCES

1. Grinfeld M and Welner M. Pill poisoned? The seasoning of medication defenses. The Forensic Echo 2(3):4–10 (1998).
2. Teicher MH, Glod C, and Cole JO. Emergence of intense suicidal preoccupation during fluoxetine treatment. Am J Psychiatry 147(2):207–210 (1990).
3. Grinfeld M and Welner M. Pill poisoned? The seasoning of medication defenses. The Forensic Echo 2(3):3–6 (1998).

4. Locy T and Pasternak D. Can drugs spark acts of violence? U.S. News and World Report 128(9):44 (2000).
5. Walsh MT and Dinan TG. Selective serotonin reuptake inhibitors and violence: a review of the available evidence. Acta Psychiatr Scand 104(2):84–91(2001).
6. Buck OD. Sertraline for reduction of violent behavior. Am J Psychiatry 152(6):953 (1995).
7. Frankenfield DL, Baker SP, Lange WR, Caplan YH, and Smialek JE. Fluoxetine and violent death in Maryland. Forensic Sci Int 64(2–3):107–117 (1994).
8. Heiligenstein JH, Beasley CM Jr, and Potvin JH. Fluoxetine not associated with increased aggression in controlled clinical trials. Int Clin Psychopharmacol 8(4):277–280 (1993).
9. Fava M, Rosenbaum JF, McCarthy M, Pava J, Steingard R, and Bless E. Anger attacks in depressed outpatients and their response to fluoxetine. Psychopharmacol Bull 27(3): 275–279 (1991).
10. Fava M, Rosenbaum JF, Pava JA, McCarthy MK, Steingard RJ, and Bouffides E. Anger attacks in unipolar depression, Part 1: clinical correlates and response to fluoxetine treatment. *Am J Psychiatry 150(8):1158–1163 (1993).
11. Fava M, Alpert J, Nierenberg AA, Ghaemi N, O'Sullivan R, Tedlow J, et al. Fluoxetine treatment of anger attacks: a replication study. Ann Clin Psychiatry 8(1):7–10 (1996).
12. Fava M, Nierenberg AA, Quitkin F, et al. A preliminary study of the efficacy of sertraline and imipramine on anger attacks in depression. NCDEU annual meeting (1995).
13. Rubey RN, Johnson MR, Emmanuel N, and Lydiard RB. Fluoxetine in the treatment of anger: an open clinical trial. J Clin Psychiatry 57:398–401 (1996).
14. Coccaro EF and Kavoussi RJ. Fluoxetine and impulsive aggressive behavior in personality-disordered subjects. Arch Gen Psych 103:1081–1088 (1997).
15. Doctors release man who tried to kill his wife. The Capital. February 24, 2001.
16. Stoll AL, Mayer PV, Kolbrener M, Goldstein E, Suplit B, Lucler J, et al. Antidepressant-associated mania: a controlled comparison with spontaneous mania. Am J of Psychiatry 151(11):1642–1645 (1994).
17. Physicians Desk Reference. Montvale, NJ: Medical Economics, 2001.
18. Tomb DA. Psychiatry for the house officer. Baltimore: Williams & Wilkins, 1981.
19. Radomski JW, Dursun SM, Reveley MA, and Kutcher SP. An exploratory approach to the serotonin syndrome: an update of clinical phenomenology and revised diagnostic criteria. Med Hypotheses 55(3):218–224 (2000).
20. Bhanji NH. Serotonin syndrome following low-dose sertraline. Can J of Psychiatry 45(10): 936–937 (2000).
21. *State of Connecticut v. Christopher DeAngelo*. 2000 Conn. Super. LEXIS 1557.
22. Gorman JM. The essential guide to psychiatric drugs. New York: St. Martin's Press, 1990: 143–144.
23. Ingram IM and Timbury GC. Side effects of Librium. Lancet 2:766 (1960).
24. Deitch J and Jennings R. Aggressive dyscontrol in patients treated with benzodiazepines. J Clin Psych 49(5):184–188 (1988).
25. Gardner RL and Cowdry RW. Alprazolam-induced dyscontrol in borderline personality disorder. Am J Psychiatry 142:98–100 (1985).
26. Bond AJ, Curran HV, Bruce MS, O'Sullivan G, and Shine P. Behavioral aggression in panic disorder after 8 weeks' treatment with alprazolam. J Affective Disorder 35(3):117–123 (1995).
27. Welner M. Drug-facilitated sexual assault. New York: Academic Press, 2001.
28. Daderman AM, Fredriksson B, and Kristiansson M. Violent behavior, impulsive decision-making, and anterograde amnesia while intoxicated with flunitrazepam and alcohol or other drugs: a case study in forensic psychiatric patients. J Am Acad Psychiatry Law 30(2):238–251 (2002).

29. American Psychiatric Association. Benzodiazepine: dependence, toxicity, and abuse. Washington, DC: American Psychiatric Association, 1990:44.
30. Kaplan HI, Sadock BJ, and Grebb JA. Synopsis of psychiatry: behavior sciences clinical psychiatry. Baltimore: Williams & Wilkins, 1994:911.
31. American Psychiatric Association. Benzodiazepine: dependence, toxicity, and abuse. Washington, DC: American Psychiatric Association, 1990:15–19, 49–57.
32. *Boswell v. State,* 610 So. 2d 670.
33. DSM–III–R. Washington, DC: American Psychiatric Association, 1987:87.
34. DSM–IV Washington, DC: American Psychiatric Association, 1994:77.
35. Maletzky BM. The diagnosis of pathological intoxication. J Stud Alcohol 37(9):1215–1228 (1976).
36. Defense of drunkenness in English criminal law. 49 LQ Rev 528, 533 (1933).
37. 30 ALR 761–762 (1924).
38. *Commonwealth v. Walker*, 283 Pa 468, 129 A 453 (1925).
39. *State v. Hall*, 214 NW2d 205 (1974, Iowa).
40. *Tackett v. Commonwealth*, 205 Ky 490, 266 SW 26 (1924).
41. *People v. Gerrior*, 155 Ill App 3d 949 (1987, 2d Dist).
42. *Burchfield v. State*, 219 Ga App 40 (1995).
43. *Commonwealth v. McAlister*, 313 NE2d 113 (1974, Mass).
44. *Jones v. State*, 648 P2d 1251, 103 S Ct 799 (1982, Okla Crim).
45. *Teeters v. Commonwealth*, 310 Ky 546, 221 SW 2d 85 (1949).
46. *State v. Rippy*, 104 NC752, 10 SE 259 (1889).
47. *Aliff v. State*, 955 S.W.2d 891.
48. *People v. Baker*, 42 Cal 2d 550 (1954).
49. *State v. Gardner*, 230 Wis. 2d 32, 601 N.W. 2d 670.
50. *Arizona v. McKeon*, 2002 Ariz. App. LEXIS 8.
51. *Bennett v. State*, 161 Ark 496 (1923).
52. Simon RI and Sadoff RL. Psychiatric malpractice: cases and comments for clinicians. Washington, DC: American Psychiatric Press, 1992:101.
53. Kaplan H and Sadock B. Pocket handbook of psychiatric drug treatment. Baltimore: Williams & Wilkins, 1993.
54. Welner M. Medication defenses: myths and realities. american psychiatric association annual meeting, May 22, 2002, Philadelphia.
55. *Miller v. Florida*, 2001 Fla. App. LEXIS 14475.
56. *Michigan v. Wilkins*, 184 Mich. App. 443.
57. Kaplan HI, Sadock BJ, and Grebb JA. Synopsis of psychiatry: behavior sciences clinical psychiatry. Baltimore: Williams & Wilkins, 1994.
58. Aubry JM, Simon AE, and Bertschy G. Possible induction of mania and hypomania by olanzapine or risperidone: a critical review of reported cases. J Clin Psychiatry 61(9):649–655 (2000).
59. Pleak RR, Birmaher B, Gavrilescu A, Abichandani C, and Williams DT. Mania and neuropsychiatric excitation following carbamazepine. J American Academy Child Adolesc Psychiatry 27:500–503 (1988).
60. Kaplan HI, Sadock BJ, and Grebb JA. Synopsis of psychiatry: behavior sciences clinical psychiatry. Baltimore: Williams & Wilkins, 1994.
61. McElroy SL, Pope HG Jr, Keck PE Jr, Hudson JI, Phillips KA, and Strakowski SM. Are impulse-control disorders related to bipolar disorder? Compr Psychiatry 37(4):229–240 (1996).
62. Chengappa KN, Vasile J, Levine J, Ulrich R, Baker R, and Gopalani A. Clozapine: its impact on aggressive behavior among patients in a state psychiatric hospital. Schizophr Res 53 (1–2):1–6 (2002).

63. Sheard MH. Effect of lithium on human aggression. Nature 230:113–114 (1971).
64. Meltzer HY. Treatment of suicidality in schizophrenia. Ann NY Acad Sci 932:44–58 (2001).
65. Physicians Desk Reference. Montvale, NJ: Medical Economics, 2001.
66. Wysowski DK, Pitts M, and Beitz J. An analysis of reports of depression and suicide in patients treated with isotretinoin. J Am Acad Dermatol 45(4):515–519 (2001).
67. Bard M and Welner M. Bad acne: guilty defendant may bring med mal. The Forensic Echo 2(3):23–24 (1998).
68. Jacobs DG, Deutsch NL, and Brewer M. Suicide, depression, and isotretinoin: is there a causal link? J Am Acad Dermatol 45(5):S168–S175 (2001).
69. Isotretinoin, no other drugs found in Florida teen pilot's body. Dermatology Times. February 2002.
70. van Riemsdijk MM, van der Klauw MM, van Heest JA, Reedeker FR, Ligthelm RJ, Herings RM, and Stricker BH. Neuropsychiatric effects of antimalarials. Eur J Clin Pharmac 52: 1–6 (1997).
71. Rouveix B, Bricaire F, Michon C, Franssen G, Lebras J, and Bernard J. Mefloquine and an acute brain syndrome. Ann Internal Med 110:577–578 (1989).
72. Speich R and Haller A. Central anticholinergic syndrome with the antimalarial mefloquine. N Engl J Med 331:57–58 (1994).
73. Stuiver PC, Lightelm RJ, and Gould TJLM. Acute psychosis after mefloquine. Lancet 2: 282 (1989).
74. Hennequin C, Bouree P, Bazin N, Bisaro F, and Feline A. Severe psychiatric side effects observed during prophylaxis and treatment with mefloquine. *Arch Intern Med 1*54(20):2360–2362 (1994).
75. *US v. Mezvinsky*, 206 F. Supp. 2d 661 (E.D. Pa 2002).
76. Benjamin M and Olmstead R. Army had 1996 Lariam warning. United Press Int'l. Aug 22, 2002.
77. Hirschfeld RM, Keller MB, Panico S, et al. The National Depressive and Manic-Depressive Association consensus statement on the undertreatment of depression. JAMA 277(4):333–340 (1997).
78. Metzner JL. Class action litigation in correctional psychiatry. J Am Acad Psychiatry Law 30(1):19–29 (2002).
79. *Perloms v. United States*, (1915, CA4 SC) 228 F 408.
80. Rosenheck R, Chang S, Choe Y, Cramer J, Xu W, Thomas J, et al. Medication continuation and compliance: A comparison of patients treated with clozapine and haloperidol. J Clin Psych 61(5):382–386 (2000).
81. Bosker G and Albrich JM. Emergency detection of adverse drug reactions in the elderly. Resident and Staff Physician (September, 1989).
82. Jansen PL. Liver disease in the elderly. Best Pract Res Clin Gastroenterol 16(1):149–158 (2002).
83. Thompson D and Pollock B. Psychotropic metabolism: gender-related issues. Psychiatric Times 47–49 (January 2001).
84. Maletzky BM. The episodic dyscontrol syndrome. Dis Nerv Syst 34:178–185 (1973).
85. Pounder DJ. The nightmare of postmortem drug changes. In: Wecht CH, ed. Legal Medicine. Salem: Buttersworth, 1993:163–191.
86. Koh A and Pizzo PA. Empirical oral anitbiotic therapy for low risk febrile cancer patients with neutropenia. Cancer Invest 20(3):420–433 (2002).
87. Tamminga WJ, Werner J, Oostehuis B, Wieling J, Wilfert B, de Liej LFMH, et al. CYP2D6 and CYP2C19 activity in a large population of Dutch healthy volunteers: indications for oral contraceptive-related gender differences. Euro J Clin Pharmacol 55(3):177–184 (1999).

Index

A

Acamprosate, alcoholism treatment, 435
ACE inhibitors, *see* Angiotensin-converting enzyme inhibitors
Acetaminophen,
   drug interactions,
      alcohol, 414–416
      overview, 359, 360
   indications and contraindications, 359
   pharmacokinetics, 358
   poisoning, 416
   preparations and dosing, 359
   toxicity, 359
Adenosine, side effects, 226
AIDS, *see* Human immunodeficiency virus
Akathisia, antipsychotic drug induction, 190, 191
Albuterol,
   adverse reactions, 548
   contraindications, 546
   inhalation administration, 538
   oral dosing, 537, 538
   preparations, 537, 538
   prophylactic treatment, 538
Alcohol,
   alcoholism treatment, 434–437
   amethystic agents, 437, 438
   blood alcohol concentration, 396, 400
   drug interactions,
      anabolic steroids, 526, 527
      aspirin, 419, 420
      barbiturates, 431, 432
      benzodiazepines,
         fatalities, 24, 25
         pharmacodynamic effects, 32–37, 432–434
      categories of interactions, 396
      cimetidine, 422–424
      cisapride, 420, 421
      erythromycin, 421
      histamine-2 receptor antagonists, 422–424
      illicit drugs, 434
      mechanisms, 396–398
      nicotine interactions, 471, 472, 474
      opioids, 136
      propoxyphene, 430, 431
      prospects for study, 439–441
      ranitidine, 421, 422
      study design, 397–399
      tricyclic antidepressants, 162
      verapamil, 421
   first-pass metabolism, 417, 418
   impairment induction, 425–427, 439, 440
   intake patterns, 395
   metabolism,
      alcohol dehydrogenase,
         inhibitors, 407–410
         isozymes, 406
         Michaelis–Menten kinetics, 406, 407
      aldehyde dehydrogenase,
         inhibitors, 411–413
         isozymes, 410
      CYP2E1,
         acetaminophen interactions, 414–416
         functions, 413, 414
   pharmacokinetics,
      absorption, 400–403
      distribution, 403, 404
      elimination, 404, 405
   tobacco smoke interactions, 475
   tolerance development, 427, 428
   toxicity, 428–430
Alfentanyl, benzodiazepine interactions, 29–31

Allopurinol,
  drug interactions, 372
  indications and contraindications, 372
  mechanism of action, 372
  preparations and dosing, 372
α-Agonists, anabolic steroid interactions, 528
α-Blockers,
  contraindications, 231
  drug interactions, 232, 233
  indications,
    benign prostatic hyperplasia, 231
    hypertension, 231
  side effects, 230–232
Aluminum, β-blocker interactions, 236
Aminoglutethimide,
  adverse reactions, 572
  contraindications, 571
  drug interactions, 572, 573
  mechanism of action, 569, 570
  metabolism, 570
  pharmacokinetics, 569
  preparations, 569
Aminophylline,
  β-agonist interactions, 554
  β-blocker interactions, 236
Amiodarone,
  β-blocker interactions, 236
  drug interactions, 226–229
  metabolism, 227
  side effects, 225, 226
Amphetamines,
  adverse reactions, 548
  anabolic steroid interactions, 527
  β-agonist interactions, 552
  contraindications, 546
  dosing, 538, 539
  indications, 538, 539
  preparations, 538
Amphotericin B, β-agonist interactions, 552
Amprenavir, drug interactions, 324
Anabolic steroids, *see also specific steroids*,
  administration routes, 505, 506
  adverse reactions, 521, 522, 524–526
  biosynthesis, 516, 517
  contraindications, 522, 523
  drug interactions,
    alcohol, 526, 527
    α-agonists, 528
    amphetamines, 527
    anticoagulants, 526
    antiretroviral drugs, 527, 528
    β-agonists, 552
    carbamazepine, 528
    clonidine, 528
    cocaine, 529
    imipramine, 529
    insulin, 526
    nonsteroidal antiinflammatory drugs, 526
    opioids, 529
    overview, 530
    oxyphenbutazone, 529
    sodium, 526
  history of study, 496, 497
  mechanism of action, 517, 518
  metabolism, 519–521
  physical properties, 500–502
  preparations, 504, 505
  stacking schedules, 507
  stereochemistry, 500
  structures, 497–499, 503
  transport, 518, 519
Anakinra,
  drug interactions, 370
  indications and contraindications, 370
  mechanism of action, 370
Anastrozole,
  adverse reactions, 572
  contraindications, 571
  drug interactions, 572, 573
  mechanism of action, 569, 570
  metabolism, 570
  pharmacokinetics, 568
  preparations, 568
Androgens, *see* Anabolic steroids
Androstenedione,
  adverse effects, 524
  contraindications, 522
  dosing, 508
  indications, 508
  preparations, 507, 508
  relative activity of drugs, 504
Angina,
  management, 254, 255
  types, 254, 255
Angiotensin-converting enzyme (ACE) inhibitors,
  drug interactions, 248, 249
  mechanisms of action, 244, 245
  pregnancy precautions, 248
  side effects,
    acute renal failure, 246
    anaphylactoid reactions, 248

Index 649

angioneurotic edema, 248
cough, 247
hyperkalemia, 246, 247
hypotension, 246
overview, 245, 246
toxicity, 248
Angiotensin II receptor blockers,
drug interactions, 250, 251
mechanism of action, 249, 250
pregnancy precautions, 250
side effects, 250
Antacids,
benzodiazepine interactions, 37–39
statin interactions, 279
Antiarrhythmic drugs,
classification, 219–221
drug interactions with amiodarone, 226–229
side effects by drug class, 221–226
Antibiotics, *see also specific antibiotics*,
benzodiazepine interactions, 54–58
Anticonvulsants, *see also specific drugs*,
benzodiazepine interactions, 51–53
opioid interactions, 136, 137
Antiepileptic drugs, *see also* Anticonvulsants,
mechanisms of action, 90
side effects, 90, 94, 95
Antifungal agents, benzodiazepine interactions, 44–47
Antimicrobials,
assays, 312
classification, 301, 303
drug interactions, *see also specific drugs*,
CYP metabolism, 310, 311
herbal supplements, 311, 312
toxicological and forensic investigations, 312, 313
microbial metabolism, 310
pharmacokinetics,
absorption, 304–306
distribution, 306
elimination, 309, 310
host–parasite considerations, 303, 304
metabolism by host, 307–309
overview, 301, 302
Antiplatelet agents,
classes, 272–275
drug interactions by class, 272–275
side effects by class, 272–275
Antipsychotics,
CYP polymorphisms in metabolism, 203, 204

drug interactions,
benzodiazepines, 201, 203
nefazodone, 199
nicotine, 203, 472
phenytoin, 200, 201
tricyclic antidepressants, 200
legal implications,
akathisia, 191
civil law, 207
cognitive side effects, 193, 194
criminal law,
competency, 205, 206
medication defenses, 206, 207
questioning of suspects, 204, 205
disability status, 207–209
drug interactions, 204
malpractice litigation, 209, 210
testamentary capacity, 210
mechanisms of action,
acetylcholine blockade, 194, 195
dopamine blockade, 188–190
neuroanatomy, 195, 196
metabolism, 198–202
side effects,
adrenergic effects, 196
akathisia induction, 190, 191
clozapine, 201, 202
cognitive side effects of dopamine blockade, 192, 193
neuroleptic malignant syndrome, 197
seizures, 198
sexual dysfunction, 194, 197, 198
sudden death and cardiac conductance, 196, 197
sugar metabolism effects, 195
tardive dyskinesia induction, 191, 192
weight gain, 195
tobacco smoke interactions, 476, 477
traditional versus atypical antipsychotics, 187
types, 18
Antipyrene,
benzodiazepine interactions, 62–64
statin interactions, 279
Antiretroviral drugs,
classes, 320
drug interactions,
additive toxicities, 328
anabolic steroids, 527, 528
benzodiazepines, 58–60
opioids, 135, 136
pharmacodynamic interactions, 323, 329
pharmacokinetic interactions,
mechanisms, 321–323
table, 324–328

Aspirin,
  adverse effects, 345
  alcohol interactions, 419, 420
  contraindications, 345
  drug interactions, 346, 347
  indications, 344, 345
  mechanism of action, 344
  pharmacokinetics, 343
  preparations and dosing, 345
  tobacco smoke interactions, 475, 476
  toxicity management, 346
Atovaquone, antiretroviral drug interactions, 324
Azathioprine,
  drug interactions, 365
  indications and contraindications, 365
  preparations and dosing, 365
Azithromycin, benzodiazepine interactions, 57

B

Barbiturates,
  alcohol interactions, 431, 432
  nicotine interactions, 472, 473
  opioid interactions, 138
Benzodiazepines,
  administration routes and dosing, 7
  alcoholism treatment, 435
  antipsychotic drug interactions, 201, 203
  criminal defense aspects, 635, 636
  development, 3, 4, 9, 10
  drug interactions,
    alcohol pharmacodynamic and pharmacokinetic interactions, 32–37, 432–434
    analgesics, 27–31
    anesthetics, 27–31
    antibiotics, 54–58
    anticonvulsants, 51–53
    antifungal agents, 44–47
    antipyrene, 62–64
    antiretroviral agents, 58–60
    cardiovascular agents, 53–55
    diflunisal, 64
    disulfiram, 64
    epidemiology studies of mortality,
      alcohol interactions, 24, 25
      motor vehicle fatalities, 27, 28
      opioid interactions, 24–26
    gastrointestinal agents, 37–44
    glucocorticoids, 64
    grapefruit juice, 60–62
    herbal supplements, 66
    modafinal, 66
    nicotine, 473
    oral contraceptives, 49–51
    paracetamol, 64
    probenecid, 64, 65
    selective serotonin reuptake inhibitors, 47–49
    theophylline, 62
  half-life, 7
  mechanism of action, 4
  metabolism,
    CYP types, 22, 23
    enzyme determination techniques, 15, 16, 18, 19, 21, 22
    overview, 10–14
  pharmacokinetics, 6, 8, 9
  plasma protein binding and distribution, 6, 8
  selective serotonin reuptake inhibitor interactions, 181
  side effects, 6
  structures, 8–13
  tobacco smoke interactions, 478
  types and trade names, 5
  uses, 4, 6, 7
β-Agonists, *see also specific drugs*,
  administration routes, 537
  adverse reactions, 547–551
  biosynthesis, 543, 545
  chemistry, 531, 532
  contraindications, 546, 547
  drug interactions, 551–555
  mechanism of action, 543, 544
  metabolism, 545, 546
  physical properties, 534–536
  preparations, 537
  stereochemistry, 532, 534
  structures, 532, 533
  uses, 531
β-Blockers,
  classification, 233–235
  drug interactions,
    amiodarone, 228
    benzodiazepines, 53–55
    overview, 236–238
  indications, 234
  metabolism, 234, 235
  side effects, 224, 225, 235, 236
  tobacco smoke interactions, 479
  types, 234
Bezafibrate, statin interactions, 277
Bretylium, side effects, 226

Index

C

Caffeine,
   nicotine interactions, 473
   tobacco smoke interactions, 478
Calcium channel blockers,
   β-blocker interactions, 236
   drug interactions,
      amiodarone interactions, 228, 229
      benzodiazepines, 53–55
      overview, 243, 244
   indications, 241, 242
   side effects,
      cardiac function, 242, 243
      overview, 242
   types, 242
Cannabinoids, opioid interactions, 139
Carbamazepine,
   adverse reactions, 94, 99, 100
   chemistry, 95, 98
   contraindications and precautions, 100
   drug interactions,
      anabolic steroids, 528
      antiepileptic drug interactions, 96
      benzodiazepines, 51–53
      non-antiepileptic drugs, 97
      overview, 100
   pharmacokinetics,
      absorption, 98
      distribution, 99
      excretion, 99
      metabolism, 99
   pharmacology, 98
   tobacco smoke interactions, 479
Carbon tetrachloride, nicotine interactions, 473
Cardiac glycosides, *see* Digoxin
Celecoxib,
   drug interactions, 361
   indications and contraindications, 360
   pharmacokinetics, 360
   preparations and dosing, 360, 361
Chloral hydrate, alcohol dehydrogenase interactions, 409, 410
Chlorambucil,
   drug interactions, 367
   indications, 366, 367
   preparations and dosing, 367
Chloroquine,
   drug interactions, 368
   indications, 367
   preparations and dosing, 367

Chlorpropamide, aldehyde dehydrogenase inhibition, 412
Cholestyramine,
   adverse reactions, 283
   contraindications, 282
   drug interactions,
      β-blockers, 236
      overview, 282, 283
   mechanism of action, 281
   pharmacokinetics, 282
Cimetidine,
   alcohol interactions, 422–424
   benzodiazepine interactions, 39–42
   β-blocker interactions, 236, 237
   nicotine interactions, 474
   opioid interactions, 136
   statin interactions, 279
Ciprofloxacin,
   benzodiazepine interactions, 56–58
   opioid interactions, 137
Cisapride,
   alcohol interactions, 420, 421
   benzodiazepine interactions, 38, 39
Clarithromycin,
   antiretroviral drug interactions, 324
   benzodiazepine interactions, 57
Clenbuterol,
   adverse reactions, 548, 549
   assays, 582
   contraindications, 546
   indications, 539
   mechanism of action, 539
Clofibrate,
   drug interactions, 280
   mechanism of action, 279, 280
   side effects, 280
Clomiphene,
   administration routes, 561
   adverse reactions, 563
   contraindications, 562, 563
   drug interactions, 563
   mechanism of action, 562
   metabolism, 562
   preparations, 561
Clonidine,
   anabolic steroid interactions, 528
   β-blocker interactions, 237
   mechanism of action, 230
   metabolism, 230
   side effects, 229
Clopidogrel,
   drug interactions, 275
   side effects, 273, 274

Cocaethylene, alcohol interactions, 434
Cocaine,
    adverse reactions, 549
    anabolic steroid interactions, 529
    β-agonist interactions, 553
    contraindications, 546
    mechanism of action, 539
    nicotine interactions, 474
    opioid interactions, 139
    selective serotonin reuptake inhibitor interactions, 181
    topical anesthesia, 539, 540
Colchicine,
    drug interactions, 371
    indications and contraindications, 371
    mechanism of action, 371
    preparations and dosing, 37
Colestipol,
    adverse reactions, 283, 284
    contraindications, 282
    drug interactions,
        β-blockers, 236
        overview, 282, 283
        statins, 278
    mechanism of action, 281, 282
    pharmacokinetics, 282
Corticosteroids, β-agonist interactions, 553
COX, see Cyclooxygenase
Cyclofenil,
    administration routes, 555
    adverse reactions, 556
    contraindications, 555
    detection,
        analytical techniques, 581–583
        blood, 579
        false positives, 584
        functional testing, 584, 585
        hair, 580, 581
        interfering factors in assays, 586
        involuntary doping, 583, 584
        saliva, 579, 580
        urine, 577–579
    mechanism of action, 555, 556
    preparations, 555
Cyclooxygenase (COX),
    inhibitors, see Nonsteroidal antiinflammatory drugs
    isoforms, 338
Cyclophosphamide,
    drug interactions, 367
    indications, 366, 367
    preparations and dosing, 367

Cyclosporin,
    drug interactions,
        amiodarone, 227
        overview, 364, 365
    indications and contraindications, 364
    preparations and dosing, 364
CYP1A2, inhibitors for study, 20, 21
CYP2A6, inhibitors for study, 20, 21
CYP2B6,
    benzodiazepine metabolism, 22, 23
    inhibitors for study, 20, 21
CYP2C19,
    benzodiazepine metabolism, 22, 23
    inhibitors for study, 20, 21
    polymorphisms and tricyclic antidepressant metabolism, 158, 163
CYP2C8, inhibitors for study, 20, 21
CYP2C9, inhibitors for study, 20, 21
CYP2D6,
    inhibitors for study, 20, 21
    polymorphisms and tricyclic antidepressant metabolism, 156–158, 163
CYP2E1,
    acetaminophen interactions, 414–416
    alcohol metabolism, 413, 414
    inhibitors for study, 20, 21
CYP3A4,
    benzodiazepine metabolism, 22, 23
    grapefruit inhibitors, 60, 61
    inhibitors for study, 20, 21
CYP3A5, benzodiazepine metabolism, 22, 23

D

Danazol,
    adverse effects, 524
    contraindications, 523
    dosing, 509, 510
    indications, 509
    pharmacokinetics, 509
    preparations, 508, 509
Delaviridine, drug interactions, 324
DHT, see Dihydrotestosterone
Diazoxide,
    adverse effects, 241
    indications, 241
    pharmacology, 241
Diclofenac,
    drug interactions, 350
    indications and contraindications, 350
    pharmacokinetics, 349, 350
    preparations and dosing, 350

Index

Didanosine, drug interactions, 324
Diflunisal,
  drug interactions,
    benzodiazepines, 64
    overview, 347, 348
  pharmacokinetics, 347
  preparations and dosing, 347
Digoxin,
  drug interactions,
    amiodarone interactions, 228
    β-agonist interactions, 552
    β-blocker interactions, 236
    pharmacodynamic interactions, 253
    pharmacokinetic interactions, 252, 253
    statins, 278
  mechanism of action, 251, 252
  pharmacokinetics, 252
  toxicity and monitoring, 253, 254
Dihydrotestosterone (DHT),
  adverse effects, 524
  dosing, 510
  indications, 510
  pharmacokinetics, 510
Dipyridamole,
  drug interactions, 273
  side effects, 272, 273
Disopyramide, side effects, 223
Disulfiram,
  alcoholism treatment, 434, 435
  aldehyde dehydrogenase inhibition, 411, 412
  benzodiazepine interactions, 64
Diuretics,
  indications, 258, 259
  loop diuretics,
    adverse events, 265, 266
    contraindications, 266
    drug interactions,
      β-agonists, 554
      overview, 266, 267
    indications, 265
    mechanism of action, 265
    metabolism, 265
  mechanisms of action, 259, 260
  renal sites of action, 260
  thiazide diuretics,
    adverse reactions, 263–265
    contraindications, 261, 262
    drug interactions,
      β-agonists, 554
      overview, 262, 263
    mechanism of action, 260
    pharmacokinetics, 261

Dobutamine,
  adverse reactions, 549, 550
  contraindications, 546
  intravenous dosing, 540
  mechanism of action, 540

E

Ebrotidine, benzodiazepine interactions, 40, 42
Efavirenz, drug interactions, 325
Endorphins,
  functions, 126, 127
  processing, 126
  types, 126
Entacapone, β-agonist interactions, 553
Epilepsy,
  epidemiology, 89
  etiology, 89
  medications, *see* Antiepileptic drugs
Ergot alkaloids, β-agonist interactions, 553
Erythromycin,
  alcohol interactions, 421
  amiodarone interactions, 229
  benzodiazepine interactions, 56–58
  statin interactions, 279
Erythropoietin,
  adverse reactions, 577
  contraindications, 576
  drug interactions, 577
  indications, 573–575
  mechanism of action, 575, 576
  metabolism, 576
  preparations, 573–575
Escherichia coli, pathogenic strains, 296, 297
Etanercept,
  drug interactions, 370
  indications and contraindications, 370
  mechanism of action, 369
  preparations and dosing, 370
Ethambutol, benzodiazepine interactions, 57
Ethanol, *see* Alcohol
Ethosuximide,
  adverse reactions, 94, 105, 106
  chemistry, 104, 105
  contraindications and precautions, 106
  drug interactions,
    antiepileptic drug interactions, 96
    non-antiepileptic drugs, 97
    overview, 106
  metabolism, 105
  pharmacokinetics, 105
  pharmacology, 105

Etodolac,
    drug interactions, 352
    pharmacokinetics, 352
    preparations and dosing, 352
Exemestane,
    adverse reactions, 572
    contraindications, 571
    drug interactions, 572, 573
    mechanism of action, 569, 570
    metabolism, 570
    pharmacokinetics, 569
    preparations, 569

F

Famotidine, benzodiazepine interactions, 40, 42
Felbamate,
    adverse reactions, 95, 112
    chemistry, 111
    contraindications and precautions, 112
    drug interactions,
        antiepileptic drug interactions, 96
        non-antiepileptic drugs, 97
        overview, 112, 113
    metabolism, 111
    pharmacokinetics, 111, 112
    pharmacology, 111
Felodipine, drug interactions, 243
Fenifibrate,
    drug interactions,
        overview, 280
        statins, 277
    mechanism of action, 279, 280
    side effects, 280
Fenoprofen,
    indications and contraindications, 356
    pharmacokinetics, 356
    preparations and dosing, 356
Fentanyl, benzodiazepine interactions, 29–31
Fibrates, see Clofibrate; Fenifibrate; Gemfibrozil
Flecainide,
    amiodarone interactions, 227
    side effects, 224
Fluconazole, drug interactions,
    benzodiazepines, 46
    overview, 325
5-Fluorouracil, opioid interactions, 137
Fluoxetine,
    benzodiazepine interactions, 47–49
    criminal defense aspects, 631–635
Fluoxymesterone,
    adverse effects, 524
    contraindications, 523
    dosing, 511
    indications, 511
    pharmacokinetics, 510
Flurbiprofen,
    indications and contraindications, 356
    pharmacokinetics, 356
    preparations and dosing, 356
Fluvoxamine,
    benzodiazepine interactions, 47–49
    opioid interactions, 136, 137
Fomepizole, alcohol dehydrogenase interactions, 409
Food-drug interactions,
    monoamine oxidase inhibitors, 150, 151
    nutritional status interactions,
        absorption effects, 389
        excretion effects, 390
        food intake, 387, 388
        metabolism effects, 389, 390
        overview, 386, 387
        weight gain, 388, 389
    opioids, 134, 135
    pharmacological aspects, 379, 380
    phases of nutrient–drug interactions,
        pharmaceutical phase, 380, 381
        pharmacodynamic phase, 384, 386
        pharmacokinetic phase, 381–384
Fructose, amethystic agent, 437, 438

G

Gabapentin,
    adverse reactions, 95, 107
    chemistry, 106
    contraindications and precautions, 107
    drug interactions,
        antiepileptic drug interactions, 96
        non-antiepileptic drugs, 97
        overview, 107
    metabolism, 107
    pharmacokinetics, 106, 107
    pharmacology, 106
Ganciclovir, drug interactions, 325
Gemfibrozil,
    drug interactions,
        overview, 280
        statins, 277
    mechanism of action, 279, 280
    side effects, 280
Gentamicin, opioid interactions, 137

Index

GHB, *see* γ-Hydroxybutyrate
Glucocorticoids, benzodiazepine interactions, 64
Gold,
    drug interactions, 366
    indications and contraindications, 366
    mechanism of action, 366
    preparations and dosing, 366
Gonadotrophin-releasing hormone,
    administration routes, 559
    adverse reactions, 559
    contraindications, 559
    drug interactions, 560
    indications, 559
    mechanism of action, 559
    preparations, 558, 559
Gout,
    acute attack management, 371
    arthritis management, 372, 373
Grapefruit juice,
    CYP inhibitors, 60, 61
    drug interactions,
        benzodiazepines, 60–62
        overview, 384, 386
Growth hormone, *see* Human growth hormone
Guanethidine, β-agonist interactions, 553

H

Haemophilus influenzae,
    diagnosis of disease, 298
    transmission, 297, 298
Halofenate, β-blocker interactions, 237
HCTZ, *see* Hydrochlorothiazide
Heparin,
    complications, 267, 268
    mechanism of action, 267
    tobacco smoke interactions, 476
Hepatitis, virus types and diseases, 298, 299
Herbal supplements,
    antimicrobial interactions, 311, 312
    benzodiazepine interactions, 66
    β-agonist interactions, 553
    opioid interactions, 135
    selective serotonin reuptake inhibitor interactions, 180
Herpes simplex virus (HSV), clinical features and management, 299
HGH, *see* Human growth hormone
Histamine-2 receptor antagonists,
    alcohol interactions, 422–424
    benzodiazepine interactions, 39–42
HIV, *see* Human immunodeficiency virus

HSV, *see* Herpes simplex virus
Human growth hormone (HGH),
    adverse reactions, 558
    biosynthesis, 557
    contraindications, 558
    drug interactions, 558
    indications, 557
    mechanism of action, 557
    metabolism, 558
    pharmacokinetics, 556, 557
    preparations, 556
Human immunodeficiency virus (HIV),
    see also Antiretroviral drugs,
    epidemiology of AIDS, 319
    management, 320, 321, 329
Hydralazine,
    dosing, 240
    indications, 240
Hydrochlorothiazide (HCTZ),
    adverse reactions, 263–265
    contraindications, 261, 262
    drug interactions, 262, 263
    mechanism of action, 260
    pharmacokinetics, 261
γ-Hydroxybutyrate (GHB), alcoholism treatment, 435, 436

I

Ibuprofen,
    drug interactions, 354
    indications and contraindications, 353
    opioid interactions, 135
    pharmacokinetics, 353
    preparations and dosing, 353, 354
IGF-1, *see* Insulin-like growth factor-1
Imipramine, anabolic steroid interactions, 529
Indinavir, drug interactions, 325
Indomethacin,
    adverse effects, 349
    contraindications, 349
    drug interactions, 349
    gout management, 371
    pharmacokinetics, 348
    preparations and dosing, 348, 349
Infliximab,
    drug interactions, 369
    indications and contraindications, 369
    mechanism of action, 369
    preparations and dosing, 369
Insulin,
    anabolic steroid interactions, 526
    β-agonist interactions, 553

Insulin-like growth factor-1 (IGF-1),
    administration routes, 560
    adverse reactions, 561
    biosynthesis, 560, 561
    mechanism of action, 561
    preparations, 560
Isoniazid,
    benzodiazepine interactions, 57
    tricyclic antidepressant interactions, 152
Isoproterenol,
    administration routes, 540, 541
    adverse reactions, 550
    β-blocker interactions, 237
    contraindications, 547
    indications, 540
Israpidine, drug interactions, 243
Itraconazole, drug interactions,
    benzodiazepines, 46
    overview, 325

K

Ketoconazole,
    amiodarone interactions, 229
    antiretroviral drug interactions, 326
    benzodiazepine interactions, 44–46
Ketoprofen,
    indications and contraindications, 356
    pharmacokinetics, 356
    preparations and dosing, 356, 357
Ketorolac,
    indications and contraindications, 353
    pharmacokinetics, 353
    preparations and dosing, 353

L

Lamotrigine,
    adverse reactions, 94, 101, 102
    chemistry, 100
    contraindications and precautions, 102
    drug interactions,
        antiepileptic drug interactions, 96
        non-antiepileptic drugs, 97
        overview, 102
    metabolism, 101
    pharmacokinetics, 101
    pharmacology, 100, 101
Lansoprazole, benzodiazepine interactions, 42–44
Leflunomide,
    drug interactions, 366
    indications and contraindications, 365

mechanism of action, 365
    preparations and dosing, 365
Legal aspects,
    antipsychotics,
        akathisia, 191
        civil law, 207
        cognitive side effects, 193, 194
        criminal law,
            competency, 205, 206
            medication defenses, 206, 207
            questioning of suspects, 204, 205
        disability status, 207–209
        drug interactions, 204
        malpractice litigation, 209, 210
        testamantary capacity, 210
    civil cases by state, 627, 628
    cross-claims by physicians or pharmacists
        against pharmaceutical companies, 616
    forensic evidence of causation reliability,
        616–627
    pharmaceutical company civil action
        case law,
        learned intermediary doctrine, 609, 610
        multiple theories of liability, 615, 616
        negligence and strict liability, 610–615
    pharmacist civil action case law,
        learned intermediary doctrine, 602–604
        reasonable care requirement, 606–608
        voluntary undertaking theory of liability,
            604–606
    physician civil action case law, 599–602
    psychotropic medications in criminal
            defense,
        benzodiazepines, 635, 636
        criminal responsibility evaluation,
            collateral witnesses, 641
            event history, 641
            laboratory testing, 641, 642
            medical history, 640, 641
            past patterns of violence, 640
        involuntary intoxication, 636–639
        Prozac, 631–635
        serotonergic antidepressants
            and agitation frequency, 634
        underlying condition in criminal
            behavior, 639
Legionnaire's disease, clinical features
    and management, 300
Letrozole,
    adverse reactions, 572
    contraindications, 571

Index

drug interactions, 572, 573
mechanism of action, 569, 570
metabolism, 570
pharmacokinetics, 568
preparations, 568
Levetiracetam,
adverse reactions, 95, 115
chemistry, 114
contraindications and precautions, 115, 116
drug interactions,
antiepileptic drug interactions, 96
non-antiepileptic drugs, 97
overview, 116
metabolism, 115
pharmacokinetics, 115
pharmacology, 114, 115
Levodopa,
β-agonist interactions, 554
β-blocker interactions, 237
Lidocaine,
β-blocker interactions, 236
side effects, 223
Lithium, selective serotonin reuptake inhibitor interactions, 181
Litigation, *see* Legal aspects
Loop diuretics, *see* Diuretics
Lopinavir, drug interactions, 326
LSD, *see* Lysergic acid diethylamine
Lysergic acid diethylamine (LSD), opioid interactions, 139

M

MAOIs, *see* Monoamine oxidase inhibitors
Maprotiline, β-agonist interactions, 555
Meclofenamate,
indications and contraindications, 357
pharmacokinetics, 357
preparations and dosing, 357, 358
Mefenamic acid,
indications and contraindications, 357
pharmacokinetics, 357
preparations and dosing, 357, 358
Meloxocam,
indications and contraindications, 358
pharmacokinetics, 358
preparations and dosing, 358
Meningitis,
chronic disease, 296
pathogens, 295, 296
Methadone,
benzodiazepine interactions, 28–31

selective serotonin reuptake inhibitor interactions, 181
uses, 129
Methanol,
alcohol dehydrogenase interactions, 407, 408
poisoning, 408
Methotrexate,
drug interactions, 364
indications and contraindications, 364
mechanism of action, 362
pharmacokinetics, 364
preparations and dosing, 364
Methyldopa, β-blocker interactions, 237
Methyltestosterone,
adverse effects, 525
contraindications, 523
dosing, 511
indications, 511
pharmacokinetics, 511
preparations, 511
Metoclopramide, opioid interactions, 135
Metoprolol, selective serotonin reuptake inhibitor interactions, 181
Metronidazole,
aldehyde dehydrogenase inhibition, 412, 413
benzodiazepine interactions, 44–46
Mexiletine, side effects, 223
Minoxidil,
dosing, 241
indications, 240
pharmacology, 240
Modafinal, benzodiazepine interactions, 66
Monoamine oxidase inhibitors (MAOIs),
β-agonist interactions, 554
β-blocker interactions, 237
depression management, 149
enzyme isoform specificity, 150
food interactions, 150, 151
narcotic analgesia interactions, 151, 152
overdose, 150
Moricizine, side effects, 224
Morphine, benzodiazepine interactions, 29, 31

N

Nabumetone,
indications and contraindications, 352
pharmacokinetics, 352
preparations and dosing, 352, 353
Naltrexone,
adverse effects, 525
alcoholism treatment, 435, 436

benzodiazepine interactions, 30
contraindications, 523
dosing, 512
indications, 512
pharmacokinetics, 512
preparations, 511, 512
Naproxen,
drug interactions, 355
indications and contraindications, 355
pharmacokinetics, 354, 355
preparations and dosing, 355
Nefazodone, benzodiazepine interactions, 47–49, 199
Neuroleptic malignant syndrome (NMS), antipsychotic drug induction, 197
Nevirapine, drug interactions, 326
Niacin,
drug interactions,
overview, 284, 285
statins, 277
indications, 284
precautions, 284
Nicardipine, drug interactions, 243
Nicotine,
drug interactions,
alcohol, 471, 472, 474
antipsychotics, 203, 472
barbiturates, 472, 473
benzodiazepines, 473
β-blocker interactions, 236
caffeine, 473
carbon tetrachloride, 473
cimetidine, 474
cocaine, 474
mechanisms,
pharmacodynamic mechanisms, 471
pharmacokinetic mechanisms, 470, 471
opioids, 474
phencyclidine, 474
tricyclic antidepressants, 472
tripelannamine, 472
pharmacology, 467, 468
replacement therapy,
adverse effects, 483, 484
components, 467
contraindications, 482
forms, 463–465
precautions, 483
prevalence of use, 465
tobacco, *see also* Smoking,
chewing tobacco, 482
components, 467
forms, 465, 466
prevalence of use, 466, 467
toxicity, 468, 469
Nifedipine, drug interactions, 243
Nimodipine, drug interactions, 243
Nisoldipine, drug interactions, 244
Nitroglycerin,
angina management, 254–256
contraindications, 258
drug interactions, 258
mechanism of action, 256, 258
side effects, 257
sublingual administration, 256, 257
tolerance, 257
Nitroprusside,
dosing, 238
mechanism of action, 238, 239, 258
metabolism, 238
monitoring, 239
side effects, 240
Nizatidine, benzodiazepine interactions, 40, 42
NMS, *see* Neuroleptic malignant syndrome
Nonsteroidal antiinflammatory drugs (NSAIDs), *see also specific drugs*,
anabolic steroid interactions, 526
classification, 337, 338
cyclooxygenase inhibitors,
adverse effects, 341, 342
analgesic effects, 341
antipyretic effects, 341
chemistry, 338
drug interactions, 342, 343
pharmacodynamics, 340, 341
pharmacokinetics, 338, 340
selection guidelines, 362
types, 338, 339
disease-modifying antirheumatic drugs,
alkylating agents, 366, 367
antimalarial agents, 367, 368
classification, 362, 363
immunosuppressive drugs, 362, 364–366
interleukin-1 antagonists, 370
tumor necrosis factor-α antagonists, 369, 370
gout management, 370–373
half-lives, 344
NSAIDs, *see* Nonsteroidal antiinflammatory drugs

Index

O

OCs, *see* Oral contraceptives
Omeprazole, benzodiazepine interactions, 42–44
Ondansetron, alcoholism treatment, 435
Opioids, *see also specific opioids*,
    abuse, 127–129
    classes, 123
    drug interactions,
        alcohol, 136
        anabolic steroids, 529
        anticonvulsants, 136, 137
        antiretroviral drugs, 135, 136
        barbiturates, 138
        benzodiazepines,
            fatalities, 24–26
            pharmacodynamic effects, 28–30, 138
        cannabinoids, 139
        cimetidine, 136
        ciprofloxacin, 137
        cocaine, 139
        endocrine drugs, 139
        5-fluorouracil, 137
        fluvoxamine, 136, 137
        food, 134, 135
        gentamicin, 137
        herbal supplements, 135
        ibuprofen, 135
        lysergic acid diethylamine, 139
        metoclopramide, 135
        nicotine, 474
        oral contraceptives, 137
        phenothiazines, 138, 139
        propofol, 138
        propoxyphene, 137
        psychoactive agents, 138, 139
        quinidine, 137
        rifampin, 136
        tricyclic antidepressants, 135
        trovafloxacin, 135
        urinary acidifiers, 137, 138
    genotoxicity, 141
    history of use, 123, 127, 128
    immunosuppression, 141
    mechanism of action, 127
    overdose,
        clinical presentation, 131, 132
        diagnosis, 132, 133
        management, 133, 134
        postmortem examinations, 141–143
    pharmacokinetics, 123–125
    physiological effects,
        cardiovascular system, 130
        central nervous system, 128, 129
        gastrointestinal system, 130
        peripheral effects, 128
        respiratory system, 129, 130
    receptors, 125, 126
    tolerance and physical dependence, 130, 131
Oral contraceptives (OCs),
    benzodiazepine interactions, 49–51
    opioid interactions, 137
    statin interactions, 278
Oxandrolone,
    adverse effects, 525
    contraindications, 523
    dosing, 513, 514
    indications, 513, 514
    pharmacokinetics, 513
    preparations, 512
Oxaprozin,
    gouty arthritis management, 373
    indications and contraindications, 357
    pharmacokinetics, 357
    preparations and dosing, 357
Oxcarbazepine,
    chemistry, 95, 98
    drug interactions,
        antiepileptic drug interactions, 96
        non-antiepileptic drugs, 97
        overview, 100
    pharmacokinetics,
        absorption, 98
        distribution, 99
        excretion, 99
        metabolism, 99
    pharmacology, 98
Oxmetidine, benzodiazepine interactions, 40, 42
Oxymetholone,
    adverse effects, 525
    contraindications, 523
    dosing, 514
    indications, 514
    preparations, 514
Oxyphenbutazone, anabolic steroid interactions, 529

P

Pantoprazole, benzodiazepine interactions, 42, 44
Papaveretum, benzodiazepine interactions, 29, 31

Paracetamol, benzodiazepine interactions, 64
Paroxetine, amiodarone interactions, 229
Penicillamine,
  drug interactions, 369
  indications, 368
  preparations and dosing, 368
Performance enhancers, see also Anabolic steroids; β-agonists; Clomiphene; Cyclofenil; Erythropoietin; Gonadotrophin-releasing hormone; Human growth hormone; Insulin-like growth factor-1; Tamoxifen,
  history of use, 493–496
  International Olympic Committee restrictions, 496
Pethidine, benzodiazepine interactions, 29, 31
Phencyclidine, nicotine interactions, 474
Phenothiazines,
  β-blocker interactions, 237
  opioid interactions, 138, 139
Phentermine, selective serotonin reuptake inhibitor interactions, 181
Phenylpropanolamine (PPA),
  adverse reactions, 550, 551
  β-blocker interactions, 237
  contraindications, 547
  dosing, 541, 542
  indications, 541
  mechanism of action, 541
Phenytoin,
  adverse reactions, 93, 94
  antipsychotic drug interactions, 200, 201
  benzodiazepine interactions, 52, 53
  β-blocker interactions, 237
  contraindications and precautions, 93
  drug interactions,
    amiodarone, 229
    antiepileptic drug interactions, 96
    non-antiepileptic drugs, 97
    overview, 94, 95
    selective serotonin reuptake inhibitors, 181
  formulations, 90, 91
  fosphenytoin as prodrug, 91
  pharmacokinetics,
    absorption, 91, 92
    distribution, 92
    excretion, 93
    metabolism, 92, 93
  pharmacology, 91
Piroxicam,
  indications and contraindications, 358

  pharmacokinetics, 358
  preparations and dosing, 358
PPA, see Phenylpropanolamine
Probenecid,
  drug interactions,
    benzodiazepines, 64, 65
    overview, 373
  gouty arthritis management, 373
Probucol,
  mechanism of action, 281
  side effects, 281
Procainamide,
  amiodarone interactions, 228
  side effects, 222, 223
Propafenone, side effects, 224
Propofol,
  benzodiazepine interactions, 30, 31
  opioid interactions, 138
Propoxyphene,
  alcohol interactions, 430, 431
  benzodiazepine interactions, 30, 31
  opioid interactions, 137
Propranolol,
  adverse reactions, 551
  contraindications, 547
  indications, 542
  mechanism of action, 542
Proton pump inhibitors, benzodiazepine interactions, 42–44

Q

Quinidine,
  amiodarone interactions, 227
  β-blocker interactions, 237
  opioid interactions, 137
  side effects, 221, 222

R

Ranitidine,
  alcohol interactions, 421, 422
  benzodiazepine interactions, 40, 42
Reserpine, β-blocker interactions, 237
Rifabutin, drug interactions, 326
Rifampin, drug interactions,
  benzodiazepine interactions, 54, 56, 57
  β-blocker interactions, 236
  opioid interactions, 136
  overview, 327
Risperidone, selective serotonin reuptake inhibitor interactions, 181

Ritonavir, drug interactions,
  benzodiazepine interactions, 58, 60
  overview, 327, 328
Rofecoxib,
  drug interactions, 361, 362
  indications and contraindications, 361
  pharmacokinetics, 361
  preparations and dosing, 361
Roxithromycin, benzodiazepine interactions, 57, 58

S

Salmonellosis, clinical features and management, 300
Saquinavir, drug interactions,
  benzodiazepine interactions, 58–60
  overview, 328
Selective serotonin reuptake inhibitors (SSRIs),
  adverse reactions, 181
  CYPs in metabolism, 177, 178
  depression management, 149, 175
  drug interactions,
    benzodiazepines, 47–49
    herbal supplements, 180
    pharmacodynamic interactions, 178, 179
    pharmacokinetic interactions, 179
    tricyclic antidepressants, 159–161, 181
  mechanism of action, 175, 176
  pharmacokinetics,
    absorption, 176
    distribution, 176, 177
    elimination, 177
    metabolism, 177
  serotonin syndrome, 149, 151, 178, 179
Sertraline, benzodiazepine interactions, 47–49
Sexual dysfunction, antipsychotic drug induction, 194, 197, 198
Smoking, see also Nicotine,
  cardiovascular disease risk, 469
  cancer risk, 469, 470
  pulmonary disease risk, 470
  drug interactions with tobacco smoke,
    alcohol, 475
    antiarrhythmic drugs, 479
    antipsychotics, 476, 477
    aspirin, 475, 476
    benzodiazepines, 478
    β-blockers, 479
    caffeine, 478
    carbamazepine, 479
    diuretics, 479
    heparin, 476
    insulin, 480
    opioids, 480, 481
    steroid hormones, 481
    tacrine, 481
    theophylline, 481, 482
    tricyclic antidepressants, 476
    warfarin, 476
Sotalol, side effects, 226
SSRIs, see Selective serotonin reuptake inhibitors
Stanozolol,
  adverse effects, 525
  contraindications, 523
  dosing, 514
  indications, 514
  preparations, 514
Statins,
  drug interactions,
    antacids, 279
    antipyrine, 279
    bile acid sequestrants, 278
    cimetidine, 279
    digoxin, 278
    erythromycin, 279
    fibric acid derivatives, 277
    oral contraceptives, 278
    warfarin, 278
  mechanism of action, 276
  side effects, 276, 277
Streptococcus, pathogenic groups, 297
Streptokinase,
  contraindications, 271
  indications, 270, 271
  pharmacology, 271, 272
Sulfasalazine,
  drug interactions, 368
  indications, 368
  preparations and dosing, 368
Sulfinpyrazone,
  drug interactions, 373
  gouty arthritis management, 373
Sulindac,
  drug interactions, 351
  indications and contraindications, 351
  pharmacokinetics, 350, 351
  preparations and dosing, 351

T

Tamoxifen,
  administration routes, 564
  adverse reactions, 565, 566
  contraindications, 565
  drug interactions, 566, 567
  indications, 564
  mechanism of action, 564, 565
  metabolism, 565
  preparations, 563
Tardive dyskinesia, antipsychotic drug induction, 191, 192
Taste perception, drug effects, 388
TB, see Tuberculosis
TCAs, see Tricyclic antidepressants
Terbinafine,
  administration routes, 543
  adverse reactions, 551
  benzodiazepine interactions, 46
  contraindications, 547
  mechanism of action, 542, 543
Testosterone,
  administration routes, 515, 516
  adverse effects, 525, 526
  contraindications, 523
  dosing, 516
  drug interactions, 530
  indications, 516
  pharmacokinetics, 515
  preparations, 514, 515
Theophylline,
  benzodiazepine interactions, 62
  β-agonist interactions, 554
Thiazide diuretics, see Diuretics
Thiopental, benzodiazepine interactions, 30
Thioridazine, tricyclic antidepressant interactions, 161
Thyroid hormone, β-agonist interactions, 555
Tiagabine,
  adverse reactions, 110
  chemistry, 109
  contraindications and precautions, 110
  drug interactions, 110, 111
  metabolism, 110
  pharmacokinetics, 110
  pharmacology, 109
Ticlopidine,
  contraindications, 274, 275
  drug interactions,
    overview, 274
    tricyclic antidepressants, 161
  side effects, 273, 274

Tissue plasminogen activator,
  contraindications, 271
  indications, 270, 271
  pharmacology, 272
Tobacco, see Nicotine; Smoking
Tocainide, side effects, 223
Tolbutamide, aldehyde dehydrogenase inhibition, 412
Tolmetin,
  drug interactions, 352
  indications and contraindications, 351
  pharmacokinetics, 351
  preparations and dosing, 351, 352
Topiramate,
  adverse reactions, 95, 108, 109
  chemistry, 107, 108
  contraindications and precautions, 109
  drug interactions,
    antiepileptic drug interactions, 96
    non-antiepileptic drugs, 97
    overview, 109
  metabolism, 108
  pharmacokinetics, 108
  pharmacology, 108
Torsades de pointes, drug induction, 227
Toxic shock syndrome (TSS), clinical features and management, 300
Tricyclic antidepressants (TCAs),
  CYP polymorphisms, 156–158, 162
  depression management, 149
  drug interactions,
    alcohol, 162
    antipsychotics, 200
    β-agonists, 555
    β-blockers, 237
    isoniazid, 152
    nicotine, 472
    opioids, 135
    selective serotonin reuptake inhibitors, 159–161, 181
    thioridazine, 161
    ticlopidine, 161
  metabolism, 154–156
  overdose,
    clinical features, 152, 153
    CYP polymorphisms and drug interactions, 162, 163
    mortality, 153
  pharmacology, 154
  structures, 152–154
  tobacco smoke interactions, 476
  toxicity, 152

Index

Tripelannamine, nicotine interactions, 472
Trovafloxacin, opioid interactions, 135
TSS, *see* Toxic shock syndrome
Tuberculosis (TB), clinical features and management, 301
Tubocurarine, β-blocker interactions, 237
Tyramine-restricted diet, 391

V

Valproic acid,
   adverse reactions, 94, 103, 104
   chemistry, 102
   contraindications and precautions, 104
   drug interactions,
      antiepileptic drug interactions, 96
      benzodiazepines, 52, 53
      non-antiepileptic drugs, 97
      overview, 104
   metabolism, 103
   pharmacokinetics, 102, 103
   pharmacology, 102
Venlafaxine, benzodiazepine interactions, 47–49
Verapamil,
   alcohol interactions, 421
   drug interactions, 244
Vigabatrin,
   adverse reactions, 95, 114
   chemistry, 113
   contraindications and precautions, 114
   drug interactions,
      antiepileptic drug interactions, 96
      non-antiepileptic drugs, 97
      overview, 114
   metabolism, 113
   pharmacokinetics, 113, 114
   pharmacology, 113
Vorozole,
   drug interactions, 572, 573
   indications, 569
   mechanism of action, 569, 570
   metabolism, 570, 571

W

Warfarin,
   adverse effects, 267, 268
   drug interactions,
      absorption effects, 268, 269
      albumin binding effects, 269, 270
      amiodarone, 228
      metabolism effects, 269
      selective serotonin reuptake inhibitors, 181
      statins, 278
   mechanism of action, 267
   tobacco smoke interactions, 476

Z

Zonisamide,
   adverse reactions, 95, 117
   chemistry, 116
   contraindications and precautions, 117
   drug interactions,
      antiepileptic drug interactions, 96
      non-antiepileptic drugs, 97
      overview, 117
   metabolism, 116
   pharmacokinetics, 116
   pharmacology, 116